Mental Health Nursing

A South African Perspective

Seventh edition

Editor:
Lyn Middleton

JUTA

> **Disclaimer**
>
> In the writing of this book, every effort has been made to present accurate and up-to-date information from the best and most reliable sources. However, the results of healthcare professionals depend on a variety of factors that are beyond the control of the authors and publishers. Therefore, neither the authors nor the publishers assume responsibility for, nor make any warranty with regard to, the outcomes achieved from the procedures described in this book.
>
> The authors and publisher have exerted every effort to ensure that drug selections and dosages set forth in this text are in accord with current recommendations and practice at the time of publication. However, readers are urged to check the package insert for each drug for any change in indications of dosage and for added warning and precautions. The information in this book is provided in good faith and the authors and publisher cannot be held responsible for errors, individual responses to drugs and other consequences.

Mental Health Nursing: A South African Perspective

First published 1992 as *Psychiatric Nursing: A South African Perspective*
Second edition 1994
Third edition 1997
Fourth edition 2004 published as *Mental Health Nursing: A South African Perspective*
Fifth edition 2010
Sixth edition 2014
Seventh edition 2020

Juta and Company (Pty) Ltd
First floor, Sunclare Building, 21 Dreyer Street, Claremont 7708
PO Box 14373, Lansdowne 7779, Cape Town, South Africa
www.juta.co.za

© 2020 Juta and Company (Pty) Ltd

ISBN 978 1 48512 469 6

All rights reserved. No part of this publication may be reproduced or transmitted in any form or by any means, electronic or mechanical, including photocopying, recording, or any information storage or retrieval system, without prior permission in writing from the publisher. Subject to any applicable licensing terms and conditions in the case of electronically supplied publications, a person may engage in fair dealing with a copy of this publication for his or her personal or private use, or his or her research or private study. See section 12(1)(a) of the Copyright Act 98 of 1978.

Project manager: Seshni Kazadi
Editor: Barbara Orpen Hathorn
Proofreader: Lilané Putter Joubert
Cover designer: Drag and Drop
Typesetter: Wouter Reinders
Indexer: Sanet le Roux

Typeset in 10.5 on 13 pt Minion Pro

Front cover photograph:
Noluyanda Mqutwana, aged 14 at the time of the photograph being taken, outside her family home in Khayelitsha on 30 January 2000. At the time, this talented ballerina was part of the Dance for All project.

Published in South Africa

The author and the publisher believe on the strength of due diligence exercised that this work does not contain any material that is the subject of copyright held by another person. In the alternative, they believe that any protected pre-existing material that may be comprised in it has been used with appropriate authority or has been used in circumstances that make such use permissible under the law.

CONTENTS

About the Authors xi
List of Abbreviations xiv

SECTION 1: Frameworks and Foundations 1

Chapter 1: The History of Mental Health Nursing 3
L R Uys and Y Havenga
Introduction 3
Mental health care in the early days 3
Mental health care in the 20th and 21st century 6
Contemporary issues in mental health nursing 14
Conclusion 18
Web resources 18
References 19

Chapter 2: A Conceptual Framework for Mental Health Nursing 22
L R Uys and A A H Smith
Introduction 22
Defining mental health 23
Defining mental health nursing 25
Nurse–MHCU relationship 26
Conclusion 35
Web resources 35
References 36

Chapter 3: Comprehensive Mental Health Care 37
L R Uys and S Arunachallam
Introduction 37
The epidemiology of mental illness in South Africa 38
Comprehensive mental health care 40
Planning programmes 50
Conclusion 57
Web resources 58
References 58

Chapter 4: Mental Health Care in the Health Care System 61
L R Uys and S Arunachallam
Introduction 61
Organisation of mental health services 62
Levels of structure and service 64
The integration of mental health care into PHC 67
Functions of mental health services in different settings 70
Human resources and training 70

Description of primary mental health care 71
Multidisciplinary teams 72
Conclusion 76
Web resources 77
References 77

Chapter 5: The Consumers in Mental Health 80
L R Uys and P D Martin
Introduction 80
The stigma associated with being mentally ill 81
Consumers' perceptions on recovery from mental illness 84
The family or 'carer' perspective 86
Other roles of consumers 93
Advocacy by consumers 95
Involvement in policy, planning and evaluation 96
Conclusion 97
Web resources 97
References 98

Chapter 6: Legal Structures in Mental Health Care Nursing 100
N Naidoo and D McQuoid-Mason
Introduction 100
The Mental Health Care Act 101
Medicines and Related Substances Control Act 124
Prevention of and Treatment For Substance Abuse Act 124
Children's Act 126
Conclusion 127
Web resources 127
References 127

Chapter 7: Ethical Dilemmas in Mental Health Nursing 128
L van Rhyn
Introduction 128
Ethical theories 129
Ethical principles in nursing and health care 132
The structure of an ethical dilemma 135
Specific ethical problems in psychiatric nursing 139
Patient rights 143
Culture-sensitive care 145
Ethics review boards and committees 145
Conclusion 146
Web resources 147
References 147

Chapter 8: Working with Cultural Diversity in Mental Health Care 149
L R Uys and N Nkosi-Mafutha
Introduction 149
Culture 149
Cultural competence 153
Diversity and cultural diversity 155
Conclusion 159
Web resources 159
References 160

SECTION 2: The Mental Health Nursing Process 163

Chapter 9: The Mental Health Care Nursing Process 165
L R Uys and A Marx
Introduction 165
Interpersonal mental health care nursing attitudes 166
Interpersonal mental health care nursing communication skills 167
The relationship between a mental health care nurse and an MHCU 172
The mental health care nurse–family relationship 175
The mental health care nursing process 176
Conclusion 177
Web resources 177
References 177

Chapter 10: Mental Health Assessment of Hospitalised or Community-based Individuals 179
G E Pietersen and L Middleton
Introduction 179
Developing a context for mental health assessment and diagnosis 181
Mental health assessment 184
Assessment formulations for healthy lifestyle functioning 200
Assessment related to different contexts 201
Specific, focused mental health assessments 202
Constructing clinical mental health nursing formulations 206
Formulating a mental health nursing diagnosis 207
Group assessment 208
Conclusion 212
Web resources 212
References 212

Chapter 11: Mental Health Nursing Interventions 214
L R Uys and Y Havenga
Introduction 214
Mental health education 214
Crisis intervention 221

Individual counselling 229
Therapeutic groups 234
Milieu therapy 241
Hospital discharge planning 248
Symptom management and relapse prevention 249
Home visits 254
Case management 255
Limit setting 259
Dealing with anger and aggression 260
Conclusion 274
Web resources 275
References 276

SECTION 3: Psychopathology and Nursing Interventions 281

Chapter 12: Nursing the Mental Health Care User with an Anxiety Disorder 283
L Middleton and G E Pietersen
Introduction 283
The anxiety response 284
Understanding anxiety as a phenomenon (an experience/happening/event) 287
Understanding anxiety from a cognitive behavioural perspective 289
Normal versus pathological anxiety 292
The experience of interacting with an anxious MHCU 301
Mental health nursing and assessment of anxiety 303
Nursing interventions related to stress/anxiousness and/or pathological anxiety 307
Psychopharmacology related to treatment of anxiety disorders 317
Conclusion 323
Web resources 323
References 324
Resources not referred to in the text 324

Chapter 13: Nursing a Person with a Mood Disorder 326
M A Jarvis and L Middleton
Introduction 326
Definitions 327
Depressive and bipolar disorders 327
Nursing interventions with MHCUs presenting with depressive features 334
Other interventions 351
Suicide 355
Bipolar mood disorders 366
Conclusion 371
References 371
Resources not referred to in the text 375
Annexure 376

WHO (five) Well-being Index (WHO-5)	377
Beck's Suicide Intent Scale	378
Suicide risk assessment	380

Chapter 14: Nursing the Mental Health Care User with Schizophrenia, Schizophrenia Spectrum and Other Psychotic Disorders 382

L R Uys and Y Havenga

Introduction	382
Diagnosis of schizophrenia spectrum and other psychotic disorders	384
Application of nursing process to assessment and diagnosis of MHCUs with schizophrenia	386
Applying the nursing process to the care, treatment and rehabilitation of MHCUs with schizophrenia	389
Conclusion	407
Web resources	407
References	408

Chapter 15: Nursing the Patient with a Substance-related Disorder 410

L R Uys and P D Martin

Introduction	410
Commonly used substances	411
Core concepts associated with patterns of substance use	414
Alcohol-related disorders	418
Other common dependence-producing substances	439
Treatment of substance-dependent people	447
Conclusion	449
Web resources	449
References	449

Chapter 16: Nursing the Patient with a Neurocognitive Disorder 452

L R Uys, L Middleton and V van Zyl

Introduction	452
Incidence and prevalence of delirium and mild and major NCDs	453
Understanding NCDs	454
The aetiology or causes of NCDs	459
DSM-5 classification of delirium and major NCDs	461
Distinguishing NCDs	463
Assessing NCDs	466
Intervening in NCDs	472
Family and carer liaison	483
Social control	487
Coping with epilepsy: principles for psychosocial nursing intervention	489
Conclusion	496
Web resources	496
References	496

Chapter 17: Nursing Care of Persons with Intellectual Disabilities 498
L R Uys, L Middleton and R Ramalisa
Introduction 498
Prevention 500
Intellectual disability 501
Assessment 505
Support for parents of children with intellectual disabilities 510
Stimulation of development 515
Teaching self-care and other skills 524
Institutional care 545
Adult persons with intellectual disabilities 547
Management of challenging behaviour 550
Conclusion 552
Web resources 552
References 553

Chapter 18: Nursing the Mental Health Care User Diagnosed with a Personality Disorder 555
A Fourie
Introduction 555
Understanding the person with a personality disorder 556
Using a transactional analysis model when treating patients with personality disorders 561
Working with MHCUs with specific personality disorders 573
Conclusion 608
Web resources 608
References 609

SECTION 4: Care of Special Groups 611

Chapter 19: People who have Experienced Trauma 613
N Nkosi-Mafutha and M Hlungwani
Introduction 613
Defining trauma and crisis 614
Normal response to trauma 616
Diagnosis of trauma and stressor-related disorders 617
Trauma counselling and interventions 623
Debriefing 627
Impact of working with victims of violence and self-care 631
Domestic violence 633
Abuse of the elderly 637
Child abuse 638
Effects of trauma on children 643
Handling disclosure about abuse 650
Helping children affected by trauma 651
Working with groups affected by trauma 657

Conclusion	661
Appendix I	661
Appendix II	668
References	676

Chapter 20: People with a Mental Illness who have Comorbid General Medical Conditions 678
A A H Smith

Introduction	678
Prevalence of comorbid medical disorders and SMDs	680
Vulnerability factors	683
Nursing assessment, treatment and management	686
Conclusion	691
Web resources	692
References	692

Chapter 21: Mental Health Nursing in the Context of Human Immunodeficiency Virus and Tuberculosis 693
J R Naidoo

Introduction	693
The relationship between HIV/TB co-infection and mental illness	694
Psychological conditions associated with HIV/AIDS and TB	696
Psychotropic drug interactions with HIV/TB	701
Conclusion	702
References	703

Chapter 22: Mental Health Nursing of Children and Adolescents 705
L van Rhyn

Introduction	705
Mental disorders in children and adolescents	706
Assessment of children with mental health disorders	724
Managing emotionally and behaviourally disturbed children	737
Conclusion	739
Web resources	740
References	740

Chapter 23: Nursing Forensic Mental Health Care Users 743
L R Uys and T Bock

Introduction	743
Historical background	744
Current legal provisions in South Africa	746
Services provided for a mentally ill offender	753
Classification of forensic psychiatric patients	754
The nurse in the observation unit	755
The nurse in the security unit	757

The conflicting role of the mental health nurse in a forensic unit	764
The forensic nurse	765
Conclusion	766
Web resources	767
References	767

SECTION 5: Appendices 771

Appendix One	773
Appendix Two	782
Appendix Three	787
Appendix Four	790
Appendix Five	793
Appendix Six	795
Appendix Seven	796
Appendix Eight	803

INDEX 815

ABOUT THE AUTHORS

Sathasivan Arunachallam obtained his bachelor's degree from UNISA, his master's degree from the University of Johannesburg, his PhD from the University of the Western Cape (UWC) and a postgraduate diploma in Advanced Psychiatry from the University of Stellenbosch. Currently he teaches postgraduate students at the UWC.

Theresa Bock obtained her PhD at North West University (NWU) in 2015. She is currently Head of Campus and Head of Department of Psychiatric Nursing Science at the Metro East Campus of the Western Cape College of Nursing. She is an experienced psychiatric nurse and was involved in compiling the curricula for the R880 year course in Psychiatric Nursing Science and the R212 curriculum for Advanced Psychiatric Nursing Science. She currently teaches both undergraduate and postgraduate students and is involved in training multidisciplinary hospital teams on the management of aggression and violence.

Alan Fourie is a clinical psychologist, Jungian analyst and senior lecturer within the Department of Psychology at Rhodes University. He has worked in a variety of healthcare settings, including Elizabeth Donkin Psychiatric Hospital, King Edward Hospital, and Entabeni and Valkenberg hospitals. He has specialised in analytical psychology and trained as a Jungian analyst through the South African Association of Jungian Analysts. His current research focus is analytical psychology and indigenous models of healing.

Yolanda Havenga obtained master's and doctoral degrees in Psychiatric Nursing from the University of Johannesburg (UJ). She has lectured Psychiatric Nursing at the then University of Limpopo (Medunsa campus) and currently lectures Psychiatric Nursing Science at the Tshwane University of Technology (TUT) where she is also the head of department. She actively supervises master's and doctoral students in Nursing Science.

Tintswalo Mercy Hlungwani holds a B Cur degree from Medunsa, a PDM in Health Management, a MSc in Mental Health and a PhD in Public Health. She is currently a senior lecturer in the division of Health and Society at the University of the Witwatersrand (Wits). She teaches Public Health in both post- and undergraduate programmes at the university. Her research interests include mental health, health promotion and interventions on social determinants of health.

Mary Ann Jarvis holds a bachelor's degree in Nursing (Honours: Mental Health), a master's degree in Nursing (Mental Health) and PhD (Nursing) from the University of KwaZulu-Natal (UKZN). Prior to her current position, her career was divided between working in acute psychiatry, wellness management in the private sector and teaching in a college setting. She is currently a lecturer at UKZN to both undergraduate and postgraduate students in the field of mental health.

Nokuthula Gloria Mafutha obtained her first master's degree in General Nursing in 2008, an Advanced Psychiatry Clinical master's degree in 2012 and her doctorate from TUT in 2017. Nokuthula joined the Department of Nursing Education at Wits in 2016 as a lecturer in General Nursing and Psychiatric Nursing.

Penelope Martin obtained a PhD at UWC. Penny is currently the clinical programme coordinator at the School of Nursing at UWC. She teaches Community Psychiatric Nursing to postgraduate nursing students. Her areas of interest are stress and coping in mental health, as well as emotional support for diverse populations.

Annemarie Marx is a senior lecturer in Psychiatric Nursing Science and Health Service Management at NWU, Potchefstroom Campus. She has been involved in teaching interpersonal skills courses and the theory of Psychiatric Nursing Science for a number of years.

David J McQuoid-Mason, B Comm (Natal) LLB (Natal) LLM (London) PhD (Natal), is a professor of Law at the Centre for Socio-Studies, UKZN, Durban; a director of Street Law South Africa; and President of the Commonwealth Legal Education Association. He was Dean of the Law School at the former University of Natal for 13 years. Professor McQuoid-Mason has conducted workshops in over 60 countries and published more than 150 articles in law and medical journals. He has written two books, co-authored 18 books (including an *A-Z of Nursing Law*, an *A-Z of Medical Law* and *Bioethics, Human Rights and Health Law*) and contributed more than 70 chapters to books. Professor McQuoid-Mason has delivered over 140 papers at national and over 220 papers at international conferences.

Lyn Middleton is the programmes director for the Training in Health Equity Network (THEnet), a global movement advocating for socially accountable transformative health workforce education. Prior to joining THEnet, Lyn was the sub-Saharan regional nursing advisor for ICAP at Columbia University and before that, worked at KZN where she taught, mentored and supervised students from across the African continent in mental health. She has a PhD in Nursing, holds honorary positions in the School of Health Sciences (Pharmaceutical Department) at UKZN, the Kamuzu College of Nursing, University of Malawi, and the Faculty of Health, Social Care and Education at Kingston University and St George's University of London. Lyn has authored and co-authored journal articles, books and training materials in the areas of health workforce education; mental health and policy; and more recently, antimicrobial resistance.

Joanne Naidoo is an associate professor of Nursing at the Nelson Mandela University (NMU) and has been engaged in academia for the past 16 years. Her research interest is in the area of HIV nursing care with a specific focus on the psycho-social aspects of people living with HIV. This is demonstrated though the peer reviewed research she has authored (see https://www.researchgate.net/profile/Joanne_Naidoo/contributions and https://scholar.google.com/citations?user=krkXOqwAAAAJ) for more information about her research).

Nerissa Naidoo obtained her LLB degree *summa cum laude* from the UKZN in 2018 and is currently pursuing her master's at Harvard University.

Elize Pietersen completed her training as a nurse at UFS, where she also obtained a master's degree in Psychiatric Nursing. She taught Psychiatric Nursing at her alma mater for a number of years, making clinical teaching her main focus. She started her clinical research career at the University of Cape Town (UCT) managing a neuro-psychiatric-genetic study that involved bipolar disorder. She obtained her PhD at UCT where she continues her clinical research career at present.

Rudo Ramalisa is a lecturer at the Vaal University of Technology (VUT). She completed her master's degree in 2014 and is currently studying towards a PhD in Nursing Science. She is a registered psychiatric nurse with the South African Nursing Council.

Amanda (Mandy) Smith worked at UKZN in the School of Nursing and Health Sciences where she also obtained her master's degree in Mental Health Nursing *cum laude*. She has been involved in mental health nursing education, and practice, for 20 years and has a special interest in serious mental illness, collaborative practice and psychosocial rehabilitation. A keen clinical practitioner and researcher, she continues to be involved in clinical practice and in developing a data-led evidence-based practice for mental health nursing. She now works for the Priory Group UK.

Lily van Rhyn obtained a bachelor's degree in Nursing from NWU, a master's degree in Psychiatric Nursing at the Pretoria University and a PhD in Child Psychiatric Nursing from the University of the Free State (UFS). She was a senior lecturer at the School of Nursing at UFS for 37 years where she developed an advanced diploma in Child Psychiatric Nursing. Her area of interest is mainly the mental health and resilience of children and adolescents in Africa.

Verna van Zyl completed her nurse and midwifery training at Otto du Plessis College, Tygerberg Hospital; psychiatric nursing at Stikland Hospital and holds a bachelor's and honours degree from UNISA. She obtained her master's degree at UWC and is currently a lecturer at Western Cape College of Nursing.

LIST OF ABBREVIATIONS

AA	Alcoholics Anonymous
AC	Adapted child
ACT	Assertive community treatment
ADHD	Attention-deficit/hyperactivity disorder
ADL	Activities of daily living
AEASA	Action on Elder Abuse South Africa
AIDS	Acquired Immunodeficiency Syndrome
ANAC	Association of Nurses in AIDS Care
ANI	Asymptomatic neurocognitive impairment
AOD	Alcohol and other drugs
ART	Antiretroviral treatment
BMI	Body mass index
BPD	Bipolar disorder
BPS	Brief Psychiatric Rating Scale
BVC	Broset Violence Checklist
CAMHS	Child and adolescent mental health services
CATIE	Clinical Antipsychotic Trials of Intervention Effectiveness
CBS	Culture-bound syndrome
CBT	Cognitive behavioural therapy
CC	Community clinic
CC	Conforming child
CE	Centre for Epidemiologica
CFI	Cultural formulation interview
CHC	Community health centre
CISM	Critical incident stress management
CL	Community level
CNS	Central nervous system
CP	Critical parent
CPI	Child Psychiatric Interview
CPM	Conspicuous psychiatric morbidity
CPMHC	Comprehensive psychiatric/mental health care
CRP	C-reactive protein
CT	Computed tomography
CVD	Cardiovascular disease
DALY	Disability-adjusted life year
DD	Developmental disorder
DHS	District health system
DL	District level
DR	Discharge report
DSM	*Diagnostic and Statistical Manual of Mental Disorders*
DSSA	Down Syndrome South Africa
DT	Delirium tremens

EAP	Employee assistance programmes
ECG	Electrocardiogram
ECT	Electroconvulsive therapy/treatment
EDL	Essential drugs list
EEG	Electroencephalograph
EPS	Extrapyramidal side effects
ETP	Educational theatre programmes
FAFOFS	Friends and Family of Schizophrenics
FC	Free child
FGA	First-generation agent
GAF	Global assessment of functioning
GBD	Global burden of disease
GDS	Geriatric Depression Scale
GI	Glycaemic index
GID	Gender identity disorder
HAD	HIV-associated dementia
HAND	HIV-associated neurocognitive disorder
HDRS	Hamilton Depression Rating Scale
HEAL	Halt Elder Abuse line
HIV	Human immunodeficiency virus
HPM	Hidden psychiatric morbidity
ICD	International Classification of Diseases
ICN	International Council of Nurses
ICNP	International Classification for Nursing Practice
LGBT	Lesbian, gay, bisexual and transgender
LMIC	Lower middle-income countries
MAOI	Monoamine oxidase inhibitor
MDD	Major depressive disorder
MEC	Member of the Executive Council
MHCU	Mental health care user
MMSE	Mini-mental state examination
MND	Mild neurocognitive disorder
MOCA	Montreal Cognitive Assessment
MRI	Magnetic resonance imaging
MSE	Mental state examination
NAMI	National Alliance on Mental Illness
NCD	Neurocognitive disorder
NCDLB	NCD with Lewy body
NDSS	National Down Syndrome Society
NGO	Non-governmental organisation
NHI	National health insurance
NHS	National Health Services
NMDA	N-methyl-D-aspartate

NNAAMI	National Network of Adult and Adolescent Children who have a Mentally Ill Parent(s)
NP	Nurturing parent
NPS	New psychoactive substances
PANSS	Positive and Negative Syndrome Scale
PDD	Persistent Depressive Disorder
PET	Positron emission tomography
PHC	Primary health care
PL	Provincial level
PM	Conspicuous psychiatric morbidity
PSR	Psychosocial rehabilitation
PTSD	Post-traumatic stress disorder
RC	Rebellious child
REM	Rapid eye movement
REPSSI	Regional Psychosocial Support Initiative
RO	Reality orientation
RtHB	Road to Health Booklet
rTMS	Repetitive Transcranial Magnetic Stimulation
SADAG	South African Depression and Anxiety Group
SAMHSA	Substance Abuse and Mental Health Services Administration
SANC	South African Nursing Counsel
SANS	Scale for the Assessment of Negative Symptoms
SAPS	Scale for the Assessment of Positive Symptoms
SAPS	South African Police Service
SASH	South African Stress and Health
SDS	Self-rating Depression Scale
SE	Supported employment
SGA	Second-generation agent
SHS	Secondary health system
SIDAS	Suicidal Ideation Attributes Scale
SMD	Serious mental disorders
SPJ	Structured professional judgement
SPS	SAD PERSONS Scale
SRQ	Self-reporting questionnaire
SSRI	Selective serotonin reuptake inhibitors
START	Strive Towards Achieving Results Together
STEP	Systematic training in effective parenting
TB	Tuberculosis
TQS	Ten Question Disability Screen
TSH	Thyroid stimulating hormone
UCT	University of Cape Town
UK	United Kingdom
UN	United Nation

UNICEF	United Nations International Children's Emergency Fund
UNODC	United Nations Office on Drugs and Crime
USA	United States of America
VC	Videoconferencing
WAS	Ward Atmosphere Scale
WCC	White cell count
WFMH	World Federation for Mental Health
WHO	World Health Organisation
YANA	You Are Not Alone

SECTION 1
Frameworks and Foundations

CHAPTER 1

The History of Mental Health Nursing

L R Uys and Y Havenga

Learning Outcomes

After studying this chapter, you should be able to:
- describe in broad terms the history of mental health nursing up to the 20th century
- identify the most important historical trends in the development of psychiatry in the 21st century
- describe how international trends have influenced psychiatry in South Africa
- identify important events in the development of mental health services and mental health nursing in South Africa.

INTRODUCTION

The history of mental health services and mental health nursing is closely related to social and scientific development and to the prevailing views and trends of society. The views and trends in mental health nursing must therefore be seen against the wider background of history.

MENTAL HEALTH CARE IN THE EARLY DAYS

The history of mental health care will be traced from the early period through to the Renaissance, the Reformation and the 19th century.

The early period up to the Renaissance

A number of civilisations flourished in ancient times and during the period before Christ. The aetiology or cause of mental illness was generally considered to be supernatural with limited distinction between medicine, magic and religion (Kneisl & Trigoboff, 2013). Methods of treatment were of a physical and religious nature. Hippocrates (460–370 BC) suggested mental illness was caused by unbalanced 'body humors': blood, black bile, yellow bile and phlegm (Kneisl & Trigoboff, 2013). Physical treatments included, among others, cold baths and bloodletting, constraint, beatings and diets (Pelletier & Davidson, 2015). The aim of some methods was to make the body so uncomfortable for the strange spirit that it would leave. An example of this would have been overheating the patient. Other times they tried to entice the spirit out of the body with beautiful music. Religious treatment concentrated on rituals. Monasteries often provided mental health care and priests played a role in treating the mentally ill (Shuttleworth, 2018).

The Reformation

The rise of science led to a more sophisticated classification of mental disorders. However, people of this time did not have a clear understanding of the causes (Kneisl & Trigoboff, 2013). Large institutions that harboured all types of people, including prostitutes, unmarried mothers and the mentally ill, were at one time a common phenomenon. Conditions in these institutions were very bad and in the late 18th century in England and France, William Tuke, Philippe Pinel and Jean-Baptiste Pussin began to separate the mentally ill from the others and to treat them with respect and compassion in a humane environment, referred to as 'moral treatment' (Kneisl & Trigoboff, 2013; Pelletier & Davidson, 2015). Moral treatment was so successful that it led to the large-scale establishment of institutions called 'asylums' or 'sanctuaries'.

The 19th century

The 19th century was marked by an increase throughout the world in the number of institutions for the mentally ill as moral treatment was replaced with custodial care. This period is often referred to as the custodial period. The concept of mental illness as a disease was developed only by the end of the 18th century, and the term 'psychiatry' was coined by a French physician in 1808 (Gillis, 2012). The cause of mental illness was largely unknown and limited treatment was available. The focus of hospitalisation was to ensure safety (especially of others) and to manage aggression. However, conditions were often non-therapeutic in nature (Gillis, 2012). In the United States of America (USA), Dorothea Lynde Dix (1802–1887), a teacher who later became a nurse, was responsible for an international effort to provide better hospital facilities for mental health care users (MHCUs). She founded and enlarged over 30 psychiatric hospitals (Kneisl & Trigoboff, 2013).

In South Africa, the first psychiatric hospitals were opened at this time. In 1818 Somerset Hospital opened and some beds were allocated for MHCUs with psychiatric conditions. Beds were limited to those admitted from far as this was the only hospital in the Cape providing mental health treatment (Gillis, 2012). To reduce the overcrowding at Somerset Hospital, the prison on Robben Island was turned into a hospital in 1836 for persons living with leprosy, the chronically ill and MHCUs (Gillis, 2012). The custodial care given there was evidently of a high standard and the 1891 report of the resident medical officer mentions the training of nurses and assistants. Robben Island was used for MHCUs in the Cape until Valkenberg Hospital opened in 1892 (Gillis, 2012). Psychiatric hospitals were, in time, erected throughout the country and legislation was passed for the management of MHCUs. The chronological establishment of psychiatric hospitals in South Africa is set out in Table 1.1. Many of these hospitals were not designed for this purpose to begin with and many of them are now more than a hundred years old, but still in use.

Table 1.1 Chronological establishment of psychiatric hospitals in South Africa

Year	Name	Place
1846	–	Robben Island
1876	Grahamstown Lunatic Asylum (later Fort England)	Grahamstown (old military barracks)
1875	Pietermaritzburg Lunatic Asylum (later Town Hill)	Pietermaritzburg (temporary building – moved to permanent building in 1882)
1883	Bloemfontein-Zielziekehospitaal (later Oranje Hospital)	Bloemfontein
1889	Port Alfred Lunatic Asylum (Later Kowie)	Port Alfred (old military barracks)
1892	Pretoria Krankzinnegengesticht (later Weskoppies)	Pretoria
1897	Fort Beaufort Lunatic Asylum	Fort Beaufort (old military barracks)
1891	Valkenberg Lunatic Asylum	Observatory, Cape Town (old reformatory)
1922	Queenstown Mental Hospital (later Komani)	Queenstown
1922	Witrand Institute	Potchefstroom
1922	Alexandra Care and Rehabilitation Centre	Cape Town
1927	Fort Napier Hospital	Pietermaritzburg (old military barracks)
1943	Sterkfontein Hospital	Krugersdorp
1946	Tara – the H Moross Centre	Johannesburg
1950	Woodside Sanctuary	Johannesburg
1951	Denmar Specialist Psychiatric Hospital (Denmar Specialist Psychiatric Hospital, 2014)	Pretoria
1962	Stikland Hospital	Bellville
1966	Bophelong Hospital	Mafikeng
1970s	Woodside special care centres	Johannesburg, Cape Town
1972	Thabamoopo Mental Hospital	Polokwane
1974	Lentegeur Hospital	Cape Town
1980	Umzimkulu Hospital	Umzimkulu
1980	Care Haven	Port Elizabeth
1984	Vista Clinic (Vista Clinic, nd)	Pretoria
1993	Life Hunterscraig Private Hospital	Port Elizabeth

Year	Name	Place
1998	Crescent Clinic	Cape Town
2000	Life Riverfield Lodge	Johannesburg
1985–2012	Akeso Psychiatric Clinics (Akeso Psychiatric Clinics, 2017)	Kenilworth, Kommetjie, Umhlanga, Bishopscourt, Pietermaritzburg, Mpumalanga, Milnerton, George, Alberton, Randburg, Parktown, Arcadia
2012	Palm Tree Clinic (Palm Tree Clinic, nd)	Cape Town

The numbers of psychiatric hospitals have increased, with the World Health Organisation (WHO) and the Department of Psychiatry and Mental Health, University of Cape Town (UCT), reporting in 2007 that South Africa had 3 460 outpatient mental health facilities, 41 psychiatric inpatient units located in general hospitals and 23 psychiatric hospitals (WHO & UCT, 2007).

MENTAL HEALTH CARE IN THE 20TH AND 21ST CENTURY

Mental health care in the 20th and 21st centuries will be looked at from both an international and a South African perspective.

International perspective

In the early 20th century the understanding and treatment of mental illnesses were greatly influenced by psychoanalysis and the work of prominent psychiatrists such as Emil Kraepelin, Sigmund Freud (Kneisl & Trigoboff, 2013) and Karl Jung (Gillis, 2012). The increase in the number of psychiatric hospitals during this time resulted in a change from small centres to overpopulated institutions where inadequate numbers of staff tried to manage MHCUs by using mechanical restraints and isolation cells. Custodial care was no longer therapeutic.

During the 1920s and early 1930s physical treatments were common and included insulin and Cardiazol convulsion therapies; electroshock and prefrontal leucotomies; and malarial-induced fever for the treatment of 'general paralysis of the insane' (Minde, 1977; Daey Ouwens et al, 2017). Most of these treatments were discontinued. However, major treatment changes took place after 1930 when it was observed that MHCUs with symptoms of schizophrenia improved after seizures. This observation led to the commencement of electroconvulsive treatment (ECT). The period of physical treatment was then followed by the use of psychotropic drugs (Minde, 1977).

The implementation of psychotropic drugs in the late 1940s and 1950s made a significant contribution to modern-day mental health treatment. The introduction of lithium in 1949 and chlorpromazine in 1955 led to much improved management of aggression and disruptive behaviours. Improved treatment of psychosis greatly increased the possibility of discharge and led to the large-scale deinstitutionalisation of MHCUs and the transfer of treatment to the community. Also, the introduction of antidepressants improved the outcome for MHCUs and shortened hospital stays (Gillis, 2012).

In 1908 a discharged MHCU, Clifford Beers (1876–1943), published a book entitled *A Mind that Found Itself*, in which he described his appalling experiences in American psychiatric hospitals. The publication of this book led to the founding of the first Mental Hygiene Society, which grew to become a national organisation within a year. It later became internationally known as the 'Mental Health Society' and was a precursor to preventative psychiatry and child guidance clinics (Parry, 2010).

In the 1950s the pressure exerted by this society – together with the help of a few influential psychiatrists and certain social scientists who, by means of a number of studies, illustrated the negative consequences of custodial care – led to a renewed focus on the social environment in which treatment takes place. This development, which was called social psychiatry, emphasised the creation of a therapeutic environment in wards and the avoidance of high fences, locked doors, restraints and isolation.

In the USA, mental health nursing was a subdiscipline developing significantly in the practical and theoretical realms from the 1950s to the 1980s. This development took place under the leadership of Hildegard E Peplau, who is regarded as the mother of mental health nursing. She played a significant role in the development of the therapeutic role and abilities of mental health nurses in American state psychiatric hospitals. She developed a model of interpersonal relationships in nursing, which was published in 1952 as *Interpersonal Relations in Nursing* (Callaway, 2002).

Another nurse who played a prominent role during the same period was Ida J Orlando, whose thorough study of the interaction between nurse and MHCU appeared in 1972 under the title *The Discipline and Teaching of the Nursing Process* (Orlando, 1972). These two mental health nurses, and many others who advocated for mental health nursing, ensured that mental health nursing content was incorporated as part of basic nurse training. Mental health nurses began to act as consultants to their medico-surgical colleagues in general hospitals, helping with the emotional problems of MHCUs, and many nurses specialised in mental health nursing. The *Journal of American Psychiatric Nurses Association* was published in the 1990s and in the beginning of the new millennium the focus was on mental health nursing care that would integrate biological, psychological, social, spiritual and environmental dimensions (Kneisl & Trigoboff. 2013).

The 1990s has been described as the 'decade of the brain' and the 'decade of recovery'. During this period the understanding of mental disorders was further expanded with an increased focus on the biological basis for mental disorders and a recovery-oriented paradigm (Kneisl & Trigoboff 2013; Piat & Sabetti, 2009).

In the new millennium the focus was on the reform of mental health care with a shortened length of stay in hospital. Increased availability and revised action of psychiatric medications and the development of diagnostic techniques have improved the possibilities for treatment (Kneisl & Trigoboff, 2013). The focus and needs of MHCUs have changed with an increased incidence of dual diagnoses such as substance-use disorders and other comorbidities. Complementary, alternative and integrative healing practices are more frequently included in mental health care and treatment (Kneisl & Trigoboff, 2013). More recently, technology has been implemented in the treatment of mental health conditions such as telepsychiatry programmes that increase access to mental health services and have the potential to improve MHCU outcomes (Lauckner & Whitten, 2015).

South African perspective

A number of issues regarding mental health care are now examined from the South African perspective. These include mental health action groups, management, quality of care, community services, legislation, the effects of apartheid and education and training.

Mental health action groups

The mental health movement also spread to South Africa. A committee was established in Cape Town in 1913 to look after the interests of people with intellectual disabilities. The activities of this committee soon spread to the mentally ill and the committee advocated for legislative provision for the management of MHCUs. This action led directly to the promulgation of the Mental Disorders Act of 1916. By 1920 the group had grown into the National Council for Mental Health. The Council moved its headquarters to Johannesburg in 1926 and, with the help of affiliated mental health societies, played an important role in the development of services such as child guidance clinics, training centres for people with intellectual disabilities and juvenile courts (Minde, 1955).

Management

Control of mental health care institutions was transferred from the Department of Health to the Department of Internal Affairs in 1909, as these institutions were not regarded as hospitals. In 1943 they were returned to the jurisdiction of the national Department of Health, while all other hospitals were by now the responsibility of the provincial administrations. This placement of psychiatric hospitals outside of the provincial departments of health led to their isolation from the mainstream of medical development and to large-scale stagnation of the services. The isolation was only broken in 1988 when psychiatric hospitals were placed under the management of the provincial administrations.

Quality of care

As was the case internationally, psychiatric hospital care in the middle of the 20th century was poor. Miss Iris Marwick was appointed correspondent to the International

Council of Nurses regarding mental health in South Africa (Marwick, 1975). Her reports began appearing in the *Nursing Record* in 1933. In these reports she sketched a picture of serious over-population, extremely poor working conditions for nursing staff and acute staff shortages. Mental health care during this period has been described as dehumanising and violent in nature. According to Jones (2012), overcrowding was a challenge with it being reported in 1948 that there were 3100 more patients than beds available in mental health institutions. Overcrowding and conditions were considerably worse for black patients than for white patients (Jones, 2012).

In this climate Miss Marwick and Dr H Moross developed Tara Hospital in the northern suburbs of Johannesburg into a progressive psychiatric hospital. Tara was originally a military hospital, but it was transferred to the provincial administration in 1946. Although it was, in effect, a psychiatric hospital, it did not admit certified (involuntary) MHCUs. The hospital could, therefore, be developed under the auspices of the provincial administration. Modern methods of treatment, such as milieu therapy, a children's clinic, an open-door policy and day care were implemented, and the hospital became the leader in the field of mental health care. The hospital had various recreational facilities and made use of a multidisciplinary team approach. Flexible visiting hours and weekend leave were introduced to enhance reintegration into the community (Jones, 2012). Champions for a new approach to mental health care, such as Maxwell Jones and John Bowlby, visited Tara Hospital and they came to be at the forefront of new ideas in mental health treatment (Gillis, 2012).

Community services
Social workers of the Mental Health Association throughout the country started to give aftercare support to MHCUs in the community in the early 1920s. The first effort by a psychiatric hospital itself to work outside the confines of the institution was made in 1953 when Tara Hospital provided the first psychiatric outpatient service and nurses conducted home visits and helped form support groups after discharge (Jones, 2012). An aftercare service for discharged MHCUs of the Tara Hospital was established. This service was so popular that, after an investigation by the Department of Health, it was extended to other metropolitan areas. This cooperation between the psychiatric hospital, local government and the Mental Health Association, as well as the active involvement of mental health nurses, established the pattern for the rapid development of community services.

Outpatient departments were developed at all the large psychiatric hospitals in the 1970s, and inpatient populations began to decline. The radical type of deinstitutionalisation, which resulted in the revolving-door syndrome of repeated discharge and readmission in the USA, was never practised in South Africa. Outpatient clinics were gradually opened throughout the country and MHCUs were carefully discharged according to their ability to lead a dignified existence outside the institution.

This dramatic change in the service necessitated a change in legislation and resulted, in 1973, in the promulgation of the Mental Health Act. This facilitated admission without isolation, as well as legalised outpatient treatment. The changing pattern is illustrated in Figure 1.1.

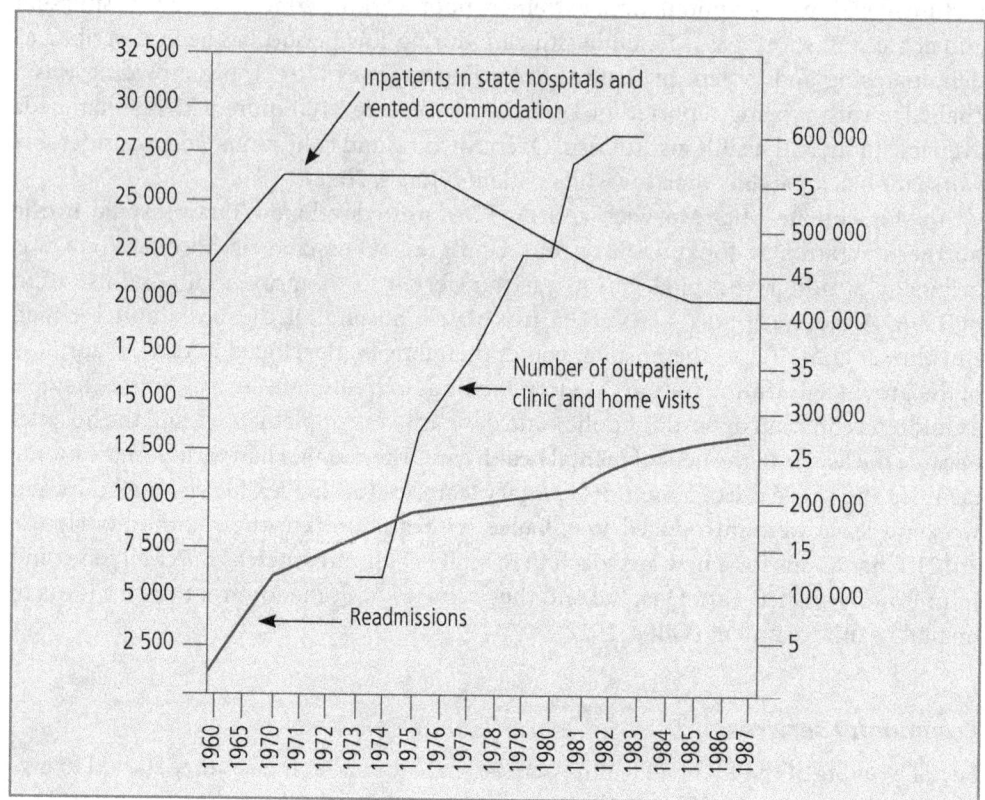

Figure 1.1 Changing patterns in South African mental health services 1960–1987

Source: Adapted from the National Health Report (Department of Health, 1989).

Legislation

Before South Africa became a Union in 1910, the supposed 'Lunacy Laws' governed psychiatric care. The first inclusive Act, the Mental Disorder and Defective Persons Act of 1916, was developed by Dr J T Dunston (Gillis, 2012). In 1961 a section was added to this Act that accommodated outpatients and free services for voluntary patients who were unable to foot the bill (Jones, 2012). A number of versions and amendments followed such as the Mental Health Act 18 of 1973 and the most recent Mental Health Care Act 17 of 2002 (Gillis, 2012). The Mental Health Care Act 17 of 2002 protects the human rights of people with mental disorders.

Apartheid

The National Party government, which came to power in 1948, placed racism on the statute book. Over the years this had a profound influence on mental health problems in the country, as well as on the development of services.

Human right violations and unfavourable practices and legislation affected the mental health of black, Indian and coloured South African groups, some of these being the Immorality Act 50 of 1927; the Immorality Amendment Act 21 of 1950 and the Prohibition of Mixed Marriages Act 55 of 1949 (Gillis, 2012). Some of the impacts of these practices included the following:

- They broke up family life by virtue of the fact that urbanisation of families was prohibited by enforcing migrant labour.
- They promoted poverty by controlling admission to the free economy, land ownership, quality education and job opportunities.
- They intensified stress in the community by the forced removal of people from familiar to strange environments; prosecution and intimidation by the enforcement of laws and race classification on an unwilling population; and by suppressing popular leadership.

Racial discrimination, political violence and exclusion due to apartheid and colonisation affected human development and impacted negatively on mental health (APA, 1979; Bantjes et al, 2017; Vogelman, 1986). The lifetime prevalence of 30 per cent for mental disorders in South Africa is high compared to a number of other countries, and substance-use disorders are particularly high in comparison (Stein et al, 2008). However, the South African Stress and Health (SASH) study, a large-scale population-based study of common mental disorders in South Africa, produced limited differences in lifetime prevalence of psychiatric disorders according to race. These results may be due to the varied definitions of race in South Africa and the other complex sociodemographic influences (Stein et al, 2008).

The quality of services offered to the various population and gender groups differed considerably as South African mental health practices were controlled by political, racial and gendered inequality (Jones, 2012). The negative positions of disadvantaged population groups naturally also influenced mental health services. The availability of services such as training centres for children with intellectual disabilities, child guidance clinics, school psychologist services and psychotherapeutic services are but a few examples. Care was mainly focused on white males, as apartheid ideologies suggested that Africans had to return to their 'traditional' way of life and be taken care of by their families. Women too had to be taken care of by their families (Jones, 2012). The APA found during a 17-day investigation of mental health services in South Africa in 1978, that black South Africans received inferior mental health care and were exposed to psychiatric practices that led to unnecessary deaths (APA, 1979).

Black MHCUs were often made to sleep on the floor, did not have sheets and were given substandard nutrition (Dhai, 2012).

There were very few black doctors, which led to an acute shortage of black psychiatrists. Until the late 1970s–early 1980s there were only white psychiatrists (Jones, 2012). Black people were also under-represented in professions such as occupational therapy, clinical psychology and social work, and this in turn hampered the functioning of multiprofessional teams in mental health services.

The creation of the Tricameral Parliament resulted in the control of mental health services, particularly community services, being divided among the three houses of Parliament. This fragmentation was not implemented to the same extent in all the provinces, but in many regions it led to a serious duplication of services, while access to their nearest service was suspended for some MHCUs. Maldistribution of staff resulted in less-than-optimal functioning of services.

In 1994 the first democratically elected government came into power. The period since then has been characterised by major changes in the health services and in society. Mental health reform also took place based on the 1997 White Paper for Transformation of the Health System. In 1997 the Mental Health Policy Guidelines were developed but limited implementation has occurred due to the low priority given to mental health and the shortage of human resources. In 2012 the Minister of Health initiated a number of health summits, including a National Mental Health Summit which involved maximum stakeholder consultation. This led to the development of the National Mental Health Policy Framework and Strategic Plan 2013–2020 (Department of Health, 2013).

Education and training

In the early 18th century, mental health nursing had a low social status in South Africa and was perceived as not suitable for a 'respectable woman'. Male orderlies were often employed in these environments. Florence Nightingale, in her correspondence with Rev Middleton Wilshire, the chaplain of Robben Island where mentally ill persons were treated, acknowledged as early as 1887 that specialised competencies were required of nurses working with the mentally ill.

Tara Hospital was a training hospital since its establishment as it had psychiatrists, psychologists, psychiatric nurses, occupational therapists, physiotherapists and social workers training there. Specialist psychiatric training was initiated at Tara Hospital, with the introduction of the Diploma of Psychological Medicine at the University of the Witwatersrand in 1949. Similar programmes at other medical schools in the country commenced thereafter. Consequently, psychiatric academic departments and full-time professorial positions were implemented at medical schools. Undergraduate psychiatry was introduced into the Bachelor of Medicine and Bachelor of Surgery (MBChB) degrees (Gillis, 2012; Jones, 2012) and postgraduate specialisations in psychiatry.

Mental health nursing training became the responsibility of the South African Medical Council in 1928, although many nurses still wrote the examination of the Royal Medico-Psychological Association of Britain until this practice was ended by legislation in 1932. In 1931 the regulations were published for two qualifications leading to registration in mental nursing and the nursing of people with intellectual disabilities. When the

South African Nursing Council was established in 1944, it took over from the Medical and Dental Council in regulating nursing education (Minde, 1977; Samson, 1978). The admission level was raised to standard eight (the equivalent of today's grade 10) in order to place mental health nursing on par with other branches of the profession. However, the numbers dropped so dramatically that the level was again lowered to standard six – now grade eight (Minde, 1977). Mental health nurses were often recruited from industrial schools. The training was poor: there were no classrooms, specific lecture periods or trained tutors.

Regulations were promulgated as far back as 1954 for a one-year programme in mental health nursing which would combine the previous two diplomas, but the programme was only implemented in the 1960s. Black mental health nurses were trained from 1958 and 1959 after all restrictions had been overcome (Minde, 1977). The first mental health nurses commenced their training as tutors in 1965, and this small group made a far-reaching contribution to the development of mental health nurse training in South Africa. Standard 10 (grade 12) was finally laid down as the minimum admission level for training in 1975. The first training school for black nurses in mental health nursing opened in 1956 and the first six black psychiatric nurse instructors registered an additional qualification with the South African Nursing Council in 1969 (Samson, 1978).

Advanced courses in mental health nursing were offered by Tara Hospital in the 1950s and at Groote Schuur Hospital in Cape Town in 1962 which led to an exceptional group of mental health nurse practitioners, but this programme was later discontinued (Gillis, 2012). During the 1970s general nurses training at the then B G Alexander College, the Witwatersrand College of Nursing, and the H F Verwoerd Hospital, Pretoria, completed practical training at Tara Hospital (Minde, 1977).

In 1970, two universities (Orange Free State and Pretoria) initiated a basic, integrated degree course that included mental health nursing, and this integrated approach was accepted as the model for all basic training in the country in 1986 when the nursing programme changed from three to four years. Based on this model, 21 per cent of the curriculum content of the four-year diploma or degree programme leading to registration as a professional nurse (in the fields relating to general, community, or psychiatric nursing care) and also as midwife (Nursing Act 50 of 1978, regulation 425) is dedicated to mental health (WHO & UCT, 2007).

The inclusion of mental health in the general nursing programme broke the isolation of mental health nursing and made it part of the broader health service. It further opened the way for postgraduate programmes in mental health nursing and the first nurses to receive clinical master's degrees in this field of nursing did so in 1976. Nursing PhDs commenced in South Africa in 1970 (Potgieter, in Coetzee et al, 2015) with 16 nursing departments/schools offering doctoral degree programmes by 2015 (Coetzee et al, 2015).

The post-apartheid era has seen the nursing profession challenged with transforming nursing education in line with, and at the pace of, the broader higher education and health sectors' transformation process in South Africa (Department of Health, 2013).

General dissatisfaction in some forums about the quality of nurses, and a view that the old curriculum framework and content was unresponsive and outdated (Armstrong & Rispel, 2015), has led to national macro-curricular changes in nursing. The Nursing Act 50 of 1978, as amended, has regulated the training of nurses in South Africa from 1990 to 2004. The Nursing Act 33 of 2005 (section 31) regulates training of the auxiliary nurse (regulation 169 of 8 March 2013); the registered nurse (regulation 171 of 8 March 2013); and the professional nurse (regulation 174 of 8 March 2013). It also makes provision for an advanced diploma in midwifery (regulation not available at time of printing) and postgraduate diplomas (regulation not available at the time of printing).

Mental health nursing in the four-year bachelor's degree (Nursing Act 33 of 2005, regulation 174) consists of comparatively less mental health content than the previous four-year comprehensive programme (Nursing Act 50 of 1978, regulation 425). The end-date for the enrolment in the four-year comprehensive programme (Nursing Act 50 of 1978, regulation 425) is 31 December 2019 (South African Nursing Council, 2016). Mental health nursing will be offered as a postgraduate diploma.

The future of mental health nursing and the preparedness of nurses to address the growing burden of mental illnesses will inevitably be influenced by these curricular changes and the fact that mental health nursing does not seem to be a popular field of specialisation. In a study conducted by Jansen and Venter (2015) in the Free State, it was reported that nursing students found mental health nursing less favourable as they feared stagnation and a loss of their nursing skills.

Of concern is the misalignment between the training of enough nurses in mental health and national strategic planning and needs. With the National Mental Health Policy Framework and Strategic Plan 2013–2020 (Department of Health, 2013) in mind, it is important that more nurses be trained in mental health nursing, so that mental health nursing knowledge and these skills may become more widely available. Nurse generalists must be able to identify and refer mental disorders commonly seen at the primary health care (PHC) level (Mkhize & Kometsi, 2008). We argue that identification and referral alone will not address the growing need for mental health services in the country.

CONTEMPORARY ISSUES IN MENTAL HEALTH NURSING

Contemporary issues in mental health care, treatment and rehabilitation that influence mental health nursing are the re-engineering of PHC, a greater focus on psychosocial rehabilitation in community psychiatric care, the recovery paradigm, and decolonisation.

Re-engineering of PHC

In the second half of the 20th century the realisation dawned on the world that hospital-centred health care services were not effective in promoting health and were far too expensive for the limited resources of many communities. In 1978, during a meeting in

Alma-Ata, Kazakhstan, the WHO adopted the declaration that PHC was the way to go in order to ensure health for all by the year 2000. This declaration resulted in the South African government's accepting as its policy a comprehensive PHC approach.

The PHC approach has important implications for mental health services. In the initial Alma-Ata declaration, psychiatric/mental health care was not included among PHC services. This oversight probably stems from the historic position of mental health as less prioritised in the health services, coupled with the fact that the declaration was adopted before the enormous growth in the science of neurology since the 1990s. It may also stem from an underestimation of the seriousness and extent of mental illness. Whatever the reasons, the advantages of including mental health care in PHC are as follows:

- Nurses and other health professionals in community settings will learn to understand mental health better, which will enable them to be positive role models in their communities, thereby combating the stigma attached to MHCUs and their families.
- Early detection and treatment in the PHC setting will be possible, so that treatment will cause the least possible disruption in the role-functioning of the MHCU.
- Even if hospitalisation is sometimes necessary, there will be a local professional involved in the procedure of admission. This will increase the involvement of the family and the local social network in the treatment of the MHCU.
- Rehabilitation will also be possible within the community in which the MHCU lives.

The South African government has been committed to implementing PHC principles. Some progress has been made, however, there are a number of challenges.

Progress

The progress that has been made towards implementing the PHC approach to mental health includes:

- The promulgation of the Mental Health Care Act no 17 of 2002 which is designed to improve access to mental health services, promote PHC services, and enhance the integration of mental health care into general health services and the development of community-based mental health services
- The development of the National Mental Health Policy Framework and Strategic Plan 2013–2020 which, among other objectives, focuses on scaling up decentralised integrated PHC services; on increasing public awareness to reduce stigma and discrimination; and on intersectoral collaboration, mental health promotion and recovery within the community (Department of Health, 2013; Stein, 2014)
- Some progress on the integration of mental health into PHC with district level health care providing emergency psychiatric service and medication management of long-term MHCUs (Petersen & Lund, 2011)
- The establishment of the National Directorate: Mental Health and Substance Abuse, Department of Health, who oversee education and awareness campaigns in mental health (Department of Health, 2013).

Limitations and challenges

Some of the limitations and challenges regarding the PHC approach to mental health care include the following:

- There is hospital-focused treatment and a treatment gap where many South Africans, especially in rural areas do not have access to mental health care, treatment and rehabilitation.
- Mental health care, treatment and rehabilitation are underfunded and under-resourced. The district health levels are allocated limited resources (Department of Health, 2013) and hospitals on regional and district health levels experience inadequate infrastructure, limited numbers of personnel and high administrative burdens related to requirements in the Mental Health Care Act 17 of 2002. They also have limited contact with review boards (Ramlall et al, 2010).
- There is an emphasis on medication management of persons with severe and chronic mental illnesses, with limited focus on mental health promotion, prevention, early detection and treatment of other common disorders (Petersen & Lund, 2011; Department of Health, 2013).
- Deinstitutionalisation occurs at a faster pace than the development of adequate and equipped community-based services and resources (Petersen et al, 2009). The consequences of deinstitutionalisation have led to an increased number of persons with mental illness living on the streets and frequent readmissions (Department of Health, 2013). One of the most recent tragic consequences has been the deaths of 144 MHCUs who were moved from the Life Esidimeni care centres to ill-equipped non-governmental organisations in 2016.
- There are limited human resources in the public sector rural PHC areas. There is a dire need for mental health nurses in these areas to which the tasks of diagnosis and prescription can be shifted. A study conducted in 2013 indicated that there were 0.68 mental health nurses per 100 000 of the population in the public sector rural PHC setting. Not enough nurses are trained to bridge the gap (De Kock & Pillay, 2016).

Psychosocial rehabilitation and the recovery paradigm

When deinstitutionalisation occurred in the 1970s (mainly internationally), MHCUs were transferred to the community without preparing the community for the influx. Mental health care professionals were still concentrated in hospitals, while most of the MHCUs were to be found within the community. Alternative housing and vocational rehabilitation services were not available in the community. Staff working in outpatient settings did not have the necessary skills to help people in this new situation. Families became the main providers of care, as MHCUs were often discharged in their care with little notice or preparation. Although MHCUs were discharged and living in the community, the situation caused as many problems as it solved and often did not lead to an improved quality of life for the MHCUs or their families.

Gradually community mental health professionals and consumers (mostly family members, but also the patients themselves) formulated their problems, developed strategies to cope with these problems and became more vocal in demanding services that satisfied their needs. This change is now called the rehabilitation era. The groups involved identified various services as essential for the care of a mentally ill person in the community. These included case management, crisis intervention, treatment, basic support, enrichment, rights protection and psychiatric rehabilitation.

A recovery-oriented rehabilitation paradigm has emerged in the past two decades (Piat & Sabetti, 2009) and is motivated by:
- research evidence and psychopharmacological developments leading to significant clinical improvement
- the rights of people living with mental illness to reintegrate and live a meaningful life within their communities (Piat & Sabetti, 2009).

The recovery-oriented rehabilitation paradigm is associated with concepts and theories of resilience, survivorship, hope, engagement, societal connectedness and autonomy (Piat & Sabetti, 2009).

Principles relating to the level of health service delivery that supports recovery are:
- integration of mental health into general health services
- intersectoral collaboration
- mental health promotion and illness prevention
- elimination of social exclusion such as discrimination and stigmatisation
- full participation and leadership by MHCUs
- mental health provider training in recovery values and practices
- cultural sensitivity and sensitivity towards human rights (Piat & Sabetti, 2009).

The move from the community psychiatric era to the rehabilitation and recovery era has not yet been completed in South Africa and a lot of work is yet to be done to integrate mental health care into PHC. The focus of most community psychiatric services is still on treatment rather than rehabilitation.

Decolonisation

Colonialism is widely associated with the notion of European countries occupying the land of indigenous persons. Cultural domination is then achieved where power and privilege befall the coloniser and widespread prejudice is present (Fay, 2016). Nursing is not untouched by colonisation. Schultheiss (2010: 151) explains the dichotomy in perspectives about the colonised history of nursing all over the world:

> *The history of nursing in the age of empire is a story of good intentions mixed with cultural chauvinism, of professional rigor mixed with condescension, of devotion and generosity shaped and often distorted by ideas of gendered and racial conventions, and of ambitious reform crushed by an inability to think beyond the bounds of imperialism.*

Those involved in mental health care need to be aware of the oppressive practices associated with colonisation and of what needs to be done in implementing decolonisation strategies (Fay, 2016). Despite some efforts that have been made towards developing a culturally sensitive approach in mental health services, mental health practice, research and education have been focused mostly on western Euro-centric paradigms. These pertain to principles of prevention and treatment of mental illness with limited use of indigenous knowledge systems (Fellner, 2016). The continued relevance of the nursing profession in general, and specifically mental health nursing, will require engagement with decolonisation procedures (McGibbon et al, 2014). Traditional educational and mental health care institutions will increasingly be required to incorporate indigenous knowledge about mental health and illness, and cultural identity into the training curricula for general and specialist mental health professionals (Thurston & Mashford-Pringle, 2015). A critical stance should be followed when considering internalised colonialised paradigms and theories in mental health nursing. The colonisation counter-narrative (McGibbon et al, 2014) in mental health care requires a deep and critical engagement with the structural determinants of mental health, social justice in mental health care, treatment and rehabilitation, and human rights in South Africa. Critical reflection on and in mental health nursing practice is required. This should involve a deep sense of awareness and a critical stance towards western worldviews and the legacy of apartheid that continue to influence mental health services, mental health nursing practice, education and research (McGibbon et al, 2014; Mulaudzi, 2016.).

CONCLUSION

To date mental health services have been shaped by many factors within as well as outside the country's borders, and this is a process that is expected to continue. Going forward and building on the lessons learned in history – a form of activism for improving mental health services for all South Africans – is imperative. Nurses are aptly positioned and are required to advocate for the protection and promotion of the rights of all people, especially those who are particularly vulnerable, like MHCUs. A collective voice to influence much-needed improvements in mental health service delivery in South Africa is required.

WEB RESOURCES

https://www.wits.ac.za/clinicalmed/departments/psychiatry/clinical-services/specialist-hospitals/
    Website of the University of the Witwatersrand gives a brief history of the Tara Moross Hospital, including some pictures of the early and current buildings.

REFERENCES

Akeso Psychiatric Clinics. 2017. *Akeso behavioural healthcare group.* https://www.akeso.co.za/ (Accessed 17 March 2018).

American Psychiatric Association (APA). 1979. 'Report of the committee to visit South Africa'. *American Journal of Psychiatry*, 136 (2): 1498–1506.

Anthony, W, Cohen, M and Frakas, M. 1990. *Psychiatric Rehabilitation.* Boston: Boston University.

Armstrong, S J and Rispel, L C. 2015. 'Social accountability and nursing education in South Africa'. *Global Health Action*, 8: 27879. http://dx.doi.org/10.3402/gha.v8.27879 (Accessed 25 August 2019).

Bantjes, J, Swartz, L and Niewoudt, P. 2017. 'Human rights and mental health in post-apartheid South Africa: lessons from health care professionals working with suicidal inmates in the prison system'. *BioMedCentral International Health and Human Rights*: 17–29.

Callaway, B J. 2002. *Hildegard Peplau. Psychiatric Nurse of the Century.* New York: Springer.

Coetzee, S K, Klopper, H C and Kim, M J. 2015. 'The quality of doctoral nursing education in South Africa'. *Curationis* 38 (1).

Daey Ouwens, I M, Lens, E, Fiolet, A T L, Ott, F A, Koehler, P J, Kager, P A and Verhoeven, M W A. 2017. 'Malaria Fever Therapy for General Paralysis of the Insane: A Historical Cohort Study'. *European Neurology*, 78: 56–62.

De Kock J and Pillay, B J. 2016. 'Mental health nurses in South Africa's public rural primary care settings: a human resource crisis'. *Rural and Remote Health*, 16: 3865.

Denmar Specialist Psychiatric Hospital. 2014. *Denmar.* http://denmar.co.za/ (Accessed 17 March 2018).

Department of Health. 1989. *National Health Report 1988.* Pretoria: Department of Health.

Department of Health. 2013. *National Mental Health Policy Framework and Strategic Plan 2013 –2020.* National Department of Health: Pretoria.

Dhai, A. 2012. 'A health system that violates patients' rights to access health care'. *South African Journal of Bioethics and Law*, 5 (1): 2–3.

Fay, J. 2016. 'Decolonising mental health services one prejudice at a time: psychological, sociological, ecological, and cultural considerations'. *Settler colonial studies*: 1–13.

Fellner, F H. 2016. *Returning to Our Medicines: Decolonizing and Indigenizing Mental Health Services to Better Serve Indigenous Communities in Urban Spaces.* DPhil, thesis. Vanvouver: University of British Colombia.

Gillis, L. 2012. 'The historical development of psychiatry in South Africa since 1652'. *South African Journal of Psychiatry*, 18 (3): 78–82.

Jansen, R & Venter, I. 2015. 'Psychiatric nursing: an unpopular choice'. *Journal of Psychiatric and Mental Health Nursing*, (22): 142–148.

Jones, T F. 2012. *Psychiatry, Mental Institutions, and the Mad in Apartheid South Africa.* New York: Taylor and Francis.

Kneisl, C R and Trigoboff, E. 2013. *Contemporary Psychiatric-Mental Health Nursing.* 3rd edition. Boston: Pearson.

Lauckner, C and Whitten, P. 2015. 'The State and Sustainability of Telepsychiatry Programs'. *Journal of Behavioral Health Services & Research*, 305–31.

Marwick, I. 1948a. 'International Congress of Mental Health'. *South African Nursing Journal*, XV(l).

Marwick, I. 1948b. 'South African Trained Nurses Association report'. *South African Nursing Journal*, November: 27 and 32.

Marwick, I. 1975. Iris Marwick – The pioneer of psychiatric nursing in South Africa. *SA Verplegingtydskrif*, 30 March.

Minde, M. 1955. 'Mental Health. Past Present and Future'. *SA Tydskrif vir Geneeskunde*, 26 November: 1124–1127.

Minde, M M. 1974. 'Mental Health Services in South Africa Part II During the British Occupation'. *South African Medical Journal*, 48 (38): 1629–1632.

Minde, M M. 1977. 'History of Mental Health Services in South Africa Part XIV. Psychiatric Education'. *South African Medical Journal*, 15: 210–215.

McGibbon E, Mulaudzi, F, Didham, P, Barton, S and Sochan, A. 2014. 'Toward decolonizing nursing: the colonization of nursing and strategies for increasing the counter-narrative'. *Nursing Inquiry*, 21 (3): 179–191.

Mkhize, N and Kometsi, M J. 2008. 'Community Access to Mental Health Services: Lessons and Recommendations'. In: Barron, P and Roma-Reardon, J (ed). *South African Health Review 2008*. Durban: Health Systems Trust.

Mulaudzi, M. 2016. 'Toward decolonizing nursing: The colonization of nursing and strategies for increasing the counter-narrative'. *Proceedings of the South African Nursing Conference, held in South Africa*, 24-26 February 2016. Pretoria: DENOSA.

Orlando, I J. 1972. *The Discipline and Teaching of Nursing Process (an Evaluative Study)*. New York: Putnam.

Palm Tree Clinic. nd. http://palmtreeclinic.co.za/ (Accessed 17 March 2018).

Parry, M. 2010. 'Voices from the past. A Mind That Found Itself: An Autobiography'. *American Journal of Public Health*, 100 (12): 2354–2356.

Pelletier, J F and Davidson, L. 2015. 'At the very roots of psychiatry as a new medical specialty: the Pinel-Pussin partnership'. *Santé mentale au Québec*, 40 (1): 19–33.

Petersen I, Bhana, A, Campbell-Hall, V et al. 2009. 'Planning for district mental health services in South Africa: a situational analysis of a rural district site'. *Health Policy and Planning*, 24: 140–150.

Petersen, I and Lund, C. 2011. 'Mental health service delivery in South Africa from 2000 to 2010: one-step forward, one step back'. *South African Medical Journal*, 101 (10): 751–757.

Piat, M and Sabetti, J. 2009. 'The Development of a Recovery-Oriented Mental Health System in Canada: What the Experience of Commonwealth Countries Tells Us'. *Canadian Journal of Community Mental Health*, 28(2): 17–33.

Ramlall, S, Chipps, J and Mars, M. 2010. 'Impact of the South African Mental Health Care Act No 17 of 2002 on regional and district hospitals designated for mental health care in KwaZulu-Natal'. *South African Medical Journal*, 100 (10): 667–670.

Samson, J P. 1978. 'Nursing education and the black nurse'. *Curationis*, 1(1): 47–55.

Schultheiss, K. 2010. Imperial Nursing: Cross-Cultural Challenges for Women in the Health Professions: A Historical Perspective. *Policy, Politics, & Nursing Practice*, 11 (2): 151–157.

Shuttleworth, M. 2018. 'Psychology and Mental Illness in the Middle Ages'. https://brewminate.com/psychology-and-mental-illness-in-the-middle-ages/ (Accessed 1 May 2019).

South African Nursing Council (SANC). 2016. *Circular 7/2016*. http://www.sanc.co.za/archive/archive2016/newsc1607.htm (Accessed 19 May 2019).

Stein, D J. 2014. 'A new mental health policy for South Africa'. *South African Medical Journal*, 104(2): 115–116.

Stein, D J, Seedat, S, Herman, A, Moomal, H, Heeringa, S G, Kessler, R C and Williams, D R. 2008. 'Lifetime prevalence of psychiatric disorders in South Africa'. *British Journal of Psychiatry*, 192(2): 112–117.

Swartz, L. 2002. Integrating services, marginalizing patients: psychiatric patients and primary health care in South Africa. *Transcultural Psychiatry*, 39 (2): 155–172.

Thurston, J M and Mashford-Pringle, A. 2015. 'Nursing and Indigenous education integration'. *Journal of Nursing Education and Practice*, 5(10): 9–15.

Vista Clinic. nd. https://www.vistaclinic.co.za/ (Accessed 17 March 2018).

Vogelman, L. 1986. *Apartheid and Mental Health.* Johannesburg: Proceedings of the OASSSA National Conference.

World Health Organisation (WHO) and University of Cape Town (UCT) Department of Psychiatry and Mental Health. 2007. *WHO-AIMS report on Mental Health System in South Africa.* Cape Town.

CHAPTER 2

A Conceptual Framework for Mental Health Nursing

L R Uys and A A H Smith

Learning Outcomes

After studying this chapter, you should be able to:
- define and discuss the concept of mental health
- define mental health nursing
- explain and implement the components of a mental health nursing practice model
- describe the process of and engage in reflective practice.

INTRODUCTION

In South Africa, mental health nursing forms part of the basic (pre-registration) education of professional nurses. The South African Nursing Council (SANC) proposed new standards that allow for the content of mental health nursing to be integrated into all nursing modules. This approach equips graduates to work as generalist nurses within decentralised, integrated health services in the country. In addition, it positions graduates to access specialist or advanced mental health nursing as a postgraduate specialisation.

Most students choosing a nursing career have a vague idea of what mental health nursing entails. Despite the national and global commitment to integrated mental health care, nurses are accustomed to a care system that separates mental and physical health, but this is gradually changing. These changes can be seen in the way that mental and physical health problems are interwoven: people with mental disorders are more likely to develop physical conditions such as diabetes, heart disease, stroke and respiratory distress; and the impact on mental health of diseases, such as human immunodeficiency virus (HIV)/acquired immunodeficiency syndrome (AIDS) or tuberculosis (TB), is known. Nurses' consideration of the impact of physical illness on the mental health of patients, and on their families, is gaining momentum as an important part of the global (WHO, 2010; 2013; 2018) and local mental health strategy (South African Department of Health, 2013). While integration of services increases accessibility and makes economic sense, it also aims to avoid the separation and stigmatisation of mentally ill persons.

The integration of mental health services within general health care services means that nurses in medical–surgical contexts will have contact with mental health care users (MHCUs) and their families as they seek help for physical ill-health concerns (see

Chapter 21). Understanding of an MHCU's struggle with mental illness seldom extends beyond mental illness stereotypes. These stereotypes include the following: that persons with mental illness are difficult, threatening, unpredictable, dangerous, incompetent, and responsible for their own illness (Baziga & Smith, 2016; WHO, 2017).

Stigma, a social 'achievement' (this means that essentially, stigma is only 'felt' if there is a power differential), was first described by Irving Goffman (1963), cited in Corrigan et al (2005), as a process that marks a person as different and 'less than'. Current understanding of stigma components and processes is that society, usually informally, agrees on negative stereotypical characteristics associated with specific labels. For example, 'schizophrenic' becomes 'schizo' and the associated meanings are consciously acknowledged in people's thought processes. The use of this label is then quickly followed by separating this individual from the 'in' group. Separation is accompanied by emotional reactions among members of the 'in' group – anger, fear, disgust, pity, guilt – that in turn result in prejudicial responses. These prejudicial responses limit social inclusion of the 'out' group, in this instance persons who have been assigned a mental illness label of schizophrenia (Baziga & Smith, 2016; WHO, 2017). In a nurse such prejudicial responses influence the nature of the nurse–patient relationship. The nurse–patient relationship is an interpersonal interaction at the core of frameworks for mental health nursing practice, which is facilitated by the nurse's clinical skills and shaped by their personal beliefs about mental health and illness (see 'Nurse–MHCU relationship'.

It is important for nursing students to explore their own reactions to their practice experience. They should also challenge their assumptions and accepted stereotypes about mental illness, so that these reactions do not render them ineffective when caring for persons with mental ill-health challenges. For the nurse who is observant, mental ill-health challenges within the current health care system could include: a postnatal mother struggling with depression, a patient in intensive care following a car accident and struggling with post-traumatic syndrome, or an MHCU post-surgery struggling with delusional beliefs. A person struggling with mental illness symptoms is in pain, and usually afraid. They have been brought up in the same society as everyone else and are aware of the negative stereotypes associated with mental illness labels. The last thing they need from helping professionals is rejection.

DEFINING MENTAL HEALTH

Definitions are objective statements which describe the meaning of a term through a process of noting definite and distinct characteristics. These identified characteristics allow for measurement and allocation to a specific category. For example, in mainstream dictionaries 'female' is defined as an adjective according to reproductive characteristics: 'denoting the sex that can bear offspring or produce eggs, distinguished biologically by the production of gametes (ova) which can be fertilised by male gametes' (Oxford Dictionary, 2018). However, modern social understandings of the term female, within the current lesbian, gay, bisexual and transgender (LGBT) climate, have more to do with subjective experiences of gender identity than with biological characteristics. This has resulted in definitive allocations to specific categories becoming problematic. Defining complex concepts that are socially constructed and dynamic in such a way that the definition remains relevant can be difficult; and mental health is such a concept.

Initial definitions of mental health focused on the absence of symptom clusters linked to a diagnosis (or label) of mental illness within diagnostic frameworks such as the DSM-5 (American Psychiatric Association, 2013). These definitions are too narrow and do not account for subjective well-being. The result is that ill health rather than health is identified as a form of measurement and the nurse focuses on secondary and tertiary prevention rather than primary prevention. Current definitions of mental health, grounded in social models of care, attempt to be more health focused and inclusive. For example, the World Health Organisation (WHO) defined mental health to be 'a state of well-being in which the individual realises his or her own abilities, can cope with the normal stresses of life, can work productively and fruitfully, and is able to make a contribution to his or her community' (WHO, 2014). The WHO added the following principles for consideration when defining this concept:

- Mental health, physical health and social functioning are interdependent and the relationship between these is complex. For example, a person is diagnosed with HIV/AIDS and experiences fear in direct response not only to the diagnosis, but also to other people's possible reactions to them. To hide any physical manifestations, the person isolates themselves with the result that they are unable to derive support from others and depression manifests. Depressive symptoms result in a loss of energy and interest in caring for oneself, with a resultant deterioration in physical health and further impaired social functioning.
- Mental health is culturally determined and linked to normative behaviour: if behaviour is 'the norm' in a specific community then it will be perceived as 'normal' by members of that community, even though another community would consider the behaviour an indication of mental ill health. For example, several communities in South Africa communicate with ancestors and behave in response to actual, or potential, direct influence of these ancestors in their life. This behaviour might not be normative in other communities.
- Mental health is not a static state in that once it has been achieved it remains unchanged and intact.
- Rather, it can be measured on a continuum were movement is influenced by internal beliefs (also known as self-concept or self-esteem) used to interpret ongoing experiences. These beliefs, about self and the world we live in, develop through interactions with others and influence how we interpret our ongoing experiences. This interpretation determines feelings experienced which in turn affect our behavioural responses.

What is evident within current mental health definitions is that mental ill health extends beyond the boundaries of the psychiatric diagnostic framework and care setting, is more than a collection of diagnosable symptoms, and influences all aspects of the person's life.

DEFINING MENTAL HEALTH NURSING

Mental health nursing is an interpersonal process in which counselling includes planned interventions that can be focused on the prevention of mental ill health, or on facilitating rehabilitation and promoting recovery.

- *An interpersonal process.* This aspect of the definition emphasises the fact that the key knowledge and skills involved in mental health nursing deal with the intrapersonal and interpersonal dynamics of human beings. It is an intensely personal human process.
- *Planned interventions.* This part of the definition makes it clear that mental health nursing is based on knowledge of human behaviour both in sickness and in health. It is not merely doing what comes naturally; it is an evidence-based, planned, controlled, targeted action on the part of the nurse.
- *Prevention of mental ill health.* This aspect of the mental health nurse's role is determined by where they work. It encompasses being aware of the risks to mental health within the environment and addressing these through *planned interventions* implemented and facilitated by the nurse's *interpersonal relationships* with individual MHCUs or groups at risk.
- *Facilitating rehabilitation.* Rehabilitation refers to psychosocial rehabilitation (PSR), a process facilitated by the mental health nurse and other practitioners, which allows the patient to articulate and pursue specific rehabilitation goals. The MHCU begins, or increases, their knowledge and understanding of their symptomatology and use of psychopharmacology with the clear purpose of continuing to live, work and participate in community life. As a process, PSR encourages empowerment through facilitating the MHCUs' ability to participate, choose and negotiate choices, and develop a sense of self-efficacy that facilitates a positive view of the future and future endeavours. At the core of PSR is recognition of MHCUs, and their family members, as experts through experience while still recognising research knowledge, and the clinical experience and skill of mental health care practitioners.
- *Promoting recovery.* While PSR facilitates a future recovery orientation within practice and service provision, recovery is in fact the achievement of the MHCU, and their family. Recovery, previously defined as clinical recovery with no symptoms, now relates to the MHCU's sense of self-efficacy that engages and guides in selecting and achieving a meaningful and productive life alongside the limitations of the illness.

Deinstitutionalisation and decentralised community mental health care, with an increasing emphasis on service-user involvement, and the MHCU's right to rehabilitation services, were first conceptualised within the South African Mental Health Care Act 17 of 2002. Local policy (KZN Department of Health, 2010) and the national strategic plans (Mental Health Strategic Plan, 2013–2020, cited in WHO,

2013) conceptualise PSR as a cost-effective modality for community-based treatment and management of mental health. At the centre of these documents are the concepts of service user–practitioner relationships, recovery and rehabilitation, recognition of a participatory process and emphasis on service-user priorities and strengths in engaging and solving their own problems. These values suggest a need to re-examine the way mental health nurses interact with patients and their families and are a call to reflective practice.

The mental health nurse is in a unique position. They are in the MHCU environment for prolonged periods of time, within different health contexts, and at different positions on the persons health care trajectory. The mental health nurse should use their unique position to engage and counsel the MHCU. The model in Figure 2.1 provides a conceptual framework for mental health nursing that illustrates core aspects of practice and guides the mental health nurse in engaging and counselling MHCUs.

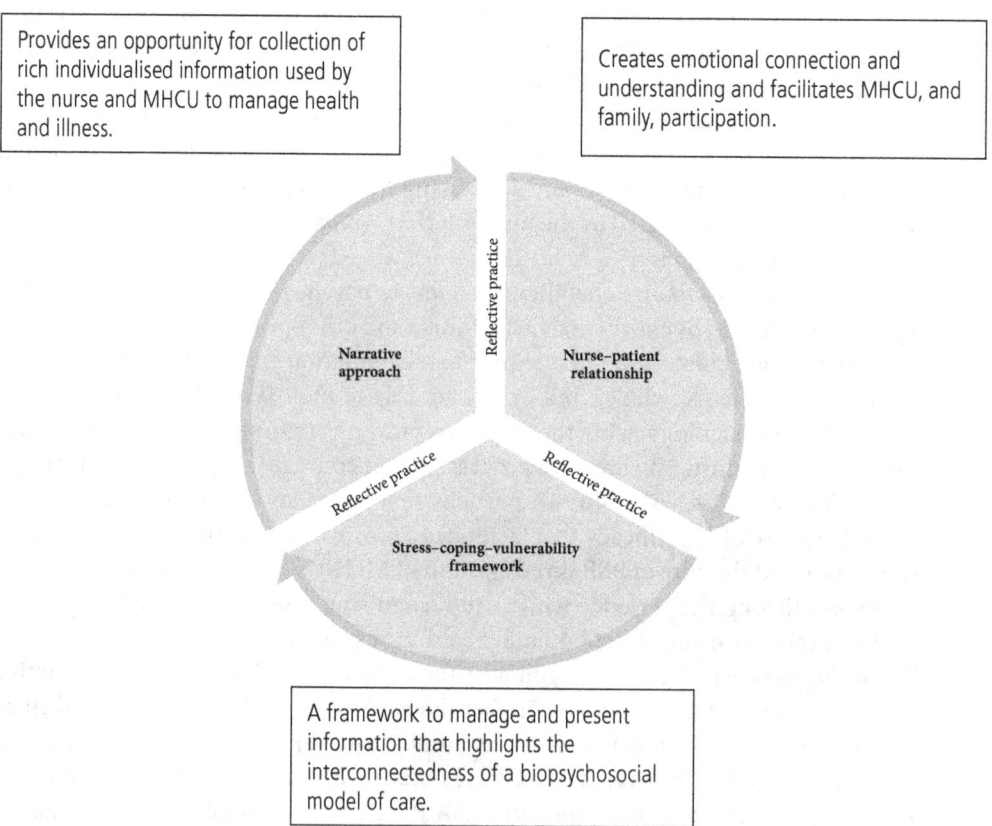

Figure 2.1 A model for the practice of mental health nursing

NURSE–MHCU RELATIONSHIP

Briefly, this relationship is the professional relationship between MHCUs, their families, and the nurse. The extent and nature of this interpersonal interaction is facilitated by the nurse's clinical skills – listening, reflecting, questioning, interpreting and explaining – and personal beliefs about mental health and illness underlying the interaction.

Despite the lack of empirical evidence that the nurse–MHCU relationship facilitates the nurse's therapeutic practice, there are extensive qualitative studies that report on perceptions from MHCUs and their families regarding the value of this relationship. Books and research studies, aimed at helping professionals such as psychologists, counsellors, nurses, report on the importance of a therapeutic alliance with the person(s) being care for. First, MHCUs want a relationship with the nurse based on understanding, human acceptance and trust. Secondly, MHCUs' active engagement with their treatment and recovery is significantly affected by interpersonal interactions that seek to recognise their opinions, expectations and experiences. Lastly, these interactions should place emphasis on the strengths of MHCUs and their families in engaging, understanding, learning and managing illness symptoms and solving their own problems. A useful place to keep up to date with the expectations that MHCUs and their families have of nurses is via service-user organisations and websites. At the end of the chapter a list of useful websites includes those for the South African Depression and Anxiety Group (SADAG); Experts by Experience, and Mind for Better Mental Health.

The defining attributes of MHCU and family participation include:

An established service user–practitioner relationship that includes a trusting, respectful and connected relationship acknowledging the importance of self-efficacy – the belief that one is capable of achieving what one sets out to do. Without this belief, most people will stop trying. Nurses should ask themselves if their style of communication suggests that the MHCU and their family are seen as competent and capable of pursuing and attaining goals aimed at living a fulfilling life, or whether the MHCU is seen as someone who is broken and incapable of being anything but ill.

Surrendering of some practitioner power that allows for choice and recognises that within current community-based models of care, MHCUs cannot be forced to follow practitioners' directives about treatment, and that a choice exists beyond the treatment site. Recognition of this fact facilitates reflection and negotiation with the MHCU, couched in the recognition of shared responsibility while the nurse empowers and supports. Evidence suggests that empowerment leads to positive MHCU mental health outcomes such as increased mental well-being, independence, self-efficacy, motivation to participate and enhanced self-esteem.

Shared information and knowledge refer first to obtaining and acknowledging the value of the opinions, expectations and experiences of MHCUs, and where appropriate, those of their families. Secondly, this refers to sharing practitioner clinical knowledge and research evidence that can inform decisions. Recognition of both parties' expertise is critical to working together and establishing rapport.

Active mutual engagement of both the nurse and the MHCU is required to facilitate participation. During an initial mental health crisis, it is possible that the MHCU's willingness to engage is linked to current struggles with specific symptoms or fears. Throughout the health–illness–health trajectory, MHCUs' ability to process information, their attitude to health care, level of trust, and what they perceive to be most important at that time, will influence participation in treatment. It is always possible for active engagement to occur. This can be during a mental illness crisis while the nurse is encouraging, listening, validating and being empathic to the MHCUs' sharing their experience of the crisis, their reality through the lens of the symptoms experienced, or their reasons for not wanting treatment. Engagement at this point has much value as this can reduce the MHCU's fear, and result in the development of trust so crucial to the nurse–MHCU relationship. It can also highlight information to be used in relapse prevention plans formulated later.

A narrative approach to communication

Narrative refers to a story, a description of events (Cambridge Dictionary, 2018). A narrative approach literally involves encouraging MHCUs, and their families, to tell their stories. This approach has replaced the style of using questioning focused on symptoms or medication such as: 'Are you eating?' 'Are you sleeping?' 'Are you taking your medication?' While it is important to gather data about vegetative functioning and medication use, valuable information is lost when specific 'bites' are sought, and this establishes the foundation for MHCUs' telling the nurse what they perceive the nurse as wanting to hear.

The core principles of using a narrative approach in interactions with the MHCU, and their family, include the following:

- There is a recognition that each person is unique – their biology, psychology and social context – and each person will have a unique experience of symptom(s) and treatment.
- This uniqueness means that each individual MHCU is an expert regarding their lives. The MHCU, rather than the nurse, decides what to talk about and where to start the story.
- The narrative (story) facilitates understanding of the problem for the nurse, the MHCU and their family.
- The nurse's role is one of curiosity, respect and participation (working with).
- The nurse uses words with care, specifically avoiding labelling the MHCU as the problem.
- The nurse listens for skills, abilities and successes within the narrative.

When nurses are encouraged to use a narrative approach and to listen to the MHCUs' stories, they often report being worried that they will miss important information. Their concerns relate essentially to their not asking the questions they would have formulated in order to write their report. This fear is unfounded. Consider that while an MHCU is telling a nurse a story about something that happened, the nurse would be able to complete a full mental status examination just by listening and clarifying:

- whether affective expression is visible
- if mood is described within the story

- how the MHCU structures sentences (form and flow of thought)
- the content of thought in the story, including, because the MHCU is encouraged to choose the story to be told, possible concerns or preoccupations. In addition, strengths and what the MHCU likes, dislikes, hopes for, and fears can be within the story
- if concentration is visible in the MHCUs' ability to remain focused on the story
- to what extent judgement is present, which will be evident within descriptions of decisions the MHCU took in the story.

The nurse can, at the end of the story, ask direct, open-ended questions to gather information they feel has not been obtained. There is nothing wrong with the nurse's checking the 'list of questions' they had before ending the interview and asking the MHCU to clarify specific information. However, if the nurse merely asks closed and specific open-ended questions they will limit the information gathered and learn little of the MHCU's life beyond the mental illness label and treatment.

Finally, one of the most valuable outcomes of a narrative approach to counselling is the opportunity to separate the MHCU from their psychiatric label. Within general health care one does not speak of a patient as being the illness, for example, 'she is cervical cancer'. Within the language of mental health illness, the MHCU is often labelled as the diagnosis: 'she is schizophrenic', not 'she has...' or 'she struggles with the symptoms of...'. This language, linked to issues of the stigma surrounding mental illness, is unconsciously used. The MHCU is left feeling 'less than others' and responsible for the illness, symptom emergence and re-emergence. This is a form of self-stigma that embraces a 'spoilt identity' – someone who is incapable, or indeed not worthy, of a fulfilling life that includes the things most people have and hope for: a place to live, love and gainful employment. While listening to the MHCU's narrative the nurse can use the opportunity to separate the person from the mental illness label.

Externalising the problem

What follows are some tips for nurses regarding the separation of the MHCU from the mental illness label, also known as externalising the problem. Recommendations include:
- Turn adjectives into nouns by using 'it' or 'the', 'the voices' rather than 'your voices'. This suggests a separate identity from the MHCU.
- Do not rush. Even if the person continues to speak of 'my depression/schizophrenia/voices', one should continue to use 'the...'.
- Try to name the symptom so that it reflects the MHCU's experience of it.
  - This objectifies the problem
  - Avoid using powerful names. While one can use 'the voices', this name suggests some power. By listening to descriptions of what, when, and where relating to the MHCUs' description of auditory hallucinations, it is possible to reduce the 'power' of the experience by the language used to describe the experience. For example, terms like 'the moaner', 'the criticiser', 'the negative one', 'the liar' could be used.

- Externalising has the added advantage of positioning the MHCU in opposition to the symptom/problem.
- Sometimes the MHCU will describe several symptoms/problems rather than one 'diagnostic label'. In such an instance, name each one.
- Listen for aspects of the story where the MHCU triumphed or won. For example, the MHCU may describe, 'My depression was so bad that I didn't want to go. I kept thinking no one will bother if I don't go, but I forced myself to go.' Amplify these events as successes, and as examples of personal strength and winning. For example, 'You won, you were stronger than "the depression" that wants to separate you from other people.' Amplify these competencies and strengths, ie the unique outcomes.

Stress–vulnerability framework

Frameworks are useful tools for helping the nurse. They are a means of organising the information that they have obtained, and also assist in looking at the interrelatedness of the information. The most useful of these frameworks is the stress–vulnerability framework, also sometimes referred to as a model; the stress–vulnerability model or stress–coping–vulnerability model. This framework has been in the public domain since the 1980s and despite variations on the name always focuses on the same three core interrelated categories of information: that *psychobiological vulnerability* interacts with the *psychosocial stressors* of daily life, with both mitigated by *protective factors*. The fourth category of information is not part of this interaction but rather the result. These are the presence, or re-emergence, of signs and symptoms of ill health. This framework allows the nurse to place information into four distinct categories: the first three are interrelated in the combined effect they have on the fourth – an increase or decrease in the emergence of symptomatology. Figure 2.2 provides a diagrammatic representation and is followed by a detailed discussion of each category and their interrelatedness.

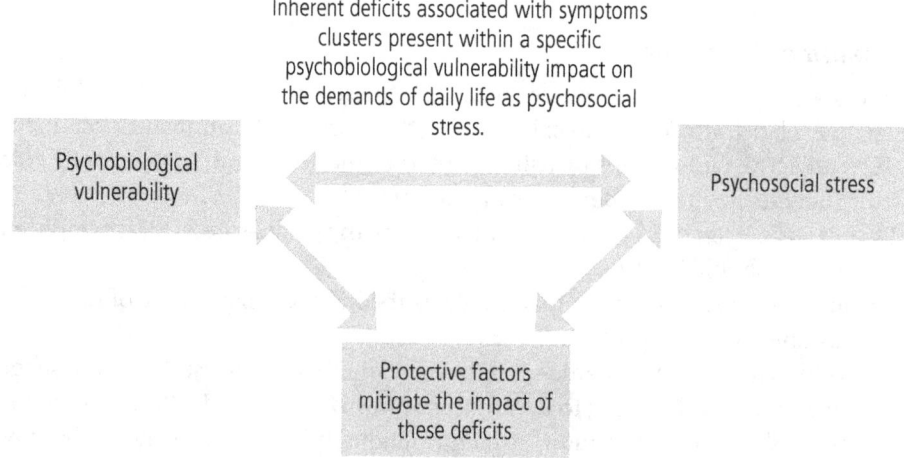

Figure 2.2 Stress–vulnerability framework

Psychobiological vulnerability

This refers to the symptom cluster or diagnostic label; the inherent neurotransmitter dysregulation associated with the specific symptom cluster. Individual symptoms impact the cognitive, emotional and physical functioning of the MHCU. These deficits associated with neurotransmitter dysregulations tend to be consistent within diagnostic labels and include, for example, the lack of energy associated with depressive illness, impaired concentration associated with schizophrenic illness, impaired impulse control associated with bipolar mood disorder, or disturbed sleep associated with almost all mental illness. The mental health nurse must look, listen and record symptoms so that this information can be used to predict and where possible mitigate their impact by implementing protective factors. These deficits, such as lack of energy associated with depression, impact on the person's everyday life. Imagine being a mother of two children under the age of five and struggling with a depressive illness. Lack of energy, an inherent deficit within a depressive illness symptom cluster, will make completing tasks associated with one's role as mother difficult and produce heightened stress levels.

Psychosocial stress

This refers to the unpleasant anxiety or fear experienced when one is attempting to engage with a task for which one does not have the resources to facilitate successful completion. In our current culture 'stress' is an overused term that has resulted in assumed understanding and little interrogation. A student nurse states they are stressed by exams, essentially not knowing if they have the knowledge to complete the task. Meeting new people produces fear because we are unsure if we have the social skills to make friends; some report stress linked to not being able to find the right outfit for an occasion. Within the context of symptom clusters relating to mental illness, the MHCU may not have the ability to engage with previously successful tasks; the concentration to study for an exam; or the ability to filter environmental stimuli within social situations to make sense of or 'keep up' with conversation(s) taking place, or the energy to complete washing or cook a meal.

As stated earlier, when gathering information through listening to the MHCU's narrative, and paying attention to visual information, the nurse can determine the existence of current symptoms. The nurse's knowledge of the different clusters of symptoms, or diagnostic labels, can help in indicating associated potential deficits associated with the MHCU's activities of daily living, both social and occupational. The narrative approach, encouraging the MHCU to tell stories about their life, enables the nurse to establish the current psychosocial context of the MHCU's life: Is the person working? In what job? What specific skill set does that job require? Are they a parent? This information enables the nurse to note actual and potential stressful situations or events based on the nurse's knowledge of deficits associated with that specific symptom cluster/diagnostic label. For example, the MHCU may be a student at university and the deficits usually associated with their symptom cluster suggest they will have cognitive difficulties that will make listening in class, ordering their thoughts, and storing new information, difficult. The nurse knows that protective factors, needed to mitigate the impact of the MHCU's symptoms, should be introduced.

Figure 2.3 below illustrates the interconnectedness of these three aspects of the framework, as applied to a schizophrenic illness.

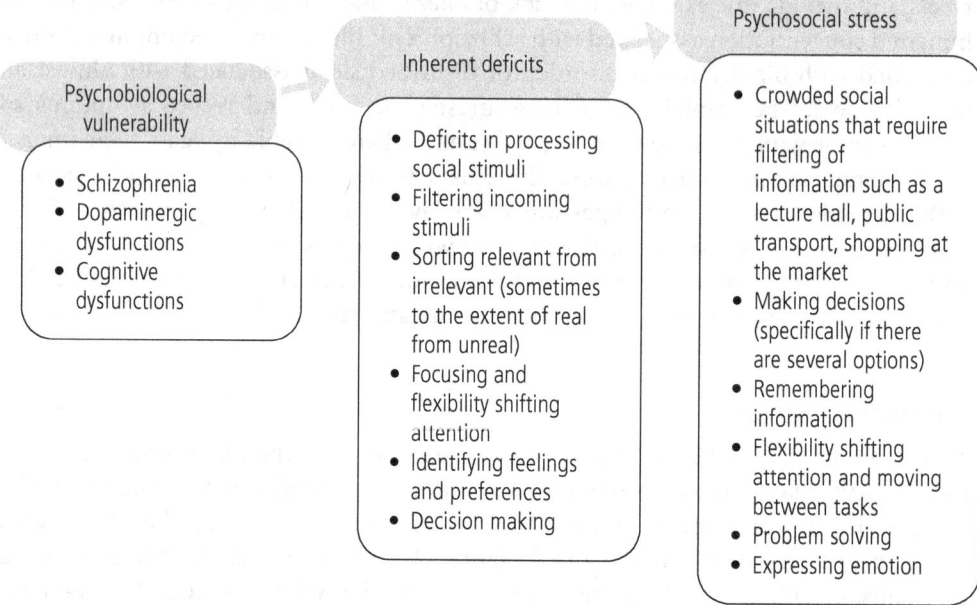

Figure 2.3 Relationship between psychobiological vulnerability and psychosocial stress as applied to a schizophrenic illness

Protective factors

These are those factors that can mitigate the impact of the deficits, inherent within the diagnosed vulnerability, on the MHCU's psychosocial functioning. These include knowledge, taught skill, practical and emotional support and psychotropic medication. This content will be included in other chapters of the book addressing specific symptom clusters/diagnostic labels. What is important for the mental health nurse to internalise is that this framework aids the nurse in their preventative practice; from information gathered through counselling of the MHCU, and their family, the nurse can introduce protective factors and monitor the emergence of symptoms to evaluate the effectiveness of their interventions.

Reflective practice

While mental health nurses obtain knowledge related to health and illness and develop skills to facilitate nursing interventions as part of their education and training programme, learning and the nurse's development of their practice extends beyond credentials.

Practice development is a dynamic process that produces changes in behaviours, skills or attitudes that are contextually relevant, and facilitated by reflection. This reflection is a process of active, purposeful thought applied to a nursing practice experience. The aim of this purposeful thought is to understand meanings and outcomes of a practice experience for all involved: MHCUs, their families and nurses and other health care practitioners. New understandings can lead to confirmation of, or new perspectives and changes in, what we do and/or how we do it.

Reflective practice requires critical appraisal of practice experiences, of those perceived as both good and bad. While reflecting on nursing practice is critical to positive outcomes in health care, it can be emotionally traumatic to review a practice experience that the nurse perceives as less effective than desired. Actively reflecting on these situations requires bravery, resilience and an understanding that one gains knowledge and skills through one's best efforts to improve nursing practice. Having said this, the process of reflective practice is first, essentially a private endeavour, the nurse choosing who they invite to participate in the process. Secondly, reflective practice highlights successful and satisfying practice experiences. To facilitate a balanced view of a practice experience, a model or format for reflection is used.

What is involved?

A model is merely a description of steps within a process, like a recipe for a chocolate cake that describes the 'ingredients required' and the 'how' or method in which they are used to get the best result. In the same way that there are many recipes (models) for a chocolate cake, there are several reflective practice models.

The most recent, by George (2018), continues to illustrate that all reflective practice models include the following common steps:

Step 1: Give a clear description of the event or situation: what was done by whom, how, and, if available, the facts and figures of the outcome.

Step 2: Explore feelings, intuition, gut reaction and emotions associated with the event or situation.

Step 3: Evaluate the experience: what you perceive to be good and bad about it.

Step 4: Review findings thus far to make sense of the incident.

Step 5: Identify what you may need to know, see, and/or understand before you handle a similar situation in the future

Step 6: Conclude what you would do if the situation arose again.

Implementing the steps

To use a reflective model effectively, there should be a written account of the practice experience and the reflective process. By recording reflections in a journal or diary, whether handwritten or computer-generated, nurses can review their writings and learn more from them. There are three important points to remember:

1. Make a habit of writing up at least one experience per day and writing up experiences on the same day they occurred.
2. Balance problematic experiences with satisfying experiences. It is important to reflect on practice one perceives as effective and producing positive outcomes.
3. Always endeavour to be open and honest with oneself. Find the authentic 'self' to do the writing. Remember, you choose if, when and what to share.

Step 1
- Split each page into three columns using the vertical line.
- Write the detailed description of the practice experience on the left side.
- Use actual dialogue wherever possible to capture the situation.

Step 2
- Use the middle column for feelings, intuition and emotional reactions.
- Align these descriptions with descriptions of events and actual dialogue. This will facilitate the clarity needed for step 4.

Step 3
- Write your evaluations of effective/less effective within the right-hand side column.

Step 4
- Read and review the description, the facts and figures relating to the event or situation.
- Review any records made about one's gut reaction and emotions at the time.
- Record the feelings and intuitions one is experiencing as one reads.
- Useful questions to ask oneself as one reads are:
  - What was I trying to achieve?
  - Why did I respond as I did?
  - What internal factors were influencing me?
  - Did my actions match my beliefs?
  - What were the consequences for the MHCU, family, other practitioners and me?
  - Do I have evidence for the consequences I outlined above?

Step 5
- At this point, if one has not done so already, it can be very useful to share one's reflections with a mentor/colleague. Their input can be invaluable in answering further reflective questions:
  - What knowledge should have informed me?
  - How can I access that knowledge now?
  - How does this connect with previous experiences?
  - Could I handle this better in similar situations?
  - Is there a specific skill I need to be effective in this situation?
  - Who has that skill set? Who can I learn from? Is there a potential mentor to guide me through this specific learning process?

Step 6
- Identify actual, and potential, consequences of changing one's response in the future.
- Spend time acknowledging what could have been done better and what improvements could be made.
- Formulate an action plan of how to respond in the future.
- Move on. One has used the experience to improve one's practice.

A strong influence on clinical practice in the 21st century is the evidence-based practice approach or data-driven practice. Evidence-based practice is 'the conscientious, explicit and judicious use of current best evidence in making decisions about the care of individual patients' (Duke University: Module 1). The evidence is gained from systematic reviews of all available literature. A good nurse will make use of both their clinical expertise and the best available external evidence; used on their own, neither of these two aspects is enough. External evidence can inform, but it can never replace individual clinical expertise. The individual clinician's expertise is that which decides if the evidence gathered is applicable to a particular MHCU and, if so, how it should be integrated into the appropriate clinical decision. Evidence-based practice builds on but can never replace clinical skills, clinical judgement and clinical experience.

CONCLUSION

Nursing is currently the most important resource within health care, specifically mental health care where other specialist practitioners can be in limited supply. In addition, the rapid growth of knowledge and research-based evidence associated with mental health and illness has resulted in a greater emphasis on, and appreciation for, mental health care and its place within global health care. Nurses are called on to integrate mental health care within general nursing and specialist nursing practice; as well as to integrate the care of MHCUs within general and specialist practice sites. General and mental health nurses need to work together to embed knowledge that results in better health care outcomes for all.

WEB RESOURCES

The world wide web (www), specifically Google Scholar, is the most potent source of reviews of current peer-reviewed research evidence. Other sites include national and global sites that promote free access such as:

http://www.who.int (World Health Organisation (WHO))

https://www.sahealth.sa.gov.au
   SA Health is a site run by the government of Southern Australia that offers information often transferrable to South Africa.

https://www.nice.org.uk/ (National Institute for Health and Care Excellence)

https://www.hindawi.com/journals/nrp/ (Open access journal, Nursing research and practice)
Service-user groups and organisations:
http://www.cqc.org.uk/ (Experts by Experience, a service user–practitioner group)
http://www.sadag.org (South African Depression and Anxiety Group)
https://www.mind.org.uk/ (Mind, a service-user group and charity)
https://guides.mclibrary.duke.edu/ebptutorialinteractive/module1

The University of Duke offers some free access tutorials, specifically one on evidenced-based practice.

REFERENCES

American Psychiatric Association. 2013. *Diagnostic and Statistical Manual of Mental Disorders*: DSM-5. 5th edition. Arlington, VA: American Psychiatric Association.

Baziga, V and Smith, A. 2016. 'In principle yes, in application, no; Rwandan nurses support for integration of mental health care services'. *African Journal of Nursing and Midwifery*, 18 (1): 170–182.

Cambridge Dictionary. 2018. https://dictionary.cambridge.org (Accessed March 2019).

Corrigan, W, Kerr, A and Knudsen, L. 2005. 'The stigma of mental illness, explanatory models and methods for change'. *Applied and Preventative Psychology*, 11: 179–190.

Duke University. 'EBP Tutorial Interactive: Module 1: Intro to EBP'. https://guides.mclibrary.duke.edu/ebptutorialinteractive/module1 (Accessed May 2019).

George, L S. 2018. 'Reflective practice – Key for lifelong learning'. *Manipal Journal of Nursing and Health Sciences*, 4 (2).

KwaZulu-Natal Department of Health. 2010. 'Policy for mental health on psychosocial rehabilitation', http://www. health.gov.za (Accessed November 2017).

Mental Health Care Act 17 of 2002. *Government Gazette*, 499, No 24024. Cape Town, South Africa.

Oxford Dictionary. 2018. https://en.oxforddictionaries.com (Accessed December 2017).

World Health Organisation (WHO). 2010. 'mhGAP intervention guide for mental, neurological and substance use disorders in non-specialized health settings'. Geneva: Author: http://www.who.int/publications/en/ (Accessed August 2010).

World Health Organisation (WHO). 2013. 'Mental health action plan 2013–2020', http://www.who.int/publications/ (Accessed January 2014).

World Health Organisation. 2017. *Fact sheet no 218. 2017*. 'Mental health problem, the undefined and hidden burden'. http://www.who.int/publications/ (Accessed January 2014).

World Health Organisation (WHO). 2014. 'Strategy on people-centred and integrated health service', http://www.who.int/publications/en/ (Accessed June 2015).

World Health Organisation (WHO). 2018. 'Management of physical health conditions in adults with severe mental disorders', http://www.who.int/publications/en/ (Accessed February 2019).

CHAPTER 3

Comprehensive Mental Health Care

L R Uys and S Arunachallam

Learning Outcomes

After studying this chapter, you should be able to:
- discuss the seriousness of mental illness as a health problem
- define and discuss recovery from mental illness
- define comprehensive health services
- differentiate between primary, secondary and tertiary prevention
- differentiate between primary, secondary and tertiary health care, and prevention
- differentiate between the health promotion approach and the high-risk approach to primary prevention of psychiatric illness
- describe the life skills approach to primary prevention
- describe the gatekeeper approach to secondary prevention, and discuss the problem of primary health care workers in terms of gatekeeping for psychiatric conditions
- define psychosocial rehabilitation and distinguish this from treatment
- describe the basic elements of rehabilitation interventions, and the major interventions used in this field
- define a psychiatric or mental health programme
- distinguish between ad hoc and rational planning and between problem-based and service-based planning
- describe the process of planning a programme
- distinguish between change forces, resistance forces and hindrance forces
- contrast and compare different methods of evaluating a mental health programme
- debate the need for programme evaluation.

INTRODUCTION

Before looking at the mental health care system it is important to understand the context and the extent of the mental health care problem. Mental illness has always been a neglected area of health care, because its economic, social and other consequences are not immediately visible. In the past, mortality figures were the most common way of estimating the seriousness of a condition. In those terms, mental illness did not look very important. Even when a person committed suicide because of depression or schizophrenia, it was not documented as morbidity of schizophrenia or depression but was reported under the heading 'suicide' (Miller et al, 2014).

More recently, a measure has been developed to estimate the seriousness of the consequences of an illness. It is called the global burden of disease (GBD) and it is measured in terms of the disability-adjusted life year (DALY). The DALY refers to the number of years during which the quality of life is impaired – in other words, the years during which a person cannot function properly due to illness. In terms of the DALY, mental illness is one of the greatest causes of hardship resulting from ill health; it was responsible for 11 per cent of the GBD in 1990 and is predicted to rise to 15 per cent by 2020 (WHO, 2003). The seriousness of the problem of mental illness is heightened by the following factors:

- Mental health problems affect a large proportion of the population. About one in five people will suffer from a mental disorder sometime in their lives (Williams et al, 2007). See Table 3.1 for some prevalence figures.
- It affects people in the prime of their lives and often cannot be cured in the short term. This is especially true of schizophrenia, one of the most serious mental illnesses, with high incidences in adolescents and young adults.
- It causes long-term disability. The adverse effects of mental illness are often worse than those of physical illness, since mental illness involves the brain, which is the centre of a person's personality and life. People with a mental illness are the most difficult group to rehabilitate in terms of vocational activity (Rossler, 2006).

THE EPIDEMIOLOGY OF MENTAL ILLNESS IN SOUTH AFRICA

The first nationally representative psychiatric epidemiological study, the South African Stress and Health (SASH) survey, found that 16.5 per cent of adults had experienced a mood, anxiety or substance-use disorder in the previous 12 months (see Table 3.1).

Table 3.1 The 12-month prevalence of adult mental disorders in South Africa

Disorder	%
Anxiety	8.1
Mood	4.9
Impulse	1.8
Substance use	5.8
Schizophrenia	1.0
Bipolar	1.0
Any anxiety, mood, impulse or substance-use disorder	**16.5**

Source: Williams et al (2007) in Department of Health (2013: 11)

The 12-month prevalence of child and adolescent mental disorders in the Western Cape was reported to be 17 per cent, based on a review of local and international epidemiological literature (see Table 3.2)

Table 3.2 The 12-month prevalence of child and adolescent mental disorders in the Western Cape

Disorder	%
Attention-deficit/hyperactivity disorder	5.0
Conduct disorder	4.0
Oppositional defiant disorder	6.0
Enuresis	5.0
Separation anxiety	4.0
Schizophrenia	0.5
Depression & Dysthymia	8.0
Bipolar disorder	1.0
Obsessive compulsive disorder	0.5
Agoraphobia	3.0
Simple phobia	3.0
Social phobia	5.0
Generalised anxiety disorder	11.0
Post-traumatic stress disorder	8.0
Any child and adolescent disorder	**17**

Source: Kleintjes et al (2006) in Department of Health (2013: 12)

The stigma attached to mental illness is almost universal and greatly increases the suffering of mental health care users (MHCU) and their families.

There are other factors mitigating against mental illnesses being taken seriously. For instance, until recently, psychiatric diagnoses were often vague and unreliable. This led to the conception that mental illness was not a 'real' illness. Newer methods of studying the brain, such as positron emission tomography (PET) scans and functional magnetic resonance imaging (MRI), and research-based diagnostic classifications (such as the DSM-5) are gradually eliminating such misconceptions.

Another factor often confusing health care workers used to the 'medical model' is the greater emphasis on the psychosocial context of illness and treatment in mental health care. Cockerham et al (2017: 4) explain why the social context of disease is important: 'In emphasizing the social context, we do not imply that social problems are the sole or even the principal cause of mental disorders.' However, a brain disorder such as epilepsy may very well be the result of a blow to the head received during civil unrest. Even if the epilepsy is the result of hereditary factors, social factors will determine whether or not the family will be able to obtain anticonvulsive treatment for the child and so avoid complications. Social factors therefore exert an influence on all illnesses and health care.

Psychological factors play an equally important role. The presentation of any disease, its progress and its outcomes, are profoundly influenced by the person who has the disease. A person suffering from schizophrenia expresses their own personality, life experience and culture in the context of hallucinations, although the hallucinations may be completely biological in nature. Eisenberg (1986) calls mental health care that does not take psychological factors into consideration 'mindless biological psychiatry', and psychological care which underestimates the influence of biological factors 'brainless social psychiatry'.

In 2001 the World Health Organisation (WHO) dedicated its annual report to mental health. In the final chapter of this report, it is said that:

only a few countries have adequate mental health resources. Some have almost none. The already large inequalities between and within countries in terms of overall health care are even greater for mental health care. Urban populations, and in particular the rich, have the greatest access, leaving essential services beyond the reach of vast populations. And for the mentally ill, human rights violations are commonplace.

This report led to the WHO's request to governments to scale up their psychiatric services.

World leaders recognise the promotion of mental health and well-being, and the prevention and treatment of substance abuse, as health priorities within the global development agenda. The United Nations General Assembly in September 2015 adopted the Sustainable Development Agenda which includes mental health and substance abuse. Particularly, Goal 3 of the 17 Sustainable Development Goals focuses on ensuring healthy lives and promoting well-being for all at all ages through prevention and treatment of non-communicable diseases, including behavioural, developmental and neurological disorders, which constitute a significant challenge for sustainable development (WHO, 2018).

COMPREHENSIVE MENTAL HEALTH CARE

The comprehensiveness of services offered to a population can be described and evaluated in many ways. One way is to say that the services should address all the health problems of persons 'from the cradle to the grave'. This approach defines comprehensiveness in terms of the recipients of the care, and more specifically in terms of the lifespan of such recipients. Another way is to look at comprehensiveness from the perspective of the process of illness. Health care can then be viewed in terms of 'from before illness comes, to after it has disabled a person'. This is the approach that we will follow in this chapter.

If a health service is comprehensive in these terms, it includes primary prevention (before illness), secondary prevention (during illness) and tertiary prevention (after illness). It is important not to confuse these concepts with the levels of health care, which are often also described as primary health service, secondary health service, and tertiary health service. These terms refer to the level of specialisation in the service and have nothing to do with the prevention level.

It is a mistake to think, therefore, that in primary health care (PHC) only primary prevention is undertaken. All levels of health care should perform primary, secondary and tertiary prevention.

Primary prevention

Primary prevention refers to reducing the incidence of disorders by preventing disorders from occurring. It is aimed at healthy people who do not yet have ways of life (lifestyles) that expose them to risk factors for mental illness. These strategies are aimed at people who are basically healthy and who seek the development of community and individual lifestyles that can maintain and enhance a state of well-being.

Primary prevention has several aims, some of which are:
- minimising the exposure of healthy people to risk factors
- increasing a person's resilience to mental illness (Baumann, 2014)
- decreasing the incidence of psychiatric morbidity in the community. This demands health promotion, which includes illness prevention.

Since primary prevention strategies are aimed at people who are essentially healthy, it is a sector of health care in which volunteers and natural community support networks can be used most successfully. This is an important part of organising primary prevention, because the steep demand for secondary prevention often prevents health professionals from giving adequate attention to primary prevention. Without this focus, it is doubtful whether primary prevention will be able to attain the goal of reducing mental illness.

Mechanisms protecting mental health

The following five mechanisms protect people from becoming mentally ill or emotionally distressed (Rutter, 1995; WHO, 2004):

1. *Those that involve a reduction in the personal impact of risk experiences.* For example, the risk that divorce holds for children can be greatly diminished by not drawing them into the conflict around the marriage break-up. Another example is that the influence of high-risk environments on adolescents can be greatly reduced if they join a positive peer group.
2. *Those that reduce negative chain reactions.* An example of this mechanism is the debriefing of a group after a traumatic experience, which breaks the chain of more and more restrictive defence mechanisms being used. Another example is teaching adolescents social skills, which allows them to deal with conflict by using humour or diversion, thus preventing escalation into violence.
3. *Those that promote self-esteem and self-efficacy.* These include not only feeling good about yourself, but also about your ability to handle life. The development of these abilities and this attitude of mind during childhood and adolescence is dependent

on secure and supportive relationships, successful taking of responsibility and successful task accomplishment, as well as coping with manageable stress.
4. *Those that open up positive opportunities.* Opportunities for education and sport, which take young people away from stressful, deprived and crime-ridden environments, fall in this category. For older people, a geographical move or the attainment of literacy may lead to new opportunities.
5. *Those that develop and maintain healthy communities.* Communities consisting of well-employed people, who live in safe environments where there is minimal violence and conflict, allow for social capital to grow and promote mental health in members of the community.

There are three approaches to primary prevention, and these need not be mutually exclusive.

The mental health promotion approach
The whole population is the possible target for mental health promotion. Throughout the individual's lifespan, facilitating the development and achievement of goals is essential in mental health (Jung-Ah Min et al, 2013)

The mental health promotion approach entails awareness of different issues throughout the different stages of life with regard to:
- children and adolescents – tobacco, alcohol, and eating habits; problematic overuse of internet or online games, social networking services and text messaging
- adults – work stress, marital relations, child rearing
- old age – health concerns, retirement, bereavement and fear.

This approach fits in well with the PHC approach, which has the total development of communities as its target. It is a multisectoral approach and involves all sectors of the public service in fulfilling the basic needs of the population. Improved housing and nutrition, clean water, basic education and literacy are the aims of this approach. Meeting these basic needs will undoubtedly result in a decrease in depression and anxiety.

High-risk approach
This approach targets individuals who may be susceptible to a specific disorder. Such people are identified on the basis of aetiological research, which describes the factors characterising those people most likely to experience the disorder (Newton, 1992).

The high-risk approach is particularly appropriate in the following circumstances:
- The important risk factors for a disorder are known (for example, negative social factors *plus* negative psychological factors greatly increase the risk of depression in women).
- The group at risk can be identified relatively cheaply and easily (for example, a brief checklist can enumerate those factors identifying women who are at risk for depression).

- The prevention strategy is too difficult or too expensive to implement for the whole population (for example, a support group for women who are at risk for depression cannot be run for all women in the country).

Most primary prevention strategies in mental health demand trained professionals and a great deal of time. This makes these interventions expensive and, in the face of an increasing scarcity of professionals, very difficult to implement on a population-wide basis. This approach is therefore very appropriate in the field of mental health.

Table 3.3 summarises those factors that could be used to draw up different prevention programmes.

Life skills approach
The life skills approach focuses on the transitions from one life stage to another, and endeavours to help people cope with the demands of each successive stage. Most people go through a predictable series of stages: preschool, school, puberty and adolescence, leaving home and young adulthood, parenting, retiring, old age. Although most people make these transitions without major problems, a life skills approach to primary prevention hypotheses that mental illness can be prevented by equipping people better to cope with the different stages. The *life skills approach*, or *anticipatory guidance*, is a teaching approach which can be used successfully with the total population (for example, putting all people due to retire through a retirement preparation course), or with the high-risk approach (for example, identifying mothers who seem to be having trouble with parenting and offering them a support-group experience).

Table 3.3 Factors to be targeted in illness prevention programmes

Antecedent	Disorder	Strategy
WOMEN - Early loss of mother (past support) - Absence of close other (current support) - Present negative relationship	Depression in women	Group or individual intervention to: - Improve self-concept - Establish new close relationships - Break free from negative relationships
MIDWIFERY SERVICE - Low birth weight - High life changes - Inability or unwillingness to care for the baby - Diffuse social problems - Marital problems - Chronic ill health	Child abuse Postpartum depression	- Referral to primary health practitioner - Telephone number and assurance of support given - A supportive discussion with mother - Support group for mothers, with or without skills teaching
THREAT For example: - Going for HIV test - Pregnancy after several miscarriages	Depression Anxiety, especially post-traumatic stress disorder (PTSD)	POST-THREAT - Counselling - Practical support

Antecedent	Disorder	Strategy
CRISIS For example: ■ Positive HIV test ■ Another miscarriage ■ Rape ■ Violence		POST-CRISIS ■ Debriefing ■ Crisis intervention ■ Environmental manipulation to ensure safety
ADOLESCENTS ■ Children who have had many different carers ■ Poor planning ■ Acting helpless ■ Poor participation in extracurricular activities	Early pregnancy Poor parenting Child abuse Anxiety depression	■ Encourage extracurricular activity ■ Life skills training programmes in high schools to improve planning and self-esteem

Source: Newton (1992)

Secondary prevention

Secondary prevention aims to decrease the prevalence of psychiatric disease through early diagnosis and effective treatment. Early detection of psychiatric illness demands a great deal of public education to make people in general more aware of the signs of mental illness. Since the education of the whole population is so expensive, the *gatekeeper approach* is often used. This means that professionals and non-professional groups who work in a helping or protecting capacity with a great number of people can be taught how to identify early signs and symptoms. For instance, teachers can be used to identify child and adolescent problems; parents can be taught about the signs and symptoms of drug abuse in adolescents; and police can be taught to identify the abuse of women and children. Gatekeepers are also taught to whom they can refer persons with possible problems (Burnette et al, 2015).

Nurses working in PHC settings also play an important role in case finding. It has been shown that 20–50 per cent of patients attending PHC clinics suffer from psychiatric morbidity. The psychiatric condition is often concealed under the cover of ill-defined somatic conditions that repeatedly bring the patient to general medical services, with no positive results. This is called *hidden psychiatric morbidity* (HPM) and should be distinguished from *conspicuous psychiatric morbidity* (CPM), such as psychosis, which is seldom missed. If undetected, the patients with HPM will either be given negative labels such as 'neurotic' and receive little attention, or a great many expensive investigations and treatments will be undertaken unnecessarily. These patients therefore increase the burden on PHC services and increase expenses, while their suffering is not alleviated.

Some studies have indicated that as many as 80 per cent of such HPM patients are not detected by PHC staff (Munk-Jørgensen et al, 1997) This is particularly true of certain African patients, who rarely present with depression or anxiety, but rather with somatic complaints. According to the South African College of Applied Psychology (2013: 1) this is because:

> *often there is not even a word for 'depression' – it's basically not deemed a real illness in the African culture. As a result, sufferers are afraid of being discriminated against, disowned by their families or even fired from work, should they admit to having a problem. There is still the perception that someone with a mental illness is crazy, dangerous or weak. Because there is often an absence of physical symptoms with mental illness, it is considered 'not real', a figment of the imagination.*

Somatic symptoms often shown by patients with HPM include weakness, dizziness, back pain, fertility problems, headache, abdominal pain and chest pain (Matteson, 2015). These symptoms often indicate the presence of real physical disease, and the confusion they cause PHC workers can therefore be understood. What makes the problem worse, however, is that in about 20 per cent of cases the psychological distress presents in patients who are actually suffering from a physical condition at the same time.

To improve the detection of HPM in PHC patients, it is recommended that PHC nurses use the self-reporting questionnaire (SRQ) for screening those patients whom they think may have a psychiatric disorder. A screening test such as the SRQ is not intended to be diagnostic, but is rather aimed at facilitating the sifting out of persons who seem to be well from those who are probably not well. This questionnaire contains 20 questions and, if the patient replies in the affirmative to eight or more questions, a full psychiatric history should be undertaken. It may be necessary to translate the questionnaire into the patient's home language. Some individuals may not answer with a 'yes' or 'no' only. In this case, the interviewer will have to interpret whether the discursive answer given by the patient indicates a positive or a negative response.

The SRQ
1. Do you often have headaches?
2. Is your appetite poor?
3. Do you sleep badly?
4. Are you easily frightened?
5. Do your hands shake?
6. Do you feel nervous, tense or worried?
7. Is your digestion poor?
8. Do you have trouble thinking clearly?
9. Do you feel unhappy?
10. Do you cry more than usual?
11. Do you find it difficult to enjoy your daily activities?
12. Do you find it difficult to make decisions?
13. Is your daily work suffering?
14. Are you unable to play a useful part in life?
15. Have you lost interest in things?

16. Do you feel that you are a worthless person?
17. Has the thought of ending your life been in your mind?
18. Do you feel tired all the time?
19. Do you have uncomfortable feelings in your stomach?
20. Are you easily tired?

(WHO, 1994; Kumbhar et al, 2012)

Tertiary prevention

Tertiary prevention is the reduction of the severity of the mental disorder and the associated disability by means of rehabilitative intervention. It is aimed at preventing the development of complications of mental illness such as loss of employment, suicide, and further functional impairment (Baumann, 2015).

Over the decades, health professionals have projected a very negative view of the chances of recovery of people suffering from serious mental illness. The dominant view, which was often passed on to MHCUs and their families, was that once you had a serious mental illness, recovery was impossible and you would therefore be living with a life sentence of mental illness. Over the last two decades, this prognostic pessimism has been widely challenged by consumers and psychiatric rehabilitation practitioners, and gradually mental health professions have reached consensus that recovery is not only possible, but probable. Recovery has two meanings:

- *Clinical recovery*. This means that the MHCU is in long-term remission, with symptoms greatly reduced or even removed, and the person is functional. Clinical recovery can be measured, and research conducted between 1975 and 2001 shows recovery rates of between 46 per cent and 68 per cent in groups of MHCUs with the diagnosis of schizophrenia (Slade et al, 2008).
- *Personal recovery*. This refers to a deeply personal, unique process of changing one's attitudes, values, feelings, goals, skills and roles so that one can live a satisfying, hopeful and contributing life, even with limitations caused by the illness (Anthony, 1993).

The process of recovery

The process of recovery is described as involving a series of stages through which the MHCU and family moves after diagnosis of a mental illness:
- *Moratorium*. The person is confused, in denial, and withdraws to protect themselves.
- *Awareness*. The first glimmer of hope of recovery is triggered by a role model, a clinician, a significant other or from within the person themselves.
- *Preparation*. The person decides to work towards recovery, finding their own pathway and doing what is necessary.
- *Rebuilding*. The working stage means that the person forges a new identity, sets new goals and strives towards them, reassesses old values and takes responsibility for managing the illness and controlling life. There is a growing acceptance of risks and setbacks.

- *Growth.* The person manages the illness, has a positive view of self and hope for the future. This is really the outcome of the process (Andresen et al, 2003).

The kind of support the person needs differs in each stage of the process. The focus on recovery has become a service philosophy in many countries, such as Scotland and Australia. Recovery-focused mental health services have 10 characteristics, described in Table 3.4.

Table 3.4 Characteristics of recovery-focused mental health services

Principle	Description
1. Self-direction	Consumers lead, control, exercise choice over, and determine their own path of recovery.
2. Individualised and person-centred	There are multiple pathways to recovery, based on the individual person's unique needs, preferences, and experiences.
3. Empowerment	Consumers have the authority to exercise choices and make decisions that impact their lives and are educated and supported in doing so.
4. Holistic	Recovery encompasses the varied aspects of an individual's life including mind, body, spirit and community.
5. Non-linear	Recovery is not a step-by-step process, but one based on continual growth with occasional setbacks.
6. Strengths-based	Recovery focuses on valuing and building on the multiple strengths, resiliency, coping abilities, inherent worth, and capabilities of the individual.
7. Peer support	The invaluable role of mutual support in which consumers encourage one another in recovery is recognised and promoted.
8. Respect	Community, system and societal acceptance and appreciation of consumers – including the protection of consumer rights and the elimination of discrimination and stigma – are crucial in achieving recovery.
9. Responsibility	Consumers have personal responsibility for their own self-care and journey of recovery.
10. Hope	Recovery provides the essential and motivating message that people can and do overcome the barriers and obstacles that confront them.

Source: Adapted from Slade et al (2008)

A health service focused on a recovery approach is not easy to achieve. In the past, a 'compliant' patient was the most prized patient – one who does as they are told, taking their medication, and not complaining nor asking for more and different treatments. In contrast, the recovery-based service values a patient who takes responsibility, makes their own decisions, and may even decide not to use certain prescribed services (Jacobson & Curtis, 2000). Unless most mental health services change radically, one will not be able to call them 'recovery-focused services'.

Recovery is hard won. Psychiatric illness is one of the most devastating illnesses one can have (Judd 1990; Gray & Vawda, 2016). The adverse effects of mental illness are often worse than those of physical illnesses. Furthermore, the risk of suicide among people with mental illness is 18 times that of the general population. This group is also the most difficult of all people with disabilities to get back to work (Brolin & Brolin 1982; Kessler & Bromet, 2013).

The seriousness of mental illness and the fact that the MHCUs are at home for the greatest part of their illness place an enormous burden on the family (Hertog & Gilmoor, 2017; Du Plessis et al, 2017). The unanticipated task of caring for a mentally ill person often totally disrupts and dominates the lives of parents and even siblings.

Rehabilitation

Intensive and sustained efforts are therefore necessary to rehabilitate persons with a mental illness. In the South African context, psychiatric services are mostly still in the de-institutional era where the focus is on treatment and not on rehabilitation. However, evidence for the positive effects of a non-specialist driven, psychosocial rehabilitation program for service users with mental illness in a low-resourced South African setting is emerging. For example, Brooke-Sumner et al (2018) found that service users participating in a structured support group in the community, and receiving ongoing medication through primary care, reported a number of benefits including:

- improvements in self-esteem and illness management
- reduced risk taking
- reduced social isolation and improved sociability
- improved financial management and involvement in income-generating activities
- increased acceptance by the community.

Psychosocial rehabilitation

Psychosocial rehabilitation involves improving the functioning of a person with a psychiatric disability in a specific environment. It is important to distinguish between rehabilitation and treatment – two processes which occur simultaneously in cases of long-term mental illness.

Table 3.5 Differences between rehabilitation and treatment

	Rehabilitation	**Treatment**
Mission	Improved functioning and satisfaction in specific environments	'Cure', symptom reduction, or the development of therapeutic insights
Causal theory	None	Based on a variety of causal theories which determine the nature of intervention
Focus	Present and future	Past, present and future

	Rehabilitation	**Treatment**
Diagnostic content	Assess present and future skills and support	Assess symptoms and possible causes
Primary techniques	Increasing skills and skills-use Increasing understanding and support Increasing resources and resource-use	Psychotherapy and pharmacotherapy

Source: Adapted from Anthony, Cohen and Farkas (1990)

Central to rehabilitation is the reintegration of the disabled person into the community. Therefore, although a range of institutions may be used in the rehabilitation process, it is essentially community based. In terms of the health care system, it would be a function mainly of PHC clinics and community health centres.

The basic elements of rehabilitation interventions can be summarised as follows:

- *Increasing skills.* This can refer to general life skills, or specific vocational skills, and may refer to skills in the MHCU or in their family. An increase in skills assists the whole network to cope better with stress and, in some instances, can prevent stress.
- *Increasing support.* Any action which can increase the support received by the MHCU and family assists in preventing breakdown and promoting health. This refers to entitlements, material assistance and psychosocial support.
- *Manipulating resources.* This may include aspects such as marketing the MHCU to a service or marketing a service to a client. But it may require negotiating changes in the service to make it more appropriate to the client. It may also mean advocating service improvement or creation.
- *Optimising symptom control.* The successful rehabilitation of the MHCU is very dependent on optimal symptom control. This is usually done through medication, although psychotherapy may play a role. Symptom control, which is adequate when staying at home, may not be suitable when working. Therefore, the rehabilitation worker must work closely with the person who is treating the MHCU.
- *Education of the general public.* Reintegration of the MHCU into society is dependent on the attitudes of the general public, and specific groups within that general grouping, such as employers. Changes in attitude need to be addressed purposefully and specifically and complement increasing support for the MHCU and their family.

The interventions that have been developed in this field or incorporated into it are listed below. These technologies form the basic building blocks of a community-based rehabilitation programme. They combine the basic elements of rehabilitation to address the needs of the MHCU, often in a specific area.

- *Psycho-education.* This means that consumers (MHCUs and their families) are taught about mental illness, its treatment and management, so that they can cope better with community-based care. In some cases, MHCUs and their families are provided with very little information, often not even a diagnosis. Vague terms such as 'nervous breakdown' are still frequently used. 'Psycho-education' refers to an intensive and responsive teaching process. It empowers the family and the patient with knowledge and skills and has been proved to make a dramatic difference to the long-term outcome for the MHCUs.

- *Case management.* This is an approach to long-term care which addresses all the needs of the disabled person and is aimed at assessing such needs, linking the person to a variety of services, and coordinating service use to achieve a successful outcome. Although there are different models of case management, it would seem that the generalist model is most appropriate in the South African situation. In this model, one person, who may belong to any of the helping professions, coordinates the treatment, without keeping strictly to professional boundaries (Levine & Fleming, 1987; Hawkins et al, 2018). It provides the consumer with the same, identifiable helper in the complex health system.
- *Skills teaching.* This is the structured teaching of life skills required in the specific social, vocational and living environment of the person with mental illness. It can be done during day programmes or group sessions.
- *Vocational rehabilitation.* This process enables the person to secure and retain suitable employment and to make satisfactory progress in the chosen field. The aim is integrated and competitive employment. This means that the person works for at least minimum wages (or better), with non-disabled co-workers, in a position which offers scope for advancement in a setting that produces valued goods and services. The favoured way of achieving this is through *supported employment* (SE). A disabled person in supported employment works in the open labour market, with ongoing support and under working conditions that have been specially negotiated (Wehman et al, 1992). An individual is placed in a work setting and a job coach works with them until they can manage. After this, visits from the coach continue, in case problems arise. Vocational rehabilitation is led by the occupational therapist.
- *Appropriate housing.* The housing of the disabled person should suit their own needs and lifestyle, and optimise social and vocational functioning. This necessitates a range of housing options, from group homes to single accommodation.

PLANNING PROGRAMMES

The nurse has an important role in developing new programmes. This includes the planning, implementation and evaluation of such programmes. Without this skill it is difficult for the nurse to lead a nursing team or to run a health service. Planning means that future actions are decided on in order to solve a present or anticipated problem or to achieve certain objectives. In health services, nurses could implement ad hoc planning or rational planning.

Ad hoc planning

In this type of planning, decisions are made only when problems have actually occurred and the decision is then made instantly, based on the information that is superficially available. An example of ad hoc programme planning would be a unit in which there are increasing problems with MHCU violence. The registered nurse in charge mentions this in a discussion with the nurse administrator and they decide to change one single room into a seclusion room. In this planning there is no thorough collection of data about the problem and no serious consideration of different possible causes or solutions. The less forward planning there is in a service, the more instant decisions have to be made every day. Since these decisions are often not good ones, they lead to increased resistance to change in the system.

Rational planning

This means that systematic data collection is done in regard to possible alternatives and probable effects are intelligently anticipated before decisions are made. Taking the above example, rational planning means that the incidents of violence would be carefully documented for a specific period, noting the type of violence, who was involved, what the context was and which interventions were used. Possible alternatives, such as increasing the opportunities for gross motor activities in the daily programmes of MHCUs, giving staff in-service training in the prevention of violence, increasing or changing medication or establishing a behaviour modification programme with the use of a seclusion room. This could be done by utilising evidence-based practice, and through local discussions and needs assessments.

In light of all this information a decision would be made involving, as far as possible, those who would actually implement the plan.

When a planner plans programmes, a wide range of factors influence the decisions to be made, but the main areas of influence are *political factors* and *clinical factors*. Idealistic nurse planners often think that only clinical factors, those which are best for the MHCUs, should be considered. That is not possible, however, since administrative factors must be taken into account, such as whether resources necessary for the implementation of a plan have been budgeted for, whether enough staff can be made available when needed for implementation, or whether agency policies allow this kind of programme.

Even when a proposed programme is administratively possible and clinically desirable, it may still be doomed by political factors. This means that powerful individuals or groups might oppose it because they see it as a threat to their interests. A planner therefore needs to look at every alternative, not only in terms of whether the programme is good for the MHCUs and whether it is administratively possible, but also in terms of whether enough support can be lobbied for it from people in power positions to get it approved. Consultation with people for whom the programme is being planned is also important, especially in community programmes. People are more likely to support the programme if they are actually involved in its planning.

The process of programme planning

Nurses encounter the task of programme planning in one of two circumstances:
1. They can be faced with a specific problem and decide to plan a programme to address the problem. For instance, a psychiatric community nurse finds that the service is continually being asked to assist with patients with long-term substance abuse who have been treated repeatedly by all the available services. None of these services wants to be involved with these patients, because they see the situation as useless and a waste of resources. Instead of continually going through the motions and getting frustrated by the lack of a satisfactory answer, the nurse decides to initiate a programme. This kind of programme planning is problem based.
2. Nurses can do programme planning for any service to which they are allocated in order to enhance the effectiveness of the service. For instance, a nurse who is put in charge of an outpatient clinic can plan to bring a range of programmes into being to ensure that the unit reaches its goals. This approach is service based.

The process of programme planning differs for the two types of approaches, although, in many respects, there are some similarities.

Problem-based programme planning

1. *Define the problem operationally* so that everybody concerned understands it in the same way. In the example mentioned above, the problem can be defined as that of people with substance/alcohol dependence who are not eligible for the main treatment, or assistance programmes for substance users because of their repeated relapses. This definition makes it clear that the patients are a problem due to their labelling by the main service and not merely due to their relapse rate. This kind of definition makes it easier to get clarity on exactly what the problem is.
2. *Do a needs assessment* to establish the extent of the problem. This includes a survey of how many patients are involved over a specific period of time and perhaps also what percentage they form of the total patient population. The severity of the problem also needs to be outlined in terms of current outcomes. What are the results of non-intervention? Sometimes a thorough needs assessment indicates that the problem is not large enough to warrant special attention, while in other cases it might underline the need for action.
3. *Survey existing services* to establish which of them currently address the problem and to what extent and in what way they do so. In order to prove that a gap exists in the service, it is essential that you thoroughly check what is already available. Sometimes relevant programmes are available, but they might not be able to cater for the numbers involved or they might be inaccessible. The survey should make all this clear.
4. *Survey similar programmes nationally and internationally.* It is not necessary to reinvent the wheel. If your service is experiencing a problem, chances are very good that some other service has had a similar problem and has experimented with solutions. Contact other services in the country and ask about the problem and

possible solutions. Do a literature review to see how it has been handled in other countries.

5. Based on all the information gathered, *develop a model* that includes:
   - the aims and objectives of the programme
   - the activities included in the programme
   - the resources necessary (cost, staff and space)
   - the time frame for the programme and
   - proposals for finding the resources.

   One would have already considered the different alternatives at this stage and would have made a selection based on clinical, administrative and political considerations. You can include different alternatives in a programme proposal. Table 3.6 gives a model of a programme in a community setting. In this table the last two elements of the programme (time frame and proposals for finding the resources) are not included.

6. Plan for the evaluation of the programme. Unless evaluation is part of the initial planning, it may be impossible to implement later, since the necessary data may not have been collected appropriately.

Service-based programme planning

1. In this case the first step is to *analyse the situation*. In a community service this includes a community profile as well as a service profile, while in an inpatient service it includes only a service profile. A service profile consists of a numerical description of the service (including admission, discharge and readmission figures, demographics of the patient population, staff figures and all other relevant statistics), as well as an anecdotal description of the main features of the service.

2. *Analyse the data* to answer the following questions:
   - Is the service addressing the most serious problems of the community or patient population?
   - Is the service sensitive to the needs around it?
   - Are there any gaps in the service?
   - Could the task be done more effectively or efficiently?

This step corresponds roughly with step 2 of the problem-based approach to planning. If problems are experienced, one should follow the steps of that approach.

Table 3.6 A model of a programme for women exposed to intimate partner violence

Programme aims
- To enable women exposed to intimate partner violence to handle the situation in a way that increases both their own and their children's well-being

Programme objectives
- To increase community knowledge of the programme

→

- To increase women's knowledge of how to improve their own and their family's health in relation to family violence
- To increase women's ability to solve problems of family violence

Activity sequence

Objectives	Activity	Resources
- Increased numbers	- Design handbill - Send to stakeholders - Organise radio interviews with all stations - Make personal contact with police and casualty wards	- Staff time - Printing cost - Graphic art cost
- Increased knowledge and skills	- Teach women about: family violence in relation to family health, community resources and legal issues	- Problem-solving skills - Staff time to prepare teaching material and to teach - Outside lecturers

- Decreased anxiety and depression
- Increased self-confidence
	- Provide social support through:
	  - encouraging extended family interviews
	  - teaching in groups, allowing exploration of feelings
		- Group time
		- Staff time for family interviews

Source: Adapted from Budgen (1987)

Implementing programmes

The implementation of anything new in a service is always a difficult task. It is not enough to have a good plan and enthusiasm. Great skill and wisdom and careful planning are imperative in order to achieve change in a system. The more bureaucratic the system, the more difficult it is to effect change.

Singh (2005) postulates that in any stable situation there is a dynamic balance between the forces *for* change and those *against* change. The process of change in such a situation consists of:

- unfreezing the forces that preserve the status quo
- implementing the change process by which the current system is changed to the future system and
- refreezing the situation, so that the new system becomes the accepted routine.

During the phase of unfreezing, efforts are made to weaken support for the status quo by raising the consciousness of people in the system about the limitations of the present situation and possibilities for change. This involves specifically strengthening the forces for change as listed in the first arrow in Figure 3.1, while at the same time decreasing the strength of the restraining forces listed in the other two arrows.

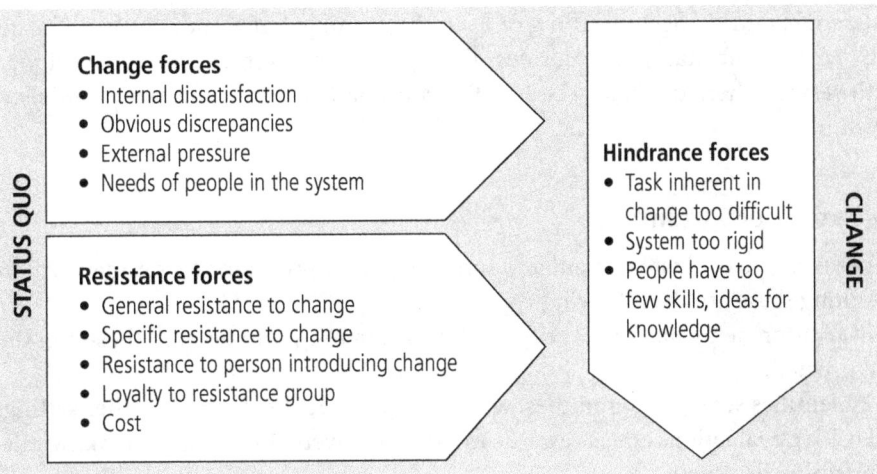

Figure 3.1 Motivating forces for change

Example

You are in charge of an outpatient unit and you would like the two registered nurses to see long-term MHCUs in groups. You could increase factors supporting change by bringing to the attention of staff information that indicates that many of the long-term MHCUs are not functioning well in the community, as well as giving them articles describing innovative group approaches to the problem. This should increase their dissatisfaction with the current system. At the same time you could involve the nurse administrator, who is supportive of the idea, in providing some external pressure. You find that the registered nurses have never had training in group therapy and that the psychologist in the unit is opposed to nurses getting involved in such therapy. To decrease the power of these opposing forces, you could organise in-service training for the nurses in group therapy. A multidisciplinary team meeting should be convened to resolve the matter.

When the system is ready to implement the change, it is important to choose an opportune time. You are setting yourself up for failure if you start something new when, for example, one registered nurse is going through a divorce, the unit is being renovated and there are workers all over the place, and the hospital is getting ready for a centenary celebration. It is also important to start on a small scale and to try out the innovation first, so that you can identify and eliminate problems.

Once the change has been implemented, you will need to ensure that it will be continued even if you leave the area. This can be done by collecting evidence of the success of the change and by giving this kind of feedback to the staff promptly and frequently. It is also important to ensure that the new behaviour is rewarded by social recognition, improved working conditions, more interesting assignments, monetary recognition or any other result that makes it worthwhile for the staff.

Most people find change unsettling or even threatening, but without change the quality of the service inevitably deteriorates. Change, as an essential part of working in a health service, therefore has to be handled with patience and sensitivity, but also with determination.

Evaluating programmes

It is necessary to evaluate current and innovative new programmes for many reasons. Among these are the following:
- Evaluation helps staff to identify weaknesses in programmes, and these can then be corrected.
- It identifies strong programmes, which can then be duplicated in other settings.
- Positive evaluations act as rewards for staff involved; they assist in making effective planning decisions.
- Results can be used to support requests for increased resources.
- Evaluation is part of being accountable for public money spent, as well as being a part of professional accountability.

Evaluation of a whole programme is not an easy task. A programme often consists of a complex series of activities that take place over a long period, frequently involving more than one service setting and a changing staff component. Furthermore, evaluation takes time and money and these commodities are always in short supply. Nevertheless, evaluation of one's own practice is an essential part of being a professional and should not be neglected.

There are four main methods of programme evaluation:
1. *Recipient judgement.* In this method the recipients of the programme are asked to evaluate the programme, usually by means of a questionnaire or an interview. This could involve MHCUs, their families or community groups. The problem with this method is that people are often dependent on the service and are therefore reluctant to criticise it, or that they give the answers that they think are expected, instead of saying what they really think. The results of this kind of evaluation may therefore not be valid.
2. *Expert judgement.* There are different ways in which a person or persons can be used to evaluate a programme. One of these is called a *peer review*, which means that those running the programme select people from outside their group or system whom they see as their peers to come in and evaluate what they have done. They supply the peer evaluators with written material on the programme and the group also conducts an on-site visit to look at programme activities. A discussion is then held between the peer evaluators and programme staff to discuss findings and recommendations. A written report is provided after the discussion. This method is often chosen by staff because they can select the evaluators and, since the evaluators are peers, they are in a similar situation to the programme staff and can evaluate with understanding.

A different form of expert judgement involves choosing a person or persons who are *expert(s)* in the field and then going through the same process as with the peer group. In this case the judges have much more knowledge and experience than the programme staff and might therefore give useful advice. However, this kind of evaluation can be very threatening to staff.

3. *Quality assurance process.* This method consists of the following steps:
   - setting standards for a programme or service
   - identifying ways in which the standards can be measured
   - doing the measurement
   - identifying problem areas and implementing remedial action
   - repeating the measurement.

   This methodology has been used extensively in nursing and is useful in that the programme is measured against standards set by the staff themselves or by a peer group. It is also more structured than the peer review and staff know in advance against which standards they will be evaluated.

4. *Research approach.* In this method the programme is evaluated by using the steps of the research process. This can be either a qualitative or a quantitative approach. In the qualitative approach an in-depth analysis of the programme is conducted by describing how it actually functions. In a quantitative approach different forms of numeric data and statistics are used to analyse how the programme is working. This could include morbidity data, utilisation statistics or need/demand statistics.

Morbidity does not include only primary impairment in the form of physical or psychological symptoms and signs, but also secondary impairment in terms of quality of life and productivity. Secondary impairment can be measured through diagnostic surveys, attitude surveys and functional assessment scales. This is a very useful method and to a certain extent it is part of every other method.

It is becoming increasingly difficult to claim that one is delivering a quality service without some form of evaluation being done. Such unsubstantiated claims are seen as both unscientific and unprofessional.

CONCLUSION

Mental health problems affect a large proportion of the population; hence the emphasis on the provision of a comprehensive mental health care service. Comprehensive mental health care includes primary, secondary and tertiary health care provided to the South African population. It also includes primary, secondary and tertiary prevention.

Mental illness usually affects people in the prime of their lives, and often cannot be cured in the short term. It can cause long-term disability throughout the lifespan of an individual, thus the need for comprehensive services. Programmes to meet the mental health needs should be planned, implemented and evaluated.

WEB RESOURCES

http://www.iapsr.org

This website belongs to the International Association for Psychosocial Rehabilitation. In the section 'PSR resources' you will find a list of topics, each leading to other sites and more information.

http://www.prosci.com/

This website has a range of tutorials on change management, for instance the 'Change management' series and the 'Effective project planning and start-up' tutorial. The site is sponsored by the Quality Leadership Centre.

http://www.uspra.org

This is the site of the US Psychiatric Rehabilitation Organisation and has very useful resources under 'articles' and also under 'resources'. Their newsletter is interesting too, although the focus is very much on the USA.

https://researchspace.ukzn.ac.za/bitstream/handle/10413/14401/Brooke-Sumner_Carolyn_2015.pdf?sequence=2&isAllowed=y

This link provides access to a doctoral thesis entitled 'Psychosocial rehabilitation for schizophrenia in South Africa'. Published in 2015, this document is a mine of information about PSR and the recovery models in the global and South African context. It details a PSR intervention for low-income and resource-poor settings.

REFERENCES

Andresen, R, Oades, L and Caputi, P. 2003. 'The experience of recovery from schizophrenia: towards an empirically validated stage model'. *Australian and New Zealand Journal of Psychiatry*, 37: 586–594.

Anthony, W. 1993. 'Recovery from mental illness: the guiding vision of the mental health system in the 1990s'. *Innovations and Research*, 2: 17–24

Anthony, W, Cohen, M and Farkas, M. 1990. *Psychiatric Rehabilitation*. Boston: Boston University.

Baumann, S E. 2014. *Primary care psychiatry*. Cape Town: Juta.

Brolin, D E and Brolin, J C. 1982. *Vocational Preparation of Persons with Handicaps*. 2nd edition. Columbus: Charles E Merrill Publishing Co.

Brooke-Sumner, C, Selohilwe, O, Mazibuko, M S and Petersen, I. 2018. 'Process Evaluation of a Pilot Intervention for Psychosocial Rehabilitation for Service Users with Schizophrenia in North West Province, South Africa'. *Community Mental Health Journal*, 54 (7): 1089–1096. doi: 10.1007/s10597-018-0318-9.

Budgen, C M. 1987. 'Modelling: a method for program development'. *JONA*, 17 (12): 19–25.

Burnette, C, Ramchand, R and Ayer, L. 2015. 'Gatekeeper Training for Suicide Prevention'. *Rand Health Quarterly*. Jul 15, 5 (1): 16.

Cockerham, W C, Bryant, W, Hamby, M A, and Oates, G R. 2017. 'The Social Determinants of Chronic Disease'. *American Journal of Preventative Medicine*, Jan, 52 (1 Suppl 1): S5–S12.

Department of Health. 2013. *National Mental Health Policy Framework and Strategic Plan 2013–2020*. Pretoria: Government Gazette.

Du Plessis, E, Koen, M P and Tlhowe, T T. 2017. Strengths of families to limit relapse in mentally ill family members. *Health SA Gesondheid*, 22 (1): 28–35.

Eisenberg, L. 1986. 'Mindlessness and brainlessness in psychiatry'. *British Journal of Psychiatry*, 148: 497–508.

Gray, A and Vawda, Y. 2016. Health Policy and Legislation. *South African Health Review 2016*. doi: 10.1093/heapol/czq021.

Hawkins, E J, Danner, A N, Malte, C A, Painter, J M, Lott, A M K and Baer, J S. 2018. 'Feasibility of a care management approach for complex substance use disorders and high acute services utilization'. *Journal of Substance Abuse Treatment*, 92: 100–108.

Hertog, T N and Gilmoor, A R. 2017. 'Informal care for people with chronic psychotic symptoms: four case studies in a San community in South Africa'. *HSC Health & Social Care in the Community*, 25 (2): 538–547.

Jacobcon, N and Curtis, L. 2000. 'Recovery as policy in mental health services: strategies emerging from the States'. *Psychosocial Rehabilitation Journal*, 23 (4): 333–341.

Jung-Ah Min, Chang-Uk Lee, and Chul Lee. 2013. 'Mental Health Promotion and Illness Prevention: A Challenge for Psychiatrists'. *Psychiatric Investigation* Dec, 10 (4): 307–316.

Judd, L L. 1990. 'Putting mental health on the nation's agenda'. *Hospital and Community Psychiatry*, 41 (2).

Kessler, R C and Bromet, E J. 2013. 'The epidemiology of depression across cultures'. *Annual Review of Public Health*, 34: 119–138. doi: 10.1146/annurev-publhealth-031912-114409.

Kleintjes, S, Flisher, A, Fick, M, Railoun, A, Lund, C, Molteno, C and Robertson, A. 2006. 'The prevalence of mental disorders among children, adolescents and adults in the Western Cape, South Africa'. *South African Psychiatric Review*, 9: 157–160.

Kumbhar, U T, Dhumale, G B and Kumbhar, U P. 2012. 'Self-Reporting Questionnaire to diagnose psychiatric morbidity'. *National Journal of Medical Research*, 2 (1), Jan–March.

Levine, I S and Fleming, M. 1987. *Human Resources Management: Issues in Case Management*. Baltimore: University of Maryland.

Matteson, W. 2015. 'Missing the diagnosis: The hidden medical causes of mental disorders'. http://www.continuingedcourses.net/active/courses/course101.php (Accessed 12 May 2018).

Miller, A, Schmidt, U, Angermeyer, M C, Chauhan, D, Murthy, V, Toumi, M and Cadi-Soussig, N. 2014. 'Humanistic burden in schizophrenia: A literature review'. *Journal of Psychiatric Research* 54: 85–93.

Munk-Jørgensen, P, Fink, J I, Brevik, O S, Dalgard, M, Engberg, L, Hansson, M, Holm, M, Joukamaa, H, Karlsson, V, Lehtinen, P, Nettelbladt, C, Stefansson, L, Sørensen, J, Jensen, L, Borgquist, I, Sandager, I and Nordström, G. 1997. 'Psychiatric morbidity in primary public health care: a multicentre investigation. Part II. Hidden morbidity and choice of treatment'. *Acta Psychiatrica Scandinavica*, 95: 1–72.

Newton, J. 1992. *Preventing Mental Illness in Practice*. London: Routledge.

Rossler, W. 2006. 'Psychiatric rehabilitation today: an overview'. *World Psychiatry*, Oct, 5 (3): 151–157.

Rutter, M. 1995. 'Psychosocial adversity: risk, resilience and recovery'. *Southern African Journal of Child and Adolescent Psychiatry*, 7 (2): 75–88.

Singh, K. 2005. *Organisation change and development*. India: University of Delhi.

Slade, M, Amering, M and Oades, L. 2008. 'Recovery: an international perspective'. *Epidemiologia e Psichiatria Sociale*, 17 (2): 128–137.

South African College of Applied Psychology. 2013. 'Mental Health in South Africa: Whose problem is it?'. https://www.sacap.edu.za (Accessed 4 March 2018).

Wehman, P, Sale, P and Parent, W. 1992. *Supported Employment*. Boston: Andover Medical Publishers.

Williams, D R, Herman, A, Stein, D J, Heeringa, S G, Jackson, P B, Moomal and Kessler, R C. 'Prevalence, Service Use and Demographic Correlates of 12-Month Psychiatric Disorders in South Africa: The South African Stress and Health Study'. *Psychological Medicine* 2007, 38 (2): 211–220.

World Health Organisation (WHO). 1994. 'A user's guide to the self-reporting questionnaire (SRQ)'. Geneva: WHO. http://whqlibdoc.who.int/HB/1994/WHO_MNH_RSF_94.8.pdf (Accessed 20 October 2017).

World Health Organisation (WHO). 2003. *Investing in Mental Health*. Geneva: WHO.

World Health Organisation (WHO). 2004. *Promoting Mental Health: Concepts, Emerging Evidence, Practice*. Geneva: WHO.

World Health Organisation (WHO). 2018. 'Sustainable developmental Goals'. https://www.who.int/mental_health/SDGs/en/ (Accessed 2 January 2019).

CHAPTER 4

Mental Health Care in the Health Care System

L R Uys and S Arunachallam

Learning Outcomes

After studying this chapter, you should be able to:
- briefly outline the district health system
- distinguish between mental health care offered at various levels of the health care system: primary health care, secondary health care, and tertiary health care
- describe how a primary mental health service should function
- demonstrate skill in consulting specialists, in referring patients to them and in using telemedicine support in primary health care settings.

INTRODUCTION

In South Africa, private and public health systems exist in parallel. The public system serves the vast majority of the population but is chronically underfunded and understaffed. The wealthier 20 per cent of the population use the private system and are far better served. Currently the Department of Health is working to establish a national health insurance (NHI) system arising out of concerns about discrepancies within the national health care system, such as unequal access to health care among different socioeconomic groups. The health services of this country have been going through major changes due to the National Health Act 61 of 2003 that provides for the establishment of the district health system (DHS). In this system, mental health care is incorporated into primary health care (PHC). The integration of mental health care into PHC is an essential strategy that is vital for providing a full range of mental health care, such as prevention and health promotion, early intervention and rehabilitation (Mugisha et al, 2017).

It is important to understand how mental health care fits into this service, and to develop the skills necessary to function adequately at the PHC level. Mental health care in South Africa is governed by the Mental Health Care Act 17 of 2002. The availability of mental health legislation is the basis of providing mental health care to the community. This valuable legislation plays a central role in the acceptance into the community of persons with mental disorders, integration of mental health at the level of PHC, the provision of care of acceptable quality and the expansion of access to care at community level (Ayano, 2018).

In South Africa mental health care is seen as part of the basic education of professional nurses aimed at equipping them to work as generalist nurses in the comprehensive health services of the country. It is expected that the professional nurse will be able to assess persons with mental health problems and manage them or to refer them onwards. From 2020 there will be a postgraduate diploma in mental health nursing offered at universities and nursing colleges, which will equip a specialist mental health nurse to assess and manage mental health clients.

ORGANISATION OF MENTAL HEALTH SERVICES

In line with recommendations from the World Health Organisation (WHO) regarding the organisation of mental health services, the South African mental health system will include a range of settings and levels of care including PHC, community-based settings, general hospitals and specialised psychiatric hospitals as illustrated in the diagram in Figure 4.1.

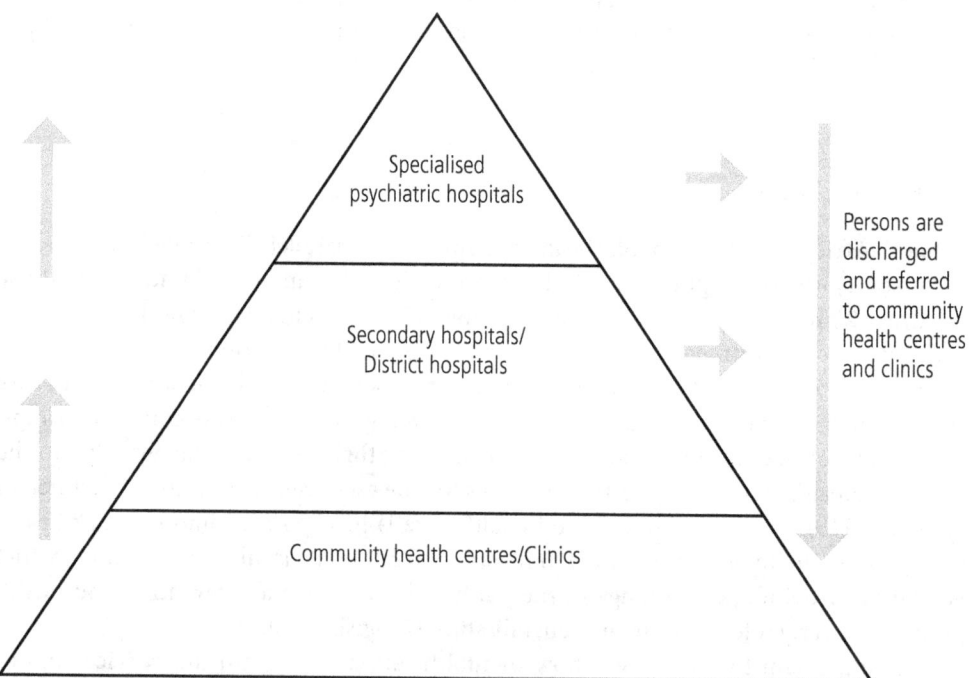

Figure 4.1 Diagram of mental health services in South Africa

Overview of the district health system

The DHS is a way of referring to a model for planning and organising a health system using the district as the basic unit.

The basic unit

A *district* is a coherent, geographically defined area in which all health services are coordinated by one district health authority, which is part of the lowest level of government. A district should be small enough to allow for effective community participation, but also large enough to allow for efficient comprehensive community and first-level hospital care in such an area.

The population (number of people) served by a district varies and is not the only determinant of district boundaries. For instance, the populations of the proposed districts for the greater Durban area vary from 100 000 to 448 000. Some districts are very densely populated, and others are more rural and difficult to access. However, a population of about 250 000 per district would be average.

Ideally, the boundaries of the health districts should coincide with administrative and political boundaries. For example, local authority election boundaries should be the same as those of districts. The boundaries delineating other sectors, such as education or policing, should also coincide with the health district boundaries. The co-determination of boundaries will facilitate the administration of multisectoral activities.

One of the basic assumptions of the DHS is that people in each district know their own situation best and should therefore have maximal autonomy in management decisions. This means that financial, staff and service decisions should be the responsibility of the staff of the local institution and not be controlled provincially. This approach will be effective only if a participatory management style is used by managers, allowing staff and the community to be increasingly involved in decision making.

The basic principles

The DHS allows for the implementation of PHC that adheres to the following principles:
- *Equity* in the services supplied to all consumers
- *Comprehensiveness* which includes intersectoral collaboration and promotive, preventive, curative, rehabilitative and multidisciplinary health services at all levels of care
- *Community participation and empowerment* which promotes community development, is accountable to the community, and engages the community in the planning, implementation and evaluation of health services
- *Affordability and sustainability* in terms of the country's resources
- *Efficiency* which means that the service should function with minimum waste and maximum goal attainment.

Responsibilities of the district health services

The district health services function according to the National Mental Health Policy Framework and Strategic Plan of 2013–2020 (Department of Health, 2013). The district health services are responsible for the following:

1. The provision of mental health promotion and prevention interventions, in keeping with national and provincial priorities
2. The inclusion of mental health in the core package of district health treatment and rehabilitation services which include:
   - routine screening for mental illness during pregnancy, and provision of counselling and referral where appropriate
   - medication monitoring and psychosocial rehabilitation within a recovery framework for severe mental illness
   - detection of mental illness and management of common mental disorders (eg, depression and anxiety disorders) in PHC clinics, and referral where appropriate
   - detection and management of child and adolescent mental disorders in PHC clinics, and referral where appropriate
3. The provision of emergency care (24 hour) and 72-hour observation services in designated district and regional hospital inpatient settings, as set out in the Mental Health Care Act
4. The conducting of mental health training programmes for all general health staff for basic screening, detection and treatment of mental health conditions, as well as referral of complex cases
5. The establishment and maintenance of mental health supervision systems for health staff at the PHC level
6. The establishment and maintenance of specialist mental health teams to support the PHC staff
7. The establishment and maintenance of referral and back-referral pathways for mental health
8. The implementation of clinical protocols for assessment and interventions at the PHC level
9. The establishment and maintenance of community-based rehabilitation programmes, through trained community health workers
10. The development of intersectoral collaboration between a range of sectors involved in mental health, through the establishment of district multisectoral forums for mental health
11. The undertaking of mental health education programmes in communities
12. Improving the capacity of district health management teams for planning, implementing, supervising, monitoring and evaluation of mental health programmes at district and community levels
13. Provision of psychotropic medication to all appropriate levels of the DHS, as determined by the essential drugs list (Department of Health, 2013).

LEVELS OF STRUCTURE AND SERVICE

This section provides information on the structure and services provided by the different levels of the health services.

Health care in each province is delivered at the community level (CL), at the district level (DL) and at the provincial level (PL).

Health care at the CL

Community services are delivered from a community health centre (CHC), or a community clinic (CC) serving a designated community, and are governed by a health committee representative of that community.

The CC is staffed by nurses, whereas the CHC at most has a basic multidisciplinary team. Most CCs render a 40-hour-per-week daytime service, while CHCs render a full-time service (24 hours, every day of the week). Table 4.1 details the proposed tasks of each level of service.

In terms of mental health care, each clinic should render a comprehensive service, including diagnosing and treating the most common mental health conditions, community-based rehabilitation, and preventive and promotive services. If a condition falls outside the capabilities of clinic staff, or if there is an intractable problem, they consult with support staff at the CHC or the district hospital, who form their support system. The CHC or the district hospital are also the two services to which they may refer patients.

Table 4.1 Tasks at the various levels of health services

Community level (CL)	District level (DL)	Provincial level (PL)
- Environmental health - Promotive and health education - Family planning - Antenatal, delivery, post- and neonatal care - Comprehensive care for children and school health - Comprehensive services for communicable and other diseases, & optometry - Treatment of common illnesses and injuries - Community rehabilitation - Community mental health - Community geriatric - Community nursing and home care - Oral health	*All the services in the first column plus:* - Planning of health services for the district - Development of CL services - Provision of essential medicines at CL - Transport for the district - Environmental health at DL - Provision of facilities - Maintenance of equipment, facilities, etc - Monitoring and evaluation of health services in the district - Health information system	- Translate national policy to provinces - Monitoring and evaluation of implementation of mental health care - Provision of sustainable budget - Working with district health managers - Consulting with stakeholders for planning and delivery of services - Facilitating intersectoral collaboration, eg with the department of social development and housing - Integration of mental health care - Expanding mental health workforce

→

Community level (CL)	District level (DL)	Provincial level (PL)
■ Accident and emergency ■ Medical social work ■ Basic laboratory and diagnostics, including X-rays ■ Health monitoring ■ Occupational health ■ Basic medico-legal services	■ Human resource development ■ Training and research ■ Cooperation with other districts ■ Ensuring cooperation within the district	■ Building capacity for mental health management ■ Establishment of a mental health directorate in each province ■ Responsible for provision of psychiatric inpatient and limited outpatient services at hospitals

Health care at the DL

Each district has a designated district hospital (level one hospital) for example, Khayelitsha district hospital, at which non-specialist inpatient services are provided, as well as the usual range of community services.

As far as mental health care is concerned, in view of the shortage of members of the multidisciplinary team, such as clinical psychologists and occupational therapists, this may be the first level at which a team of 'specialists' could be made available for referral and consultation.

Health care at the provincial level (PL)

According to the National Health Act 61 of 2003, the provincial departments of health are responsible for the provision of all hospital services. This includes hospitals at levels one, two, three and four.

Provincial hospitals (level three hospitals) provide the final referral service for the whole province, where a wider range of specialties and subspecialties is available. Forensic psychiatry will probably be handled mainly at this level.

Level 4 hospitals are those that supply a service on a national level, for example Groote Schuur Hospital, which supplies a heart transplant service to the whole country. It is envisaged that the various provinces will supply different national services.

Health care services and psychotropic medication

Essential psychotropic drugs should be provided and made constantly available at all levels of health care. According to the National Mental Health Policy Framework and Strategic Plan 2013–2020 (Department of Health, 2013: 29):

- All psychotropic medicines, as stipulated on the standard treatment guidelines and essential drugs list (EDL), will be available at all levels of care, including at PHC clinics.
- Drug interactions with other medications will be carefully monitored in all treatment of mental disorders.
- Routine screening and treatment of physical illness in all consultations for people with mental illness will be implemented.

- The use of psychotropic medication should be carefully monitored and evaluated, in line with broader quality improvement mechanisms in the Department of Health.

THE INTEGRATION OF MENTAL HEALTH CARE INTO PHC

The government's health plan, under the heading 'Mental Health', proposes 'improved integration of mental health care, including mental disorders, especially at primary level' (WHO, 2001). This is in line with the recommendations of the WHO (2001), which say that 'governments should take all necessary steps to improve mental health care at every organisational level, but especially at CL, through integration with the PHC system, supervision being provided by more skilled personnel and referral services being available for the more difficult types of cases'.

Integrating specialised health services such as mental health services into PHC is one of the WHO's most important recommendations (WHO, 2001).

The provision of mental health services in PHC includes diagnosing, treating and management of people with mental health disorders; developing plans regarding the prevention of mental health disorders; promoting mental health. It also involves ensuring that PHC staff are able to utilise fundamental psychosocial and behavioural science skills, for example, interviewing, counselling and interpersonal skills, in their daily work in order to improve general health outcomes in PHC (WHO, 2008).

Advantages of integration

According to the WHO (2007), this integration will have the following advantages:
- There will be a reduction in stigma for people with mental disorders and their families, as attending a PHC service is not associated with any specific health condition. For example, a person may attend because of hypertension, diabetes or a mental health condition.
- There will be improved access to care as integrated care helps to improve access to mental health services and treatment of comorbid physical health conditions such as hypertension and diabetes.
- There will be improved prevention and detection of mental disorders as PHC workers are professionals who are the first level of contact for individuals, family and community with the national health system. Most important is equipping these PHC workers with mental health skills to promote mental health and prevent mental disorders.
- Treatment and follow-up of mental disorders will be in place as people who are diagnosed with a mental disorder are often unable or find it difficult to access any treatment for their mental health problems. By providing mental health services at PHC services, more people can receive treatment because of the 'close to home' services. It is also more cost effective as people do not have to travel long distances, and there are fewer language and cultural barriers because the staff should be from local communities.

- Another positive effect is reduced chronicity and improved social integration for the person with the mental disorder and their family as they will not be treated far from their homes. This will result in productivity at home and enhance societal integration which could improve the likelihood of recovery.
- There will be greater protection of human rights as there is less likelihood of being admitted to a psychiatric institution which is often associated with human rights violations. Those receiving care at a PHC centre are less likely to experience discrimination from their community.

Differences in accessibility of facilities and resources

The following three points outline the wide-ranging differences that exist between the nine provinces in the accessibility of facilities and resources for mental health:

1. In some settings, psychiatric services are still provided by a specialised psychiatric team, which visits primary health clinics on specific days or at specific times. This is mainly in outlying and rural areas. This team consists of psychiatric trained nurses and sometimes a medical doctor and social worker. The team is based at a psychiatric hospital. As soon as a psychiatric patient is classified as 'chronic stable', they are transferred to the comprehensive service and are no longer seen by specialists (Western Cape Government 2007). In other settings, community health nurses offer the psychiatric service, but at specific times. Not all of these nurses have psychiatric training, and no other special training has been provided to them.
2. In the past, the PHC level service used to be involved with supplying the patient with psychiatric medication, assessing the effectiveness of the medication and organising admission when necessary. The social worker could assist in obtaining disability grants for the patients. No case finding, rehabilitation or primary prevention activities were involved. The narrow focus on medication without counselling left major needs of patients unattended (Swartz, 2002).
3. When a new patient comes to the clinic, they are referred to a hospital in some instances. From there they may be sent to a psychiatric hospital in the province or put on medication by the local medical doctor. This may involve travelling long distances from an outlying area, or a long period of hospitalisation far from home.

Challenges in incorporating mental health care into PHC

The problem is therefore how to transform the current system into one where comprehensive psychiatric/mental health care (CPMHC) will be incorporated into every PHC setting. The challenges related to this transformation are numerous:
- Financing is crucial to integrating mental health care into PHC, which in a low- and middle-income country like South Africa is challenging (Davies & Lund, 2017)
- The current staff may not have the necessary skills and knowledge to cope with the task. According to SA Nursing Council (SANC) statistics for 2016, only 42 per cent of nurses registered with this council have a registration in mental health/

psychiatric nursing, and in some provinces (Mpumalanga) it is as low as 34 per cent (SANC, 2016). Furthermore, most of the nurses with mental health nursing training received their training in psychiatric hospitals and their skill in community-based approaches is limited. According to the SANC (2016), in 2008 only 51 per cent of the nurses of the country were registered and the training of the other categories of nurses covered little or no psychiatric content.

- If nurses have to make diagnoses and put patients on medication, there should be legal provision for these tasks. The Nursing Act 33 of 2005 (section 56) makes provision for certain nurses to assess, diagnose, prescribe treatment, keep and supply medication for prescribed illnesses and health related conditions. The Medicines and Related Substances Control Amendment Act 94 of 1991 makes provision for regulations to be made authorising nurses to do this; these regulations have not been promulgated.
- The current PHC system is inadequate as it is. Adding new responsibilities to an already overloaded service is a challenge.
- District hospitals, which should provide the back-up for the community-based service, themselves seldom provide quality psychiatric care. Bartlett et al (2011) point out that all over Africa psychiatric hospitals are understaffed, far from the homes of patients, and give only traditional custodial and chemical treatment. This is also true of a few of South African hospitals.
- Lund and Flisher (2002) identified many problems undermining the psychiatric services, such as the patient-to-staff ratio currently in the government sector. Using statistics from the population census of 1996, they found that the staff/bed ratio for the country was 0.3 staff per bed. The ratio of community psychiatric service staff to daily patient visits for the country was 0.6.
- Health care workers often have a negative attitude towards psychiatric patients and their care, and this may make it very difficult to obtain their cooperation with regard to the proposed changes. Mavundla and Uys (1997) surveyed the attitudes of nurses in a general hospital towards psychiatric patients and found that 90 per cent of them held negative views.
- It might be difficult to convince policy makers of the importance of putting additional resources into psychiatric/mental health care. Popular causes, such as maternal and child services, or more dramatic problems such as human immunodeficiency virus (HIV)/acquired immunodeficiency syndrome (AIDS), are often regarded as greater priorities. Furthermore, the broadening of the definition of mental health has allowed the focus to shift from the people with serious mental illness to those with social problems. In a country where social problems are widespread, the temptation to use skilled professionals to deal with these is great.

This shift means that even less attention is available for those people living with serious mental illness and their families.

FUNCTIONS OF MENTAL HEALTH SERVICES IN DIFFERENT SETTINGS

The National Mental Health Policy Framework and Strategic Plan 2013–2020 (Department of Health, 2013: 22) specifies various functions that should be performed by mental health services in different settings. These settings include community mental health services, general hospitals and specialised psychiatric hospitals. The different functions are outlined in Table 4.2.

Table 4.2 Functions of mental health services in different settings

Settings	Functions
1. Community mental health services	<ul><li>Community residential care</li><li>Day-care services</li><li>General health outpatient services at PHC clinics</li><li>Specialised mental health support</li></ul>
2. Psychiatric services at general hospitals	<ul><li>Inpatient units for admissions of mentally ill persons for all categories</li><li>Provision of 72-hour assessments</li><li>Psychiatric wards must be designated in terms of the Mental Health Care Act</li></ul>
3. Specialised psychiatric hospitals	<ul><li>Provision of inpatient and limited outpatient services</li><li>Function as centres of excellence in providing training; supervision; support to secondary and primary health services</li><li>Provision of subspecialist services like forensic psychiatry and child and adolescent services</li></ul>

This table makes it clear that nurses at all levels need to be involved in mental health care.

HUMAN RESOURCES AND TRAINING

According to a study by Lund et al (2000), a comprehensive mental health service for 100 000 members of the population needs 38 hospital beds, and 24 psychiatric nurses, two occupational therapists, three social workers, two clinical psychologists and four psychiatrists. Of the 24 nurses, 17 should work in hospitals, and seven in ambulatory care, while one should be a manager. These calculations are based on a WHO model.

The National Mental Health Policy Framework and Strategic Plan 2013–2020 (Department of Health, 2013: 28–29) specifies that:
- All health staff working in general health settings will receive basic mental health training, and ongoing routine supervision and mentoring.
- The expansion of the mental health workforce will be actively pursued by all provincial departments of health.
- A task-shifting approach will be used in the development of the mental health workforce, whereby trained non-specialist workers deliver evidence-based psychosocial interventions, with supervision and support from specialists.

- Capacity will be developed for staff in the National Directorate: Mental Health and Substance Abuse, and (for) the provincial mental health coordinators in policy development, planning, service monitoring and the translation of research findings into policy and practice.
- At the DL, non-health related public sector workers and civil society partners, including user-led service providers who can contribute to mental health care in the district, will have access to basic in-service training in mental health.

DESCRIPTION OF PRIMARY MENTAL HEALTH CARE

In order to address the needs of consumers at the PHC level, a comprehensive approach involving primary, secondary and tertiary prevention strategies is essential. A focus only on primary medical care, or on secondary prevention, will not address the needs of most consumers.

Primary mental health care is part of PHC services. Primary mental health care should be provided by community health workers and primary care nurses and doctors. Nurses should be trained and updated in the early detection, diagnosis, treatment and referral to higher levels of care (Baumann, 2015).

These PHC practitioners therefore have to be skilled in the process of identifying which people they can help and who should be referred to the secondary health system (SHS).

It is accepted that at PHC clinics nurses will be the only professionals available for the next decade, while at CHCs there might be additional staff members such as a social worker or doctor. They may act as consultants to clinic staff. The secondary health care back-up team for the PHC service providers will mainly be based at the district hospital level. It is hoped that at this level at least a specialist psychiatric nurse, a social worker and an occupational therapist will be available. These people act as *consultants* to the PHC staff and not as supervisors. They are also the expert team to whom the PHC staff refer patients.

Primary mental health care and needs of communities

The needs of communities with regard to primary mental health care include the following:
- *Control of serious mental illness.* This is the greatest perceived need of communities. The priority given to treating the severely mentally ill is seen as a strong point in the services of developing countries (Jacob & Coetzee, 2018).
- *Mental health rehabilitation* is a further aspect of the comprehensive mental health service. Persons suffering from severe and persistent mental illness require rehabilitation in many ways. The goal of mental health rehabilitation is to help individuals to develop the emotional, social and intellectual skills that are needed to live, learn and work in the community with the least amount of professional support. Psychiatric rehabilitation comprises two intervention approaches. The first

approach aims at developing the individual's skills in interacting with demanding situations. The second approach is geared towards the development of environmental resources to reduce possible stressors. Most mentally ill persons need a combination of both approaches (Rössler, 2006).
- *Case finding.* Case finding, a strategy for targeting resources at individuals or groups who are suspected to be at risk for mental health problems, is an important task that should be done at the PHC level. Unless the at-risk individuals or groups are identified and helped appropriately, unnecessary suffering and inappropriate interventions will result. The National Institute for Mental Health in the USA also identifies client identification and outreach as an essential component of a comprehensive, community-based mental health system. Case finding is important for increasing coverage of mental health care in low- and middle-income countries (Mark et al, 2017).
- *Primary prevention.* Mental health prevention is viewed as intervening to *minimise* mental health challenges by addressing contributing factors of mental health problems before a specific mental health problem has been identified in an individual, group, or population of focus like children and adolescents. The ultimate goal should be to reduce the number of future mental health problems in the population (Miles et al, 2010).

MULTIDISCIPLINARY TEAMS

Multidisciplinary teams, which are comprised of staff who vary in their educational and professional experiences, bring together diverse perspectives, expertise, and skills to mental health care. Multidisciplinary teams have become commonplace across mental health settings and are widely considered fundamental to health service delivery. Some of the benefits of multidisciplinary team models include improved consumer health outcomes and functioning, enhanced quality of life, reduced costs, and utilisation of health services (Kutash et al, 2014).

Nursing students become accustomed to interprofessional education as they encounter students of other disciplines in their classes such as social work, psychology, occupational therapy, medicine and pharmacy. This should make easier collaborative working with other health professionals once they have qualified. The goal of interprofessional collaboration is to help prepare future health professionals for enhanced team-based care of patients and improved population health outcomes (Interprofessional Education Collaborative, 2016).

Consultation

One of the ways in which multidisciplinary teams can work is through consultation. The term *consultation* can be understood in many ways. According to Miller-Keane and O'Toole (2003), consultation is a discussion by two or more health care professionals about diagnosis or treatment in a particular case or the provision of expert advice and counselling by an individual with specialised knowledge.

The consultant is a specialist, and the consultee asks for the consultant's help with regard to a current work problem which they are experiencing and which they have decided falls within the other's area of specialisation. In the DHS, the consultee will usually be the PHC nurse, and the consultant will be one of the multidisciplinary team members at the SHS level. Consultation is an empowering process due to the following factors:

- The consultant accepts no direct responsibility for the interventions which the consultee finally undertakes. The patient remains the responsibility of the consultee.
- The consultee remains free to accept or reject the advice of the consultant.
- The consultant engages in the process not only to help with the current problem, but also to increase the knowledge and skill of the consultee. The need for consultation should therefore gradually decrease.

Consultation is not supervision. The secondary health service staff are not the supervisors of the PHC staff. The PHC staff are also not there to evaluate the performance of the PHC staff. This allows PHC staff to use the consultants without fear of jeopardising their positions.

A consultant may offer helpful clarification, diagnostic formulations, or advice on treatment. In order for the consultant to give the best possible advice, the consultee must provide all the relevant information. At the same time, the consultee should remember that the consultant also has other work to do, so the consultation should take up the least time possible. It is important, therefore, to prepare carefully for a telephonic consultation, so that all the information is available, and the consultee knows exactly what they want.

When the nurse plans to consult a specialist, it is also important to decide which of the multidisciplinary team members will be the most appropriate, for instance:

- a diagnosis or medication problem: psychiatrist or psychiatric nurse
- a counselling or behavioural problem: psychologist or social worker
- a financial or legal problem: social worker.

Referral

Another area in which multidisciplinary teams are involved is referral.

Referral means that the nurse transfers responsibility for the patient's care to another institution or person. There are different reasons for a referral, for example:

- The patient does not fit into any of the psychiatric diagnoses with which the practitioner is familiar.
- The patient is not responding to treatment, even after an adjustment of medication. In this case, the PHC practitioner may consult a specialist on the case first, especially if a telephone is available, before the patient is referred to a hospital.

- The patient requires assistance which the PHC centre is unable to deliver, for example a patient who needs to see a social worker about a child-care grant.
- The patient is a danger to themselves or to others and cannot be contained in a community setting, for example a suicidal patient.

When doing a referral, a standardised form may be used. This should be addressed either to the doctor or the appropriate professional. A copy of the referral letter should be kept in the patient's file. The following components are essential to a referral:
- patient's name
- referring clinic/service
- person making the referral
- diagnosis of the patient (if available)
- treatment the patient is currently receiving
- the reason for the referral, for example: 'The patient does not seem to be responding to the medication and continues to report symptoms as bad as those suffered two months ago when treatment was initiated.'
- what is requested, for example: 'Please admit and stabilise on effective medication.'.

When a patient is referred back to the service that had previously done the referring, a reply letter or form should be sent by the SHS team member who dealt with the patient. This should include:
- the findings, or the type of treatment that was given
- whether they did what was requested and if not, why not
- any advice for further management that may be required by the PHC provider.

Telemental health

Telemental health (telepsychiatry) is another area which involves multidisciplinary teams. Telemental health is a subset of telemedicine and involves the provision of remote and rural mental health care services (usually via an audio/video secure platform) by psychiatrists, psychologists, social workers, and nurses. Most services involve assessment, therapy, and/or diagnosis (Quashie, 2015).

Videoconferencing (VC) is live, interactive two-way audio and video communication using a wide range of VC systems. These systems connect two health sites using either phone lines or the internet. The quality of the connection between two sites is dependent on the available bandwidth capacity, measured in bytes per second (bps), at the sites used to transfer video and audio between them. If the bandwidth is not adequate, the sound or video picture is too slow to be effective (Chipps et al, 2012b). If the hospital has a dedicated, functioning VC venue, nurses can consult with a mental health specialist at another VC site such as an academic hospital or a central hospital (Chipps et al, 2012c). Various mobile applications are now also available for VC consultations and this is suitable for smaller settings (such as PHC clinics) where there is adequate bandwidth. In South Africa, PHC clinics have not yet formally been linked using VC.

Most international telemental health services have been implemented to link psychiatric hospitals or psychiatric consultants with mental health clinics or outpatient clinics in general hospitals (Chipps et al, 2012a). A number of district and regional hospitals in South Africa have dedicated teaching and telemedicine VC, which can also be used for telemental health (Chipps et al, 2012d)

Some situations in which telemental health VC consultations have been effective are (Chipps et al, 2012a):
- mental health tele-education sessions
- mental health assessments and clinical interviews
- medication management
- psychotherapy/cognitive behavioural therapy
- multidisciplinary team management
- consulting with a mental health expert involving:
  - mentoring
  - assessing and diagnosing mental health patients
  - obtaining an ongoing medication review by a treating psychiatrist
  - ongoing management of care plans including treatment follow-up and review of an existing patient.

Telemental health VC consultations are contraindicated in the following situations where a patient:
- is unwilling or unable to sit in front of the camera (Pineau et al, 2006)
- refuses this treatment modality
- is violent, unstable or impulsive
- is at immediate risk of suicide or is an immediate danger to others
- requires special monitoring not available at your site
- experiences specific symptomatology that could be exacerbated by the use of video and audio
- has hearing, visual or cognitive deficits (Pineau et al, 2006).

The following is based on the *Practice Guidelines for Videoconference-based Telepsychiatry in South Africa* (Chipps et al, 2012b). When doing a telemental health consultation, these need to be in place at the hospital or clinic and at the consulting site:
- dedicated and tested VC set-ups, including VC software
- a booking system for VC consultations (Frueh et al, 2000)
- locally adapted guidelines for VC consultations for mental health care users (American Telemedicine Association, 2009).

When participating in a telemental health VC consultation, the practitioner needs to do the following (Chipps et al, 2012b):
1. Identify the responsible local clinician
2. Book the session in advance:
   - make sure that the patient has been assessed for suitability for telemental health
   - submit relevant documentation to VC participants regarding the patient at least one day prior to the consultation
3. Before the session make sure this takes place:
   - provide a full explanation to the patient of the purpose of the consultation, procedure and technical aspects of process, for example camera placements and microphone, presence of technician
   - acquire the informed consent, in writing and signed, of the mental health service user/family/guardian (as per local policy)
   - all staff and persons present must be informed of all people participating in the consultation by name, position and responsibility
4. During the session, ensure that:
   - the patient is introduced to all participants in consultation
   - the patient is interviewed by the consultant
   - there is a discussion with the patient and the local responsible clinician
   - there is confirmation of treatment and management suggestions
5. After the session there should be:
   - documentation of key decisions on the patient's file (local site)
   - a record of the clinical consultation (virtual site)
   - completion of a telemental health audit record.

CONCLUSION

The target for the South African health services has been set. It is clear that an accessible, effective service for all communities in this country is what we are aiming for. However, we are just at the beginning of the journey to achieving this goal. Our reaching it is heavily dependent on whether the nurses in primary health care settings are assisted, encouraged and able to master the skills and knowledge they will need in order to implement comprehensive PHC, and on whether policies are put in place to support their work. These are crucial to the success of the whole plan.

WEB RESOURCES

http://www.who.int/en/
> This useful website belongs to the World Health Organisation. Try 'Health Topics' with its comprehensive list of topics and information (fact sheets), each with associated links. The 'Publications' section provides a catalogue and a summary of world health reports.

http://www.health.gov.za/
> This is the website of the South African government, and you will find very useful information there. The Department of Health website offers a wide range of documents, as well as facts and statistics.

https://portal.dmh.mo.gov/
> If you want to see what a totally different health system looks like, look at what the Missouri Department of Mental Health in the USA has to offer. Their services are described on this site, including their suicide resources.

http://www.tmhguide.org/
> This is a resource for developing, implementing and using mental health services with the aid of videoconferencing (VC).

REFERENCES

AETMIS. 2006. *Agence d'évaluation des technologies et des modes d'intervention en santé*. Telehealth: clinical guidelines and technical standards for telepsychiatry. Report prepared by Pineau et al (AETMIS 06-01). Montréal: AETMIS, xxii-72.

American Telemedicine Association. 2009. 'Evidence Practice for Telemental Health'. www.americantelemed.org/docs/default-source/standards/evidence-based-practice-for-telementalhealth. pdf?sfvrsn=4 (Accessed 14 February 2018).

Ayano, G. 2018. 'Significance of mental health legislation for successful primary care for mental health and community mental health services: A review'. *Afr J Prm Health Care Fam Med*, 10 (1).

Bartlett, P, Jenkins, R and Kiima, D. 2011. 'Mental health law in the community: thinking about Africa'. *International Journal of Mental Health Systems*, 5: 21.

Baumann, S E. 2015. *Primary care psychiatry. A practical guide for Southern Africa*. Cape Town: Juta.

Chipps, J, Brysiewicz, P and Mars, M. 2012a. 'Effectiveness and feasibility of telepsychiatry in resource constrained environments? A systematic review of the evidence'. *African Journal of Psychiatry*, 15 (4): 235-243.

Chipps J, Ramlall, S and Mars, M. 2012b. 'Practice guidelines for videoconference-based telepsychiatry in South Africa'. *African Journal of Psychiatry*, 15 (4): 271-282.

Chipps, J, Ramlall, S and Mars, M. 2012c. 'A Model for Telepsychiatry for South Africa'. *African Journal of Psychiatry*, 15 (4): 264-270.

Chipps, J, Ramlall, S, Madigoe, T, King, H and Mars, M. 2012d. 'Developing telepsychiatry services in KwaZulu-Natal – an action research study'. *African Journal of Psychiatry*, 15 (4): 255-263.

Davies, T and Lund, C. 2017. 'Integrating mental health care into primary care systems in low- and middle-income countries: Lessons from PRIME and AFFIRM'. *Global Mental Health*, 4, E7. doi: 10.1017/gmh.2017.3.

Department of Health. 2013. *National Mental Health Policy Framework and Strategic Plan 2013-2020*. Pretoria: Department of Health.

Frueh, B C, Deitsch, S E, Santos, A B, Gold, P B, Johnson, M R, Meisler, N, Magruder, K M and Ballenger, J C. 2000. 'Procedural and methodological issues in telepsychiatry research and program development'. *Psychiatric Services,* December, 51 (12): 1522–1527.

Interprofessional Education Collaborative. 2016. *Core competencies for interprofessional collaborative practice: 2016 update.* Washington, DC: Interprofessional Education Collaborative.

Jacob, N and Coetzee, D. 2018. 'Mental illness in the Western Cape Province, South Africa: A review of the burden of disease and healthcare interventions'. *South African Medical Journal* 2018, 108 (3): 176–180. doi: 10.7196/SAMJ.2018.v108i3.12904.

Kutash, K, Acri, M, Pollock, M, Armusewicz, K, Serene Olin, S C and Hoagwood, K E. 2014. 'Quality Indicators for Multidisciplinary Team Functioning in Community-based Children's Mental Health Services'. *Administration and Policy in Mental Health*, Jan, 41 (1): 55–68.

Lund, C and Flisher, A J. 2002. 'Staff/bed and staff/patient ratios in South African public sector mental health services'. *S A Medical Journal*, 92 (2): 157–61.

Lund, C, Flisher, A L, Lee, T, Portens, K and Robertson, B. 2000. 'A model for estimating mental health service needs in South Africa'. *SA Medical Journal*, 90 (10): 1019–1024.

Mark, J D, Jordans, A, Brandon, A, Kohrt, B, Nagendra, P, Luitel, C, Crick Lund, D, Ivan, H and Komproe, E. 2017. 'Proactive community case-finding to facilitate treatment seeking for mental disorders, Nepal'. *Bulletin of the World Health Organization.* 95 (7): 481–544.

Mavundla, T R and Uys, L R. 1997. 'The attitudes of nurses towards mentally ill people in general hospital settings in Durban'. *Curationis,* 20 (2): 3–7.

Mental Health Care Act 17 of 2002. *Government Gazette*, No 24024.

Miles, J, Espiritu, R C, Horen, N, Sebian, J and Waetzig, E. 2001. *A public health approach to children's mental health: A conceptual framework.* Washington, D C: Georgetown University Center for Child and Human Development, National Technical Assistance Center for Children's Mental Health.

Miller-Keane and O'Toole, M. 2003. *Miller-Keane Encyclopedia & Dictionary of Medicine, Nursing, and Allied Health.* 7th edition. Elsevier. https://www.elsevier.com/books/miller-keane-encyclopedia-and-dictionary-of-medicine-nursing-and-allied-health/miller-keane/978-0-7216-9791-8 (Accessed 6 June 2018).

Mugisha, J, Abdulmalik, J, Hanlon, C, Petersen, I, Lund, C, Upadhaya, N, Ahuja, S, Shidhaye, R, Mntambo, N, Alem, A, Gureje, O and Kigozi. F. 2017. 'Health systems context(s) for integrating mental health into primary health care in six Emerald countries: a situation analysis. *Int J Mental Health Systems*, 11: 7.

Nursing Act 33 of 2005. *Government Gazette*, No 767.

Pineau, G, Moqadem, K, St-Hilaire, C, Perreault, R, Levac, E, Hamel, B, Obadia, A and Caron, L. 2006. (see AETMIS) RANZP Position Statement #44 The Royal Australian and New Zealand College of Psychiatry: Adopted 1999.

Quashie, R. 2015. 'The Boom in Telemental Health. Posted in Health Information Technology, Telehealth and Telemedicine', uncategorised in EPSTEIN BECKER & GREEN, P C. http://www.techhealthperspectives.com (Accessed 24 July 2017).

Rössler, W. 2006. 'Psychiatric rehabilitation today: an overview'. *World Psychiatry*, Oct, 5 (3): 151–157.

South African Nursing Council. 2016. *Statistical Returns for the Calendar Year 2016.* Pretoria: SANC.

Swartz, L. 2002. 'Integrating services, marginalising patients: psychiatric patients and primary health care in South Africa'. *Transcultural Psychiatry*, 39 (2): 155–172.

Western Cape Government. 2007. *Comprehensive plan for the implementation of healthcare 2010.* Cape Town: Western Cape Government.

World Health Organisation (WHO). 2001. 'New understanding, new hope'. *The World Health Report 2001 Mental Health*. Geneva: WHO.

World Health Organisation (WHO). 2007. *Integrating mental health services into primary health care*. Geneva: World Health Organisation. http://www.who.int.mental_health/policy/services/en/index.html (Accessed 18 September 2018).

World Health Organisation (WHO). 2008. 'What Is Primary Care Mental Health? WHO and Wonca Working Party on Mental Health'. *Mental health in family medicine*, 5.1: 9–13.

CHAPTER 5

The Consumers in Mental Health

L R Uys and P D Martin

Learning Outcomes

After studying this chapter, you should be able to:
- discuss the problem of stigmatisation associated with mental illness and how this can be addressed in communities in South Africa
- identify the factors associated with engaging with treatment to promote recovery from mental illness, as perceived by consumers
- describe the stages through which the family of a mentally ill person has to pass
- compare the models families use to explain mental illness and how these influence their coping strategies
- describe how families can assist a mentally ill family member towards recovery
- debate the value of support groups for consumers and describe how these can be formed and maintained
- describe the advocacy role of consumers.

INTRODUCTION

Stigmatisation associated with mental illness is pervasive and not only affects the persons who suffer from a mental disorder, but also their families, friends and communities in which they live. In South Africa, policy such as the National Mental Health Policy Framework and Strategic Plan 2013–2020 (Department of Health, 2013) alludes to the plight mental health consumers face because of their diagnosis. The effects of such a diagnosis include neglect, rejection by family and peers, social exclusion due to the stigma, abuse and violation of their basic rights which are enshrined in the Constitution of South Africa.

Consumer movement organisations have emerged to address the problems that mental health care users (MHCUs) and families face. The influence and strength of these organisations have increased greatly since the dawn of the community psychiatric era. Since the change in approach that resulted in MHCUs spending most of their time outside of hospitals – many of them in the care of their families – families have organised themselves to address their common problems. At the same time, MHCUs themselves have become more active participants in the treatment and rehabilitation process, and this has led to groups of MHCU consumers forming support groups. Strictly speaking, only those persons who have been or who are being treated in the mental health system can be regarded as consumers. However, families are often so closely involved in this process that they can also be seen as consumers of mental health care.

As a result of the acceptance of the recovery approach as a foundation of the mental health policy in many countries and states, it is now often a legal requirement that consumers should have a greater role in policy, planning and service delivery. In South Africa, the mental health review boards in each province (as stipulated by the Mental Health Care Act 17 of 2002), play a key role in advocating for the needs of MHCUs to uphold and protect their human rights. A community person must serve on the board (Mental Health Care Act). There are also a few consumer and family associations in some provinces which are run by non-governmental organisations (NGOs) such as the Mental Health Federation.

The involvement of mental health consumers in their care, treatment and rehabilitation necessitates health workers' understanding of the problems that they and their families face as they navigate a health care system in which mental health care has not been fully integrated.

THE STIGMA ASSOCIATED WITH BEING MENTALLY ILL

There are many first-hand accounts of persons who have experienced the suffering of mental illness. Such reports, appearing in the popular press, in professional journals, and in book form, greatly enrich our understanding of this illness and the stigma associated with it.

South African literature does not contain many such accounts, although there are a few (Egbe et al, 2014). The story of Lily Moya is a particularly poignant account of an MHCU in one of the psychiatric hospitals in South Africa. It describes the correspondence between Lily, a young girl from the Transkei who had great dreams and ambitions, and Dr Mabel Palmer, administrator at the University of Natal. The correspondence stretches over three years and allows us to get to know the vivid person that Lily was before mental illness claimed her and turned her into a grey figure in a back ward. Here, for instance, is Lily's description of her experiences as a substitute teacher at the age of 15 at a village school in Ncambele in 1949 (Marks, 1987: 10):

> It was a great shock to me that I should teach. The Principal teacher was quite amazed – he did not know that I was so small, indeed, the students are very big in that school ... Just imagine how I nearly lost my senses, and how I shivered from toe to hair when I found myself standing in front of such big students, very old indeed for such classes ... What would you have done if you would have been myself? Would you have gone to the classrooms or ran back home? This incidence [sic] brought a great change to this prolonged monotonous life ...

But the orphaned Lily could not find the support she needed, and the stress and alienation of her life became too great. By 1951 she was acutely depressed and, after seeking help from traditional healers, she was admitted to Sterkfontein Hospital, where she was diagnosed as having schizophrenia. She spent the next 25 years of her life in psychiatric hospitals before the deinstitutionalisation policy released her in 1976.

The experience of having a mental illness is one of the most frightening and alienating experiences a person can endure. While every other life experience can be 'managed' or 'coped with' by means of one's mental powers, in this case the brain itself is the centre of the problem, making management and coping so much more difficult. While the person looks physically healthy, and life circumstances may even be positive, the whole fabric of their personality and life is undermined by the insidious processes in the mind.

What makes the experience even more difficult is the stigma attached to people suffering from these conditions. The word *stigma* comes from the mark branded on a slave and refers to an imputation which stains or scars a person's reputation. In other words, it is a label that brands a person in a negative way in the eyes of society. Society regards people with mental illness as dangerous, not always physically, but in a more nebulous way. Those who are mentally ill might make people uncomfortable, act strangely, and do not react to people in a predictable manner. Other members of society see them as 'weak'. They should 'pull themselves together' and all will be well. They are 'ungrateful to be depressed when they have so much to be grateful for'. Or they are 'lazy – a big young man lying around all day doing nothing!'.

All these perceptions are based on a lack of knowledge and understanding of what mental illness is and how it is treated. But the perceptions are not easy to combat, since people avoid what they do not understand, and they often do not want to know. Their misconceptions are often also fed by the media, which stereotypes mentally ill persons as violent. For instance, Roberts et al (2013) reported that 40 per cent (n=277) of all newspaper articles, which mentioned mental illness over a period of two decades, alluded to mentally ill individuals with reference to violent crime rising from 12 per cent to 18 per cent.

This is part of the reason why many MHCUs and their families are socially shunned, and why persons with mental illness cannot find work, housing or friends. This vicious cycle keeps on repeating itself: the person has symptoms of the mental illness and feels strange and weird. People react to them in an exaggerated way because of the symptoms, but also because of the stigma. This reinforces the MHCU perception that they are not acceptable, deepening the suffering and withdrawal.

Specific measures have been taken to decrease the stigma. A consumer's initial contact with health care services following involuntary admission may be primary health care clinics to ensure that they are treated and stabilised in their communities within the shortest possible time. They also obtain their psychiatric medication at the primary health care clinics. This is advantageous because they are referred to medical doctors should they require medical care for physical illness. The approach is called a 'one-stop shop'.

The stigma associated with MHCUs is common in South Africa. In a qualitative study conducted in the North West Province, Egbe et al (2014) depicted four major themes related to the stigma experienced by an MHCU. These included:

1. service users' experiences of the stigma and discrimination – externalised stigma from family and community

2. causes of psychiatric stigma – beliefs and traditions perpetuated stigma and discrimination
3. impact of stigma – negative impact on consumers
4. discrimination towards service users and suggestions to combat stigma – need for education and training.

More disconcerting is that these authors alluded to the stigma associated with MHCUs as being perpetuated by health care workers (professional nurses, lay counsellors, and auxiliary social workers).

The stigma associated with mental illness goes beyond mere attitudes. A recent consensus by the World Psychiatric Association highlighted that South African medical aid schemes and their benefit systems were discriminatory against people diagnosed with mental illnesses (Depression and Anxiety Support Group, 2017). In a survey of 10 medical aid companies, they found that only two did not discriminate against mental illnesses. Discrimination involved problems such as not paying for hospitalisation resulting from suicide attempts or providing no cover for substance-abuse disorders. Some medical aids expected MHCUs to pay 50 per cent of the cost of hospitalisation upfront, while others penalised MHCUs for not obtaining authorisation prior to admission despite the fact that the MHCU might have been psychotic on admission.

The importance of stigmatisation is highlighted in the National Mental Health Policy Framework and Strategic Plan 2013–2020, where an intersectoral role and responsibility to mental health promotion and prevention refer to the inclusion of mental health literacy in the curriculum. This is for the purpose of increasing awareness and reducing discrimination and stigmatisation.

Does a psychiatric diagnostic label increase stigmatisation?

Three views on this matter can be taken into consideration:
1. Having a diagnostic label is good, since it provides information to those affected and allows them to make informed decisions and manage their illness.
2. It also allows the person to be recognised as sick and to benefit from the privileges of the sick role, such as being excused from going to work and taking care of others.
3. However, a diagnostic label is a labelling process that leads to negative stereotypes of the mentally ill and to discrimination and increased suffering.

The view of an advocacy group in the USA, the National Alliance on Mental Illness (NAMI, nd), which disapproves of euphemisms, is relevant. They hold that even if a psychiatric diagnosis leads to stigmatisation, it should be given for the purpose of providing information to those affected and the stigma should be addressed by other means (NAMI, nd).

In a systematic review of the stigma associated with mental illness in the USA (Parcesepe & Cabassa, 2013), perceptions of dangerousness varied according to the mental disorder. People with schizophrenia and alcohol abuse were perceived as being more likely to be a danger to themselves and others compared to people diagnosed with depression. Stigmatising actions such as social distance, which alludes to the exclusion of people in a variety of social settings (refusing to live next door to a person with a mental illness), were greater when there was a diagnosis of mental illness than when people had physical illnesses. The conclusion is therefore that schizophrenia is associated with being dangerous while mental illness leads to alienation.

To address the stigma associated with mental illness, the South African Mental Health Policy Framework and Strategic Plan 2013–2030 has a key objective to increase public awareness about mental health and to reduce the stigma and discrimination associated with mental illness.

CONSUMERS' PERCEPTIONS ON RECOVERY FROM MENTAL ILLNESS

South Africa has adopted a recovery model for mental illness. This includes an approach to mental health care and rehabilitation which asserts that hope and the restoration of a meaningful life are possible, despite serious mental illness. Recovery focuses on restoring self-esteem and identity while fostering and attaining meaningful roles in society (South African National Department of Health, 2013).

Over the last two decades, MHCU consumers of mental health services have expressed some very definite views regarding the process of recovery. One such view is about staying in control of their lives (optimal level of functioning) rather than returning to premorbid levels of functioning. This approach focuses on resilience and control over problems that they encounter and how they manage their lives. It is important that health care workers take note of their unique perspective.

Dixon et al (2016) conducted a review on various evidence-based, recovery-oriented treatment techniques which improved MHCU outcomes. These emerging techniques have been used by consumers to enhance their experience of mental health treatment and to promote recovery. These include attitudes and interpersonal focus; and emerging innovations towards recovery.

Attitudes and interpersonal focus

This approach involves:
- A therapeutic alliance which focuses on the quality of the relationship between the health care worker and the consumer. Consumers who are able to form good relationships with the health care worker are more likely to remain on treatment with a positive recovery outcome.
- Person-centred care which involves a comprehensive approach to understanding and responding to the consumer (MHCU and family), bearing in mind their history, needs, strengths, hopes and dreams for recovery, support needed and outcomes with regard to quality of life. The consumer's culture, background and goals are incorporated in the treatment approach towards recovery.

Emerging innovations towards recovery

Technology, such as the internet, smartphone apps and social media, is important in improving engagement with consumers, as information and support from mental health care services can be expanded through the use of this technology. Peer-support networks may assist consumers who stigmatise themselves and have a need for role modelling.

The strategies identified here emphasise the need to remain abreast of technology but one should never forget the role that others (families, communities and stakeholders) play in promoting recovery in people diagnosed with a mental illness.

While people with physical illnesses in the form of chronic diseases – like hypertension – are not viewed as being ill, mental illness is viewed differently which gives the impression that recovery is not possible. This in turn leads to a downward spiral of no hope which negatively impacts on recovery. The process of recovery has evolved over the years. Parker (2014) asserts that there is a new understanding of recovery according to which recovery is seen as a journey as opposed to an endpoint. This journey begins when the mental health problem is recognised, followed by the empowering realisation that recovery is about the whole person and not just the illness.

The USA's Substance Abuse and Mental Health Services Administration (SAMHSA) has a Recovery Support Strategic Initiative which identifies four dimensions supporting recovery from mental illness (SAMHSA, 2011). These include:

- *Health*. This involves overcoming or managing one's disease or symptoms – for example, abstaining from the use of alcohol, illicit drugs, and non-prescribed medications if the mental illness is related to a substance-abuse problem. When in recovery, informed, healthy choices that support physical and emotional well-being are made.
- *Home*. This means having a stable and safe place in which to live.
- *Purpose*. This has to do with participating in meaningful daily activities, for example being employed, attending school, volunteering at organisations, and taking care of family – thus being independent, having an income and the resources to participate in society.
- *Community*. This involves maintaining relationships and social networks with others that are deemed supportive, provide hope and friendship.

The consumer organisation, Schizophrenics Anonymous, has devised a programme to help cope with this serious illness, based on the steps devised by Alcoholics Anonymous. The steps are:

1. *I surrender*. I admit that I need help; I cannot do it alone.
2. *I choose*. I choose to be well. I take responsibility for the choices that I make.
3. *I believe*. I believe that I have great inner resources and I will try to use these resources to help myself and others.
4. *I forgive*. I forgive myself for the mistakes that I have made. I also forgive and release everyone who has injured or harmed me in any way.

5. *I understand*. I understand that erroneous self-defeating thinking contributes to my problems, failures, unhappiness, and fears. I will work towards a more constructive belief system.
6. *I decide*. I make a decision to turn my life over to the care of God, as I understand him, surrendering my will and false beliefs (Recovery-World, nd).

The active role of the MHCU in the process of recovery is clearly demonstrated in these steps. Most of these things cannot be done for the MHCU – the process is totally dependent on the MHCU themselves.

An MHCU often has to accept some level of dependence on their family for care. This is not easy nor is it uncontested. Pernice-Duca (2010) found that MHCUs often acknowledge the care with great gratitude, but they also point out issues of coercive treatment, and issues of independence versus dependence. There is growing recognition that patients are not only receivers of care, but also give care. Not only do they give care to other MHCUs in consumer-run services, but they care for their own families. For instance, they might phone regularly to reduce the worry of their families about them, or they might look after another family member for short periods to free up a primary caregiver.

THE FAMILY OR 'CARER' PERSPECTIVE

The families of people with mental illnesses usually shoulder the greatest part of the burden of caring for them. In a study conducted by McCann et al (2015) on 30 primary caregivers of people with a mental illness, findings alluded to caring being a difficult and demanding responsibility which affects caregivers adversely: emotionally, physically, socially, financially, and their lifestyle in general. However, carers in the study developed resilience in caring and this helped to sustain them in their caring role, thus enabling them to maintain their well-being. Other studies (Shah et al, 2010) have shown that the burden which this creates for the family is significant. However, the fact remains that the family is the main resource for the person suffering from mental illness. Families act as caregivers, they support other families with similar problems, they teach and educate other consumers and the public at large, they participate in research and they advocate for improved services both for the individual and for MHCUs in general (Mokgothu et al, 2015).

Caregiving in the African context is usually a family affair with multiple caregivers, a system that allows the primary caregiver times of relief from caring. Seloilwe (2006) describes the three levels of decision making practised in a family with a mentally ill member. First, certain decisions are made by the caregiver in charge of the daily life of the MHCU; secondly some will be the prerogative of the most powerful person (usually the one who provides the finances), and thirdly some decisions will be made through consultation with the whole family.

Stages of caregiving

Howard (1994) identified the following stages experienced by mothers of persons suffering from serious mental illness. These stages were confirmed in an African population by Seloilwe (2006).

Stage 1: Perceiving a problem

At this stage the parent or spouse realises that something is wrong with the person concerned. Slowly they come to see that the problem is serious and is not going 'to go away'. In some cases, this stage takes months, but in exceptional cases it can go on for years. The family then goes into a crisis with the shock of a 'breakdown' or the first hospitalisation or a similar drastic event, which confirms all their fears.

Stage 2: Searching for solutions or for help

During this stage the families search for information and assistance. They have to learn to use a totally different assistance network, often one that is poorly developed and difficult to access. They grapple with episodes of illness, and they suffer acutely from the emotional stress of the process through which they and their loved one are passing. Often families are given very little information, even to the extent of never being given a diagnosis for the problem, but only vague statements about a 'nervous breakdown'. In the African setting, traditional healers and faith healers are often the first outsiders consulted, and the western health services are only consulted if there is no improvement.

Stage 3: Enduring the situation

This stage is similar to the previous one, but the family is more focused. They often have a diagnosis by this time, and they have a better idea of what they have to deal with. Many a time they obtain their information from personal experience and a few user-support groups. They very seldom obtain their information from the health system. It is still a very distressing phase, during which the family reaches out to one another, to friends, co-workers, health care providers and religious leaders for assistance and support. They also continue to give care to the MHCU. Seloilwe (2006) calls this phase 'endless suffering'.

Stage 4: Surviving the experience

Survival is linked to acceptance. It is often triggered by the knowledge that serious mental illness is biological and not caused by bad mothering or personal weakness. This decreases the guilt and increases support and understanding. It is a time of hope and of determination in the face of ongoing stress. The family also experiences ongoing grief over the 'loss' of their old life, and of the person who the MHCU was and could have been.

Understanding these stages could assist health workers in providing appropriate support to families. It could also help families to understand their own feelings.

The burden of caregiving

Families looking after a family member with a mental illness usually do this due to the emotional bond between them – because they perceive it as their duty, because they feel guilty and often just because they don't have a choice. Continuous, long-term caregiving leads to significant stress that is often referred to as the 'family burden' or the 'caregiving burden'.

The caregiving burden includes the following dimensions:
- *Symptom-specific burden.* This is the impact of the specific problems of the MHCU, which demand supervision and assistance. An example is that an MHCU might not be able to, or be unwilling to, manage their own medication and the family member has to take charge of this aspect of care.
- *Social burden.* This is the impact on social relationships of the mentally ill person's presence. For instance, the presence of a mentally ill brother who has to live with his married sister has many implications for the social relationships in her family.
- *Emotional burden.* This is the impact of the care experience on the mental and emotional well-being of the caregiver, for instance an elderly mother becoming worried and afraid of her adult son who tends to be aggressive during acute episodes of illness.
- *Financial burden.* This is the financial cost to the family of caregiving, such as providing food, transport and housing (Pazvantoglu et al, 2014).

The burden of caregiving should be recognised by the health team, and families should be supported in order to reduce the burden.

Ways in which families explain mental illness

The way people deal with something depends on how they understand and explain it; this is also true of the way in which families deal with mental illness. For example, religion and spirituality sometimes play a significant role in the lives of people with schizophrenia. Non-medical explanations from MHCUs and their families about their illness include that they were ill because they had been bewitched and were possessed by evil spirits (Napo et al, 2012).

Patel (1995) conducted a review of the literature on explanatory models to explain the beliefs about mental illness, with a specific focus on concepts, classification and models of causality and phenomenology in 11 sub-Saharan African countries. A brief explanation of the focal points follows:
- *Concepts.* The holistic view of illness experiences incorporated a distinction between the mind and the body.
- *Classification and aetiological models of mental illness.* Disease causation and classification are intimately related to traditional religious beliefs. Religious beliefs are shared by many African people. Three beliefs about the cause of illness include
  - all things that happen have a cause
  - some things that happen to people are caused intentionally, for example, birth and drought

– the cause can be determined by divine intervention, reasoning and empirical judgement and memory.

The general belief is that both physical and mental illness have external causes. Witchcraft is seen as an important cause of illness and adversity. Illness on the other hand is classified both aetiologically and phenomenologically. In order to classify a mental illness, the type and severity of the behavioural disturbance is used. A cause for the illness is usually given as it provides meaning to the patients for the illness experience. Illness is usually classified as normal or abnormal with the normal illness being treated with biomedical and traditional methods. Abnormal illness is related to traditional beliefs of misfortune, supernatural forces, illness caused by others or the behaviour of the person or family for which the person must seek the assistance of the traditional healer.

- *Phenomenology of mental illness.* Illnesses with marked behavioural disturbances are described as being similar to an acute psychotic illness. Some behavioural disturbances include tearing clothes, talking to oneself, and poor self-care. Phenomenology is used by the traditional healer to understand the nature of the illness for which there is always a cause.

Guidelines for families living with a family member who is mentally ill

There are three pillars that can guide families living with a person who has a serious mental illness.

Create an environment with low stress

It is clear that stress plays a major role in the process of mental illness. It is therefore important for families to identify sources of stress for the MHCU and to try to eliminate or limit such sources. It is important to remember that all people have different stress levels, and one should therefore not assume that what one might find stressful is also stressful to someone else. The following strategies to decrease stress may be useful.

- *Keep to a predictable schedule.* This decreases decisions and adjustments and seems to have a calming effect on people in emotional distress.
- *Develop appropriate expectations.* Considerable stress can result when families expect more of the MHCU than they can manage. Many families do not understand that the lack of motivation, a feature of many mental illnesses, is not laziness. They cling to the expectation they had of the person during the premorbid period and fail to adapt. Expectations should therefore be low, and the MHCU's tolerance should be tested gradually. This means having less rather than more: fewer activities, fewer people, fewer expectations, and fewer demands. Sometimes the MHCU themselves may have high expectations; the family must then caution the MHCU to take small steps towards the ultimate goal, or to postpone big projects.

- *Speak simply and clearly.* Since people with mental illnesses often have problems processing information, they find it difficult to follow long, loud, rapid and complicated sentences. Speaking in short, simple sentences, slowly and clearly, may be all that is necessary. With a highly agitated MHCU, it might also be necessary to listen quietly, without correction and interruption.
- *Plan for stressful situations.* This is often the best policy to avoid stressful situations. However, this is not always possible with essential activities such as going for a job interview or writing a test. In such cases families can reduce the stress by preparing the MHCU for the situation. An MHCU needs to know what to expect and should be well prepared for their role in the procedure. They should be allowed plenty of time to enter the situation, for instance leaving for the interview in good time. They should even be allowed to retreat temporarily if necessary.
- *Avoid over-involvement.* Although families mean well, MHCUs often cope better if the family manages to keep some distance between them. Families find that the more they approach the MHCU, the more the person withdraws. Constant enquiries and 'hovering' increase stress. Families should therefore try to limit face-to-face contact, and make sure that they develop outside interests to take their minds off the MHCU and give them time by themselves.
- *Deal actively with one's own stress.* Families often experience feelings of guilt, anger and anxiety, which can be transmitted to the MHCU. It is therefore important that families find positive and active ways of decreasing these negative feelings in themselves. Support groups can play a very important role in this regard, as can time away from the MHCU.

Managing disturbing behaviour successfully

In a study of black families caring for members suffering from schizophrenia, most families described passive, withdrawn behaviour and violent behaviour as the most difficult to deal with (Molefe, 2009). Withdrawn behaviour sometimes meant withdrawal even from the family but, in other cases, the MHCUs put enormous social demands on family members, since they were the MHCU's only 'friends'. Violence and aggression were often directed at family members and this kept families living in fear. The third set of behaviours mentioned was delusions, especially persecutory delusions aimed at the family.

In addition, people with mental illnesses present with an array of behaviours which include but are not limited to:
- lack of motivation
- problematic eating/sleeping behaviours
- difficulty completing tasks
- isolation from others
- poor financial management.

The following interventions may be useful to families trying to deal with disturbing behaviour resulting from mental illness:

- *Persistent inactivity.* Some families deal with this problem by leaving the MHCU to their own devices. This is not a good solution in the long term, since it does not enhance social reintegration. A more useful approach is to plan a schedule of a few simple activities and then to add others later as the MHCU manages to keep to the schedule. One could start with self-care activities and add household tasks later. The MHCU should understand clearly what is expected, and the family should insist on adherence without lecturing or nagging. Rewards can be used to promote activities. If the MHCU continues to be lethargic, it may be necessary for the family to talk to the treatment team about adjusting the medication. However, the family must also be careful not to assist the MHCU when it is not necessary, since this reinforces the helpless role.
- *Refusal of treatment.* It may be very difficult for families to intervene when an MHCU who is obviously in need of treatment refuses either to go to the clinic or to take the medication. A discussion with the treatment team may be useful, since they may be able to initiate and maintain medication treatment through home visits. Serobatse, Du Plessis and Koen (2014) have found that home visits are extremely effective in improving treatment involvement. Changing to intramuscular medication instead of oral tablets may also prove useful. Another approach the treatment team could follow is to participate in a course involving MHCU and family education, especially with other consumers. This approach has a very positive effect on treatment utilisation.
- *Aggressive behaviour.* Aggressive behaviour can be very difficult to handle and is disruptive of home life. The first step in managing such behaviour is to analyse the circumstances of the violence, since the precursors to violence influence the way in which one should deal with it.
    - First, in the case of aggressive behaviour, it must be remembered that people who are mentally ill sometimes have legitimate grievances and may have valid reasons for getting angry. One should therefore listen to what they say and find out what their anger is all about.
    - Secondly, in cases where the violence is the result of a relapse, the MHCU should display other symptoms which indicate an acute phase of the illness. In such cases intervention with medication and/or hospitalisation is indicated.
    - A third reason for aggression could be that the MHCU is using threats or aggression to get their own way. If people tend to be intimidated by the MHCU, and to give in to demands, things can only get worse. In such cases the following steps should be followed:

    Step 1: Convene a meeting of family and health workers during a calm period and decide which demands will no longer be accepted.

    Step 2: Tell the MHCU in a calm way what will not be tolerated and what the consequences will be if they act aggressively. The consequences should be appropriate to the type of aggression: for example, mild acting out

can be followed by a loss of privileges, while serious aggression may lead to being forced to leave home.

Step 3: Be fully prepared to carry out the plan when the confrontation comes. Have telephone numbers ready, people ready to assist, and do not try to bluff.

Step 4: Evaluate how well the plan worked and change it if necessary. Do not expect everything to change at once but keep on trying.

- A fourth reason for aggression is that the person loses control over themselves. An MHCU often finds self-control very difficult and lashes out when cornered. They are not trying to manipulate others as in the previous category, but simply cannot control themselves. The following steps are useful in such cases:

Step 1: Learn to identify the signs that show that the person is beginning to lose control.

Step 2: Give the MHCU space by suggesting that the issue be discussed later. Give the person physical space as well; do not touch or approach them.

Step 3: Preserve your own safety, especially if the person remains very agitated. Phone for help, lock a door, stay outside or call neighbours.

Step 4: When things are calmer, discuss the issue and do not give in just to keep the peace.

Promoting social reintegration and rehabilitation

In the long run it is not enough simply to try to deal with and prevent problems. One also has to consider the quality of life of the mentally ill family member and try to promote functioning in the usual social roles which their age prescribes.

One of the goals a family can set is to try to enlarge the life experience of the MHCU. A first step could be to involve the MHCU in daily activities, or to share a hobby or pleasurable activity. This might stimulate further interest and involvement. People have different strengths and, if the strengths of the MHCU can be identified, these can provide the springboard to a richer life. An interest in music could be used to motivate the patient to join a music appreciation course or a small band; an interest in animals could lead to involvement in an animal shelter. Often the most difficult part is to get the MHCU to take the first step. Sometimes taking the first step with them may help, while at other times a group activity might be more acceptable. Convincing the MHCU just to 'try it once', and allowing the inherent reward of the activity to prompt further participation, could also prove successful.

Another important area of endeavour is the encouragement of independent life skills. Although the patient may currently be living with the family, this situation may not always be possible or ideal. It is therefore important that an effort be made over time to improve the MHCU's functioning in areas such as management of own finances, personal hygiene and maintaining an acceptable environment. These are skills that can be learnt if a systematic and MHCU-centred approach is used. When working with the family member, it is important to remember that the person is still an adult, notwithstanding the severe disability the mental illness may have caused. Patronising remarks about 'being good' or 'pleasing Mom' are not appropriate for adults. Scolding, nagging or moralising also seldom has the desired effect. Respect and positive comments, which build self-respect, are more likely to succeed.

OTHER ROLES OF CONSUMERS

Under the influence of the recovery movement, consumers are involved in mental health services in multiple ways. Their involvement is often a legal requirement, but even in countries where this is not the case, it is a powerful tool for service improvement.

Support groups for consumers

The most effective support groups are grassroots organisations of consumers (families, MHCUs or both) that organise and govern themselves (WHO, 2003). Although professionals may have initiated some of these groups, it is important for consumers to take charge to ensure the survival of the group when professionals leave and to make certain that the group addresses the needs of the members.

The growth of support groups over the last two decades has its roots in the community psychiatric movement, as well as in the self-help ideology which is part of the primary health care approach. Consumers have come to be recognised as equal partners of health workers in all aspects of care provision. Peer support occurs when people who have shared experiences draw on this experience to offer emotional and practical support to one another to manage their illness (Trachtenberg et al, 2013).

Functions of support groups

In the USA, support groups started small and then grew to formidable organisations. The organisation NAMI has over 100 000 members, while other support groups render extensive consumer-run services with enormous budgets. In South Africa, the South African Depression and Anxiety Group (SADAG) is Africa's largest mental health support and advocacy group. SADAG has over 40 000 members and more than 200 support groups in South Africa which include outreach groups in remote rural areas. The activities carried out by the support groups are aimed at people with mental illnesses such as depression, bipolar mood disorders, post-traumatic stress disorder, obsessive compulsive disorder, anxiety, trauma, sleeping disorders, schizophrenia, teen suicide and substance abuse. These support groups are run by MHCUs for MHCUs.

Activities include but are not limited to:
- social and recreational activities
- protection or advocacy efforts on behalf of individual consumers
- advocacy efforts on behalf of all persons with psychiatric disability
- assistance with activities of daily living

- provision of information
- therapeutic interventions, for example skills teaching; counselling
- fundraising.

Three levels of needs have been identified by NAMI and the organisation advises that support groups should try to address all three of these levels at each meeting:

1. *Head out of the sand.* On this level a consumer or family has just begun to accept the mental illness. They are still shocked and grieving and may be denying the reality at times. They need support and education from the group to deal successfully with this stage.
2. *Learning to cope.* The second level refers to families and MHCUs who have lived with mental illness for some time. They have been frustrated by the lack of information and help and disgusted by the stigmatisation. They are tired of the struggle and angry at the system. They need continued support and further information, as well as assistance and encouragement to work towards independence for the mentally ill person.
3. *Change.* At this level families who have accepted the illness and have learnt to cope; they may now want to do something to improve the services or change the system. They need to be involved in social action, policy making, lobbying and other activities which could bring about change.

Starting a support group

One consumer (family or MHCU) or one professional can start a support group. Asking service providers such as clinics, private practitioners and hospitals to hand out letters of invitation to consumers may prove successful. Social media platforms such as Facebook and WhatsApp can be used to advertise support groups and recruit members.

Once a few consumers have been identified, a date, time and place can be set for the first meeting. It is important to find an accessible place for the meeting and to set a convenient time. A Saturday or Sunday might be the most appropriate for many people, as long as the venue is accessible by public transport even on a Sunday. A family home might be the best place to meet if the group is small. If people have telephones, it would be a good idea to give them an encouraging call the day before the meeting. Using a bulk cell phone messaging system (WhatsApp message system) for communication is well worth the effort, since most people in South Africa have mobile phones and this system is more economical than phone calls.

The group should be run by the consumers themselves; they should begin by structuring themselves by electing a chairperson, secretary and treasurer. A name may also be chosen. NAMI recommends that a group choose a name that does not use a euphemism for mental illness, so as to fight the stigma. The group then decides on goals and a mission and may later develop a complete constitution. Early on, the group members should exchange names, addresses and phone numbers, so that they can form an accessible support network for one another.

It is important that the business part of the meeting be kept short, so that there is enough time for sharing and caring. Consumers are encouraged to share their problems and experiences, while others support and assist with empathy, information and even concrete assistance.

Groups usually meet once a month, and deal with business, support and information. Later in the life of the group, social action will be included. At that stage more frequent meetings may be necessary. The following factors ensure the growth of a strong support group (Fieldhouse et al, 2017):

- *Give all members a sense of ownership of the group*. Listen to their ideas; use them, involve them in activities, and address their needs.
- *Ensure a rapid turnover of leadership*. A diversity of leaders leads to diverse activities and to the development of people.
- *Create an appropriate structure*. Structures such as membership requirements, a committee, an annual general meeting, a bookkeeping system and a bank account are essential for a fully functioning group.
- *Have regular meetings* with interesting speakers discussing diverse topics.
- Keep on trying to *broaden the membership base and participation*. Recruitment should be an ongoing activity.
- Try to *build continuity on the committees* by staggering the terms of office. In this way, the committee members will never all be new and inexperienced.
- *Establish committees* to work on specific issues such as stigmatisation, housing, socialisation education and recreation.
- *Hold different kinds of meetings at different times*. These could include general meetings with a speaker, an open house at a new facility, an outdoor meeting, a workshop, or a forum.
- *Produce a brochure* on your group as soon as possible, even if it consists of only one typed page. This can be used in recruitment and in obtaining financial support.
- *Give credit* where and when credit is due.
- *Hold an annual evaluation and planning meeting*, so that the group stays on track.

ADVOCACY BY CONSUMERS

(Also read 'Advocating for service improvements' in Chapter 11)

Advocacy means to 'plead in support of' something or somebody. Advocacy has become one of the main tasks of consumer groups worldwide and is usually aimed at legislators (politicians) and top administrators in the services. The National Mental Health Policy Framework and Strategic Plan 2013–2020 alludes to the role the Department of Health will play in engaging the consumer and family associations in mental health policy development and implementation, in addition to planning and monitoring of services (South African National Department of Health, 2013). Consumers must be involved in decision making.

The methods of advocacy

A newsletter can be a useful tool for communicating with political representatives and other opinion formers. It need not be long, but there should be a focus on policy issues and on the needs of consumers.

Testifying at public hearings, in front of parliamentary committees, and at commissions is another useful method. At first one may not have the required skills, but the first-hand stories of consumers are powerful tools and can have an impact which scientific documents lack.

Letters can be written to local newspapers, politicians and administrators. Letters should be short and to the point and, even if a whole group decides to write about a single topic, each should use their own words. Petitions or group letters are not as effective.

The media can play an important role in airing topics that need attention. Groups should get to know health reporters at local papers, and presenters of health programmes on radio. Television is a difficult medium to access but also a powerful one.

Serving on boards is an important way of putting consumers in positions of power. Psychiatric hospitals are all required by law to have hospital boards, and it would be useful for consumer groups to ensure that they are represented on these bodies. In the near future, clinics will also be setting up committees and districts will have health committees. All these bodies could do with a mental health consumer representative. An interview with a representative or administrator is often a very effective way of dealing with an important issue. Identify and keep to a few important issues, so that the interview does not become a general gripe session. Make sure of the facts about all these issues and decide what the person should do about each one. Select as main spokesperson an articulate member of the consumer group who can speak with confidence. They should, however, involve the other members of the delegation strategically. A diverse group of consumers (for example, parents, siblings, patients, spouses) will have greater impact. Usually delegations number about five people.

INVOLVEMENT IN POLICY, PLANNING AND EVALUATION

Service providers should promote the involvement of consumers in the process of decision making in areas of service delivery, service planning and development, training and the evaluation of services. Both MHCUs and their families have a unique perspective on care needs and provision, and they should be active partners with adequate power in the process of planning and evaluation.

Mechanisms for the involvement of consumers are the following:
- Develop empowerment workshops to train consumers in activism and advocacy.
- Make clear policy on the process of consumer involvement, in order to convey transparently to consumers their rights and responsibilities in this matter.
- Involve consumers in planning committees when developing new services, where they should be supported to take part as equal partners.

- Have consultative meetings with consumers at different points during the planning or evaluation process.
- Appoint consumer consultants to facilitate the process of involving consumers. A consumer consultant is a consumer who has been trained to represent the group and has a network of consumers on whom they can call for input.
- Involve consumers as fieldworkers for needs assessments and service evaluations.
- Conduct in-depth interviews with consumers to explore their experience of using existing services.
- Develop a structure to support consumers in creating their own consumer-participation activities, such as consumer action groups on certain issues like housing (Tambuyzer et al, 2011).

None of these mechanisms will work unless the mental health service creates a supportive environment for consumer participation. The attitudes of health professionals have been seen as a major barrier to consumer involvement – they seem to doubt that consumers add value to the process. Nurses, due to their numbers in the system and their close relationships with consumers, are well placed to change these perceptions.

Finally, experience has shown that individual consumers vary in their ability and willingness to become involved. Consumers should not be viewed as a homogeneous population, and opportunities for training and for participation should be individualised.

CONCLUSION

A mental health team that leaves out consumers is a weak team. Consumers are a force to be reckoned with – either for good, towards support and recovery, or for bad, towards alienation and defeat. Consumers, both MHCUs and their families, need to be seen as team members. Their activities require emotional and material support from the formal health sector.

WEB RESOURCES

http://www.sadag.org

The South African Depression and Anxiety Group (SADAG) is the largest non-profit organisation aimed at MHCU advocacy, education and destigmatisation of mental illness in the Africa. SADAG manages a 16-line counselling and referral call centre for MHCUs and families affected by mental illness.

http://home.vicnet.net.au/~nnaami/

This website belongs to the National Network of Adult and Adolescent Children who have a Mentally Ill Parent/s (NNAAMI) in Australia. It has many first-person stories, chat lines and information for families and professionals.

REFERENCES

Dixon, L B, Holoshitz, Y and Nossel, I. 2016. 'Treatment engagement with individuals experiencing mental health illness: review and update'. *World Psychiatry*, 15 (1): 13–20.

Depression and Anxiety Support Group. 2017. 'Are South African mental health patients having their constitutional rights contravened?', www.sadag.org (Accessed December 2017).

Department of Health. 2013. *National Mental Health Policy Framework and Strategic Plan 2013–2020*. Pretoria: National Department of Health: 1–60.

Egbe, C O, Brooke-Sumner, C, Kathree, T, Seloilwe, O, Thornicroft, O and Petersen, I. 2014. 'Psychiatric stigma and discrimination in South Africa: perspectives from key stakeholders'. *BMC Psychiatry*, 14: 191.

Fieldhouse, J, Parmenter, V, Lillywhite, R and Forsey, P. 2017. 'What works for peer support groups: learning from mental health and wellbeing groups in Bath and North East Somerset'. *Mental Health and Social Inclusion*, 21 (1): 25–33. doi: 10.1108/MHSI-11-2016-0032.

Howard, P B. 1994. 'Lifelong caregiving for children with schizophrenia'. *Archives of Psychiatric Nursing*. 8 (2): 107–114.

Marks, S. 1987. *Not Either an Experimental Doll: The Separate Worlds of Three SA Women*. Pietermaritzburg: University of Natal Press.

McCann, T V, Bramberg J and McCann, F. 2015. 'Family carers' experience of caring for an older parent with severe and persistent mental illness'. *International Journal of Mental Health Nursing*. 24 (3): 203–12. doi: 10.1111/inm.12135.

Mental Health Care Act 17 of 2002, as amended. Pretoria: Government Printers.

Molefe, S. 2009. 'Families' experiences with schizophrenia', Unpublished master's dissertation (unpublished M Arts research project, University of Stellenbosch, Cape Town. Durban).

National Alliance on Mental Illness (NAMI). nd. 'National Alliance on Mental Illness'. www.nami.org (Accessed June 2019).

Napo F, Heinz, A and Auckenthaler, A. 2012. 'Explanatory models and concepts of West African Malian patients with psychotic symptoms'. *Eur Psychiatry*, 27 (Suppl 2): S44–9.

Parcesepe, A M and Cabassa, L J. 2013. 'Public Stigma of Mental Illness in the United States: A Systematic Literature Review'. *Adm Policy Mental Health*, 40: 384–399.

Parker, J. 2014. 'Recovery in mental health'. *South Africa Medical Journal*, 104 (1): 77

Patel, V. 1995. 'Explanatory models of mental illness in Sub-Saharan Africa'. *Soc Sci Med*, 40 (9): 1291–1298.

Pazvantoglu, O, Sarisoy, G, Boke, O, Aker A A, Ozturan, D D and Unverdi, E. 2014. 'The dimensions of caregiver burden in schizophrenia: the role of patient functionality'. *The Journal of Psychiatry and Neurological Sciences*, 27: 53–60.

Pernice-Duca, F. 2010. 'Family network support and mental health recovery'. *Journal of Marital Family Therapy*, 36 (1): 13–27.

Recovery-World. nd. 'Schizophrenia 6 Steps for Recovery'. https://recovery-world.com/Schizophrenia-6-Steps-for-Recovery.html (Accessed June 2019).

Roberts, E, Bourne, R and Basden, S. 2013. 'The Representation of Mental Illness in Bermudian Print Media, 1991–2011'. *Psychiatric Services*, 64 (4): 388–388.

Seloilwe, E S. 2006. 'Experiences and demands of families with mentally ill people at home in Botswana'. *Journal of Nursing Scholarship*, 38 (3): 262–268.

Serobatse, M B, du Plessis, E and Koen, M P. 2014. 'Interventions to promote psychiatric patients' compliance to mental health treatment: A systematic review'. *Health SA Gesondheid*, 19 (1): Art. #799.

Shah, A J, Wadoo, O and Latoo, J. 2010. 'Psychological Distress in Carers of People with Mental Disorders'. *British Journal of Medical Practitioners*, 3 (3): a327.

South Africa. 2002. The Mental Health Care Act, no. 17 of 2002. Pretoria: Government Printers.

Substance Abuse and Mental Health Services Administration (SAMHSA). 2011. *News Release 12/22/2011*, 'SAMHSA announces a working definition of "recovery" from mental disorders and substance use disorders'. http://www.samhsa.gov/newsroom/advisories/1112223420.aspx (Accessed 18 July 2017).

Tambuyzer, E, Pieters, G and Van Audenhove, C. 2011. 'Patient involvement in mental health care: one size does not fit all'. *Health Expectations*, 17: 138–150

Trachtenberg, M, Parsonage, M, Shepherd, G and Boardman, J. 2013. *Peer Support in Mental Health Care: Is it good value for money?*. London: Centre of Mental Health.

World Health Organisation (WHO). 2003. 'The mental health context'. Geneva. WHO.

CHAPTER 6

Legal Structures in Mental Health Care Nursing

N Naidoo and D McQuoid-Mason

Learning Outcomes

After studying this chapter, you should be able to:
- outline the broader legal context within which mental health nurses practise
- explain the most important terms used in the Mental Health Care Act 17 of 2002
- compare and contrast the various ways in which a person may be admitted to a psychiatric hospital
- explain the procedure to be followed when a mental health care user (MHCU) has been mechanically restrained, secluded or subjected to electroconvulsive treatment
- explain the procedure to be followed when an MHCU has absconded
- discuss the rights to which an MHCU is entitled in terms of the Mental Health Care Act
- identify situations in which disclosure of otherwise confidential information is permitted
- discuss the Choice on Termination of Pregnancy Act 92 of 1996 and Sterilisation Act 44 of 1998 as amended, with specific reference to their importance to mental health nursing practice and obtaining informed consent
- explain the provisions of the Medicines and Related Substances Control Act 101 of 1965 as amended, which provides guidelines to psychiatric nurses regarding the possession, supply, administration and prescription of medicines
- explain the provisions of the Children's Act 38 of 2005 as amended, which have implications for psychiatric nursing practice.

INTRODUCTION

Psychiatric nursing in South Africa is governed by the following laws:
- the Constitution of the Republic of South Africa, 1996, which guarantees, among others, the right to life, the right to dignity, the right to physical and psychological integrity, the right to privacy, the right of access to healthcare services and the right not to be refused emergency medical treatment
- the National Patients' Rights Charter of 2002, a policy developed by the Department of Health to realise these constitutional rights
- the Nursing Act 33 of 2005
- the National Health Act 61 of 2003
- the Health Professions Act 56 of 1974, as amended

- the Mental Health Care Act 17 of 2002, as amended
- the Criminal Procedure Act 51 of 1977, as amended
- the Medicines and Related Substances Control Act 101 of 1965, as amended
- the Children's Act 38 of 2005, as amended
- the Choice on Termination of Pregnancy Act 92 of 1996, as amended
- the Sterilisation Act 44 of 1998, as amended.

These Acts are discussed with reference to the sections governing the practice of psychiatric nurses. However, the Constitution, the Patients' Right Charter, the Nursing Act and the National Health Act will not be discussed in detail, as they serve to provide a broader context. Mental health nurses should keep abreast of the professional requirements of nurses and instances in which legal liability may arise.

THE MENTAL HEALTH CARE ACT
Overview

The Mental Health Care Act 17 of 2002, read with its regulations, governs mental health care services in the country, including the practice of psychiatric nursing. The Act provides a more comprehensive, human rights-based approach to the provision of mental health care services than is provided by the now-repealed Mental Health Act 18 of 1973.

The purpose of the Mental Health Care Act is to:
- provide for the care, treatment and rehabilitation of persons who are mentally ill
- set out the different procedures to be followed in the admission of such persons
- establish review boards in respect of every health establishment and determine their powers and functions
- provide for the care and administration of the property of mentally ill persons
- repeal certain laws
- provide for matters connected therewith.

The Act aims to regulate mental health care services in a manner that:
- makes the best possible mental health care, treatment and rehabilitation services available to the population equitably, efficiently and in the best interests of MHCUs within the limits of the available resources
- coordinates access to mental health care, treatment and rehabilitation services to various categories of MHCUs
- integrates the provision of mental health care services into the general health services environment.

Definitions of main terms used in the Act

The main terms and their definitions, which are used in the Mental Health Care Act, are listed in this section.

Mental health care user (MHCU)

This term refers to a person receiving care, treatment and rehabilitation services or using a health service at a health establishment aimed at enhancing the mental health status of a user, state patient or mentally ill prisoner. Where the person concerned is under the age of 18 years or is incapable of taking decisions and in certain circumstances, the term may include the following people as having a corresponding meaning to MHCU:
- a prospective user
- the person's next-of-kin
- a person authorised by any other law or court order to act on that person's behalf
- an administrator appointed in terms of the Mental Health Care Act
- an executor of a deceased person's estate.

Mental health status

This refers to the level of mental well-being of an individual, as affected by physical, social and psychological factors, and which may result in a psychiatric diagnosis.

Mental illness

This is a positive diagnosis of an illness related to mental health in terms of accepted diagnostic criteria. It is made by a mental health care practitioner who is authorised to make such a diagnosis.

Severe or profound intellectual disability

This refers to a range of intellectual functioning extending from partial self-maintenance under close supervision, together with limited self-protection skills in a controlled environment through limited selfcare and requiring constant aid and supervision, to severely restricted sensory and motor functioning and requiring nursing care.

Rehabilitation

This is a process that facilitates an individual attaining an optimal level of independent functioning.

Health establishment

This is an institution, facility, building or place where persons receive care, treatment and rehabilitation assistance, diagnostic or therapeutic interventions or other health services, and includes facilities such as community health and rehabilitation centres, clinics, hospitals and psychiatric hospitals.

Medical practitioner
This is a person registered as such in terms of the Health Professions Act 56 of 1974, as amended.

Mental health care practitioner
This is a psychiatrist, registered medical practitioner or nurse, occupational therapist, psychologist or social worker who has been trained to provide prescribed mental health care, treatment and rehabilitation services.

Mental health care provider
This is a person providing mental health care services to MHCUs. The term includes mental health care practitioners.

Head of health establishment
This is a person who manages the establishment concerned.

Mental health review board
This is a body established by the Member of the Executive Council responsible for health services in a province in terms of section 18 of the Mental Health Care Act.

Rights and duties relating to MHCUs
The Mental Health Care Act requires that the best interests of the MHCU must be upheld. The Act sets out the rights of MHCUs and the duties of mental health care providers. These rights and duties do not exclude the rights and duties which the relevant persons or institutions have in terms of any other law.

Rights to life, dignity and access to health care services
The constitutional rights to life, dignity, physical and psychological integrity, privacy and access to health care services of every MHCU must be respected. The Esidimeni tragedy in Gauteng that resulted in the death of 143 MHCUs was due to the neglect of these rights (McQuoid-Mason, 2018).

Every MHCU must be provided with the care, treatment and rehabilitation services that improve the mental capacity of the user to develop to their full potential, and that facilitate their integration into community life. The services provided must be proportionate to their mental health status, and should intrude as little as possible into the constitutional rights of patients, to give effect to the appropriate care, treatment and rehabilitation. The following of proper procedures regarding the obtaining of consent is fundamental to this.

Consent to care, treatment and rehabilitation services and admission to health establishments

A health establishment or health care provider may provide care, treatment and rehabilitation services to or admit MHCUs only if:
- the users have consented to the care, treatment and rehabilitation services or to admission
- there has been authorisation by a court order or a review board or
- due to mental illness, any delay in providing care, treatment and rehabilitation services or admission may result in: (a) the death or irreversible harm to the health of the users; (b) the users inflicting serious harm to themselves or others; or (c) the users causing serious damage to or loss of property belonging to them or others.

The Act stipulates that in the emergency circumstances referred to above, the health care provider, or health establishment providing the services, must report this in writing, in the prescribed manner, to the relevant review board. The provider or establishment may not continue to provide the services for longer than 24 hours unless an application for voluntary, assisted or involuntary services is made within the 24-hour period.

Consent to treatment or operations for illness other than mental illness

An MHCU who is capable of giving informed consent to treatment or an operation, must decide whether or not to have the treatment or operation. Informed consent means that the user must:
- have knowledge about the treatment or operation
- an understanding and appreciation of the consequences of the treatment or operation and
- have voluntarily consented to all the consequences of such treatment of operation.

The National Health Act 61 of 2003 provides that health care providers must give every health care user the following information when obtaining an informed consent:
- The user's health status except in circumstances where there is substantial evidence that the disclosure of the user's health status would be contrary to the best interests of the user
- The range of diagnostic procedures and treatment options generally available to the user
- The benefits, risks, costs and consequences generally associated with each option
- The user's right to refuse health services and explain the implications, risks, obligations of such refusal.

The health care provider must give the user the information in a language that the user understands and in a manner which takes into account the user's level of literacy.

Consent by children or on behalf of children to treatment or operations for illness other than mental illness

In terms of the Children's Act 38 of 2005, a child over the age of 12 may consent to their treatment if they are of sufficient maturity and have the mental capacity to understand the risks, benefits, social and other implications of the treatment. Such a child may only consent to a surgical operation if, in addition to the above, they are duly assisted by their parent or guardian. The provisions of the Choice on Termination of Pregnancy Act 92 of 1996 apply when children seek a termination of pregnancy.

The parent, guardian or caregiver of a child may consent to medical treatment of the child if the child is:
- under the age of 12 years or
- over the age of 12 years but is of insufficient maturity or is unable to understand the benefits, risks and social implications of the treatment.

Parents or guardians may consent to a surgical operation on the child if the child is:
- under the age of 12 years or
- over 12 years old but is of insufficient maturity or is unable to understand the benefits, risks and social implications of the operation.

The superintendent of a hospital, or the person in charge of the hospital may consent to the medical treatment of, or a surgical operation on, a child. Such consent may be given if:
- the treatment or operation is necessary to preserve the life of the child or to save the child from serious or lasting physical injury or disability
- the need for the treatment or operation is so urgent that it cannot be deferred for the purpose of obtaining the consent that would otherwise have been required.

The Minister may consent to the medical treatment of or surgical operation on a child who is unable legally to consent if a parent or guardian:
- unreasonably refuses to give consent or to assist the child in giving consent
- is incapable of giving consent or of assisting the child in giving consent
- cannot readily be traced or
- is deceased.

The Minister may also consent to the medical treatment of or surgical operation on a child if the child unreasonably refuses to give consent.

In all cases, the High Court as the upper guardian of all minors may give consent if nobody else can be found. Applications for such consent in urgent cases can be made at very short notice after office hours or on weekends to the duty judge at their home.

Consent in terms of the Mental Health Care Act

The Mental Health Care Act 17 of 2002 provides that if a registered medical practitioner deems an MHCU incapable of giving informed consent, then a curator, spouse, parent, child over the age of 18, adult brother or sister, partner or associate may consent to the treatment or operation. Informed consent must be obtained in accordance with the current statutory requirements.

The head of the health establishment may consent to the treatment or operation if:
- none of the persons mentioned above is available and attempts at locating them have been unsuccessful, and this is confirmed in writing
- the head of the health establishment is satisfied that the most appropriate intervention is to be performed, after discussion on the alternatives available
- the treatment or operation is recommended by the medical practitioner who will perform it.

Special consent provisions for termination of pregnancy and sterilisation

In terms of The Choice on Termination of Pregnancy Act 92 of 1996, different situations apply and these are outlined in the following section.

Termination of pregnancy – abortion

The Choice on Termination of Pregnancy Act provides that a termination of pregnancy (an abortion) may only take place with the informed consent of the pregnant woman. In cases where a woman is severely mentally disabled to such an extent that she is completely incapable of understanding and appreciating the nature or consequences of a termination of her pregnancy, her pregnancy may be terminated upon the request of, and with the consent of, her natural guardian, spouse or legal guardian. If such a person cannot be found, then the request and consent of her *curator personae* (a person appointed by the High Court to make decisions for her) will suffice. In addition, the consent of two medical practitioners, or a medical practitioner and a registered midwife who has completed the prescribed training course, is required.

The pregnancy may only be terminated within the first 12 weeks of the gestation period, or from the 13th up to and including the 20th week of the gestation period if a medical practitioner, after consultation with the pregnant woman, is of the opinion that:
- the continued pregnancy would pose a risk of injury to the woman's physical or mental health or
- there exists a substantial risk that the foetus would suffer from a severe physical or mental abnormality or
- the pregnancy resulted from rape or incest or
- the continued pregnancy would significantly affect the social or economic circumstances of the woman.

At any time during the pregnancy of such a woman, two medical practitioners, or a medical practitioner and a registered midwife who has completed the prescribed training course, may consent to the termination of her pregnancy after consulting her natural guardian, spouse, legal guardian or *curator personae*. After the 20th week of pregnancy, they may only do so if they are of the opinion that the continued pregnancy would pose a risk of injury to her health or life or there exists a substantial risk that the foetus would suffer injury or from a severe physical or mental abnormality. The termination of the pregnancy shall not be denied if the natural guardian, spouse, legal guardian or *curator personae* refuses to consent to it.

In the first 12 weeks of the gestation period, the termination may be performed by a registered midwife who has completed the prescribed training course. Thereafter, it may only be performed by a medical practitioner.

Sterilisation

In terms of the Sterilisation Act 44 of 1998, for sterilisation to be performed on any person who is incapable of consenting, or incompetent to consent, a request must be made to the person in charge of the hospital by, and with the consent of, the parent, spouse, guardian or curator of such person. The person in charge of the hospital must, upon the request, convene a panel which will consist of a psychiatrist (or a medical practitioner if no psychiatrist is available), a psychologist or a social worker, and a nurse. The panel must consider all relevant information, including that the person is 18 years of age (unless the physical health of the person is threatened), and that there is no other safe and effective method of contraception except sterilisation. The sterilisation may only be performed if the panel approves the request.

The patients must be mentally disabled to such an extent that they are incapable of:
- making their own decision about contraception or sterilisation
- developing mentally to a sufficient degree to make an informed judgement about contraception or sterilisation
- fulfilling the parental responsibility associated with giving birth.

Unfair discrimination

The Mental Health Care Act expressly outlaws unfair discrimination of MHCUs on the grounds of their mental health status. It also entitles every MHCU to standards of care, treatment and rehabilitation equivalent to those applicable to any other health care user.

Exploitation and abuse

Every health care provider or health establishment must ensure that MHCUs are protected from exploitation, abuse and any degrading treatment; are not subjected to forced labour; and that care, treatment and rehabilitation services are not used as punishment or for the convenience of other people. The Mental Health Care Act places a duty on any person, including a psychiatric nurse, who witnesses the abuse of an MHCU, to report it to the relevant review board by completing the MHCA02 form. (The form is to be found as an annexure to the Mental Health Care Regulations of 2003).

Alternatively, they may lay a charge with the South African Police Services who will investigate the matter and take appropriate action. Thereafter, the person laying the charge must notify the review board of the charge in writing.

Caution

Mental health care providers must be particularly careful to ensure that they follow the provisions of the Mental Health Care Act and its regulations when dealing with MHCUs who are subjected to mechanical restraints, seclusion or electroconvulsive treatment. This is to ensure that MHCUs are not abused.

Nurses as advocates for their patients should ensure that the proper procedures are always followed as 'superior orders' is no defence if the subordinate knows that what is being done is wrong and unlawful – even if ordered to do so by a superior official or doctor. In such cases the nurse should report the matter to their line manager and refuse to engage in unlawful conduct.

Mechanical restraints

The Mental Health Care Act defines 'mechanical means of restraint' as 'any instrument whereby the movement of the body or any of the limbs of a user are restrained or impeded' (Regulation 1). According to Regulation 31 (1), mechanical means of restraint may not be used during the transfer of a MHCU or within a health establishment unless psychological or other means of calming, physical means of restraint or seclusion are inadequate to ensure that the MHCU does not harm themselves or others. Regulation 36 (2) states that any mechanical means of restraint in order to administer pharmacological treatment must only be used for as short a period as is necessary. And in terms of Regulation 36 (3), while an MHCU is under restraint, they must be subject to observation as prescribed by the psychiatrist or registered medical practitioner and such observations should be recorded in the clinical notes. A register must be kept of mechanical means of restraint and must be signed and completed by the relevant registered medical practitioner. Furthermore, Regulation 36 (4) states that the form of mechanical restraint, the time period used, the times when the MHCU was observed and the reason for administering such means of restraint must be outlined by the psychiatrist or registered medical practitioner in the register. Regulations 36 (5) and 36 (6) state that reports on mechanical means of restraint must be sent quarterly to the review board on the MHCA48 form and that mechanical means of restraint may not be used as punishment.

Seclusion

Regulation 37 (1) defines 'seclusion' as the isolation of an MHCU in a space where their freedom is restricted. Seclusion may only be used to contain severely disturbed behaviour, which is likely to cause harm to MCHUs themselves, others or property, and may not be used as punishment. According to Regulation 37 (2), while a user is secluded, they must be subjected to observation as prescribed by the psychiatrist or a registered medical practitioner and such observation must be recorded in the clinical notes.

According to Regulation 37 (3), the time period that the MHCU needs to be secluded and the reason for the seclusion must be outlined and must be recorded in the relevant register by the registered medical practitioner, and daily reports must be given to the head of the health establishment. Regulation 37 (4) states that reports on the seclusion must be sent to the review board quarterly on Form MCHCA 48.

Electroconvulsive treatment

Regulation 33 (1) states that electroconvulsive treatment must be conducted by a psychiatrist or a registered medical practitioner with special training in mental health and may only be carried out under a general anaesthetic together with a muscle relaxant. In terms of Regulation 33 (2), no MHCU may have more than one electroconvulsive treatment carried out in a 24-hour period and such treatment may not be administered more frequently than on alternative days.

Regulation 33 (3) provides that the head of the provincial department must consent to electroconvulsive treatment in a health establishment under the auspices of the state or a private health establishment. According to Regulation 33 (4), a health establishment that wishes to perform electroconvulsive treatment must apply in writing and shall be authorised by the provincial head of department concerned.

Regulation 33 (5) states that whenever electroconvulsive treatment is performed, a register kept for such purpose must be signed and completed by the relevant psychiatrist or registered medical practitioner and a transcript of the register must be submitted by the health department concerned to the review board on a quarterly basis in the MHCA 47 form in the annexure to give effect to section 19(1)(b) of the Act. Section 19(1)(b) deals with the powers and functions of the review board including the consideration and monitoring of decisions about the treatment of mentally ill patients.

Determinations concerning mental health status

A determination concerning the mental health status of any person must be based on factors exclusively relevant to that person's mental health status, or for the purposes of giving effect to the Criminal Procedure Act 51 of 1977, and not on the basis of a person's socio-political or economic status, or cultural or religious background or affinity. Evidence may only be presented in court that is directly relevant to the mental health status of an accused person in order to determine an accused's fitness to stand trial, or capacity to have formed an intent to commit a crime. For instance, prosecutors may not lead evidence on what accused persons sent for observation said about how they committed the crime to the psychiatrist or psychologist who examined them. Such prosecutors may only lead evidence about whether such accused persons are fit to stand trial or had the criminal capacity to commit the crime – not how they committed it.

Disclosure of information

It is illegal and unethical for mental health care providers to disclose any information that they are obliged to keep confidential in terms of any other law, for example, the National Health Act. Our courts have recognised that the special relationship of trust and confidence between mental health care providers and MHCUs is essential to ensure the effective provision of care, treatment and rehabilitation services. Patient confidentiality, however, is not absolute and may be breached in the circumstances mentioned below.

Situations where MHCUs are a danger to themselves or others

The head of the national or a provincial Department of Health, or the head of a health establishment, may disclose such information if failure to do so would seriously prejudice the health of the MHCU or of other people. Additionally, the mental health care provider may also temporarily deny MHCUs access to information contained in their health records, if disclosure of such information is likely to seriously prejudice such users, or result in the users conducting themselves in a manner that may seriously prejudice them or the health of other people.

Situations where there is a statutory duty to report

In certain instances, there is a statutory duty on the mental health care provider to disclose information about the MHCU – otherwise such provider is legally required to keep such information confidential. The Children's Amendment Act 41 of 2007 places a statutory duty on nurses who reasonably conclude a child has been abused or neglected, to report such abuse or neglect to a child protection agency or the provincial Department of Social Development. Additionally, the Criminal Law (Sexual Offences and Related Matters) Amendment Act 32 of 2007 obliges any person with knowledge or a reasonable belief that a sexual offence has been committed against a child or mentally disabled person, to report such knowledge or reasonable belief to a police official immediately. A failure by a psychiatric nurse to disclose such information will result in the imposition of a fine or imprisonment.

Giving evidence in court

When psychiatric evidence is essential to the administration of justice, the courts have permitted its use notwithstanding the right to confidentiality of the MHCU. Psychiatric nurses may be called to give evidence regarding the mental health status of the MHCU:
- in proceedings for the hospitalisation of a patient in a mental institution
- where the patient puts their mental condition in issue as part of a claim or defence
- where an accused is committed to an institution for forensic observation
- where it is necessary to establish the mental capacity of a person who has made a contested will

- in child custody suits, where the court is satisfied it is in the best interests of the child and justice for the evidence of psychiatric treatment to be led.

In terms of the Children's Act, a children's court, for the purposes of deciding a matter before it or any issue in the matter, may order, if necessary, that certain officials, including psychiatric nurses, carry out an investigation to establish the circumstances of:
- the child
- the parents or a parent of the child
- a person who has parental responsibilities and rights in respect of the child
- a caregiver of the child
- the person under whose control the child is
- any other relevant person.

Psychiatric nurses may further be required by the court to present the findings of such investigations to the court, by testifying before the court or submitting a written report to the court.

Limitation on intimate adult relationships

The head of a health establishment, subject to the conditions applicable to the provision of services in health establishments, may limit the intimate relationships of adult MHCUs only if, due to mental illness, the ability of the user to consent to these relationships is diminished. It is unethical and illegal for mental health care providers to enter into intimate adult relationships with MHCUs.

Right to representation

An MHCU is entitled to a representative, including a legal representative, when:
- submitting an application
- lodging an appeal
- appearing before a magistrate, judge or review board, subject to the laws governing rights of appearances at a court of law.

An indigent MHCU is entitled to state-funded legal aid in respect of any proceeding instituted or conducted in terms of the Mental Health Care Act, subject to any conditions fixed by Legal Aid South Africa Board in terms of the Legal Aid South Africa Act 39 of 2014.

Discharge reports

The head of a health establishment must issue a discharge report to the user who was admitted for the purposes of receiving care, treatment and rehabilitation upon their discharge, by way of the MHCA03 form.

Personal property

The Mental Health Care Act outlines the procedure for dealing with the property of mentally ill persons, or persons with severe or profound intellectual disability. Upon application, the Master of the High Court may appoint an administrator to care for and administer the property of a mentally incompetent person. The application must be made in writing, by a person over the age of 18, under oath or solemn affirmation, and must include proof that a copy of the application has been submitted to the person who is the subject of the application attached. The application must:

- set out the relationship of the applicant to that person. If not related, the reason why the spouse or next-of-kin did not make the application must be set out as well. If the relatives were not available to make the application, the applicant must set out the steps taken to establish their whereabouts before making the application
- include all available mental health-related medical certificates or reports relevant to the mental health status of the person and their capacity to manage their property
- set out the grounds on which the applicant believes that the person is incapable of managing their property
- state that the applicant had seen the person within seven days immediately before submitting the application
- state the particulars of the person and their estimated property value and annual income
- state the particulars and contact details of persons who may provide further information on the mental health status of the person who is the subject of the application.

Under certain circumstances, the Master of the High Court may appoint an administrator immediately or appoint an interim administrator if the case requires investigation. The Master must, in writing, advise the applicant and person who is the subject of the application of their decision with reasons. If the application fails, the decision of the Master can be appealed against, and, if successful, an order of the High Court can be obtained declaring the person to be incapable of managing their property, and that an administrator is to be appointed in respect of such affairs.

Knowledge of rights

Every health care provider must, before administering any care, treatment and rehabilitation services, inform the MHCU in an appropriate manner of their rights, unless they have been admitted under the emergency circumstances as provided for in the Act.

Types of facilities available

The following types of facilities are available for MHCUs:
- *Psychiatric hospitals.* Health establishments that provide care, treatment and rehabilitation services only for users with mental illnesses.
- *Care and rehabilitation centres.* Health establishments that provide for the care, treatment and rehabilitation of people with intellectual disabilities.
- *Home visits:* Mental health care providers may visit homes and places of employment, within their area of operation, of people deemed to be mentally ill or intellectually disabled, if such a home visit is required for the care, treatment and rehabilitation of the MHCU.
- *Community care.* The regulations to the Mental Health Care Act make provision for community programmes and health establishments run by, among others, organs of state, volunteer groups and non-profit organisations. Services that may be provided by these organisations include medical care, counselling, support groups and other services which would assist the recovery of the MHCU to optimal functioning. Care must be taken to ensure that such establishments are properly accredited and regulated to prevent a reoccurrence of the Esidimeni tragedy (see the section 'Rights to life, dignity and access to health care services').

All health establishments must provide the MHCU with the appropriate level of care, treatment and rehabilitation required by their professional scope of practice. If the services required by the MHCU falls outside the health establishment's professional scope of practice, the health establishment concerned must refer the MHCU to a health establishment that provides the appropriate level of care, treatment and rehabilitation needed.

A health establishment may not cause an MHCU to receive psychiatric medication for more than six months, unless authorised by a mental health care practitioner who is designated to provide medication and review psychiatric treatment.

Mental health care providers and health establishments must provide their services in a manner that facilitates community care of MHCUs.

Mental health review boards

The Act provides for the establishment of mental health review boards to oversee health establishments providing mental health care, treatment and rehabilitation services in a province. The Member of the Executive Council responsible for health services in that province must appoint three to five South African citizens to sit on the review board, who must include a mental health care practitioner, a magistrate, attorney or advocate, and a member of the community concerned.

The review board is given the task, among other duties, of:
- considering appeals against decisions of the head of a health establishment
- making decisions with regard to assisted or involuntary MHCUs

considering periodic reports on the mental health status of MHCUs (section 19(1)). The review board may, when performing its function, consult or obtain representations from any person or body with expertise (section 19(2)).

Types of MHCUs

There are different types of MHCUs, including voluntary, assisted and involuntary MHCUs; emergency MHCUs and state patients.

Voluntary MHCUs

A 'voluntary' MHCU is a person who understands and consents to the provision of appropriate care, treatment and rehabilitation services by the health establishment. In terms of the Children's Act, minors over the age of 12 years old who are of sufficient maturity and mental capacity to give informed consent to medical treatment may do so. In the case of voluntary health care users, the MHCU makes the application for admission to a mental health establishment, while the discharge is effected by the mental health care provider.

Assisted MHCUs

An 'assisted' MHCU is a person who is incapable of making an informed decision because of their mental health status and who does not refuse the health interventions.

Admission procedure
A written application for care, treatment and rehabilitation services must be made to the head of the health establishment concerned by way of the MHCA04 form. The spouse, next-of-kin, partner, associate, parent or guardian of the MHCU may only make the application provided they have seen the user within seven days before making the application. However, if the user is below the age of 18 years old on the date of the application, the application must be made by the parent or guardian of the user. The application may only be made by a health care provider if the spouse, next-of-kin, partner, associate, parent or guardian of the user is unwilling, incapable or not available to make the application.

Where a health care provider makes the application, they must state:
- the reasons why they are making the application
- what steps were taken to locate the relatives of the user in order to determine their capability or availability to make the application
- the grounds on which they believe that care, treatment and rehabilitation services are required
- the date, time and place where the user was last seen by them within seven days before the application is made.

On receipt of the application, the head of the health establishment must cause the MHCU to be examined by two mental health care practitioners. The mental health care practitioners concerned must not be the persons making the application, and at least one must be qualified to conduct physical examinations. The practitioners must submit their written findings on the completed examination to the head of the health establishment by way of the MHCA05 form. The report must state whether there is a reasonable belief that the MHCU is suffering from a mental illness or severe or profound mental disability, and requires care, treatment and rehabilitation services for their health or safety, or for the health and safety of other people. It must also include a determination on whether the MHCU is incapable of making an informed decision on the need for care, treatment and rehabilitation services, and whether the user should receive the assisted services on an inpatient or outpatient basis.

If the findings of the two medical practitioners differ, the head of the health establishment must cause the MHCU to be examined by another mental health care practitioner. The head of the health establishment may only approve the application if the findings of two medical practitioners concur that the conditions for assisted care, treatment and rehabilitation exist. They must give notice of their decision to the applicant by way of the MHCA07 form, and within seven days send a copy of the application to the relevant review board for confirmation of their decision.

The review board must within 30 days of receipt of the application documents, investigate the incapacity of the MHCU to make a decision, and the circumstances under which the user is receiving care, treatment and rehabilitation services. They will then report on their findings to the head of the relevant provincial department and request the head of the health establishment to continue the provision of services, or to discharge the user according to accepted clinical practice.

Periodic review of assisted MHCUs
The head of the health establishment must request a psychiatrist or registered medical practitioner to review the mental health status of the assisted MHCU by six months from the commencement of care, treatment and rehabilitation services. A mental health care practitioner must then conduct a second review 12 months after the first one. The mental health status of the assisted MHCU must then be reviewed every 12 months thereafter, provided that every alternate review is conducted by a psychiatrist or registered medical practitioner. The review must:
- state the capacity of the MHCU to express themselves on the need for care, treatment and rehabilitation services
- state whether there are other care, treatment and rehabilitation services that are less restrictive or intrusive on the right to movement, privacy and dignity of the user
- make recommendations regarding a plan for further care, treatment and rehabilitation services.

A summary of the report must be submitted to the review board, which will decide on the review. If the review board decides the assisted MHCU must be discharged, all care, treatment and rehabilitation services must be stopped according to accepted clinical practices, and the user must be discharged from the health establishment if admitted, unless the user consents to further services. The head of the health establishment must comply with the review board's decision.

Recovery of capacity of assisted MHCUs to make decisions

The head of the health establishment, at any time after approving the application, may have reason to believe from personal observation, information obtained, or representations by the user, that the MHCU has recovered the capacity to make informed decisions. The head must then enquire from the user whether the user is willing to continue with the care, treatment and rehabilitation services. If the MHCU consents to further interventions, the user becomes a voluntary MHCU. If the MHCU is unwilling to continue with the interventions, and the head of the health establishment is satisfied that the user is no longer suffering from the mental illness or disability identified by the medical practitioners upon their admission, the head must discharge the user immediately.

However, if the user is still suffering from the mental illness or disability, the head of the health establishment must, in writing, inform the applicant and the user's health care providers that they may make an application within 30 days of receipt for the involuntary care, treatment and rehabilitation of the user. If no application is made within 30 days, the user must be discharged.

Involuntary MHCUs

An 'involuntary' MHCU is a person who is incapable of making an informed decision on the need for care, treatment and rehabilitation services, and is unwilling to submit themselves for the receipt of these services. Mental health care providers may only provide involuntary MHCUs with care, treatment and rehabilitation services if there is reasonable belief that the MHCU has a mental illness. The illness must be of such a nature that the user is likely to inflict serious harm on themselves or others, or the services are necessary to protect the financial interests or reputation of the user.

Admission procedure

A written application for involuntary care, treatment and rehabilitation services must be made to the head of the health establishment concerned by way of the MHCA04 form. The spouse, next-of-kin, partner, associate, parent or guardian of the MHCU may only make the application if they have seen the user within seven days before making the application. The parent or guardian of the user must make the application, if the user is below the age of 18 years old on the date of the application. A health care provider may only make an application if the spouse, next-of-kin, partner, associate, parent or guardian of the user is unwilling, incapable or not available to make the application.

Where a health care provider makes the application, they must state:
- the reasons why they are making the application
- what steps were taken to locate the relatives of the user in order to determine their capability or availability to make the application

- the grounds on which they believe that care, treatment and rehabilitation services are required
- the date, time and place where the user was last seen by them within seven days before the application is made.

On receipt of the application, the head of the health establishment must cause the MHCU to be examined by two mental health care practitioners. The mental health care practitioners concerned must not be the persons making the application, and at least one must be qualified to conduct physical examinations. The practitioners must submit their written findings on the completed examination to the head of the health establishment in the MHCA05 form. The report must state whether there is a reasonable belief that the MHCU has a mental illness of such a nature that the user is likely to inflict serious harm on themselves or others, or the services are necessary to protect the financial interests or reputation of the user. It must also include a determination on whether the mental health user is incapable of making an informed decision on the need for care, treatment and rehabilitation services, and whether the user must receive these services.

If the findings of the two medical practitioners differ, the head of the health establishment must cause the MHCU to be examined by another mental health care practitioner. The head of the health establishment may only approve the application if the findings of two medical practitioners concur that the conditions for assisted care, treatment and rehabilitation exist. They must give notice of their decision to the applicant in the MHCA07 form.

If the head of the health establishment approves the application, the head must admit the MHCU to the health establishment or refer the user to a health establishment with the appropriate facilities, within 48 hours of the approval. The head of the health establishment must then request a registered medical practitioner and another mental health practitioner to assess the physical and mental health status of the user for a period for 72 hours. The practitioners must also consider whether involuntary care, treatment and rehabilitation should continue, and whether these services should be provided on an inpatient or outpatient basis. The practitioners must submit their findings to the head of the health establishment in the MHCA06 form within 12 hours after the expiry of the 24-hour period.

The mental health establishment must discharge the user immediately if the mental health status of the user does not warrant involuntary mental health services, unless the user consents to the continuation of care, treatment and rehabilitation. The head of the health establishment must discharge the mental health user if the head is of the opinion that the user requires involuntary mental health services on an outpatient basis. In such cases, the establishment must discharge the user subject to their complying with the prescribed conditions of their outpatient care, treatment and rehabilitation. The head of the mental health establishment must thereafter inform the review board in the MHCA09 form.

If the user requires involuntary mental health services on an inpatient basis, the head of the health establishment must, within seven days of the expiry of the 72-hour period, submit a written request for such in the MHCA08 form to the review board for approval. If a psychiatric hospital admits a mental health user, such hospital must keep, care for, treat and rehabilitate the user. If a health establishment which is not a psychiatric hospital admits the user, the user must be transferred to a psychiatric hospital for their care, treatment and rehabilitation pending the review board's decision.

Periodic review of involuntary MHCUs
The head of the health establishment must cause the mental health status of the involuntary MHCU to be reviewed by a psychiatrist or registered medical practitioner sixth months from the commencement of care, treatment and rehabilitation services, and a second review must be undertaken 12 months after the first one by a mental health care practitioner. The mental health status of the user must then be reviewed every 12 months thereafter, provided that every alternate review is conducted by a psychiatrist or registered medical practitioner. The review must:
- state the capacity of the MHCU to express themselves on the need for care, treatment and rehabilitation services
- state whether the MHCU is likely to inflict serious harm on themselves or other people
- state whether there are other care, treatment and rehabilitation services that are less restrictive or intrusive on the rights to movement, privacy and dignity of the user
- make recommendations regarding a plan for further care, treatment and rehabilitation services.

A summary of the report must be submitted to the review board, which will decide on the review. If the review board decides that the involuntary MHCU must be discharged, all care, treatment and rehabilitation services must be stopped according to accepted clinical practices, and the user must be discharged from the health establishment if admitted, unless the user consents to further services. The Registrar of the High Court must be notified in writing of such a discharge. The head of the health establishment must comply with the review board's decision.

Emergency MHCUs
Care, treatment and rehabilitation services may be provided without the consent of users if, due to mental illness, any delay in providing these services or admission may result in: (a) death or irreversible harm to the health of the users; (b) the users inflicting serious harm to themselves or others; or (c) the users causing serious damage to or loss of property belonging to themselves or others. The health care provider or health establishment who assesses the user must submit a report to the relevant review board using the MHCA01 form. If the user does not consent to care, treatment or rehabilitation within 24 hours after the assessment is conducted, the user must be discharged unless an application for involuntary provision of services is made.

State patients
State patients are MHCUs designated as such by a court directive issued in terms of section 77(6)(a)(i) and section 78(6)(b)(i)(aa) of the Criminal Procedure Act 51 of 1977. According to these sections, a judge is required to order an accused charged with committing an offence involving serious violence, who is incapable of understanding the proceedings, to be admitted to a psychiatric hospital pending a judge's decision. Additionally, if the court finds that an accused committed an offence involving serious violence, but due to mental illness or intellectual disability at the time of committing the act cannot be held criminally responsible, the court must order the accused to be admitted to a psychiatric hospital.

Admission procedure
When a court issues an order such as those detailed above, the registrar or clerk of the court must send a copy of the relevant official *curator ad litem* (a person appointed by the High Court to bring or defend legal action on behalf of the mentally ill person). The head of the detention centre must then send a copy of the order to the head of the national Department of Health within 14 days, requesting that the state patient be transferred to a designated health establishment. The head of the national Department of Health must determine an appropriate health establishment for the state patient and ensure arrangements are made to effect the transfer in the MHCA23 form. The head must then notify the *curator ad litem* and the head of the detention centre, who must within 14 days of receipt of such notice, ensure the state patient is transferred to the specified health establishment.

Leave of absence
The head of a health establishment may, in writing, grant leave of absence to a state patient from the designated health establishment, in the MHCA27 form. The written notice of leave must state the commencement and return date of the state patient to the health establishment, and the terms and conditions to be complied with during their period of leave, which cannot exceed six months at a time. The notice must be submitted to the head of the national Department of Health.

The head of the health establishment may, at any time during the period of leave, direct that the state patient return to the health establishment, if the head of the health establishment has reason to believe the state patient has not complied with the terms of leave. If a state patient fails to return on the stipulated return date, the patient will be deemed to have absconded.

Periodic review of mental health status of state patients
The head of the health establishment must cause the mental health status of the state patient to be reviewed by a psychiatrist or registered medical practitioner six months from the commencement of care, treatment and rehabilitation services, and a second review must be carried out 12 months after the first one by a mental health care practitioner. The mental health status must then be reviewed every 12 months thereafter,

provided that every alternate review is conducted by a psychiatrist or registered medical practitioner. The review must make recommendations on:
- a plan for further care, treatment and rehabilitation
- the merits of granting leave of absence
- the discharge of the state patient.

A summary of the report must be submitted to the head of the national Department of Health, the official *curator ad litem*, and the administrator, if appointed.

Discharge of state patients
The following persons may apply for the discharge of a state patient:
- the state patient
- an official *curator ad litem*
- an administrator
- the head of the health establishment at which the state patient is admitted
- the medical practitioner responsible for administering care, treatment and rehabilitation services to the state patient
- a spouse, an associate or a next-of-kin of the state patient
- any other person authorised to act on behalf of the state patient.

Written application must be made to a judge in chambers, in the MHCA30 form, if the applicant is an official *curator ad litem* or administrator, or in the MHCA29 form for other applicants. After consideration of the application, the judge may order that the state patient:
- remain a state patient
- be reclassified and dealt with as a voluntary, assisted or involuntary MHCU
- be discharged conditionally
- be discharged unconditionally.

If the judge orders the state patient to be discharged conditionally, the order must specify the terms and conditions of the discharge, and the period of the conditional discharge. The head of the health establishment from which the state patient was conditionally discharged must cause the state patient to be monitored at such health establishment. Alternatively, the head must arrange for another health establishment to monitor the state patient if the conditions require the state patient to present themselves for care, treatment and rehabilitation services. The person monitoring the state patient must submit a written report to the head of the health establishment relating to the terms and conditions of the discharge, every six months from the date of the conditional discharge, and at the end of the conditional discharge period.

If at the end of the conditional discharge period, the head of the health establishment is satisfied that the state patient has fully complied with the terms and conditions of their discharge, and their mental health status has not deteriorated, the head of the health establishment must unconditionally discharge the state patient immediately. The head must inform the state patient, the registrar and official *curator ad litem* accordingly.

If, after consideration of the periodic reports by the person monitoring the state patient, the head of the health establishment has reason to believe that the state patient has not fully complied with the terms and conditions of their discharge, or the mental health status of the state patient has deteriorated, they may apply to the registrar for an order amending or revoking the conditional discharge.

State patients themselves may apply to a judge in chambers for an amendment to the conditional discharge, or for an unconditional discharge, after six months from the date of the conditional discharge, and at no less than six months intervals at a time.

Mentally ill prisoners
Admission procedure

If it appears to the head of a prison, through personal observation or information provided, that a prisoner may be mentally ill, the head of the prison must cause the mental health of the prisoner to be enquired into by a psychiatrist. Where a psychiatrist is not readily available, a registered medical practitioner and mental health care practitioner may conduct the enquiry. A written report of their findings must be submitted to the head of the prison.

If the person conducting the enquiry believes the mental health status of the prisoner is of such a nature that appropriate care, treatment and rehabilitation services can be provided in the prison, the head of the prison must arrange for the provision of those services to the prisoner. However, if it is found that the prisoner will require the services of a health establishment designated in terms of the Mental Health Care Act to provide care, treatment and rehabilitation services to mentally ill prisoners, the head of the prison must request a magistrate to cause an enquiry to be held into the mental health status of the prisoner and whether transfer to a health establishment would be appropriate.

The magistrate must commission two health practitioners, at least one of whom must be a psychiatrist, psychologist or medical practitioner with special training in mental health, to enquire into the mental health status of the prisoner. If it is recommended that the prisoner be transferred to a health establishment, the magistrate must issue a written order to the head of the prison to arrange such transfer according to the procedure set out in the Mental Health Care Act. If it is recommended that the care, treatment and rehabilitation services in the prison are appropriate for the prisoner, the magistrate must issue a written order to the head of the prison to take the necessary steps to ensure such treatment is provided.

Periodic review of mental status of mentally ill prisoners

The head of a health establishment must cause the mental health status of a mentally ill prisoner to be reviewed by a psychiatrist or registered medical practitioner every six months from the date on which the mentally ill prisoner was received at the health establishment. The review must:
- Specify the mental health status of the mentally ill prisoner

- Set out recommendations regarding a plan for further care, treatment and rehabilitation of the mentally ill prisoner
- Set out recommendations regarding the merits of returning the mentally ill prisoner to the prison from which they were transferred.

The head of the health establishment must submit a summary of the report to the review board, relevant magistrate, administrator if appointed, and head of the relevant prison.

Recovery of mentally ill prisoners

If the head of the health establishment has reason to believe, from personal observation or through information obtained, that the mentally ill prisoner has recovered from the mental illness to such an extent that the prisoner no longer requires care, treatment and rehabilitation services, the head of the health establishment must compile an appropriate discharge report. The head must advise the head of the prison that the prisoner is ready for discharge and inform the magistrate in writing. The same procedure applies where a mentally ill prisoner has recovered to the extent that the prisoner can receive appropriate care, treatment and rehabilitation services at the prison.

Expiry of term of imprisonment

A mentally ill prisoner must be released from prison or the health establishment at which they are being detained upon expiry of the term of imprisonment to which they were sentenced. However, at least 90 days before the expiry of the term of imprisonment, application may be made to the head of the health establishment where the mentally ill prisoner is detained, for the continued care, treatment and rehabilitation of the mentally ill prisoner as an assisted or involuntary MHCU. Additionally, at least 30 days before the expiry of the term of imprisonment, application can be made to a magistrate for the continued detention of a mentally ill prisoner, pending the outcome of an application for assisted or involuntary care, treatment and rehabilitation.

Intervention by South African Police Services

Apprehension of mentally ill persons

A member of the South African Police Service (SAPS) may have reason to believe, from personal observation or from information obtained from a mental health care practitioner, that a person because of their mental illness or severe or profound intellectual disability is likely to inflict serious harm to themselves or others. The SAPS member must then apprehend the person and arrange for them to be:
- taken to an appropriate health establishment administered under the auspices of the state for assessment of their mental health status
- handed over into custody of the head of the health establishment or any other person designated by the head of the health establishment to receive such persons.

If a mental health practitioner, after the assessment, is of the view that the person apprehended is likely to inflict serious harm to themselves or others due to their mental illness or severe or profound intellectual disability, that person must be admitted for a period not exceeding 24 hours. This must be done so that application may be made for involuntary care, treatment and rehabilitation of the person. If the mental health practitioner is of the view that the person is unlikely to cause harm, or if no application is made within the 24-hour period, the person must be released immediately.

Absconding of MHCU

If an MHCU has absconded or is deemed to have absconded or if the user has to be transferred under any section of this Act, the head of the health establishment may request assistance from the SAPS to:
- locate, apprehend and return the user to the health establishment concerned or
- transfer the user in the prescribed manner.

If a state patient or mentally ill prisoner absconds, the head of the health establishment *must* notify and request assistance from the SAPS. The SAPS must comply with any request for assistance regarding an MHCU who has absconded.

When requesting assistance, the head of the health establishment must inform the SAPS of the estimated level of dangerousness of the MHCU. The MHCU may be held in custody at a police station for a period not exceeding 24 hours to effect the return or the transfer in the prescribed manner. A member of SAPS may use such constraining measures as may be necessary and proportionate in the circumstances, when apprehending a person or performing any function in terms of this Act.

If a state patient absconds, the head of the health establishment must notify the relevant registrar or clerk of the court concerned, and the official *curator ad litem*, within 14 days of notifying the SAPS. If a mentally ill prisoner absconds, the head of the health establishment must also notify the relevant magistrate and head of the relevant prison within 14 days of notifying the SAPS.

Maximum security facilities

The head of a health establishment may submit a request in writing to the relevant review board for an order for transfer of an MHCU to a health establishment with maximum security facilities if the user has:
- previously absconded or attempted to abscond
- inflicted or is likely to inflict harm on others in the health establishment.

The review board may not approve the request:
- in order to punish the MHCU concerned
- it is not satisfied that the mental health status of the user warrants a transfer to maximum security facilities.

MEDICINES AND RELATED SUBSTANCES CONTROL ACT

Medicine schedule	Where is it available and what do you need to know?	Example
Schedule 0	On the shelf at a general shop	Simple analgesics like aspirin
Schedule 1	Over the counter at a pharmacy; a sale record must be kept	Antibacterial and antifungal skin creams
Schedule 2	Over the counter at a pharmacy; a sale record must be kept	Cough and cold preparations
Schedule 3	Prescription only; available from the pharmacy dispensary – can be repeated for six months	Medicines for hypertension and diabetes
Schedule 4	Prescription only; available from the pharmacy dispensary – can be repeated for six months	Anti-infectives like antibiotics and antivirals
Schedule 5	Prescription only; available from the pharmacy dispensary – repeats stipulated	Psycho-active medicines like sedatives and anti-depressants
Schedule 6	Prescription only; available from the pharmacy dispensary	Narcotic painkillers
Schedule 7	Controlled substances	Drugs like cannabis and heroin
Schedule 8	Strictly controlled substances	Amphetamine, dexamphetamine and nabilone

PREVENTION OF AND TREATMENT FOR SUBSTANCE ABUSE ACT

The Prevention of and Treatment for Substance Abuse Act 70 of 2008 refers to 'service users' instead of 'MHCUs' as in the Mental Health Care Act. However, psychiatric nurses play a role in the treatment of these users. The Act provides that community-based services must consist of a multidisciplinary team, including a nurse or mental health practitioner registered with the relevant body. The director-general may also appoint a nurse as the manager of a public treatment centre or public halfway house.

Types of service users

Types of service users include voluntary and involuntary service users, and children.

Voluntary service users

A voluntary service user is a person who consents to and submits themselves to a treatment centre for treatment, skills development and rehabilitation services. Such a user is entitled to the appropriate services.

Application for admission of a voluntary service user may be made by:
- the voluntary service user
- any person acting on behalf of the voluntary service user
- if the voluntary service user is a child, the parent or guardian of that child.

The application must be accompanied by a social worker's report regarding the applicant's social circumstances, as well as any medical or psychiatric report that the manager of the treatment centre deems necessary.

Involuntary service users

An involuntary service user is a person admitted to a treatment centre upon being:
- Convicted of an offence and has, in addition to or in lieu of any sentence in respect of such offence, been committed to a treatment centre or community based treatment service by a court
- Committed to an inpatient treatment centre by way of a court order after such court has held an enquiry
- Transferred from a prison, child and youth care centre, alternative care or health establishment.

Application for a court order for admission of an involuntary service user can be made by a social worker, community leader or person closely associated with such a person. The applicant must submit a sworn statement is submitted to a public prosecutor by a social worker, alleging that the involuntary service user is within the area of jurisdiction of the magistrate's court to which such prosecutor is attached and is a person who is dependent on substances and:
- is a danger to himself or herself or to the immediate environment or causes a major public health risk
- in any other manner does harm to their own welfare or the welfare of their family and others
- commits a criminal act to sustain their dependence on substances.

Summons must then be served on the contemplated service user, and a magistrate will conduct an enquiry into whether the contemplated service user does require involuntary treatment and rehabilitation. The magistrate may order that the contemplated service user be admitted to a treatment centre for a period not exceeding 12 months.

Children

In terms of the Children's Act, if a court finds a child is addicted to a dependence-producing substance and is without any support to obtain treatment for such dependency, the court may order the child to be admitted to an inpatient or outpatient treatment centre.

Leave of absence and release on license

A service user may not leave the treatment centre unless they have been granted a leave of absence, are released on license or discharged. The manager of the treatment centre may grant a service user a leave of absence for such a period and subject to conditions prescribed by the manager. If the service user fails to comply with the conditions, the manager may cancel the leave and direct that he or she returns to the treatment centre. If the service user fails to return upon direction or on the stipulated return date, he or she is deemed to have absconded.

The manager of the treatment centre may also release a service user on license subject to conditions the manager may stipulate. The service user will remain under the supervision of a social worker until the license expires, is cancelled or they are discharged.

The manager of a treatment centre may revoke an involuntary service user's licence and direct that he or she returns to the treatment centre if the management structure has reason to believe that such service user:
- Is failing to comply with any of the conditions of his or her release
- Has not proved himself or herself capable of adjusting properly to community life.

If the service user fails to return to the treatment centre after being recalled, he or she is deemed to have absconded.

Service users who have absconded are dealt with in the same manner as MHCUs who have absconded in terms of the Mental Health Act, and must be brought before a magistrate for an enquiry.

CHILDREN'S ACT

In terms of the Constitution and the Children's Act 38 of 2005, the best interests of the child are of paramount importance in any matter concerning them. The Act also provides that in any matter concerning a child with a disability, including a mental disability, due consideration must be given to:
- Providing the child with parental care, family care or special care as and when appropriate
- Making it possible for the child to participate in social, cultural, religious and educational activities, recognising the special needs that the child may have
- Providing the child with conditions that ensure dignity, promote self-reliance and facilitate active participation in the community
- Providing the child and the child's caregiver with the necessary support services.

As previously mentioned, if a health practitioner, such as a nurse, reasonably concludes that a child has been abused or neglected, they must report such abuse or neglect to a child protection agency or provincial Department of Social Development.

CONCLUSION

South African law is comprehensive in its protection and regulation of mental health care, but mental health care providers, including mental health nurses dealing with MHCUs, must properly apply the law for its objectives to be achieved. To this end, such mental health care providers are required to function according to the law, and to keep up to date with any new developments, amendments and regulations as part of their continuing professional development.

WEB RESOURCES

As resources, all the policies, Acts and regulations discussed in this chapter may be accessed at www.gov.za

REFERENCES

McQuoid-Mason, D. 2018. 'Esidimeni deaths: Can the former MEC for health and public health officials escape liability for the deaths of the mental health patients on the basis of obedience to "superior orders" or because the officials under them were negligent?' *South African Journal of Bioethics and Law,* 11(1): 5–7.

List of Acts referred to in this chapter
Children's Act 38 of 2005
Children's Amendment Act 41 of 2007
Choice on Termination of Pregnancy Act 92 of 1996
Criminal Law (Sexual Offences and Related Matters) Amendment Act 32 of 2007
Criminal Procedure Act 51 of 1977, as amended
Health Professions Act 56 of 1974, as amended
Legal Aid South Africa Act 39 of 2014
Medicines and Related Substances Control Act 101 of 1965, as amended
Mental Health Care Act 17 of 2002
National Health Act 61 of 2003
Nursing Act 33 of 2005
Prevention of and Treatment for Substance Abuse Act 70 of 2008
Sterilisation Act 44 of 1998, as amended

CHAPTER 7

Ethical Dilemmas in Mental Health Nursing

L van Rhyn

> **Learning Outcomes**
>
> After studying this chapter, you should be able to:
> - have an understanding of the different ethical theories
> - apply a specific theory to an ethical dilemma
> - describe virtue ethics
> - discuss relational ethics
> - differentiate between the ethical principles
> - describe the structure of an ethical dilemma
> - integrate into your practice the ethical problems relevant to psychiatric nursing
> - implement cultural sensitivity in the management of ethical issues
> - understand the ethics of research.

INTRODUCTION

Not all dilemmas in life are ethical – an ethical dilemma occurs when moral claims about what is right and wrong come into conflict. An ethical dilemma may be defined as:
- a problem for which there is apparently no satisfactory solution or
- a situation in which a choice must be made between two equally unsatisfactory alternatives.

Questions such as the following arise: 'What ought I to do?' 'What are the advantages and disadvantages of this decision or action?' 'To whom does it apply?' An example of an ethical dilemma can be observed in a situation in which something considered to be 'good' is not necessarily 'right'. Conflict arises between two moral values – virtue and duty.

Ethical dilemmas arise out of health care situations where the answers to questions about which actions are 'right' or 'wrong' are often unclear. Ethical dilemmas exist at the nurse/patient/family level of interaction, in the hospital as well as in the community, and also at the policy-making level of institutions and communities.

Ethics incorporates choices and conflict relating to health care problems, for instance a long lifespan versus freedom from pain; full versus partial disclosure of information; the rights of individuals versus the rights of the community.

An example of an ethical dilemma is as follows: Shaun is a 25-year-old man who has suffered from schizophrenia for the past six years. He was hospitalised for five years but has been treated as an outpatient for the past year. He has been prescribed with antipsychotic medication twice a day. He lives with his parents and goes to the sheltered workshop (where he functions well) every day from 8:00 to 12:00. In the afternoons he works at home at his hobby of making wooden toys, which he sells. Sometimes he goes to town with his mother; she does not work. He has a girlfriend with whom he spends some evenings and weekends. He has no other friends.

For the past month Shaun has been causing problems: he has withdrawn from his parents and girlfriend and no longer wants to go to the sheltered workshop. Some days he does not want to get out of bed. His personal hygiene has deteriorated and when his mother remonstrates with him, vehement arguments ensue. He talks to himself at times. He has also lost interest in his hobby. His parents suspect that he has stopped taking his medication, although he assures them that he does take it. His mother takes him to the outpatient department for a follow-up examination, where a decision must be taken about readmitting him. Shaun is opposed to admission and his parents are uncertain, as they feel that it will be detrimental to his rehabilitation, but they find it difficult to cope with his present behaviour.

The dilemma is whether Shaun should be admitted against his will, or whether his parents' view should be ignored or considered and Shaun kept at home. This is a difficult question for many reasons and it is this kind of problem that is classified as an ethical dilemma. In essence, the ethical dilemma is whose rights/needs should be ignored or considered by the mental health team to decide whether Shaun should be admitted or not. He does not want to be admitted but the question is whether he is capable in his current mental health state to decide for himself.

ETHICAL THEORIES

Ethical theories and reasoning do not solve ethical dilemmas. However, they do suggest ways in which questions may be structured in order to make a decision. Each ethical theory judges the actions and the rules on which the actions are based.

Utilitarianism

Utilitarianism is sometimes seen as a form of teleological ethics, which studies the purpose of things. Utilitarianism focuses on the consequences of actions – on what can bring the greatest amount of happiness or the least harm to the largest number of people. It is, therefore, concerned with the end-product of actions. It is a community-oriented theory in which all people are seen as equal. Consequences for future generations, as well as for other living individuals and groups, are taken into account.

Utilitarianism can be either act-utilitarianism or rule-utilitarianism. In other words, the 'rightness' of an act or the 'rightness' of a rule is judged by the consequences brought about by the act or the rule. Pera and Van Tonder (2011: 42) argue that the trouble with either form of utilitarianism is that it makes an action good only because of its consequences and ignores the role that motives or intentions might play. Two additional problems with utilitarianism are that it is difficult to assess the levels of happiness likely to be yielded by either individual action or general rules and that the happiness of the greater number may in fact involve the unhappiness of the minority.

Egoism

People with an egotistical approach search for solutions that will be to their own benefit. An egotistical solution decided upon by a nurse need not necessarily be to the advantage of the mental health care user (MHCU), since the MHCU is not the primary concern. Nurses with this standpoint will make decisions that are the most advantageous to themselves and will not consider the MHCUs, their families or anyone else.

Professional nurses who function from an egotistical framework will select environments where, for example, they do not have to attend to MHCUs with human immunodeficiency virus (HIV)/acquired immunodeficiency syndrome (AIDS) or other infectious diseases, since that may endanger themselves. This kind of approach has no place in nursing.

Deontology

Deontology believes that both the action itself and the relevant principles and rules that are being applied are important. Examples of rules or principles are: never lie; never do to others what you do not want done to yourself. The philosopher Kant's formulation of the principle of universality states that one must act in terms of a specific basic principle only if it can be applied in all other similar situations. According to Kant, it is duty, as prescribed by a rule or principle that determines the moral value of an action. If you have done what the rule prescribes, you have acted morally or ethically.

This means that people are not subject to the will of others, but are subject only to their own will on condition that it is rational and respects the law (rules or principles). Kant considers autonomy, freedom, dignity, self-respect and respect for individual rights to be important value principles.

Act-deontologists are committed to the principle of universality. There are no criteria, standards or guiding principles. One simply gathers all the facts and then makes a decision. An act is 'right' simply by virtue of its being chosen and by the commitment to universality. Rule-deontologists hold that standards of right or wrong consist of specific rules such as keeping promises and never telling a lie.

The Christian approach

The fundamental convictions of the biblical faith of Christianity are the beliefs in creation, the fall of humankind, redemption and fulfilment. Within this framework, Christians 'read' their situation. For Christianity the highest purpose in life is that the kingship of God be proclaimed over every sphere of creation. Christianity stresses that order in society depends on obedience to the normative structures of creation ordained by God for marriage, the family, the state and the church. Human beings are created in the image of God, and in Christianity the focus is predominantly on normative obedience to God and the duties that emanate from this. Christianity has much in common with other monotheistic religions (Judaism and Islam) and much of what is said about Christianity is also true of the approach of these religions.

The essential feature of the Christian approach is love. The term 'love' has little to do with a sentimental feeling. Love is an attitude rather than a feeling. Love is respect for people, taking people to heart and treating them as people. When one understands that the opposite of love is not hate but indifference, the true meaning of love in ethics becomes clear. Love applies to the total person in all their relationships. (For instance, MHCUs should not be regarded as total entities in themselves only – their families should be included.)

Every major religion has an ethical system, and adherents to each faith are therefore influenced by the ethics of their religion. It is important for the nurse to explore the religious beliefs of MHCUs and their families, since it will facilitate understanding of their different ethical perspectives. They may be influenced strongly by the ethics supported by their religious beliefs.

Virtue ethics

Virtue ethics, sometimes called character ethics, represents the idea that individuals' actions are based upon a certain degree of innate moral value. Aristotle suggests that although people have different character traits, all have the capacity to learn or cultivate those that are important to morality.

Virtues refer to excellence in character. Virtues are an integral part of one's identity. Where moral obligations are external to the person and are imposed on the person, virtues are intrinsic to the individual. Virtue ethics addresses the sort of person somebody should be, namely a moral person and not the duties of an individual.

There are four focal virtues that are more pivotal than others in characterising a virtuous person, namely:
1. *Compassion.* Compassion is the ability to imagine oneself in the situation of another. It is furthermore an emotional response of deep tenderness and a desire to relieve the pain and suffering of others. It is so important to realise that many times the patient's need for a compassionate and caring presence outweighs the need for technical care. Nurses need to be careful, however, that compassion does not impede their ability to make objective decisions.
2. *Discernment.* The virtue of discernment is related to the concept of wisdom. It gives us insight into appropriate actions in given situations. Discernment requires sensitivity and attention attuned to the demands of a particular context. For example, a discerning nurse will recognise when an MHCU needs comfort and reassurance rather than privacy.
3. *Trustworthiness.* Trust forms the basis of successful and effective health care relationships. The trusting relationship between a nurse and an MHCU serves as the

core for ethical decision making (Pera & Van Tonder, 2011: 114). In practical terms, trustworthiness is accounted for in the reputation they have among co-workers.
4. *Integrity.* Integrity is perhaps the cardinal virtue. It means 'soundness', 'reliability', 'wholeness and integration of moral character'. It also refers to our continuing to follow moral norms over time. Integrity is compromised when the nurse acts inconsistently or in a way that is not supported by professed moral beliefs.

Ubuntu

Although Ubuntu is not an ethical theory, it provides, within the African context, a broad philosophical stance on which African ethics of virtue could be founded. Ubuntu is an African worldview on life. It represents the collective consciousness of the people of Africa and consequently provides the base from which to derive virtues. Some of the virtues that are fundamental to Ubuntu are respect, dignity, compassion, empathy, care, solidarity, consideration, patience and kindness.

Relational ethics

According to Bergum and Dosseter (2005), health care ethics is grounded in relationships between:
- care providers and patients
- patients and their families
- theorists and practitioners
- nurses themselves
- nurses and the other members of the team.

Although the context of these relationships varies, they are nurtured and sustained by their reliance on dialogue and mutual concern. It is the relationship itself that supports and informs ethical reflection and decision making.

As a practice, relational ethics looks at the way people relate to one another in various roles, namely how they relate as health care practitioner, MHCU, team member, teacher, student and friend. Such a focus attends to both who one is, as well as what one does, as ethical actions are put into practice, moment by moment.

ETHICAL PRINCIPLES IN NURSING AND HEALTH CARE
Autonomy

Autonomy expresses respect for the unconditional worth of an individual and respect for individual thought and action. In the case of individual adults an autonomous person is someone who is capable of making a rational and informed decision on their own behalf, but it does not mean that they have the right to do whatever they want or to disobey laws and regulations.

Respect for autonomy is binding on all health professionals and should be adhered to unless it is overridden by another moral principle of greater weight or standing. It may not always be possible to allow MHCUs such as the mentally disabled or psychotic persons to make their own choices. The obligation to prevent harm to others or to benefit the MHCU is perceived as having greater weight than the obligation to respect autonomy.

In some rural African communities and religious groups, individuals might not be regarded as autonomous and the research needs to respect this traditional practice without disregarding the human rights of potential participants.

Beneficence

This principle requires nurses to act in ways that benefit MHCUs and has three major components:
1. do or promote good
2. prevent harm
3. remove evil or harm.

Nurses operate under the principle of beneficence whenever they help MHCUs who cannot decide for themselves or who are incapacitated or incompetent. Protecting MHCUs from harming themselves because of thoughts, feelings or behaviours that lead to self-harm is done in a spirit of beneficence.

Non-maleficence

The principle of non-maleficence is related to beneficence. The principle requires nurses to act in such a manner as to avoid causing harm to MHCUs. Included in this principle are deliberate harm, risk of harm and harm that occurs during the performance of beneficial acts. It also means avoiding harm as a consequence of doing good. In such cases the harm must be weighed against the expected benefit. For example, sticking a needle into a child for the purpose of causing pain is always bad – there is no benefit. Giving an immunisation, on the other hand, while causing similar pain, results in benefit; that of protecting the child from serious disease.

Veracity

The term veracity relates to the practice of telling the truth. Truthfulness is widely accepted as a universal virtue. Nursing literature promotes honesty as a virtue and truth telling as an important function of nurses. Ethicists disagree about the absolute necessity of truth telling in all instances. The question is whether the truth is sometimes harmful. It may also be questioned whether it is acceptable to deceive a patient in order to prevent unnecessary suffering.

Truth telling engenders respect, open communication, trust and shared responsibility. It is promoted in all professional codes of nursing ethics.

Confidentiality

Confidentiality is the ethical principle that requires non-disclosure of private or personal information with which one is entrusted. Confidentiality is the only facet of patient care mentioned in the Nightingale pledge. The ability to maintain privacy in one's life is an expression of autonomy. The capacity to choose what others know about us, particularly intimate personal details, is important because it enables us to maintain dignity and preserve a measure of control over our own lives. Thus, maintaining confidentiality of patients is an expression of respect of persons and, in many ways, is essential to the nurse–patient relationship.

A dilemma that sometimes confronts health professionals is that they may find themselves in the position where they have made two contradictory promises: to protect confidential information and to obey the law that requires reporting. For example, the Children's Act requires that child abuse be reported. The health professional could, however, be convinced that reporting the abuse would hamper the parents' willingness to accept treatment. The professional could believe that they have a duty to the client rather than the society and could be convinced that it would be immoral and harmful to report the case.

One viewpoint is that health care professionals have a 'right' to break confidences in some circumstances, but they do not have a 'duty' to do so. According to Botma et al (2010: 18) it is a breach of confidentiality when information is willingly or unintentionally shared with an unauthorised person. There are, however, clear legal duties to divulge confidential information when necessary, such as reporting gunshot wounds, contagious diseases and child abuse.

Confidentiality has been complicated by technological advances in record keeping and the storage and reproduction of material (photocopying, computer storage, CDs and DVDs). The situation can become even worse if all the team members do not handle confidential information in the same manner. Patients' notes are usually available to all the members of the multidisciplinary team and to students of the various disciplines. There are questions around what type of information an individual team member should share with the rest of the team and when it should be shared. A further issue is how carefully sensitive information is handled within the multidisciplinary team.

Justice

Justice relates to fair, equitable and appropriate treatment in light of what is due or owed to persons, recognising that giving to some will deny receipt to others who might otherwise have received these things. Within the context of health care ethics, the relevant application of the principle focuses on distribution of goods and services. It is impossible for all people to have everything they might want or need. One of the primary purposes of governing systems is to formulate and enforce policies that deal with fair and equitable distribution of scarce resources.

There are three basic areas of health care that are relevant to questions of distributive justice. First, what percentage of our resources should reasonably be spent on health care? Secondly, recognising that health care resources are limited, which aspects of health care should receive the most resources? Thirdly, which MHCUs should have access to the limited health care staff, equipment and so forth?

In making decisions of distributive justice, one must ask the question, 'Who is entitled to these goods and services?' Some of the ways that people have historically made these decisions are:
- to each equally
- to each according to need
- to each according to merit
- to each according to social contribution
- to each according to the person's rights
- to each according to individual effort
- to each as you would be done by
- to each according to the greatest good to the greatest number (Brink et al, 2012).

Nurses seldom make such decisions as individuals. They may be involved in making such decisions in teams, for instance when developing a policy. They might also become involved in challenging policies which do not adhere to the principle of distributive justice.

Fidelity

The ethical principle of fidelity is often related to the concept of faithfulness and the practice of keeping promises. On another level, the principle of fidelity relates to loyalty within the nurse–patient relationship. Though fidelity is the cornerstone of a trusting nurse–patient relationship, most ethicists think there are no absolute, exceptionless duties to keep promises – that, in every case, harmful consequences of the promised action should be weighed against the benefits of keeping the promise.

Fidelity is also a value that extends to the team or the service within which the nurse works. Without loyalty to one's team members and one's employer, the trust, which is essential for good service delivery, might be undermined.

THE STRUCTURE OF AN ETHICAL DILEMMA

When one is confronted by an ethical dilemma, it is useful to analyse the dilemma by looking at three elements: situational facts, decision-making questions, and underlying ethical theories. The facts are always evaluated within the value system of the nurse (and others involved) and within the time available to make the decision.

The personal and professional value systems of the decision makers and those who will be affected by the decision are based on these three elements. For instance, one person may believe that death is the worst thing that can happen to anyone, while someone else in the same situation may consider a handicapped life to be the worst alternative should there be a choice. Other values that could be important to nurses are obedience to a professional code and the patient's own choice.

Time is another dimension in the clarification of dilemmas. Some dilemmas demand immediate action. If more time is available, there is a better opportunity for evaluating information and considering and discussing alternatives with those involved.

Situational facts

The following questions should be asked in order to establish a database to guide decision making:
- Who are the people involved? What is the nature of their involvement?
- What is the proposed action; what is the action about which a decision has to be made?
- What is the context of the proposed action?
- What is the purpose of the proposed action?
- What other alternatives or choices are available?
- What are the possible implications or consequences of the proposed action for all concerned?

The application of these questions is illustrated in the following example.

Example 1: Individual level application and analysis

Aletta is a 16-year-old girl with a slight intellectual disability. She lives with her parents. She has an IQ of 65 and was, at first, in a special class in a normal school, but she made no progress and now attends a training centre for people with intellectual disabilities, where she is doing very well. She is well groomed and at first glance looks like any other teenager. At home she does household tasks and is generally responsible and thorough in the performance of her duties. Her parents have no problems with her and she socialises well with two girlfriends. Aletta has been menstruating for the past two years and her parents are worried that she might fall pregnant. They have spoken to her about this, but she does not appear to understand very well. She would like to marry and have children and does not realise the concomitant implications and responsibilities. She requires help with hygiene during her periods.

Her parents are considering a hysterectomy and have consulted you for guidance.
- In this case, the parents, Aletta, a mental health nurse, and the gynaecologist should be involved in making a decision.
- The proposed action is a hysterectomy.
- The context is a girl of 16 who is well adapted and socialised and living in a stable home environment. She has normal life expectations and lacks insight into her limitations.
- The objectives of the action are to ensure that Aletta does not have a baby for whom she cannot take responsibility, and to stop her menstruating, which is difficult for her to manage.
- Other alternatives are:
  - putting her on a depo-contraceptive which will prevent pregnancy and menstruation
  - teaching her the necessary skills which will enable her to handle menstruation and to deal responsibly with sexual needs (Müller et al, 2016).

- The possible implications of the proposed action include all the dangers involved in major surgery; anger and distrust from Aletta; and irresponsible sexual behaviour, since she will still lack understanding.

All these factors should be taken into account and any decisions that are made must be tested against the ethical principles discussed earlier.

Decision-making facts

Although information is an essential component in the consideration of an ethical dilemma, decisions cannot be made purely on the grounds of information. Some guidelines for decision making are:
- Who is to make the decision – the doctor, the nurse, the patient, the family or a committee? Why?
- For whom is the decision to be taken? Is it for oneself, or for others?
- What criteria should be used – social, legal, judicial, physiological, economic, psychological or others? Why?
- What degree of consent must be obtained from the patient – free, forced or none?
- Which moral principle, if any, will be reinforced or denied by the proposed action – self-determination, love, justice or autonomy? (Newcombe, 2010).

Ethical principles

The last task in the structuring of an ethical dilemma is to begin reasoning about ethical theories or positions in order to examine alternatives. The limitations of a specific theory must always be considered in such reasoning. In this section, an example is explored.

Example 2: Systems-level application and analysis: Esidimeni event

What happened?
In October 2015 the Member of the Executive Council (MEC) for Health in Gauteng announced the termination of the contract between the Department of Health and Life Esidimeni. Around 2 000 people, who were receiving highly specialised chronic psychiatric care, were to be removed out of Life Esidimeni to families, non-governmental organisations (NGOs) and psychiatric hospitals providing acute care. From March to June 2016 mental healthcare users were discharged from Life Esidimeni in large numbers. Not one of the NGOs had a legal licence.

A total of 144 patients died of cold, hunger, dehydration and general lack of care (Dhai, 2018).

Why were patients moved?
The two reasons given by government for the move were to save money and to deinstitutionalise patients into the community. Neither reason held up (Child, 2017).

The removal of people led to many patients ending up in hospital, which was about five times more costly per patient per day. The Gauteng Department of Health was warned by the National Department of Health and psychiatrists that deinstitutionalisation could only take place with appropriate preparations.

→

This incident shocked the whole of South Africa and it was devastating to see and hear on the media how these patients were treated. Let us try to analyse some of the ethical principles which were involved during this tragedy.

Ethics principles involved
At least three principles are involved.
1. Justice
   Justice has to do with equality and fairness. In the milieu of health care, justice is the process in which individuals are treated fairly and equally resulting in the highest standard of physical, mental and social well-being. The Health Ombudsman who presided over the hearings relating to the Esidimeni event found that the NGOs could not even provide basic health care to patients who required highly specialised chronic psychiatric care. Additionally, the investigation found that in the process of moving patients, and in the aftermath thereof, several human rights were violated – specifically the rights to health, life and dignity resulting in a great injustice to society's most vulnerable group (Ferlito & Dhai, 2017).
   Justice also concerns democracy and the distribution of power. The application of justice in the health care sector by the state must lead to a better society but this was not evident in the events around the Life Esidimeni tragedy. Recipients of health care have specific rights with regard to its delivery, and these rights (life, health and dignity) are interlinked with principles of ethics (autonomy, informed consent, beneficence and non-maleficence). The state therefore has an obligation to ensure that its actions will always be for the benefit of society and that it will steer away from activities that could harm society.
2. Autonomy
   Autonomy is described as a rudimentary ethical principle in health care. It is the right of individuals to make choices about their own health issues. Individuals also have the right to be involved in the decision-making process pertaining to their health care. The concept of *informed consent* is closely linked to autonomy. Patients have the right to be informed about their treatment and care, and the right to give consent before any treatment can begin. However, autonomy and persons with mental illness pose a moral challenge. These individuals do not always have the cognitive ability to make sound judgements regarding their health and are therefore sometimes impaired with regard to the consent process. Even in these cases, however, patients should still be included as far as possible in the decision-making process.
   The notion of autonomy is also promulgated by law. Section 12(2) of the Constitution, the Mental Health Care Act 17 of 2002 (Chapter 3) and the National Health Act 61 of 2003 (Chapter 2) deal with autonomy and informed consent. Family members had the legal authority to provide consent on behalf of the patients at Life Esidimeni. This included giving consent for patients to be transferred – but they were not involved in this decision (Ferlito & Dhai, 2018).
3. Beneficence and non-maleficence
   Beneficence requires that the patient's interests be put first – that is balancing benefits (interests) against risk and cost. Non-maleficence means to do no harm.
   The character of beneficence rests on three values, namely *preventing* the infliction of unnecessary pain, *preventing* mortality and *preventing* the incapacitation of others. In the case of non-maleficence, the three values are *do not* kill, *do not* cause unnecessary pain and *do not* incapacitate others. Clearly all these six values were infringed in the Life Esidimeni tragedy. The patients and their families suffered unnecessary and preventable pain. There was utter disrespect for their dignity and welfare (Khaas, 2018).

SPECIFIC ETHICAL PROBLEMS IN PSYCHIATRIC NURSING

According to Burston and Tuckett (2013) nurses working with long-term mentally ill people in the community may experience moral stress. Moral stress usually occurs when one knows the right thing to do, but institutional or environmental constraints makes it nearly impossible to pursue the right course of action. This is a kind of ethical problem most nurses will find very familiar. It happens in many situations and presents differently in each case. However, there are also a few widely recognised issues in mental health care which are common enough to demand attention.

Stigmatisation

The list of stereotypes associated with psychiatric diagnostic categories is well known. Equally familiar are the consequences to people with these diagnoses. People labelled as drug addicts, psychotics, paranoids, 'crazies', 'schizos' and so on acquire a discredited social identity because of the character flaws often associated with these labels. To many people in the community, the labels used to stigmatise MHCUs suggest that they are dangerous, immoral, and that they disregard society's values. It is important to consider how and when psychiatric nurses, while advocating humane treatment for MHCUs, indirectly contribute to discrediting an MHCU social identity by participating in the arbitrary use of oppressive labels.

The ethical dilemmas created by stigmatisation are many. For instance, the nurse might want to keep secret the fact that the MHCU has had a psychiatric problem, while at the same time exacerbating the stigma by indicating through this behaviour that it is something that needs to be kept secret, because it is shameful. The nurse might want to support the MHCU in getting a job but may be conflicted about not disclosing the psychiatric history, thereby making it impossible to offer on-the-job support, which could increase the chances of successful vocational rehabilitation.

Involuntary admission

According to the Mental Health Care Act, one of the ways a person can be admitted to a psychiatric hospital is through involuntary admission.

Competent patients have the right to decide whether to accept or reject proposed nursing care, hospitalisation or treatment. Patients thought to be incompetent are denied this right (Appelbaum & Grisso, 1988: 1635; Dastidar & Odden, 2011: 8). According to Appelbaum and Grisso, the following factors must be considered when deciding whether a patient is competent to make an informed decision:
- the ability of the MHCU in communicating the choices to be made
- the ability of the MHCU in understanding relevant information, such as the difference between types of admission (the ability to understand what is communicated to them)
- the ability of the MHCU to appreciate the situation and its consequences.

While a person sometimes understands the words, they might not be able to understand implications and consequences. This has to be particularly tested in an interview, by eliciting the MHCU's conception of the illness, the need for and consequences of treatment, and the motives of others who are involved. The MHCU must be able to manipulate information rationally, using logical processes to compare benefits and risks.

Without an adequate assessment of competence, the MHCU's rights in treatment options can easily be overlooked.

Clinicians are sometimes accused of depriving patients of their freedom. The question, however, is, 'Which freedom?' Are the freedom of movement and of association the most important freedoms? These freedoms may be taken away only if the MHCU no longer experiences personal freedom. What they do not have cannot be taken away. What they are deprived of is taken away precisely for the sake of their personal development, which has been impaired by a particular condition. However, it is often difficult to decide which patients no longer have personal freedom or integrity of personality and therefore qualify for compulsory treatment.

There are different philosophical points of view about forced admission. The issue at stake is the individual's ability to take responsible decisions and the risk to self and others is questioned. The fact that judgement is clouded by disease is recognised by psychiatrists worldwide. In practice, however, the forecasting of danger to the patient and others creates serious problems. Such a decision is both a professional one (to decide what the possible risk is) and an ethical one (to decide whose rights are going to be put at risk, those of the community or those of the individual).

The implications of being involuntarily admitted are manifold. Involuntary MHCUs are admitted to a psychiatric hospital against their will, they are treated without their consent, they cannot manage their own financial affairs or sign contracts and they forfeit state pensions. The severe curtailment of the patients' basic human rights demands that doctors and nurses exercise their powers in this regard with the utmost care. Patients' rights should be given back to them as soon as possible. The more dependent patients are, the greater the responsibility of caregivers to treat them with respect (Janse van Rensburg, 2014).

Chapter 30 of the Mental Health Care Act deals with the rights and obligations of MHCUs. Two other aspects of the Act that protect involuntary patients' rights are:
1. seventy-two-hour assessment and subsequent provision of further involuntary care, treatment and rehabilitation in the case of an application for involuntary care
2. mental health review boards.

(Refer to Chapter 6 on Legal Structures in Mental Health Nursing.)

Electroconvulsive treatment
Electroconvulsive therapy (ECT) is used to good effect in cases of severe depression, puerperal psychosis, schizophrenia (especially the catatonic type) and hypomania that is resistant to medication. In South Africa, more MHCUs in the private sector than in the public sector receive ECT and not all provinces offer this treatment. The ECT utilisation rate in South Africa is similar to that of countries like India and Poland but

less than that of some higher income countries (Benson-Martin, 2015). The treatment entails the administration of an electric shock to the brain of 70–130 volts for 0.1–1.0 seconds. It is performed under general anaesthetic and the only side effect is transient loss of memory of recent events. The amnesia may become permanent if the treatment is repeated too often, but such misuse is rare because South Africa follows internal guidelines for administration.

This method of treatment is considered by some people to be dehumanising. Criticism of this treatment is mainly due to misrepresentations and ignorance. It is at present regarded as the last expedient in a treatment regimen after other forms of therapy have proved to be ineffective.

Informed consent must be sought for ECT. The procedure must be explained to the MHCU and their family, and written consent must be obtained from either the MHCU or their family once it has been ensured that they understand the purpose, nature and implications of the treatment.

Drugs that alter consciousness

Pharmacological agents are often used in psychiatric practice to:
- normalise a negative mood (for example, antidepressants)
- calm an anxious person or promote sounder sleep (for example, sedatives and narcotics)
- suppress psychotic symptoms (for example, neuroleptics).

Criticism of these drugs in professional circles relates to the hazards of addiction, the treatment of symptoms rather than the disease itself, and the suppression of the patient's personality.

The use of certain narcotics and sedatives may lead to drug dependency. Drug dependency is a condition of physical and psychological dependence on a substance that may lead to withdrawal symptoms if the substance is withheld. More and more of the substance must be taken to obtain the desired effect. Drug dependency has a negative effect on physical and psychological health and on normative behaviour.

Tranquilisers, sedatives and neuroleptics suppress feelings and thoughts, as well as consciousness of reality, and therefore the user's personality. These drugs are, of course, taken specifically because they suppress certain negative feelings and thoughts.

People with an intellectual disability

People with an intellectual disability are often admitted to care and rehabilitation centres for life. In such cases, the chronic restriction of freedom may lead to the dehumanisation of the patients. This in turn results in phenomena such as regression, aggression and inappropriate sexual behaviour.

Dehumanisation often takes the form of denial of the basic rights of people with an intellectual disability. These rights are:

- The right to live as normal a life as possible, for example the right to relationships, holidays, a normal routine for every day or week and recognition of personal events such as birthdays
- The right to privacy
- The right to be treated as a unique individual with one's own needs
- The right to be treated with dignity
- The right to utilise opportunities to develop one's potential (Roos, 2016).

The South African Schools Act 84 of 1996 governs the education of intellectually disabled children and endeavours to provide inclusive education for such children. This is seldom possible for the more profoundly affected children. Such children are the most vulnerable in terms of the protection of their human rights, especially the right to an environment that is of reasonable quality.

Setting professional boundaries

One of the issues with which nurses sometimes have problems is the setting of boundaries for their own involvement with MHCUs. In psychiatric nursing, nurses work with the same MHCU over long periods of time, getting to know them very well and very intimately.

Furthermore, many of them need social contact, and value their relationships with the nurse very highly. In these conditions it may not be surprising that nurses sometimes overstep the boundaries of a professional relationship to one that is more social, personal and even sexual. The following professional guidelines are important in ensuring that nurses act in the interest of the MHCU, and do not allow their own needs to intrude in a professional situation. It is a violation of professional boundaries for a nurse to:
- date or become a roommate of a current MHCU
- date or become a roommate of a former MHCU when met in a professional situation
- share personal information with an MHCU or discuss personal problems with a patient
- keep secrets of the MHCU from the treatment team
- share personal pictures of self with an MHCU
- use information obtained as a nurse to contact an MHCU to pursue a social relationship
- give to or receive gifts from an MHCU
- smuggle restricted items (for example, potentially addictive substances and medication) to an MHCU in a residential setting
- take photographs of an MHCU or their home or living quarters using a mobile phone.

It is the nurse's responsibility to set limits for all their professional relationships. To prevent such problems, it is important that nurses outline the boundaries of the nurse–MHCU relationship overtly for MHCUs and for themselves. This makes it less likely that the boundaries will be threatened in future. However, if a nurse is in a situation where they are having trouble keeping within professional boundaries with a specific patient, it is important that this be discussed with a trusted supervisor or colleague. Nurses are all human, and feelings are sometimes difficult to control. However, crossing these boundaries reflects badly on the nurse, and may be detrimental to the MHCU and the nursing profession.

PATIENT RIGHTS

Although the Department of Health has published a Patient Rights' Charter (Department of Health, 2003), it does not refer specifically to people with a mental illness or disability. The rights and duties relating to MHCUs can be seen in Chapter 3 of the South African Mental Health Care Act. In 1989 the World Federation for Mental Health (WFMH) published a *Declaration of Human Rights and Mental Health*. This document emphasises the place of mental health in achieving basic human rights. It also states that 'the fundamental rights of persons who are labelled, or diagnosed, treated or defined as mentally or emotionally ill or distressed, shall be the same as those of all other citizens' (WFMH, 1989). It then goes on to list a wide-ranging set of rights. This group is not the only one to address the rights of persons with mental illness. Amnesty International and the World Health Organisation (WHO) have produced similar documents. In South Africa the guidelines given in the South African Mental Health Care Act are used to protect the rights of MHCUs.

Eight Batho Pele principles (Local Government Action, 1997) were developed in South Africa to serve as acceptable policy and legislative framework regarding service delivery in the public service, which includes psychiatric hospitals. These principles are aligned with the constitutional ideals of:
- promoting and maintaining high standards of professional ethics
- providing service impartially, fairly, equitably and without bias
- utilising resources efficiently and effectively
- responding to people's needs
- rendering an accountable, transparent and development-oriented public administration.

The principles of Batho Pele are:
- consultation
- setting service standards
- increasing access
- ensuring courtesy
- providing information
- openness and transparency
- redress
- value for money (Local Government Action, 1997).

Right to treatment in the least restrictive setting

The idea of least restrictive setting or least restrictive alternatives has become an important component of both the deinstitutionalisation and patient rights movements. The term 'least restrictive setting' generally refers to the placement of patients in the therapeutic setting that will provide care while allowing maximum freedom. It also means providing for the least amount of limitation or interference in an individual's thoughts and decision making, physical activity and sense of self as necessary to provide for safety.

This principle of caring for the psychiatric MHCU in the least restrictive environment possible, is enshrined in the mental health legislation of many countries. It demands that a person is not kept in a psychiatric hospital when a general hospital admission is feasible; that they are not kept for five days when three days is possible, and that they are not admitted involuntarily if another alternative is possible.

A least restrictive setting for a person with a cognitive disorder might not be a psychiatric hospital but a frail care unit in a retirement centre. However, such facilities might be in short supply, making placement decisions more difficult.

Right to refuse medication

The right of the individual to refuse treatment is acknowledged by the National Health Act 61 of 2003, section 6(1)(d). An MHCU may refuse medication for many reasons. Symptoms such as delusions and denial may cause the refusal. An MHCU who refuses medication is often sicker than those who comply. Nurses should judge each situation on an individual basis. Criteria that may justify coerced treatment are as follows:

- The MHCU must be judged to be dangerous to self or others (Osafo et al, 2012).
- It must be believed by those administering treatment that the treatment has a reasonable chance of benefiting the MHCU.
- The MHCU must be judged to be incompetent to evaluate the necessity of the treatment.

Even if these three conditions are met, the MHCU should not be deceived but should be informed regarding what will be done, the reasons for it and its probable effects.

The rights of children and adolescents

In South Africa a person under the age of 18 years is seen as a minor (Children's Act 38 of 2005). As a minor, the person is considered legally incompetent. Children may therefore be admitted to a psychiatric hospital involuntarily or by the process of assisted admission. When the user is below the age of 18 years old on the date of the application, the application must be made by the parent or guardian of the user (see Chapter 5, Section 27 of the Mental Health Care Act). Fortunately, the psychiatric treatment of the majority of children in South Africa happens outside psychiatric hospitals, namely in outpatient clinics, day care centres and private practice. Even in these situations minors often do not decide by themselves to go for psychiatric help. Mostly schools, parents or members of a multiprofessional team will refer the child and the adolescent for help. An example is a social worker who will refer a child who comes from chaotic home conditions and suffers from a substance-related disorder.

The nurse's relationship regarding the child's rights includes using interventions that protect the child, supporting the family's decision-making ability while supporting the child's best interests and ensuring that the child is treated fairly. Although minors may not legally refuse treatment, a method by which the therapist/nurse can acknowledge a minor's need to have control is the ethical means of asking the child/adolescent for informal assent or agreement to treatment. Information regarding treatment should be given to children on a level they can understand. Giving minors the opportunity for assent and choices when possible provides empowerment and results in fewer power struggles between the nursing staff and the patient. This sets the stage for positive relationships with the therapist by providing the child with an opportunity to develop decision-making skills and may result in increasing their openness to treatment.

Adolescents may be developmentally able to give consent and, if interested, should be given an opportunity to sign a consent form along with the parent or guardian.

CULTURE-SENSITIVE CARE

The nursing profession has to provide care that is meaningful and sensitive to the needs of patients of all cultures. It is important that mental health nurses:
- recognise their own cultural orientation
- understand the importance of the MHCU's perspective
- develop communication skills in order to analyse the MHCU's perspective
- identify issues which influence the provision of care to people of different cultures.

ETHICS REVIEW BOARDS AND COMMITTEES

The submission of a research proposal for review by a committee or board is a policy that protects researchers and research participants. The members of the committee will consider every aspect of the proposed research, including the ethical aspects. Permission may be granted or refused to carry out the research or recommendations regarding specific changes to the research proposal by the committee members if they are not satisfied that it is in accordance with the established scientific and ethical guidelines.

Research ethics

The primary aim of research into health-related issues, namely the improvement of the quality of life of individuals and groups, situates research within the realm of the ethical: doing what is good and right. The ethical component of a research project constitutes the caring component of that research. Divided loyalty can exist between obligation towards science and the persons involved as 'subjects'. This situation is aggravated in cases where the researchers and participants were previously (or are currently) involved in a close, though professional, and therapeutic relationship.

Certain research interventions, such as experimental drug testing and interviews on sensitive issues, create vulnerability in participants. If this is not handled in an ethical manner, it not only endangers the patient and the professional integrity of the researcher, but may actually undermine the scientific integrity of research results (Amugune & Verster, 2016).

Both vulnerability and potential for exploitation increase when autonomy is diminished, as in the case of children, intellectually disabled persons, persons diagnosed with mental health problems, psychiatrically ill patients or patients dependent for treatment on the researchers. Vulnerable communities are characterised by one or more of the following:
- limited economic independence
- inadequate protection of human rights
- belonging to a group that is stigmatised or discriminated against
- inadequate understanding of scientific research
- limited availability of health care and treatment options
- impaired ability of individuals in the community to provide informed consent (Cleary et al, 2016).

In seeking ethical approval and informed consent for a research project, participants should be fully informed about the following aspects:
- purpose of the research
- methodology
- duration of the study
- nature of the participation expected
- the way in which the results will be used and disseminated
- the identity of the researcher(s) and fieldworkers
- possible side effects and detrimental aspects
- risk–benefit ratio
- the manner in which confidentiality and privacy will be secured
- financial implications – whether or not participants will be remunerated (Jacobs & Van Jaarsveldt, 2016).

The scientific integrity and competence of the researcher is of utmost importance.

CONCLUSION

The modification of a person's behaviour, whether it be psychotic, socially unacceptable, overdependent or destructive, is inherent in the interventions of psychiatric nurses, but when is behaviour 'sick'? Who determines the criteria for mentally ill behaviour? What are these criteria? According to whose standards – those of the patient, the therapist, the community – are decisions made to change behaviour? What factors play a role in the causation of this behaviour? Are these factors considered when the behaviour is altered?

The alteration of behaviour is not necessarily immoral in itself, but many ethical questions, which nurses dare not ignore, arise in the process.

WEB RESOURCES

http://www.health.gov.za/ OR http://www.health24.com
> Department of Health, South Africa (2003). The Patients' Rights Charter is given on this site. The policy guidelines regarding the 72-hour assessment of involuntary patients can also be found on this website.

http://hdl.handle.net/10755/243553
> One can learn about moral distress in a visually attractive and practical way.

unpan1.un.org, 24.07.2012 > The Health Research Policy in South Africa

https://www.ukessays.com/essays/nursing/legal-and-ethical-issues-in-mentalhealth nursing-nursing-essay.php?vref=1. A case study to learn how to critically appraise an ethical dilemma

https://wfmh.global > WFMH declaration on mental well-being and human rights

REFERENCES

For Acts, see South Africa

Appelbaum, P S and Grisso, T. 1988. 'Assessing patients' capacities to consent to treatment'. *The New England Journal of Medicine,* 319 (25): 1635–1638.

Amugune, B K and Verster, G C. 2016. Knowledge and attitude of postgraduate students in Kenya on ethics in mental health research. *South African Journal of Bioethics & Law,* 9 (2): 65–68.

Benson-Martin, J J and Milligan, P D. 2015. 'A Survey of the Practice of Electroconvulsive Therapy in South Africa'. *The Journal of ECT,* 31 (4): 253–7.

Bergum, V and Dossetor, J. 2005. *Relational Ethics: The Full Meaning of Respect*. Maryland: University Publishing Group.

Botma, Y, Greeff, M, Maluadzi, F M and Wright, S C D. 2010. *Research in Health Sciences*. Cape Town: Heinemann.

Brink, H, Van der Walt, C and Van Rensburg, G. 2012. *Fundamentals of Research Methodology for Healthcare Professionals*. Cape Town: Juta.

Burston, A S and Tuckett, A G. 2013. 'Moral distress in nursing; contributing factors, outcomes and interventions'. *Nursing Ethics,* 20 (3): 312–324

Child, C. 2017. 'Why did Esidimeni happen?'. *Sunday Times,* 9 October 2017.

Cleary, M, Siegfried, N, Walter, Escott, P and Walter, G. 2016. 'Super research or super-researched?: When enough is enough'. *Issues in mental health Nursing,* 37 (5): 380–382.

Dastidar, J G and Odden, A. 2011. 'How do I determine if my patient has decision-making capacity?'. *The Hospitalist*, August: (8).

Department of Health, 2003. 'Patients' Rights Charter'. http://www.health.gov.za (Accessed 15 June 2019).

Dhai, A. 2018. 'The Life Esidimeni tragedy: Moral pathology and an ethical crisis'. *The South African Medical Journal,* 108 (5): 382–385.

Ferlito, B A and Dhai, A. 2017. 'The Life Esidimeni tragedy: A human-rights perspective'. *The South African journal of Bioethics & Law,* 10 (2): 52–55.

Ferlito, B M and Dhai, A. 2018. 'The Life Esidimeni tragedy: Some ethical transgressions'. *South African medical Journal,* 108 (3): Editorial.

Jacobs, A C and Van Jaarsveldt, D E. 2016. 'The character rests heavily within me: Drama students as standardized patients in mental health nursing education'. *Journal of Psychiatric and Mental Health Nursing*, 23 (3–4): 198–206.

Janse van Rensburg, A B R. 2014. 'South Africa Society for Psychiatrists guidelines for the integration of spirituality in the approach to psychiatric patients'. *South African Journal of Obstetrics & Gynaecology*, 20 (4): 133–139.

Khaas, T. 2018. 'Esidimeni tragedy was a failure of the duty of care'. *City Press,* 25 March 2018.

Local Government Action. 1997. 'The Batho Pele Principles'. http://localgovernmentaction.org.dedi6.cpt3.host-h.net/content/batho-pele-principles (Accessed 15 June 2019).

Müller, A, Röhrs, S, Hoffman-Wanderer, Y and Moult, K. 2016. '"You have to make a judgment call". Morals, judgments and the provision of quality sexual and reproductive health services for adolescents in South Africa'. *Social Science & Medicine*, 148: 71–78.

Newcombe, P. 2010. 'Evolving fairness in research on human subjects'. *Journal of Child and Adolescent Psychiatric Nursing*, 23 (3): 123–124.

Osafo, J, Knizek, B L, Akotia, C S and Hjelmeland, H. 2012. 'Attitudes of psychologists and nurses towards suicide prevention in Ghana'. *International Journal of Nursing Studies*, 49 (6): 691–700.

Pera, S and Van Tonder, S. 2011. *Ethics in Healthcare.* 3rd edition. Cape Town: Juta.

Roos, J L. 2016. 'Genetic and family counselling for schizophrenia: Where do we stand now?' *South African Journal of Psychiatry,* 22 (1). doi: 10.4102/sajpsychiatry.v22i1.831 (Accessed 10 April 2018).

South Africa. Children's Act 38 of 2005.

South Africa. Mental Health Care Act 17 of 2002.

South Africa. National Heath Act 61 of 2003.

South Africa. South African Schools Act 84 of 1996.

South Africa. The Constitution of the Republic of South Africa. Act 108 of 1996.

World Federation for Mental Health (WFMH). 1989. *Declaration of human rights and mental health.* https://wfmh.global (Accessed 15 June 2019).

CHAPTER 8

Working with Cultural Diversity in Mental Health Care

L R Uys and N Nkosi-Mafutha

Learning Outcomes

After studying this chapter, you should be able to:
- define culture, cultural competence and diversity, and explain the importance of these concepts in mental health care
- describe Giger and Davidhizar's cultural phenomena, using a familiar culture as an example
- describe how people usually respond when confronted by human diversity
- demonstrate respectful engagement when working with people from different cultures
- decide how to respond to different cultural values and behaviour when caring for a person from a different cultural group
- discuss the influence of culture on the presentation, diagnosis and treatment of mental illness.

INTRODUCTION

South Africa has a population of about 56 million people of diverse origins, cultures, languages and religions. The population consists of Nguni-speaking people (isiZulu, isiXhosa, isiNdebele, isiSwati); Sesotho-speaking people (Sepedi, Setswana and Sesotho); the Xitsonga-speaking people (VaTsonga); Tshivenda-speaking people (vaVhenda); and people who speak English and Afrikaans. Additionally, the growing numbers of asylum seekers, refugees and immigrants from anglophone, francophone and lusophone countries on the African continent contribute to South Africa's cultural diversity. Nurses and nursing students in South Africa reflect this diversity and bring their own beliefs about life and health and health care, which are shaped by their cultural backgrounds, to their daily interactions with others.

CULTURE

Culture significantly influences the way people define health, and ideas about when medical advice is needed and what an illness might be. A society's culture refers to the learned, shared and transmitted values, beliefs, norms and patterns for behaviour which are characteristic of a social group, and which guide this group's thinking, decisions and actions in patterned ways, everyday (Cai, 2016). Culture can also be viewed as an integrative pattern of human behaviours. It includes knowledge, beliefs, art, morals, laws, customs and any other habits of the group and is created by the group themselves.

Culture in the form of indigenous knowledge has mostly been transmitted verbally, and little is recorded (Cumes, 2013). Indigenous is understood in the sense of something being 'traditional' or 'vernacular' by other people of different cultures. Indigenous people practise and protect a body of knowledge and skills that encompasses meaning, belief systems, livelihoods and expressions which distinguish them from other groups. Culture is passed on through generations and is shared by all members of the same cultural group. The culture of a group is never static, but changes and transforms due to interactions with technology, the environment and other cultures (Andrews & Boyle, 2002; Allen, 2010).

The significance of culture in mental health nursing cannot be overlooked because appropriate nursing care is impossible without integrating and considering the culture of the patient and their family. Knowledge of cultures other than your own is gradually built over time, based on interest and exposure. In some settings mental health nurses are involved with clients from so many cultures that 'knowing' each culture intimately will be almost impossible. However, cultural awareness is possible. Giger and Davidhizar's (2008) Transcultural Assessment Model identifies six cultural phenomena to consider when working with people from different cultures. These might form a useful framework for cultural awareness:

1. Communication, both verbal and non-verbal
2. Time perception
3. Space perception
4. Social organisation
5. Environmental control; the ability to control the environment
6. Biological variation, including dietary preferences.

These six phenomena are explained in more detail in the following sections. African culture is used to illustrate the differences between African culture and the dominant western culture in relation to this framework.

Communication

Every culture has its own way of communicating. This involves body posture, voice quality, intonation and even humour. What is polite in one culture may be considered rude in another. Here are a few important aspects of respectful communication with African people:

- *Greetings.* From an African traditional perspective, the person who initiates the greeting plays an important role. The person of higher status (for example, the chief) greets first and the other person then responds in a respectful manner, such as with a bow. In the therapeutic relationship pertaining to the mental health care practitioner and user, the mental health care practitioner is the person of higher status and should therefore greet first.

- *Voice.* Some people will speak up even when near others in order to make it clear to anyone in the vicinity that they are not gossiping.
- *Gestures.* Certain gestures may interfere with the trust relationship between the mental health care practitioner and user – for example, holding your hands behind your back while speaking to the mental health care user (MHCU). The MHCU should be able to see the practitioner's hands, to allay certain fears that the practitioner is holding 'bewitching' medication behind their back. Negative gestures, such as pointing at someone with a finger, are perceived as disrespectful. To some, making eye contact with your elder can be a sign of disrespect.
- *Initiating.* When a person enters an office or consulting room, they may show respect by sitting down immediately without greeting (since this shows respect for the nurse as having higher status).

Time perception

In many traditional cultures, social time is more important than clock time. Social time refers to the ordering of social processes, for instance a time for prayer, a time for planning, and a time for dancing. Clock time refers to either the duration of something (a period of time such as a one-hour meeting) or a point in time (10:00). For traditional cultures, encountering another person always means 'greeting time', whether or not they have time for such a greeting in terms of clock time. This example also illustrates another characteristic of traditional time perception – it is oriented to the present rather than to the future. What is occurring at this moment is more important than a future engagement.

Space perception

Personal space refers to the proximity to others that is tolerated or preferred by the members of a culture. The African culture is collectivist, not individualist in nature, and people are used to and like close physical proximity.

Social organisation

In the African traditional way, the human being is viewed as a collective being (*umntu ngumntu ngabantu*: a person is a person through other people). A human being is seen as part of a family, which includes the extended family. A person is also seen as part of the community in which they grew up, as well as a part of the ethnic group to which they belong. Humanity is based on collectivism. *Ubuntu* (humanity in the African context), is interpreted as a collective concept of mercy, care, compassion, tolerance and fairness. *Ubuntu* is not only a value but a virtue of those who practise it.

Many African traditional cultures are vertical cultures, which means that there are clear and multiple hierarchies. For instance, not only are men higher on the hierarchy than women, but the elderly are higher than the young and certain families are higher than others. A horizontal culture is characterised by greater equality in communication and relationships.

Traditional cultures are tighter in the social control they exert over their members, with people having less personal freedom to choose their own ways of living. In traditional cultures, norms and rules must be respected. For instance, gender roles are quite strict and difficult to negotiate.

Ancestors are believed to be very influential in the African traditional worldview.

To those who believe in this practice, ancestors are also responsible for the explanation of the meaning of existence. According to this belief system the ancestors possess the capacity to continue having an influence on the fortunes of their nearest living blood relatives (Adamo, 2011). They can communicate with them, warn them against dangers and guide their steps; they act as mediators between the living and God (Adamo, 2011).

While a cultural group shares a belief system and the practices of that belief system, one can never assume that everybody in the group adheres to the total package.

Environmental control

In the model this refers to beliefs about health and illness, health practices and values. Illness in the African traditional belief system encompasses relations between God, ancestors and the universe (Mokgobi, 2014). For example, when there is misunderstanding between God and the spiritual world, a sacrifice is performed as a ritual to rekindle the relationship (Adamo, 2011). If something (illness) occurs and it cannot be explained and understood, clarity is sought and it is through the process of divination that the spiritual forces behind a calamity can be determined. A diviner is therefore consulted to determine the cause of illness and to prescribe medication for different physiological, spiritual and psychiatric conditions (Mokgobi, 2014). On being consulted, they try to find a spiritual cause for the health problem, for instance by throwing bones or by listening to the ancestors in order to prescribe a remedy.

African people may consult both western and African health care providers concurrently because their culture is essentially inclusive, allowing for different (often contradictory) beliefs to be held simultaneously (Adamo, 2011). Natural and supernatural exist in the African context and both health care systems are consulted to clarify the 'how', 'where', 'when' and 'why' of their illness. Consulting the traditional health care provider clarifies especially the 'why' and 'who' of an illness. It is therefore critical to understand cultural views in ill-health because the experience and interpretations of illness and misfortune can be culture dependent.

For African people there is often a difference between naturally occurring illness (for instance measles), and those conditions only Africans get (for example *ufufunyana* = like schizophrenia), which are viewed and understood culturally. This is because the knowledge of the traditional healer is gained experientially and not through scientific methods (Cumes, 2013). This differentiation is especially important in psychiatric care. For example, a health care provider with a western (biomedical) approach will see schizophrenia as having a chemical or biological basis while a traditional healer will look at ancestors and witchcraft as possible causes.

Biological variation

Culture is often linked to ethnicity or race. As an identifying characteristic, race is very controversial due to political and sociological uses of the word. According to Little et al (2016) ethnicity can be described as 'the idea of societal groups, marked especially by shared nationality, tribal affiliation, religious faith, shared language, or cultural and traditional origins and background' while race is concerned with biological variations. Africans share a dark skin (although the variations are great) and their biological inheritance influences their susceptibility to specific diseases. Seeing people only as members of a certain group (whites, blacks, Muslims) is a kind of tyranny, since such labels do not allow the individual to be known (Johnson & Munch, 2009).

Most people like their own culture best. However, when people believe that their own culture or ethnic group is superior to that of others and have an overriding concern about race, this is called ethnocentrism. Bennet (2013) explains that ethnocentrism is the view that one's own group is the centre of everything, and this is based on familiar standards of that specific group. The manifestation of ethnocentrism is xenophobia, the fear of outsiders.

Xenophobia can be reduced by understanding that all groups have a cultural dimension. Moreover, nurses need to promote the health and well-being of all people, including immigrants. Patients' rights and the Refugee Act 130 of 1998 (section 27(g)) make it clear that refugees have the same rights to access of basic health care services as South African citizens. During the provision of health care, the mental health nurse would need to be cognisant of the laws and ensure that the patient's rights are not violated.

The consequences of xenophobia to an individual include physical, emotional and post-traumatic stress. It is therefore the mental health nurse's responsibility to identify these effects by communicating with the client effectively (without being judgemental) and by providing care appropriately. In most cases these patients might need shelter, referral to social workers and other community resources. The nurse can also play a role in providing information on where to get help other than health services and educate people at the health facility about the impact of xenophobia on an individual.

CULTURAL COMPETENCE

Campinha-Bacote (2002: 181–184) describes cultural competence as 'the process in which the healthcare professional constantly attempts to accomplish the skill to effectively work within the cultural context of a client'. The context refers to the client's family, individual or community. Furthermore, becoming culturally competent is a process, requiring reflection and action as the mental health nurse encounters culturally diverse individuals. Reflection is essential in the provision of effective, ethical and client-centred mental health nursing care to the South African population. The goal of a culturally competent mental health nurse is to understand the experience and the uniqueness of the individual for whom they are providing care.

In the journey of becoming culturally competent, the mental health nurse needs to ask themselves the right questions as they strive for cultural competency. This can be achieved by using the Campinha-Bacote (2002) mnemonic 'ASKED', which consists of self-examination questions regarding one's awareness, skill, knowledge, encounters and desire. This involves the following dimensions:

- **A**sked: Are you aware of your own biases and prejudice towards other cultures and have you made an in-depth exploration of your own culture?
- **S**kill: Do you know how to conduct a cultural assessment in a sensitive manner?
- **K**nowledge: Do you know about the worldviews of different cultures and the field of bioecology (the relationship among different living organisms and their environment)?
- **E**ncounters: Do you have sacred encounters with people from different cultures other than yours and are you committed to resolving cross-cultural conflicts?
- **D**esires: Do you want to be culturally competent?

Standards of practice for promoting cultural competence

As there is an increased migration of nurses and of the population globally, there is a dire need for culturally competent nurses. In an effort to reduce inequities in health care, a panel of experts for global nursing and the American Academy of Nursing, together with members of the Transcultural Nursing Society, identified 12 standards of practice for promoting cultural competence that can be adopted by nurses globally (Giger et al, 2007). These 12 standards are summarised below:

1. STD 1 Social Justice: Mental health nurses should be able to promote social justice for all patients. They should be able to provide fair treatment without prejudice regarding economic status, ethnicity, race or sexual orientation, and should advocate for their clients.
2. STD 2 Critical reflection: Mental health nurses need to know their own values, beliefs, heritage and culture in order to provide culturally competent mental health nursing care. This is beyond self-awareness; the nurse examines their own belief system that can hinder mental health nursing care that involves being culturally competent.
3. STD 3 Knowledge of culture: The mental health nurse needs to gain an understanding of other people's perspectives, traditional values, practices and family systems of culturally diverse individuals. This enables the mental health nurse to be aware of variables that need to be considered while providing mental health nursing care.
4. STD 4 Culturally competent practice: Mental health nurses need to use cross-cultural knowledge and culturally sensitive skills in implementing mental health nursing care that is culturally congruent.

5. STD 5 Cultural competence in health care systems and organisations: The provision of structure and resources is the responsibility of the health care system, particularly in meeting the language requirements and unique needs of their clients.
6. STD 6 Patient advocacy and empowerment: Mental health nurses should be able to recognise the effect of the health care policies, delivery systems and resources on clients and they should empower and advocate for their clients.
7. STD 7 Multicultural workforce: The multidisciplinary teams in the health care systems should be representative of the population they serve.
8. STD 8 Education and training in culturally competent care: The education and training of nurses should promote and provide culturally congruent health care.
9. STD 9 Cross-cultural communication: It should be noted that effective communication demonstrates respect and dignity.
10. STD 10 Cross-cultural leaders: Mental health nurses need to have the ability to influence individuals, families, communities, and the population in order to achieve positive outcomes of culturally competent care.
11. STD 11: Policy development: Mental health nurses need to be empowered with skills and knowledge to work with public and private organisations, professional associations and communities to establish standards for the comprehensive implementation and evaluation of culturally competent care.
12. STD 12 Evidence-based practice and research: Mental health nurse researchers should investigate and test interventions that may be most effective in alleviating inequalities in health outcomes.

It is important to note that cultural competence is the provision of respectful, sensitive and meaningful care to individuals, families and communities of diverse cultures, leading to better welfare abilities to face outcomes of illness (Gebru & Willman, 2010).

DIVERSITY AND CULTURAL DIVERSITY

Diversity concerns the ability to identify and respect other people's uniqueness for the benefit of the MHCU, family, and the community. Diversity can be viewed as a range of group members' characteristics and demographic features, such as age, gender, race, nationality, professional background and expertise. Diversity is also evident in health teams and the mental health nurse therefore needs to be able to work with MHCUs and co-workers to achieve quality mental health care outcomes. Diversity awareness recognises the importance of continuous effort in identifying differences within and among cultural groups (Jeffreys, 2008). Diversity self-awareness occurs as a mental health nurse is able to recognise how differences or similarities influence patient care as well as teamwork (Jeffreys, 2008).

One of the ways in which the mental health nurse can recognise cultural diversity is through asking the MHCU about the supplementary medication (herbs/traditional) that they use for the same illness about which they are consulting. This will make the MHCU feel respected as an individual. Another example of how mental health nurses may show respect for cultural diversity is by asking MHCUs on admission about their dietary preferences specifically related to their culture or religion.

The issues of diversity awareness and self-awareness are important regarding co-workers. For example, using any language other than English (which is mostly used in the South African health care system) when handing over patients' reports could lead to poor patient outcome and poor teamwork. Furthermore, knowing and respecting one another's cultures is crucial.

Misunderstandings could occur without this knowledge. For example, a young professional nurse who comes from a cultural background where they do not look an elder in the eye could be found to be dishonest by a mental health nurse from a different culture where a person is expected to look directly into the eyes when communicating.

In mental health, cultural diversity is critical as the interpretation of what is known to be an illness can be culturally specific. For example, among the traditional isiXhosa the syndrome *isimnyama eskoli* refers to the experience of being unable to read or see a book, having headaches, sore and red eyes, and may include dizziness, heart palpitations, weakness and hearing difficulties. The dominant psychiatric biomedical model categorises many of these symptoms as 'anxiety' in the context of pressure to perform academically. It is therefore important for the nurse to try and understand the MHCU's culture and not to undermine any culture, because many people who use health care services might still view their illness from a cultural perspective.

Some authors suggest that one should just accept all cultures as being equal and allow each person to act according to their cultural beliefs and value systems. That is not so easy. What does the nurse do when a cultural practice might be harmful to the health of the clients? An example of this could be when family members request that an MHCU be discharged so that they can be trained as a traditional healer because they believe their illness is a calling by the ancestors.

A model of culture care theory

The Leininger Sunrise Model represents the structure of culture care theory by describing the relationship between anthropological and nursing beliefs and principles (Leininger, 2006). The cultural care worldview focuses on knowledge about individuals' family groups and communities in a diverse health care system. The nurse needs to consider the patient's physical, spiritual and cultural needs in order to achieve desired health outcomes. According to Leininger (2006) this can be accomplished through cultural preservation, maintenance, and cultural care repatterning. These terms are explained below:

- *Maintenance/preservation.* This requires the mental health nurses' provision of support for cultural practices, such as employing acupressure or acupuncture for anxiety and pain relief prior to medical interventions.
- *Negotiation/accommodation.* This requires the mental health nurse to support the MHCUs and their family members in carrying out cultural activities that do not pose threats to the health of the MHCUs or any other individual in the health care setting.

- *Cultural restructuring.* This refers to nurses' efforts to deliver MHCU-centred care by helping MHCUs modify or change their cultural activities. Cultural restructuring is suggested only when certain cultural practices may cause harm to the MHCU or those in the surrounding environment.

Cultural diversity in the workplace

Cultural diversity should not only be the mental health nurses' responsibility, but the health care system also needs to create an environment which promotes a multicultural workplace. Jeffreys (2008: 40) wrote about multicultural workplace 'COMPETENCE' and described it as follows:

- **Caring:** Caring about own and co-worker's cultural values and beliefs is the first step towards multicultural workplace competence.
- **Ongoing:** Diversity awareness and sharing among co-workers fosters a workplace climate that openly embraces diversity and encourages dialogue. Ongoing awareness promotes a workplace climate which openly encourages diversity and dialogue.
- **Multidimensional:** Aspects of multicultural workplace 'COMPETENCE' include cognitive (knowledge), practical (communication skills) and affective (attitudes) dimensions.
- **Proactive:** With cultural dialogue, discussions can take place about preventing emotional pain, cultural insensitivity and conflict.
- **Ethics:** All health professionals are always bound to practising in an ethical manner and to treating patients with respect regardless of their cultural backgrounds. It is also required of health professionals always to advocate for patients.
- **Trust:** Trust is an essential component for building a multicultural workplace and begins with self-disclosure and respect for diverse values.
- **Education:** Formal education is required for cultural competence and can be achieved by inviting an expert in the field to teach about cultural diversity and competency.
- **Networking:** Health professionals need to learn about various cultures as this will help them to be culturally competent and to be more culturally sensitive.
- **Confidence:** Cultural learning should be realistic and nurses and health professionals need to avoid being over-confident or under-confident.
- **Evaluation:** There should be continual appraisal of outcomes achieved and appraisal of strategies that were implemented. This will provide guidance for future innovations within the multicultural workforce.

In mental health and illness management and care, culture has a central place. Culture influences the way in which illnesses present, the psychiatric disorders a person suffers from, and the help-seeking and help-giving behaviours of people involved. It has been shown that cross-cultural misdiagnoses are common, and these might be related not only to lack of cultural sensitivity and awareness, but also to poor translation and lack of understanding of symptom presentation in another group.

Cultural presentations of illness

The presentation of mental illness differs from culture to culture. Culture shapes the behaviour of people, including their behaviour in health and illness. This is also affirmed in the DSM-5 where it is acknowledged that all forms of distress are locally shaped; therefore the cultural identity of the person needs to be assessed first. This means that a person who is depressed will express this disease in a culturally appropriate manner, and not in a universal manner. For instance, in some languages it is difficult to express feelings such as 'sad', 'depressed', 'lonely' or 'unhappy'. In these cultures, one can expect that people will not verbally express such feelings, but that they will find different, often somatic, ways of expressing them.

Some illnesses are only found in certain cultural groups. The DSM-5 was developed in the USA, while a similar diagnostic system, the International Classification of Diseases (ICD) originate in Europe (WHO, 1992). Both describe mental disorders that are universal, such as schizophrenia, depression and intellectual disability. However, the most recent DSM manual, the DSM-5, identified and described several *culture-bound syndromes* (CBSs) which are closely or even exclusively associated with a particular population or culture.

A CBS is usually an acute, brief, reactive psychosis or hysteria, which is situational and has a good prognosis. A CBS is often serious enough to lead to a diagnosis of psychosis and admission to a psychiatric hospital. A study on CBS (Niehaus et al, 2004) found that a number of CBSs are also seen in the population of South Africa. Some 38 per cent of patients admitted to a psychiatric hospital with psychiatric diagnoses had CBSs. Some examples of the CBSs found in these groups were:

- *Idliso* or *umeqo*. This is called 'rootwork' in the DSM-5. Spells (roots) are placed on a person causing all kinds of emotional and psychological symptoms. In the Xhosa culture the process of cancelling the spell is called *qubula*. A belief in such spells is common in many cultures.
- *Amok*. This is a dissociative episode, usually seen in men, characterised by a period of brooding after some perceived slight or insult, followed by a violent outburst of aggression. This is sometimes seen as part of being called to become a *sangoma*, in which case it is called *ufunfunuana*.
- *Thwasa*. This is called 'Shin-Byung' in the DSM-5, a syndrome in which the person initially complains of anxiety and somatic problems, and in later stages is possessed by ancestral spirits. People with *thwasa* usually complain of palpitations and insomnia and will not eat.
- *Uthandazeli or sangoma*. Called a 'spell' in the DSM-5, this is a trance-like state during which the person is said to communicate with the dead and the person's personality and voice changes. In the Xhosa culture this state is part of being a *sangoma*, while the *uthandazeli* is a cadre of prophets linked to African churches.

But CBSs are not only found in the African population. Among the white population, the syndromes of anorexia nervosa and anorexia bulimia are widely considered to be CBSs (Flaskerud, 2000). Both are eating disorders found mainly in young white women. The condition called chronic fatigue syndrome, which is mainly seen in white people, may also be termed a CBS, and has many symptoms in common with CBSs in other cultural groups. Some CBSs are also found among the Indian population of South Africa. One of these is *dhat*, which is characterised by weakness, fatigue, sexual dysfunction, and a preoccupation with semen loss (Ranjith & Mohan, 2006). It is clear from these descriptions that the CBSs are embedded in the religious and cultural beliefs of the group, and unless one has knowledge of these practices, the conditions will be misunderstood. Khort et al (2013) identified several CBS symptoms, such as *koro*, whereby a man fears that his penis will retract into his body and 'brain fog', common in West Africa, where sufferers experience headaches and a worm crawling in their heads. 'Brain fog' is similar to *ode-ori*, a Nigerian cultural concept of distress. Zimbabweans refer to *kufungisisa* which is the experience of thinking too much that can lead to physical pain of the heart.

If these symptoms are presented by MHCUs, the mental health nurse should be able to verify the symptoms with the family to determine whether they are considered normal (culture bound) or abnormal.

Treatment and culture

All treatment and care approaches must be adapted to the culture of the MHCU. For instance, in African culture, direct advice is acceptable and even expected, while in western culture a more non-directive approach is often followed in counselling. In a culture where the individual is seen as inherently part of a group, including the family might be more important than in individualistic cultures.

CONCLUSION

There are few aspects of life that are as interesting as getting to know another culture and tracing the influence on mental health and mental illness on that specific culture. With the increasing globalisation of nursing, nurses may ultimately work anywhere in the world, and with the growing migration into South Africa of people from all over the globe, nurses need to prepare themselves to work with cultures with which they are not familiar.

WEB RESOURCES

World Health Organisation (WHO). 2013. 'Traditional Medicine Strategy'
  http://www.searo.who.int/entity/health_situation_trends/who_trm_strategy_2014-2023.pdf?ua=1
https://msu.edu/course/sw/850/stocks/pack/u02/cltsyndr.pdf
  Information about culture-bound syndromes can be found on this website.
Global Nursing and Health. 2010. 'Standards of Practice for Culturally Competent Nursing Care. Executive Summary'. https://tcns.org/wp-content/uploads/2018/03/Standards_of_Practice_for_Culturally_Compt_Nsg_Care-Revised_.pdf.

REFERENCES

Adamo, D T. 2011. 'Christianity and the African traditional religion(s): The postcolonial round of engagement'. *Verbum et Ecclesia*, 32 (1): 1–10.

Allen, J. 2010. 'Improving cross-cultural care and antiracism in nursing education: A literature review'. *Nurse Education Today*, 30 (4): 314–320.

Andrews, M M and Boyle, J S. 2002. *Transcultural Concepts in Nursing Care*. 4th edition. Philadelphia: J B Lippincott Co.

Bennett, M. 2013. *Ethnocentrism/Xenophobia Multicultural America: A multimedia encyclopaedia* Entry in C. Cortes, Editor. New York: Sage.

Cai, D Y. 2016. 'A concept analysis of cultural competence'. *International Journal of Nursing Sciences*, 3 (3): 268–273.

Campinha-Bacote, J. 2002. 'The process of cultural competence in the delivery of health care services: A model of care'. *Journal of transcultural nursing*, 13 (3): 181–184.

Cumes, D. 2013. South African indigenous healing: how it works. *Explore: The Journal of Science and Healing*, 9 (1): 58–65.

Flaskerud, J H. 2000. 'Ethnicity, culture, and neuropsychiatry'. *Mental Health Nursing*, 21 (1): 5–29.

Gebru, K and Willman, A. 2010. 'Education to promote culturally competent nursing care – a content analysis of student responses'. *Nurse Education Today*, 30 (1): 54-60.

Giger, J N and Davidhizar, R E. 2008. *Transcultural Nursing. Assessment and Intervention*. St Louis: Mosby Year Book.

Giger, J, Davidhizar, R E, Purnell, L, Harden, J T, Phillips, J and Strickland, O. 2007. 'American academy of nursing expert panel report: Developing cultural competence to eliminate health disparities in ethnic minorities and other vulnerable populations'. *Journal of Transcultural Nursing*, 18 (2): 95–102.

Jeffreys, M, 2008. 'Dynamics of diversity. Becoming better nurses through diversity awareness'. *NSNA Imprint*: 36–41.

Kohrt, B A., Rasmussen, A, Kaiser, B N, Haroz, E E, Maharjan, S M, Mutamba, B B, De Jong, J T, and Hinton, D E. 2013. 'Cultural concepts of distress and psychiatric disorders: literature review and research recommendations for global mental health epidemiology'. *International Journal of Epidemiology*, 43 (2): 365–406.

Johnson, Y M and Munch, S. 2009. 'Fundamental contradictions in cultural competence'. *Social Work*, 54(3): 220–231.

Leininger, M. 2002. 'Culture care theory: A major contribution to advance transcultural nursing knowledge and practices'. *Journal of transcultural nursing*, 13 (3): 189–192.

Leininger, M M. 2006. 'Culture care diversity and universality theory and evolution of the ethnonursing method'. *Culture care diversity and universality: A worldwide nursing theory*, 2: 1–41.

Little, W, McGivern, R and Kerins, N. 2016. *Introduction to Sociology – 2nd Canadian Edition*. BC Campus.

Mokgobi, M G. 2014. 'Understanding traditional African healing'. *African Journal for Physical Health Education, Recreation and Dance*, 20 (Supplement 2): 24–34.

Niehaus, D J H, Oosthuizen, P, Lochner, C, Emsley, R A, Jordaan, E, Mbanga, N I, Keyter, N, Laurent, C, Deleuze, J F and Stein, D J. 2004. 'A culture-bound syndrome "amafufunyana" and a culture-specific event "ukuthwasa": differentiated by a family history of schizophrenia and other psychiatric disorders. *Psychopathology*, 37 (2): 59–63.

Ranjith, G and Mohan, R. 2006. 'Dhat syndrome as a functional somatic syndrome: developing a sociosomatic model'. *Psychiatry: Interpersonal and Biological Processes*, 69 (2): 142–150

Shezi, E N & Uys, L R. 1997. 'Culture bound syndromes in a group of Xhosa with psychiatric disorders'. *Curationis*, 20 (2): 83–86.

World Health Organisation (WHO). 1992. *The ICD-10 Classification of Mental and Behavioral Disorders*. Geneva: WHO.

SECTION 2
The Mental Health Nursing Process

CHAPTER 9

The Mental Health Care Nursing Process

L R Uys and A Marx

Learning Outcomes

After studying this chapter, you should be able to:
- systematically manage the problems of a mental health care user (MHCU)
- describe and cultivate basic interpersonal attitudes essential in mental health care nursing
- discuss interpersonal mental health care nursing attitudes, empathy and communication skills
- describe and demonstrate the therapeutic interaction skills of the mental health care nurse
- discuss the obstacles that may occur during the therapeutic relationship.

INTRODUCTION

Nursing care, irrespective of the setting, always involves relationships. Engaging in relationships between the mental health care nurse and the MHCU is the foundation of quality nursing care. Compassion, empathy, trust and respect are the heart of the therapeutic engagement. This type of engagement leads to satisfied MHCUs, better health care outcomes, safer care and happier health care professionals. Therapeutic engagement helps give voice to the MHCU's opinions, knowledge and information about their situation and forms the basis for a shared understanding of outcomes. At the same time, the quality of therapeutic engagement from some students declines through the progression of studies and many students and experienced health care workers are insensitive to the emotions and experiences of their health care users.

Worldwide, students and professionals from nursing, medical and other health professions are voicing their concerns about the poor quality of care in mental health settings and problems with compassion and professionalism. While there are explanations for the lack of compassion that relate to education and social issues, the health system, and individuals themselves, mental health care nurses are also responsible for what they feel, say and do and for how they interact with health care users on a day-to-day basis. Since quality mental health care nursing relies heavily on the quality of the nurse's interpersonal attitudes and skills, it is essential that the nurse builds, continually reflects upon, and demonstrates helping and MHCU-oriented attitudes in a systematic process of care.

INTERPERSONAL MENTAL HEALTH CARE NURSING ATTITUDES

The following attitudes, as elucidated by Carl Rogers in the 1960s in his development of person-centred therapy, involve the mental health care nurse by means of which the nurse communicates care to the MHCU. It is hypothesised that any of the user's personal growth, psychological and emotional well-being are facilitated by a therapist who demonstrates warmth, caring and a non-judgemental understanding. The basic attitude of the mental health care nurse towards an MHCU is made up of congruence, empathy and acceptance and these are underpinned by the nurse's own self-awareness.

Congruence, also known as 'genuineness', is when the MHCU can feel the genuine interest and caring of the mental health care nurse. The MHCU feels safe in the nurse's environment. An example of congruence is when a person is happy, it shows on their face and in their eyes and verbally it will be acknowledged.

Empathy means putting oneself in another person's shoes as if those shoes were one's own. This means that one must be able to identify the affective message (emotion) in the other person's communication. Empathy is shown by reflecting emotions as perceived by the mental health care nurse to the MHCU. Four major emotions are happiness, anger, fear and sadness, although each of these subdivides into many subtle nuances. Table 9.1 gives examples of words from the main groups of emotions one can use to convey empathy.

Table 9.1 Empathy functioning scale

Happiness	Anger	Fear	Sadness
excited	hateful	doubtful	disappointed
glad	bored	frightened	hopeless
happy	guilty	guilty	hurt
in love	angry	anxious	left out
pleased	accused	worried	miserable
proud	wanting to get even	incapable	put down
relieved	frustrated	apprehensive	sad
satisfied	sarcastic		unhappy
grateful			worthless
capable			discouraged

The mental health care nurse communicates this empathic understanding of an MHCU by means of reflecting the experience. This can occur at different levels, which are known as levels of empathy.

- Primary-level empathy means that the mental health care nurse reflects an initial and basic understanding of what the MHCU feels as shared by the MHCU (Egan 1982: 88), for example:
    - MHCU: I'm so glad to be back where all my family and friends are.
    - Mental health care nurse: Being at home in these familiar surroundings makes you feel secure.

- Advanced-level empathy refers to how the mental health care nurse may reflect not only what the MHCU implicitly states about themselves, but also what the user implies or leaves only half-stated or expressed. The mental health care nurse may even intuitively become aware of what the user does not reveal or say about themselves, for example:
  - MHCU: I've been having a lot of trouble with my car. It really isn't running well at all these days; the exhaust has fallen off and the ignition has also just broken.
  - Mental health care nurse: I wonder if you might be feeling like that broken car, unable to get going and perform well ...?

Unconditional positive regard is a further concept developed by Carl Rogers (1951), which involves basic acceptance and support of a person regardless of what the person says or does, especially in the context of client-centred therapy. In the mental health care nurse–MHCU relationship, thoughts, feelings and experiences are worked through to acceptance and/or tolerance.

INTERPERSONAL MENTAL HEALTH CARE NURSING COMMUNICATION SKILLS

Through the use of communication skills and interpersonal mental health care nursing attitudes (outlined in the previous section), the mental health care nurse aims to show empathy. This is done by exploring the experiences of the MHCU and encouraging the user to ventilate feelings (see Table 9.1) through reflecting and then discussing these feelings. Communication skills that can be used include assertive behaviour, clarifying, confrontation, focusing, listening, probing, questioning and reflection of feelings. These will be outlined in the sections that follow.

Assertive behaviour

Assertive behaviour is based on an assertive view of self and others. This behaviour is based on, but not limited to, the following 'assertiveness rights':
- the right to have opinions and feelings and stand up for these
- the right to say 'no' or 'yes' without feeling guilty
- the right to decide what to do with own body, time and property
- the right to make mistakes and take responsibility for them
- the right to ask for what you want
- the right to be treated with respect
- the right to be listened to.

If one believes one has to be right all the time, or that others have to approve of what one says or does all the time, or that others always come first and one is last, it is almost impossible to act in an assertive manner. One of the central techniques used in an assertive communication style is the 'I-message'. An 'I-message' consists of the four Rs:

Report. You describe exactly what is happening in a non-blaming manner.
Example: Pat, over the last two weeks you have twice taken my textbooks from my room without asking me.

Relate. You relate or explain how this is affecting you, using 'I', not 'You'.
Example: I felt angry when I needed them, and they were not there and this wasted my time.

Request. You ask in concrete terms for what you need to be changed.
Example: Please do not remove books unless you have asked me before the time.

Result. You spell out the positive and negative results if the change is made or is not made.
Example: I can then plan my work so that we can both use the books. Otherwise, I will have to lock my room.

The same incident will be handled as follows in an aggressive manner: 'Pat, you are really making me furious by forever stealing my stuff from my room. If you cannot keep your hands off my books and stuff, then please stay out of my room!'

An acquiescent person might say (using a soft tone of voice): 'I was late with my assignment today, because I could not find my midwifery textbook last night.' See Table 9.2 for examples of the above.

Table 9.2 Contrasting assertive, aggressive and acquiescent behaviour

Behaviour	Aggressive	Assertive	Acquiescent
Aim	To dominate others	To share thoughts and feelings	Not to rock the boat
Characteristics of message	You-messages, accusing, sarcastic, absolutes (eg always, never, ought to)	I-messages Specific	Does not take a stand, gives no personal opinion
Non-verbal behaviour	Frowns, raises voice, stares down the other	Level look, neutral facial expression, clear voice	Looks down, fidgets, talks softly, frequent smiling, speaks hesitantly
Beliefs	I know best Others are fools How dare they	I have equal rights to others It is important to share thoughts and feelings I have a right to refuse	Others know better than I do I cannot refuse I cannot hurt them

→

Behaviour	Aggressive	Assertive	Acquiescent
Results	Gets isolated from others Problems remain for others	Feels good about self Problems often get solved Gets closer to others	Blames others Manipulates to get what they want Gets angry and hurt, but hides it Problems remain

Unless nurses master assertiveness, they will find it difficult to cope with interpersonal situations with colleagues and MHCUs. It is often the case that MHCUs need to be assertive and the mental health care professionals should be role models.

Clarifying

Clarifying involves making sure that the MHCU is understood, and that the message is heard as it is meant. This can be done by asking questions, by making a summary, or by saying, for example, 'I hear that you say you are happy, but you are hitting the chair.'

Confrontation

Confrontation is an action on the part of the person who is confronting. This then stimulates the person who is being confronted to reflect on or change some aspect of behaviour. Although this kind of interaction is usually unpleasant, it can be extremely beneficial in the long run. There can be discrepancies in the following areas regarding:
- Unrecognised strengths, where there is an underestimation by the person of themselves
- Unrecognised weaknesses, where there is an overestimation by the person of abilities in a specific area
- The real intent of the MHCU, where this is distinguished by words or other means. An example is the user who keeps on promising to stop using alcohol but actually continues to abuse it.

Confrontation is more effective when persuading the confronted person to examine their own behaviour if:
- it focuses on behaviour rather than on motivation, since behaviour is observable and less vague than motivation
- it is done within a healthy, meaningful relationship
- it is done with the motivation of promoting growth in the person and not in anger, or to punish or to humiliate
- it is done empathically or
- it slows down the pace of the interaction between the persons and hence allows issues to be explored in a more moderate, regulated fashion.

Focusing

Here the mental health care nurse directs the attention and the conversation of the MHCU to the topic of discussion and focuses on the detail that is happening. Focusing may reduce the MHCU's confusion and distress by enabling them to address manageable aspects of an overwhelming issue, rather than becoming entangled in an incoherent array of thoughts and feelings. However, it must be noted that, when directing the MHCU to a topic of discussion, they should not be forced to talk about problems that provoke too much pain. In such a case, the mental health care nurse could, for example, simply reflect, 'This seems too difficult to talk about', or an MHCU who is talking rather generally about a 'problematic relationship with the doctor' might be enabled to focus on this concern if the mental health care nurse were simply to say, 'Problematic …?' in a gentle, enquiring tone.

Listening

The mental health care nurse listens to the verbal and the non-verbal messages that the MHCU is giving. The mental health care nurse listens to whether the MHCU conveys powerful and meaningful feelings and thoughts, like 'I am angry'. Non-verbally, the mental health care nurse will observe body language, gestures, facial expressions that accompanies the verbal messages, or at times will only observe the non-verbal message.

Paraphrasing

This is the use of other words to reflect to the MHCU that they are being heard and that the mental health care nurse is attempting to understand the message. The message should be heard without prejudices, stereotyping and assumptions. For example, the MHCU talks about being treated in a specific way and the mental health care nurse reacts with, 'In other words, you are irritated when you are treated like a child'.

Probing

Probing involves asking clarifying questions which may indicate to the person that one needs further information on a particular issue. Probing questions asked too soon or too often tend to guide the person along certain lines or bring the MHCU to a realisation or conclusion desired by you, but which is ultimately not theirs.

Questioning

This is the asking of questions with specific goals in mind, for example
- to obtain information
- to maintain control of the conversation
- to express interest in another person
- to clarify a point

- to explore the personality
- to understand difficulties somebody might have
- to test another's knowledge
- to encourage further thought.

How questions are asked is also important and there are several ways in which this can be done. Closed questions are those that typically involve a 'yes' or a 'no' as an answer. This type of question does not elicit ongoing conversation and the person waits for another question, so these questions are good for testing understanding or obtaining biographical data. However, a misplaced closed question can kill the conversation and lead to awkward silences, so these are best avoided when a conversation is in full flow.

Open questions elicit conversation and give the person time to tell their story. Open questions are good for developing an open conversation and finding out more detail, for example, finding out the other person's opinion or issues.

Reflection of feelings

During the conversation the feelings and thoughts of the MHCU are reflected back to them. This shows that the mental health care nurse is listening and understanding what the problem is. It helps the MHCU to focus their thoughts and encourages talking about the problem. Reflection of feelings is not questioning the MHCU.

In learning this skill initially, it is useful to start with the words, 'You feel ...' For example, if the MHCU says, 'The tree fell over the road again!' the mental health care nurse may reflect, 'You feel angry that this has happened again.'

Although the task of reflecting the MHCU's feelings may seem rather simple, the mental health care nurse is likely to encounter some difficulty in developing this skill. There are several different aspects that are important to take into account when reflecting the MHCU's feelings. These involve varying the style of reflecting, timing, depth, use of minimal verbal responses and silence.

Varying the style of reflecting

In reflecting the MHCU's feelings, it is important that this should be done in a natural and genuinely warm way, so that the user does not experience the mental health care nurse's responses as monotonous and stilted. Thus, the mental health care nurse should not start every reflection with 'You feel' once they have mastered the skill, but instead should learn to vary the style of reflecting, for example by saying, 'You feel sad', 'I hear that you are angry'.

Timing

It is important to determine the MHCU's readiness before reflecting their feelings. This implies many things:

- One waits for the MHCU to finish a sentence and for a reasonable amount of time to elapse before making a reflection, thus giving the user adequate time to hear the reflection.
- One does not have to reflect every feeling that the user experiences in the therapeutic relationship.
- On the other hand, it is also ineffective to let the MHCU deliver a long monologue in trying to reflect every feeling that has been experienced during that time.

Depth

It is important to determine the MHCU's ability to receive reflections before going ahead and reflecting feelings to them. An MHCU is often not ready to hear how sad, angry or anxious they are and might experience such reflections as anxiety provoking and threatening. This is especially true in the initial phase of a therapeutic relationship when it is important to be tentative in reflecting feelings. It may be appropriate simply to make a mental note of what the user may be feeling without reflecting at all.

Use of minimal verbal responses

To allow the MHCU to carry on talking and reflecting on feelings, the mental health care nurse will make use of gestures like nodding of the head or will verbally encourage the MHCU by saying 'hhmm'. This gives the indication that the mental health care nurse is listening and following the conversation.

Silence

Using silence is a powerful way of asking questions and giving the person with whom one is conversing a chance to gather their thoughts. Most people feel the need to talk to fill the silence in a conversation and thus could answer unasked questions.

THE RELATIONSHIP BETWEEN A MENTAL HEALTH CARE NURSE AND AN MHCU

The relationship between the mental health care nurse and an MHCU depends on a range of factors, such as the personality and characteristics of each of them, the time they have spent and will spend together, the objectives of the contact and situational factors. According to different authors, there are three types of mental health care nurse–MHCU relationships. The essence of the differences lies in the levels of intimacy involved. Table 9.3 shows the different levels of the relationships and a brief outline of these different relationships follows.

The clinical/instrumental relationship is appropriate when the mental health care nurse sees the MHCU for a short time, for a minor or routine matter. The therapeutic/protective level is appropriate for most users being cared for in a hospital or in a long-term outpatient setting. In the connected/reciprocal relationship the mental health care nurse and MHCU see each other as persons in the first instance and their roles as mental health care nurses and MHCUs as secondary. This type of relationship usually develops over time and not with all MHCUs.

Table 9.3 Three levels of mental health care nurse–MHCU relationships

	Clinical/ instrumental	**Therapeutic/ protective**	**Connected/ reciprocal**
Type of knowing	General (case) knowledge	General and more specific MHCU knowledge	Case, MHCU and person knowledge
Listening	Content	Content and obvious feeling	Content and underlying feeling
Understanding	External view of the clinical situation	External and some internal user response	Primary internal, from MHCU's perspective
Exploring	Factual data	Factual data and the user's perception of the immediate situation	Personal meanings, both regarding the situation and the effect on the user's life
Intervening	Explanations and factual information Reassuring presence and manner	Sharing information Mobilising resources	Sharing own interpretations Providing support Concrete and specific feedback

Source: Adapted from Stein-Parbury (2000: 40)

All relationships develop through a number of stages, although not all pass through every stage. Table 9.4 summarises the tasks and stages in each stage. It is important that the mental health care nurse be aware of how the relationship is progressing and whether goals are being met.

Table 9.4 Tasks and stages of mental health care nurse–MHCU relationships

Phase 1 Pre-interaction phase	Prepare for the initial meeting with the MHCU.
Pre-interaction phase Tasks	Gather information regarding the MHCU from file, family and other mental health care professionals. Examine own feelings, fears, anxieties which might affect a working relationship with the MHCU. For example, if there is a history of rape, this might bring out certain fears or anxieties in the nurse.

Phase 2 Orientation phase	Set up an initial meeting between the mental health care nurse and the MHCU.
Orientation phase Tasks	Create an environment where trust and rapport will be established. Discuss the expectations and responsibilities of the mental health care nurse and the MHCU. Gather information to form a strong database and identify the MHCU's strengths and limitations. Formulate the nursing diagnosis. Set mutually accepted goals. Explore feelings of both the mental health care nurse and the MHCU.
Phase 3 Working phase	Here the therapeutic work of the working phase will be accomplished.
Phase 3 Working phase Tasks	Build on the trust and rapport that was built in the orientation phase. Practise the problem-solving methods that suit the MHCU. As the anxiety levels rise, help the MHCU overcome the resistance and other less effective behaviours in response to the discussions of painful issues. Do continued assessment of progress towards the set goals.

There are a number of obstacles that might occur in a mental health care nurse–MHCU relationship. The first is that the user might not be willing to engage in a relationship with the mental health care nurse, or the nurse might be unwilling to engage with the user. A mental health care nurse who dislikes an MHCU might be unwilling to admit it, since it is against the principles of nursing. The mental health care nurse might then ignore these feelings, rationalise them or overcompensate for them. These feelings should be acknowledged and discussed with a colleague or supervisor. If a user dislikes the mental health care nurse, it might be possible for another nurse to establish a therapeutic relationship with the user. However, if it is a general dislike related to the illness of the MHCU, patience and respect are the only options for building and maintaining a therapeutic relationship.

A second obstacle might be that the relationship becomes social instead of professional. A professional relationship does not mean a distant, formal relationship. It only means that one keeps in mind the therapeutic and care goals and works towards these. A social relationship has no therapeutic or care goals and may therefore be superficially friendly or focus on non-threatening topics. While this might be comfortable for both the MHCU and the mental health care nurse, it may leave the user without the professional assistance needed. Social chatting, which is called pathic communication, is free and aimless and is loaded with emotional agreement. It is a social ritual and when a person does not engage in this kind of communication, they are often seen as rude. The usual greeting ritual of 'How-are-you-I-am-fine-and-you-I-am-also-OK' is a good example where both participants agree to a superficial exchange without much meaning. Mental health care nurses have to use therapeutic communication, and the therapeutic relationships should also develop to address the needs of the MHCU.

Thirdly, an MHCU might transfer feelings and thoughts about significant others onto the mental health care nurse. Patterns in these relationships will be repeated in the therapeutic relationship and will have to be managed by the mental health professional. For example, if an MHCU had an overbearing father and the mental health care worker was an older male, the MHCU would fall back on the cowering manner of communicating that had been used with the MHCU's father. Countertransference on the other hand is the mental health care nurse's reaction to the MHCU. Here the mental health care nurse's ability to assess the relationship with the MHCU is confused. Some behaviours are unconsciously used in an attempt to replay conflict with significant others, for example pointing fingers in a parental way when speaking, or giggling at a remark from the MHCU.

Finally, the mental health care nurse might become over-involved with the MHCU. In such a case, the mental health care nurse reacts emotionally, becoming either a personal friend or a rescuer taking responsibility for the user's problems. In these cases, the mental health care nurse loses control over themselves and the relationship, and thus can no longer empower the MHCU or give professional assistance. The mental health care professional should set the boundaries of the therapeutic relationship with the MHCU. An example of this would be the mental health care nurse determining the space between their chair in the interview room and that of the MHCU.

When patients were asked to describe the nurse–patient relationships they had experienced in a Canadian health setting, they described two different processes: the one was the process with 'a few good nurses' and the other was the process with the nurses 'who do more harm than good' (Coatsworth-Puspoky et al, 2006). The 'few good nurses' show warmth and interest initially and give the patient hope. They explore the patient's feelings and assist them with problem solving and say goodbye when the patient leaves to go home in a manner that produces closure. The 'poor nurses' withhold their support from the start and when the patient asks for assistance, the nurse gives the impression that they see this as manipulative or attention seeking. This kind of nurse actively seeks to avoid the patient and ignores their needs and even acts in a rude or condescending manner. The conclusion of this kind of relationship leaves the patient wondering why they were treated in this manner.

THE MENTAL HEALTH CARE NURSE–FAMILY RELATIONSHIP

The mental health care nurse does not only build a relationship with the MHCU, but also with the family or primary caregivers. This relationship is built using the same competencies as those of the mental health care nurse–MHCU relationship, but it has its own challenges.

When the family experience stress during acute episodes of illness of the user, they appreciate the availability and support of health professionals. The availability (presence) of the health professional should include early contact with the family, early information about the condition of the MHCU, treatment options and protection during frightening events. The support includes listening to the family in order to assess their burden, maintain contact and validate them as people and as carers (Gavois et al, 2006). During periods when the user is not acutely ill, the mental health care nurse needs to provide opportunities for sharing, so that the treatment and rehabilitation teams coordinate their efforts with that of the family, and information and planning are shared between the teams and the family. As the user moves towards recovery, the mental health care nurse should focus on empowering the family with information. Counselling the family members separately or in a group, encouraging them to join a support group, and making sure that they grow in their understanding, might assist them in their contact with the user.

THE MENTAL HEALTH CARE NURSING PROCESS

The mental health care nursing process, a systematic approach to mental health care, has become an institution in nursing. The mental health care nurse commences with the assessment of the user or group and makes a nursing diagnosis. This is followed by the planning and implementation of care. Evaluation takes place throughout the process and this can lead to further assessment, a revision of the diagnosis, new plans and additional actions.

However, more needs to be said about nursing classification systems. Such classification systems exist to guide nursing diagnoses, nursing actions and nursing outcomes. The most comprehensive classification system is the International Classification for Nursing Practice (ICNP), which includes all three aspects. It was developed by the International Council of Nurses and published in 2001. Classification systems were developed to establish a common language for describing nursing practice, in order to enable comparison across time and space and to promote research and quality management.

A nursing diagnosis can be defined as a problem or issue that is the focus of nursing interventions. According to the North American Nursing Diagnosis Association's 1982 diagnostic system, it always involves a response to a problem. A diagnosis in this system involves a two-part statement: the actual problem, the aetiological factors and the defining characteristics. The phrases 'related to' and 'evidenced by' are useful in linking the identified problem with the causes and the characteristics. An example of this type of diagnosis might be: impaired social interaction (actual problem) related to a lack of appropriate social skills and confidence (aetiological factors) evidenced by having no friends and taking part in no social activities involving others (defining characteristics).

In the case of a problem that is only a risk and not an actual problem, the diagnosis has only two parts, namely the problem and the risk factors. An example of this type of diagnosis could be in the following form: risk of impaired social interaction related to these risk factors – long hospitalisation, low motivation, limited income.

The ICNP (ICN, 2001) identified several components to a nursing diagnosis, which also act as outcome classification. The following seven components form part of nursing actions:

1. *Action.* Counselling is an example
2. *Target.* The entity affected by the action, for example the whole person
3. *Means.* The instruments, services used or provided, for example group therapy
4. *Time.* Time intervals of the actions, for example weekly until discharge
5. *Topology.* The anatomical region in relation to the median or the total where it occurs, for example the whole person
6. *Location.* The anatomical region of the body, for example the whole person
7. *Routes.* The pathway through which a nursing action is performed, for example oral if medication; or whole person if therapy.

This is a very comprehensive approach to nursing actions and guides the way for record keeping in mental health care.

CONCLUSION

The skilled mental health care nurse is one who practises the three basic interpersonal attitudes consistently and who uses interpersonal competencies and skills in a systematic way to assess, plan interventions and assist MHCUs within a mental health care nurse–MHCU relationship. This is indeed the core of mental health care nursing.

WEB RESOURCES

http://www.psychological-hug.com
    This website was developed by Dr Lawrence Bookbinder and has very useful information about empathy. It gives you an example of an empathetic conversation and provides links to other sites on the topic.

http://www.nanda.org
    This is the website of the North American Nursing Diagnosis Association (NANDA), where you can find the most recent information about their nursing diagnostic taxonomy.

http://www.icn.ch
    This is the website of the International Council of Nurses (ICN) and it links to the ICNP classification system. The ICN invites you to submit views, participate in research and get involved in other ways.

hhttps://quizlet.com
    Website that discusses the phases of the therapeutic nurse–client relationship.

REFERENCES

Coatsworth-Puspoky, R, Forchuk, C and Ward-Griffin C. 2006. 'Nurse–client processes in mental health: recipients' perspectives'. *Journal of Psychiatric and Mental Health Nursing*, 13: 347–355.

Egan, G. 1982. *The Skilled Helper*. California: Brooks/Cole.

Gavois, H, Paulsson, G and Fridlund, B. 2006. 'Mental health professional support in families with a member suffering from severe mental illness: a grounded theory model'. *Scandinavian Journal of Caring Science,* 20: 102–109.

International Council of Nurses. 2001. *International Classification for Nursing Practice.* Geneva: ICN.

Rogers, C R. 1951. *Client-centered Therapy: Its Current Practice Implications and Theory.* Boston: Houghton Miffen.

Stein-Parbury, J. 2000. *Patient and person. Developing interpersonal skills in nursing.* 2nd edition. Sydney: Harcourt.

CHAPTER 10

Mental Health Assessment of Hospitalised or Community-based Individuals

G E Pietersen and L Middleton

Learning Outcomes

After studying this chapter, you should be able to:
- elicit specific psychopathologies during a mental health assessment
- identify and interpret characteristics of psychopathologies assessed
- account for all indicators related to patterns of current level(s) of functioning in a mental health care user (MHCU)
- assess the spectrum of lifestyle functioning of the MHCU, with specific reference to cultural and/or religious background
- determine the MHCU's position on the continuum of lifestyle functioning
- differentiate between the use and value of alternative mental health assessment methods
- specify problems identified, formulate nursing diagnoses and design a scientific justifiable nursing care plan.

INTRODUCTION

An inevitable universal question regarding mental health assessment, distinct from an unwavering psychiatric assessment and irrespective of the setting (hospitalised or community-based, rural or urban), is whether psychopathology could be viewed as something that is merely situated on a continuum called normality. On the one hand, the issue concerning the continuum of normality introduces the difficulty in distinguishing mental disorders from shades of normality, and on the other hand, it alludes to the danger of over diagnosing psychopathology and mental disorders.

Although much progress has been made in terms of research regarding the brain, in fields related to neuroscience, the aetiology (cause or set of causes) and pathogenesis (manner of development) of mental disorders remain elusive. Assessment of mental disorders should not be conducted as if brain pathology per se underpins these disorders.

Mental health disorders are predominantly categorised (diagnosed) on the basis of signs and symptoms (syndromes). Laboratory tests, for most medical conditions (as opposed to a mental health diagnosis), serve to substantiate a syndrome. However, no biomarkers (molecular evidence) exist as a basis on which a psychiatric/mental health diagnosis can be concluded.

Mental health nursing assessment involves a particular interest in the person exhibiting the psychopathology (or psychiatric diagnostic label) as opposed to a mere biological (biomedical model) explanation for the MHCU's emotions, behaviour and thought processes. Mental health nursing assessment aims to identify accurately aspects of the MHCU's emotions, behaviour and thought processes that are dysfunctional and that require interventions. Assessment is not about listening for what is *wrong* but rather for what is *missing*, the presence of which will make a difference to the MHCU's performance, experience and ultimately, quality of life. Key during a mental health assessment is to listen for concerns the MHCU has and to deliver reliably on what matters to the MHCU. Assessment is consequently grounded in a holistic view of the MHCU. Such a view encompasses physical, social, spiritual and psychological aspects of human beings. Assessment based on a holistic view informs what is in the best interest of the MHCU when planning appropriate and scientific nursing care interventions. Furthermore, holistic mental health nursing incorporates all nursing practice and has the healing of the whole person at issue.

Mental health nursing assessment should be standard operating practice for all nurses, irrespective of the category of care. Such assessment should thus be implemented effortlessly by any nurse and in any health care setting. Similar to taking a temperature or blood pressure, mental health nursing assessment should become second nature, and an instinctive everyday practice, for any nurse. A notion that only MHCUs referred to a psychiatric clinic/hospital have mental health problems, or that they are the only ones with a mental health diagnosis, is disingenuous. In fact, a timeous mental health nursing assessment, at whichever health care setting the MHCU reports to, could prevent unnecessary suffering of the MHCU, including those who are in contact with the MHCU.

Mental health nursing assessment typically involves interrogating all aspects of living. Such assessment goes beyond reflecting on the current mental health syndrome (signs and symptoms) presented by an MHCU, as these not only overlap greatly with one another, but also with what sometimes could be deemed normal. This boundary, between what is considered as normal and what is a mental health disorder, is problematic. Increasingly problems of everyday living are being considered mental health problems. The skill related to mental health nursing assessment is, in the first instance, to identify persons with normal variations in emotion, thought and behaviour to avoid an inappropriate or unnecessary mental health diagnosis. Such an unfortunate diagnosis can ultimately lead to stigmatisation and even worse, to unnecessary or inappropriate treatment. A skilful mental health nursing assessment forms the basis of nursing interventions addressing the whole person.

Another 'boundary' when conducting a mental health nursing assessment is to consider the contribution of non-mental health conditions or medical treatments, which are related to the mental health concerns of an MHCU, and vice versa. Some medications used in the treatment of human immunodeficiency virus (HIV)/acquired immunodeficiency syndrome (AIDS) and tuberculosis (TB), for instance, are known to activate or aggravate signs and symptoms that could be construed as underlying mental health disorders. In these cases, a thorough assessment is required to establish whether:

- The MHCU possibly experienced a treatment-induced psychopathological adverse event
- An underlying mental health disorder was triggered as a result of the condition or treatment received
- The MHCU indeed had a mental health condition that was undiagnosed at the time when treatment of the medical condition was initiated. However, this could be a typical chicken-or-egg situation as the 'boundary' is not always evident.

In summary, a skilled mental health nurse assessment is grounded in a theoretical framework that incorporates a holistic worldview. For most professions, including the nursing profession, mental health assessment is predominantly based on a biomedical model despite the vast array of models and theoretical frameworks on which the content, and context, of mental health assessment could be based.

DEVELOPING A CONTEXT FOR MENTAL HEALTH ASSESSMENT AND DIAGNOSIS

The thought process applied during a mental health assessment is historically derived from a biomedical understanding of mental health and mental illness. This model has as its starting point a 'disease–cure' understanding of mental health and mental illness. Psychosocial factors are considered, but only in as much as they relate to the underlying (biological) disease process. The biomedical assessment framework therefore focuses on identifying the presence of specific symptom clusters for the dual purposes of mental health diagnosis and treatment. A different model, the biopsychosocial model, is an appealing alternative to the biomedical model. Furthermore, some might argue that it is important to treat people's distress, as would be the emphasis when applying the bio-psychosocial model (Beckett, 2017; Deacon, 2013).

Historically, knowledge-generating values, traditionally associated with the scientific process of medicine, constructed psychiatry and mental illness as a medical problem. Notions of objectivity, truth, logic and reason underpin this highly ordered process of assessment, problem-statement generation, solution seeking, intervention and evaluation.

While the biomedical approach may suit the 'disease–cure' discipline of psychiatry, it has not necessarily served the best interests related to a mental health nursing practice. Mental health nursing is usually characterised as a caring rather than a curing profession. Emphasis is furthermore given to the needs of the 'whole person' and, within each subsystem of wholeness, to developing strengths and remedying deficits. It stands to reason that the 'whole person', or even aspects of it, is often difficult to put into practice in settings where a biomedical model prevails.

A biomedical approach to care consequently mirrors the delivery of mental health nursing care, as nursing practice is based on the biomedical approach in many mental health clinics and hospitals. Although this approach is important, it is only one aspect of mental health nursing practice (see Table 10.1).

There are, however, other aspects that form part of a holistic approach which, if considered as part of the assessment process, might be essential to quality holistic care. A skilled mental health nurse assessor could use the same amount of time, when doing a holistic assessment, as it would take when probing the routine questions associated with a biomedical model. Questions such as the following could not only elicit typical biomedical model concerns but also provide the MHCU with an opportunity to discuss aspects of living generally: How are you? Any problems? How do you experience your medication? Do you have any side effects? How are you eating/sleeping? How are you getting on with people at home? What do your daily activities while living at home involve? An assessment of social and spiritual aspects, regarding the person's background, cultural upbringing and practices, should also be contextualised and treated with sensitivity (Seddigh et al, 2016).

The stress–vulnerability perspective regarding the course and outcome of mental health and illness

The stress–vulnerability perspective provides a practical view on the relationship between the course and outcome of mental health and illness. It offers a framework within which to ground both the biomedical and psychosocial 'whole person' dimensions of mental health nursing assessment. Furthermore, it allows for applicable professional intervention.

According to this perspective, mental health and illness result from interactions related to four factors:
1. Basic vulnerabilities
2. Environmental stress
3. Personal and environmental protectors
4. An underlying neurological or psychological vulnerability which impacts mental health and the development of mental illness. Examples of vulnerabilities are genetic predisposition, damage or alteration to the anatomical and/or physiological and chemical systems of the neurological system and psychological vulnerabilities such as a disturbance in sense of self.

Vulnerability is triggered and indicators related to mental health or illness emerge when environmental *stressors* overwhelm or exceed the protective effects of the person's personal *coping* skills, and environmental and personal resources (*protective factors*). The person may further develop a functional disability if symptoms persistently interfere with their ability to function effectively in the different roles and tasks expected of a person within a given family and social environment.
- *Stressors* are defined as transient or ambient events that demand adaptive changes from the individual and that challenge the individual's existing coping and competence. Stressors could include a range of events, situations and experiences which the individual perceives as stressful.

- *Coping* refers to the process of striving to master environmental stressors or challenges. People draw on personal coping behaviours and environmental resources in striving to cope. Defence mechanisms, cognitive patterns and coping strategies are aspects of coping.
- *Protective factors* are personal and environmental resources which act as a buffer against the effects of stress on vulnerability.
- *Personal protectors* include self-competent beliefs about self, healthy cognitive patterns, competency in illness management, medication management, problem solving, activities of daily living, managing emotions, interpersonal relations, vocational or work-related tasks and a sense of hope, mastery, love and belonging.
- *Environmental protectors* are resources outside of the MHCU and which confer some degree of protection against stress. These are supportive family members, friends and supportive work and living environments; the availability of illness management training programmes for family members and MHCUs; skills training programmes for any or all of the activities associated with each of the patterns of healthy lifestyle functioning, for example budgeting, cooking, starting a conversation, using a taxi, finding a job; facilitated access to sustainable supportive networks, including access to physical health care, entitlement (grant) and social welfare resources; the presence of professional attitudes and behaviour which demonstrate respect and regard for the MHCU and family; the availability of professional mental health or psychiatric services including counselling, regular and competent psychiatric symptom assessment and diagnosis reviews, and ongoing medication monitoring and psychosocial rehabilitation.

Because of the multitude of factors involved in a dynamic stress–vulnerability system, it is difficult to be precise about what degree of change in stressors or protectors will initiate a trajectory towards moderated mental health, form a basis of mental illness or be causative of relapse in an individual at a particular point in time. However, the effects of vulnerability and stressors on symptoms, coping and functional abilities are lessened by the presence and action of personal and environmental protective factors that exist within the person and their environment. The goal of professional intervention is therefore to assist the person in engaging with the process of coping with temporary mental health concerns or recovery from mental illness by increasing and sustaining the presence and action of a range of protective factors in their lives.

Implications for mental health nursing assessment
When using the stress–vulnerability model in mental health nursing assessment, the following guidelines should be taken into account:
- A holistic personal and family history is necessary to identify the presence of basic vulnerabilities and the impact of these on the emotional, behavioural and thought processes (ie, the functioning) of the person.

- A full history of the MHCU's presenting problem and mental health or mental illness pattern, together with an outline of the possible stressors preceding the emergence or worsening of symptoms, is necessary.
- A thorough assessment of the person's functional abilities is necessary to understand the impact that the mental health indicators, or symptoms associated with mental illness, may have on the person's lifestyle functioning.
- A thorough assessment of the presence and action of the personal and environmental protective factors at work in the MHCU's life is necessary to determine strengths and limitations that could be the focus of intervention.

The implications of the stress–vulnerability model suggest that both a deficit and a strengths-related assessment of the MHCU are needed in order for a biomedical and a mental health nursing assessment and diagnosis to be developed. A brief outline of how they could be integrated in practice is given in the next section.

MENTAL HEALTH ASSESSMENT

The assessment of human behaviour and motivation is a complex process. Furthermore, from the perspective of the MHCU, an individual's mental health history is a personal and frequently painful life story. The interpersonal process central to mental health assessment thus tries to balance the 'telling of a life story' with the need for specific and concrete pieces of information about mental health and mental illness. This need, for the MHCU, may be only a fragment of a larger, more comprehensive account of a life narrative.

Mental health assessment is thus a conversational space in which the nurse and the MHCU, through the process of asking and answering questions, jointly recreate a particular aspect or version of the MHCU's life story. At the time when this conversation occurs a particular version of the MHCU's overall life experience is being highlighted, namely the mental health or mental illness experience or process. Highlighting the mental health story of the MHCU is important to elicit valid clinical data. The more engaged the nurse is in the life story of the MHCU, the more valid the clinical data and consequently the mental health diagnosis.

From a clinical point of view, validity refers to the accuracy of the information, that is, whether the nurse is eliciting information intended to be extracted. For example, if the nurse greets the client with, 'Hello, how are you today?' and then takes the MHCU's response, 'I am very well, thank you,' as a measure of the MHCU's affect, it is likely that this data about the affect could be invalid. There are many reasons for the likelihood of the response being invalid. One is that social norms dictate that people prefer to respond with a positive remark when asked how they are. Another is that the MHCU might be reluctant to provide a true response based on previous experiences when asked the same question. Scepticism might be part of the reluctance. A further common reason why the response could be invalid is the MHCU might fear the consequences of relaying the true nature of their affect. The consequences could be that they would be given additional medication or kept under observation. Merely taking what the MHCU says about how they are at face value might be grossly inaccurate.

Furthermore, a premise underlying this assessment – that affect and mood are the same – is incorrect. Affect can be defined as:
- a physical expression of an emotional state
- being short-term and
- caused by specific events.

Mood can be defined as:
- a pervasive and sustained state of emotion
- long term and
- usually caused by non-specific events.

Expression of affect involves facial expression, pitch of voice and use of hand or body movements. Mood could influence a person's perception of the world.

The scope and focus of this chapter are on mental health nursing assessment as applicable to any health care setting in which the nurse encounters MHCUs, such as a general hospital or community-based settings that could be in rural or urban areas. It is thus important to distinguish between mental health assessments, irrespective of the setting of the health care service, and the need to apply an assessment to reach a psychiatric diagnosis.

Assessment for a psychiatric diagnosis

An assessment for a psychiatric diagnosis has clearly defined terms and descriptions which need to be applied cautiously and correctly for the assessment to have diagnostic and treatment validity. The most widely used psychiatric diagnostic classification systems are the *Diagnostic and Statistical Manual of Mental Disorders* DSM-5 (APA, 2013; Morrison, 2014), which has been harmonised with the diagnostic system of the World Health Organisation (WHO), and the International Classification of Diseases (ICD) (WHO, 2018). Some professionals refer to both these classification systems when finalising a psychiatric diagnosis. These systems describe each mental disorder according to diagnostic criteria which in turn are derived from the best available scientific evidence. Mental disorders are then classified into a category, based mainly on:
- The stage of development during which the mental disorder appears, with neurodevelopmental disorders described first and neurocognitive disorders, which appear later in life, described last
- Whether the main symptoms of the disorder are 'internalising' (presenting mainly with emotional and somatic symptoms) or 'externalising' (presenting mainly in behavioural and substance-abuse symptoms).

Nevertheless, worldwide, the DSM classification is mostly used. A need existed for classification that minimised confusion and that created consensus among mental health professionals. Since the categories of the DSM are not necessarily evidence based, a more multidimensional approach was recommended. This means that great weight should be given to the experience and reports of the individual MHCU. The DSM-5 does recommend the use of instruments such as the Level 1 Cross Cutting Symptom Measure (1CCSM). The 1CCSM is a screening tool that asks the MHCU to report on 13 main domains such as depression, anger, anxiety, suicidal ideation and substance use, and consists of 23 questions. This may then indicate the need for further investigation.

It is essential that the cultural context of mental conditions be understood, since this may affect the expression, understanding and course of the conditions. The DSM-5 therefore recommends a cultural formulation interview (CFI) which has been tested for usefulness and acceptability, albeit based on Latin American cultures. It leads the clinician to assess five aspects of cultural formulation, including the cultural identity of the MHCU, the cultural conceptualisation of the distress experienced and cultural features of stress and vulnerability.

In contrast, the WHO Disability Assessment Schedule (WHODAS 2.0), which is used for all illnesses and not only for psychiatric MHCUs, is a 36-itemised, self-administered questionnaire allowing MHCUs to report on their own functioning, including aspects such as mobility, learning a new task and concentration (WHODAS 2.0).

These are the assessment tools that are mostly used. However, in addition, there are a vast number of assessment tools that were developed regarding specific aspects relating to mental health or psychiatric conditions. These range from articles, books and other formats (online material) that disseminate such information. Furthermore, the WHO intentionally implemented the 'mhGAP intervention guide for mental, neurological and substance use disorders in non-specialised health settings (mhGAP)' to advance straightforward mental health assessment and interventions in low- to middle-income countries (WHO, 2010).

Irrespective of the particular psychiatric assessment and diagnostic tool used, valid psychiatric data can be collected within a few minutes or over a longer period. There are two levels of assessment: information gathering during initial contact with an MHCU in order to determine immediate needs; and information gathering over time in order to collect information and form a valid data base. This is for the purposes of developing an assessment from which a differential diagnosis can be made, so that the diagnosis can be used for planning decisions and most significantly, for developing an evolving and compassionate understanding of the client.

Mental health assessment interview

A comprehensive, MHCU-oriented mental health assessment necessitates the construction of a thoroughly planned interview which incorporates more than a question and answer format about psychiatric symptoms. Such planning involves a conversational space wherein the MHCU's lifeworld and accounting regarding mental health or mental illness are made visible.

A complete mental health assessment interview consists of the following three parts:
1. *The MHCU's history.* The natural course of the disorder, including biological factors, the social history and functioning, personal history, previous mental health concerns, mental status, personality and stress factors
2. *The MHCU's mental condition.* Information about the MHCU's present psychological functioning
3. *The MHCU's physical condition.*

These three parts of mental health assessment are not separate entities and it is expected that there will be overlapping information, depending on the course of the interview. Although it is suggested that an interview is planned, the format of the assessment should mostly follow the natural, congruent flow of events as they occurred for the MHCU. 'Planned' thus refers rather to the nurse being clear about all aspects of the mental health assessment that need to be covered.

Furthermore, the mental health assessment report, which the nurse writes, should follow a certain format. This format serves as a tool the nurse uses post-interview to organise the information into a clear, coherent picture reflective of the MHCU's life story.

When interviewing a MHCU for a mental health assessment, a nurse should think of themselves as a 'therapeutic detective' finding the 'facts' (symptoms and problems), and examining the feelings, behaviours and thoughts associated with the 'facts'. This means exploring the mental health concerns of the MHCU in terms of:

- *Frequency*, for example: 'How often do you hear the voices in a day/week?'
- *Duration*, for example: 'When did the voices first start?' If the MHCU cannot remember, ask: 'Do you have any children?' If yes, ask: 'How old is the last-born? How old was the last-born when you first fell ill/heard the voices/had strange thoughts?' If no children, ask: 'How old are you? How old were you when the trouble started?'
- *Context or situation*, for example: 'In what situations are the voices more troublesome/less troublesome?'
- *Content*, for example: 'What do the voices say?'
- *Feelings*, for example: 'How do you feel when you hear the voices?'
- *Behaviours*, for example: 'What do you do when you hear the voices?'

The purpose of exploring each mental health concern in such detail is to reach an informed mental health diagnosis. The diagnostic criteria for most mental health concerns relate to:

- The length of time the MHCU had the mental health concern(s). For example, for a concern related to being depressed the MHCU must have displayed behaviour typical of depression for a period of at least two weeks (WHO, 2010).

- How often the MHCU experiences the symptoms in a day/week. For example, for the diagnosis of major depression the MHCU must experience specific symptoms (such as a depressed mood, loss of interest or pleasure) most of the day and nearly every day.

Without this kind of exploration, it is almost impossible to reach an accurate, applicable diagnosis for which appropriate interventions could be planned. However, not all MHCUs would require as detailed an interview as discussed. The nurse should tailor the interview according to the extent of the mental health concerns of the MHCU (see Table 10.1).

Table 10.1 Information gathered during a mental health assessment interview may be organised in the following way.

Assess the following	Information to be elicited during mental health assessment	Points to consider
Identifying/ demographic	<ul><li>Name</li><li>Sex</li><li>Age</li><li>Race</li><li>Marital status</li><li>Occupation</li><li>Address</li><li>Religion</li><li>Previous admissions</li></ul>	
Main complaint	The key aim of eliciting the **main complaint** of the MHCU is to determine: <ul><li>the biggest concern of the MHCU</li><li>what the MHCU considers to be the actual reason for the consultation/referral</li><li>what the nurse should focus their diagnosis/interventions on in the first instance</li></ul>	<ul><li>What the MHCU says and what the nurse knows about the problem do not always correspond</li><li>Sometimes the MHCU's discussion of the problem sounds realistic, but there is no mention of the real reason for the interview</li><li>If the information was not given by the MHCU, record from whom it was obtained</li></ul> Give a concise exposition of the problem or reason for the consultation or referral. Describe the main complaint and present the problem in your OWN words. Listen to HOW the MHCU presents the problem. Listen to WHAT the MHCU says about the problem.

→

Assess the following	Information to be elicited during mental health assessment	Points to consider

History of present problem	▪ Describe the present symptoms
	▪ State whether change occurred suddenly or gradually
	▪ Name the precipitating stress factor at the commencement of the mental health concern or illness
	   – 'How long have you had the symptom/complaint?'
	   – 'What made you decide to seek help?'
	   – 'What problems resulted in admission to hospital/visit to the clinic?'
	▪ Determine whether there is a relationship between physical and psychological symptoms
	▪ Determine when the symptoms were first noticed, the severity of the symptoms and whether they are always present or occur sporadically
	▪ Determine whether the MHCU obtains secondary gain from the illness
	▪ Determine how the symptoms influence social functioning:
	   – school
	   – work
	   – church
	   – community
	   – use of free time
	   – sexual activities
	▪ Determine the MHCU's sources of support and present strong points
		Give a concise history in chronological order of the development and course of the mental health concerns (symptoms or behaviour) for which the MHCU seeks help.

Biological and/or genetic	As applicable and appropriate regarding the presenting mental health concern(s)	There is evidence to suggest that hereditary factors play a role in mental illness. However, this does not mean that a person with a family history of mental health concern or illness will become ill

Assess the following	Information to be elicited during mental health assessment	Points to consider
Personal history	▪ Developmental ▪ Psychosocial ▪ Personal	▪ This information provides insight into the origin and course of the mental health concern(s) or disturbance ▪ The reason for taking a personal history is to obtain a precise picture and historical perspective of the MHCU's developmental process. This information furthermore helps the nurse to understand the nature of the mental health concern(s) and what they mean to the MHCU. ▪ Finding out about the person's personal history helps to identify factors that have made the person vulnerable to developing mental health concern(s). ▪ The more vulnerability factors are present in the person's history, the greater the likelihood of their becoming ill in times of stress, particularly if the person feels that they the necessary skills to cope with the stress. ▪ Note throughout the interview whether there are spontaneous lapses of memory regarding personal history and whether there are emotions associated with the phase of life: pain, stress, and conflict.
Developmental history		

Prenatal history	Pregnancy and birth:
	▪ abnormalities during birth
	▪ birth injuries
	▪ planned or unplanned infant
	
	Early childhood (birth to three years of age):
	▪ Feeding habit:
	  – bottle-fed
	  – breast-fed
	  – feeding problems	

Assess the following	Information to be elicited during mental health assessment	Points to consider
Early development	▪ When were developmental milestones reached? ▪ Note any indication of unfulfilled needs, separation anxiety, and maternal deprivation ▪ Toilet training: feelings associated with toilet training ▪ Symptoms of behavioural problems: thumb-sucking, tantrums, head-bashing, nightmares, bed-wetting, nail-biting and masturbation ▪ Personality as a child: shy, restless, overactive, withdrawn, nagging, friendly, not interested in sport, play pattern ▪ Early or recurrent dreams or fantasies	
Mid-childhood (3 to 11 years of age)	▪ School history: feelings regarding school, adjustment, sexual identification, relationships, nightmares, phobias, enuresis, pyromania, cruelty to animals and punishment	
Late childhood (puberty to adolescence)	▪ School history: relationship with teachers, specific aptitudes, extramural activities, grades passed; connect problems or symptoms with other school periods ▪ Social relationships: good friends, leader or follower, popularity, participation in gangs or groups, idealised figures, patterns of aggression, passivity, anxiety, antisocial behaviour ▪ Cognitive and motor development: learning ability and motor skills ▪ Learning problems: effect on the child	

→

Assess the following	Information to be elicited during mental health assessment	Points to consider
	▪ Emotional and physical problems: nightmares, phobias, masturbation, enuresis, running away from home, crime, smoking, use of drugs and alcohol, anorexia, bulimia, weight problem, feelings of inferiority	
Adulthood	▪ Occupational history: training for occupation, number of jobs and duration of service, job changes, present job; note ambitions, conflict situations and relationships with authority figures, peer group and subordinates ▪ Social relationships and activities: note intellectual and physical interests, depth of relationships with the same and opposite sex and the duration and quality of relationships ▪ Adult sexuality ▪ Premarital relationships ▪ Marital history: role played by spouse during courtship, age when married, family planning ▪ Attitude to pregnancy and attempts, number of children and ages: note any problems in any area of sexuality. ▪ National service: note any malfunctioning during national service	
Psychosocial history		
Early psychosocial factors	Exploring the psychosocial history can help to determine the person's prognosis. For example, people with a long premorbid history (level of functioning before the onset of the illness) of inadequate social, sexual and occupational adjustment are more	Persistent, negative early childhood experiences may result in the development of a poor self-concept which is not 'strong' enough to weather the stresses of life. A negative self-concept is evident in the early personality of the child, the way they

Assess the following	Information to be elicited during mental health assessment	Points to consider
	likely to have a poorer prognosis than those whose history shows that they fitted in at school, showed no behavioural problems, had friends, got on well with people, completed their education and were able to hold down a job.	perform at school, relate to other people, and behave in social and other situations.
Psychosexual history	▪ From whom was psychosexual information obtained? ▪ Concept of sexuality ▪ Sexual experiences	
Religious background	▪ Type of religion in family ▪ Own involvement	
Family history		
	▪ Composition of the family (note the MHCU's response when the family is discussed) ▪ Physical and emotional health ▪ Genetic hereditary patterns in the family ▪ Economic circumstances ▪ Occupation of parents ▪ Relationships in the family ▪ Parents' personalities	▪ Provide information about family customs, child-rearing methods and present support systems ▪ If the MHCU is unable or unwilling to give information, obtain permission to get information from other family members and sources ▪ The information supplied by the MHCU and that obtained from other sources may differ. The information should therefore be checked with someone

A mental health nurse who requires more or additional information about the MHCU could consult any of the multidisciplinary team members or check laboratory test results (Table 10.2).

Table 10.2 Information required during a mental health assessment and potential sources of this information

	Dr	SW	OT	PT	DT	RN	Psych	Spouse	Fam	Empl	MHCU file	Lab
Reason for referral	✓	✓				✓	✓	✓	✓	✓	✓	
Main complaint	✓	✓				✓	✓	✓	✓		✓	

	Dr	SW	OT	PT	DT	RN	Psych	Spouse	Fam	Empl	MHCU file	Lab
PREVIOUS MEDICAL HISTORY												
Medical conditions + treatment received	✓					✓		✓			✓	
Presentation(s) related to complaints	✓	✓				✓	✓	✓	✓		✓	
CURRENT MEDICAL SITUATION												
Medical/physical condition	✓					✓		✓	✓		✓	✓
Signs and symptoms/psychopathology	✓					✓	✓	✓	✓		✓	
Treatment/medication(s)	✓					✓		✓			✓	
Diet					✓	✓		✓			✓	
HISTORY												
Personal	✓	✓				✓	✓	✓	✓		✓	
Family	✓	✓				✓	✓	✓	✓		✓	
Work	✓	✓	✓			✓	✓	✓	✓	✓	✓	
Marital		✓				✓	✓				✓	
Premorbid personality		✓				✓	✓	✓	✓		✓	
Socioeconomic background		✓				✓		✓	✓	✓	✓	
Cultural or religious beliefs/practices	✓	✓				✓	✓	✓	✓			
Legal matters		✓				✓	✓	✓	✓	✓	✓	
FUNCTIONALITY												
Functioning at industrial/occupational therapy			✓								✓	
Ability to perform physical activities			✓	✓		✓					✓	
Functioning in hospital ward/in community						✓	✓				✓	

→

	Dr	SW	OT	PT	DT	RN	Psych	Spouse	Fam	Empl	MHCU file	Lab
Response to nursing care (hospital/community)						✓					✓	
INVESTIGATION(S)												
Special investigation(s) performed/planned	✓		✓	✓	✓	✓	✓				✓	✓
OTHER												
Differential diagnosis	✓					✓	✓					

Dr: Doctor; SW: Social worker; OT: Occupational therapist; PT: Physiotherapist; DT: Dietician; RN: Registered nurse; Psych: Psychologist; Fam: Family; Empl: Employer; Lab: Laboratory results

A thorough assessment of previous mental health concerns or illnesses could elicit information that has bearing on the current mental health status the MHCU (Table 10.3).

Table 10.3 Summary of information regarding previous concerns and various dimensions that constitute mental health

	Dimensions constituting mental health			
Previous aspects that inform current mental health status	**Emotional/mental/behavioural**	**Psychosomatic***	**General medical**	**Neurological#**
Symptomatology	✓	✓	✓	✓
Type of treatment	✓	✓	✓	✓
Duration of concern/illness	✓	✓	✓	✓
Effect of treatment	✓	✓	✓	✓
Compliance to treatment	✓	✓	✓	✓
Health care facilities used	✓	✓	✓	✓

*Psychosomatic disorders include, but are not limited to, hay fever; rheumatoid arthritis; ulcerative colitis; asthma; hyperthyroidism; gastrointestinal discomfort; recurring colds; and skin disorders.
Neurological disorders include, but are not limited to, cranio-cerebral trauma; convulsions; and tumours.

Assessment of an MHCU's mental status

An MHCU's mental status, irrespective of where the person is at the time of assessment on a continuum of 'normality' or disease, is evaluated mainly by observation. Disease or 'abnormality' is mostly defined by the following criteria: (a) deviance; (b) distress and (c) disability or maladaptive behaviour. Evidence related to these criteria could be on a spectrum ranging between 'normal' and disease (see Figure 10.1) A mental status assessment elicits evidence of functionality or dysfunctionality and assists in the identification of aetiological factors leaning towards psychopathology.

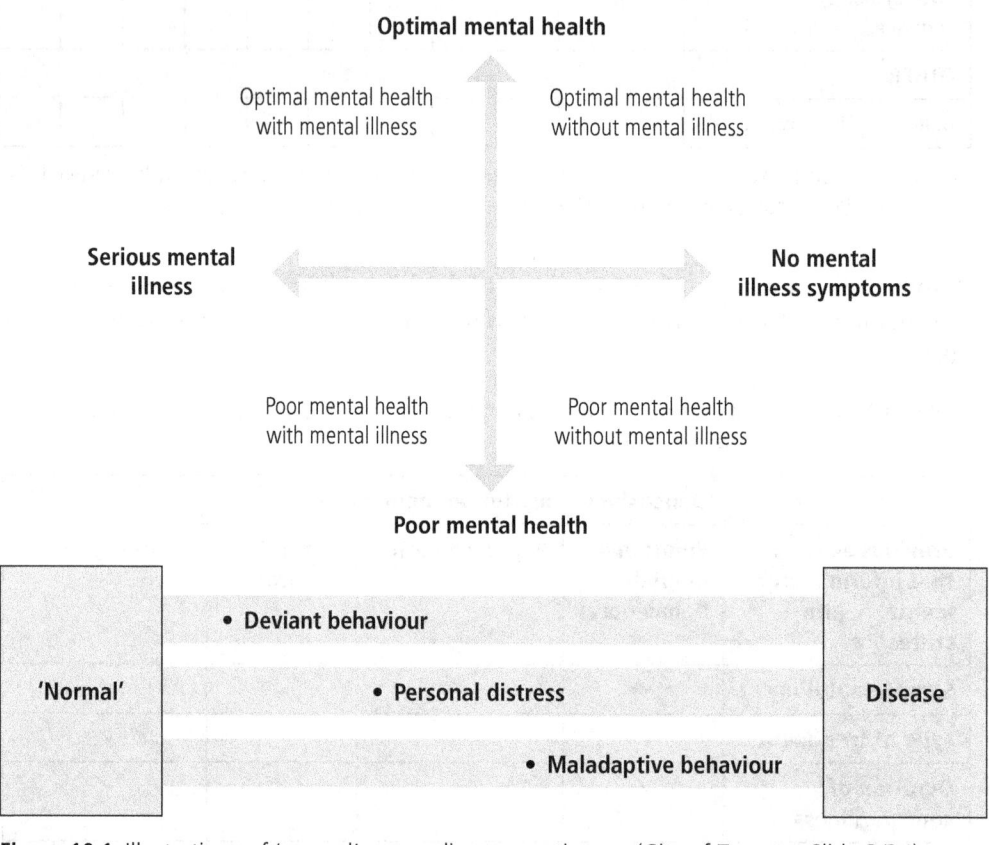

Figure 10.1 Illustrations of 'normal' versus disease continuum (City of Toronto; Slide 3/34)

The success and validity of the information gathered when assessing the mental status of a person is closely associated with the way in which the interviewer approaches the MHCU as the person may regard some of the questions as strange or absurd.

Classification of psychopathology that may be identified during assessment of mental status is shown in Table 10.4.

Table 10.4 Classification of psychopathology

Area	Normal findings	Abnormal findings
General description		
Appearance	Neat, clean	Slovenly, unkempt, neglected, wears excessively bright or dull colours, dirty clothes Anxious, panic-stricken, apathetic, confused, uncomfortable, over-expression of male/female characteristics
	Normal weight for height Normal skin colour	Overweight/underweight Flushed, cyanotic
Conduct, psychomotor activity	Maintains eye contact	Looks at floor, ceiling Mannerisms, gestures, stereotypes, echopraxia, clumsiness, tic, rigidity, wariness, hyperactivity, pugnaciousness
	Normal gait	Unsteady on feet, drags feet, stoops
Speech	Speech can be followed, is relaxed, flowing conversation, logical sequence, clear volume, tone of voice congruent with content of conversation, normal reaction time, adequate vocabulary	Very slow/too rapid Slurred speech, stuttering Too loud/too soft, mumbles Impaired/exaggerated Pressured speech, emotional, monotone, echolalia
Attitude during interview	Cooperative, pays attention, interested, frank	Defensive, hostile, playful, evasive, guarded, seductive, intrusive
Sensorium and cognition		
Level of consciousness	Lucid, alert	Drowsy, confused, stuporous, unconscious, lethargic, in fugue state
	Follows simple instructions	Unable to follow simple instructions
Orientation	Oriented to time, place, person If in hospital, knows length of stay Behaves as if aware of here and now	Disoriented to one/all three areas (time and/or place and/or person)
Attention, concentration	Maintains attention, concentration during interview	Cannot maintain attention, concentration during interview
	Able to do 100–7–7–7 with ease	If too difficult, try simple task: 4×9; 5×4

→

Area	Normal findings	Abnormal findings
Memory	Both short-term and long-term memory good	Short-term and/or long-term memory impaired/absent Impairment concealed by: ■ confabulation ■ denial ■ circumlocution depending on whether registration, retention, recall of memory is impaired
Long-term memory	Data about childhood – important events, neutral information	
Short-term memory	Past few days – What did the MHCU do yesterday? What did the MHCU have for breakfast/lunch/dinner?	
Immediate retention and recall	Ability to repeat six figures after interviewer and, after a few minutes' conversation about something else, to repeat same figures; ask MHCU to repeat your name (level of anxiety and concentration are tested in this way)	
Intelligence	Average/above average	Subnormal/intellectual disability
Note level of formal education, self-education; note ability to function at level of basic aptitude; test ability to calculate; test general knowledge; ask questions about level of education, cultural background		
Affect	Appropriate for situation	Labile, exaggerated, fluctuates during day/interview, depressed, euphoric, anxious, agitated
Thought processes		
Form	Logical, reasonably to the point, clearly understandable, flows comfortably	Autistic, thought block, circumlocution, confabulation, flight of ideas, loose associations, neologisms, perseveration, tangential thought, word salad
Content	Credible, socially and culturally appropriate	Delusions, themes – somatic, ritualistic, destructive, defensive, paranoid
Cognitive processes		
Abstract thought	Capable of abstract thought, explains symbolic meaning of idiom correctly	Concretises, explains meaning of idiom concretely
Insight, judgement	Understands realities of illness/health situation	No/deficient insight into illness/health situation
Perception		
	Correct observation of surroundings	Illusions Hallucinations

Assessment of MHCU's physical condition

A physical examination is performed by the doctor or nurse. Medical conditions, which the MHCU presents with at the time of the physical examination, could be contributing to the mental health of the MHCU. However, some physical conditions could be unrelated to the MHCU's current mental health.

Special examinations

To finalise the mental health assessment and diagnosis it is sometimes necessary to initiate or request one, or more, special examination(s). Investigations typically requested are summarised (Table 10.5) but are not restricted to these tests. Requests for special investigations are defined by the mental health problems presented by the person.

Table 10.5 Special investigations, and professionals who mostly conduct/request investigations during a mental health assessment

Test requested		Psychologist	Social worker	Medical doctor	Occupational therapist
Biochemical	Liver			✓	
	Renal			✓	
	Thyroid			✓	
	Vitamin (B12)			✓	
Endo-crinology	QQ TRH stimulation test			✓	
	Dexamethasone suppression			✓	
Electroencephalographic				✓	
Computer tomography of the brain				✓	
Neuro-psychological	Weschler	✓			
	Grassi	✓			
	Bender gestalt	✓			
Psychometry		✓		✓	
Personality	Rorschach	✓			
	TAT	✓			
	MMPI	✓			
Psychosocial report			✓	✓	
Occupational therapeutic evaluation				✓	✓

The major benefit of requesting biomedical tests is early detection of risk factors or underlying physical conditions related or unrelated to mental health. Furthermore, results produced from conducting these tests allow for more effective treatment, including early discontinuation of treatment if required. Not only will the MHCU benefit physically but the need to investigate social, spiritual, cultural and psychological indicators for the MHCU's condition will be highlighted. These same principles would apply regarding neurophysiological and personality tests even though these tests are not biological in nature. However, no test can confirm, or rule out a mental health condition. A thorough, holistic assessment is required.

ASSESSMENT FORMULATIONS FOR HEALTHY LIFESTYLE FUNCTIONING

Supporting and facilitating healthy lifestyle functioning (or functioning to the best of one's ability within the given constraints and resources) is the aim of mental health nursing. This assessment differs from a mental health assessment in that it is concerned not only with symptoms but also with eliciting information about healthy and unhealthy patterns of lifestyle functioning, and the actual and potential needs which are evident in these patterns.

A lifestyle functioning assessment is an integral aspect of a comprehensive mental health assessment since it is from this data that clinical formulations about social, occupational, family and personal functioning are made. However, MHCU histories are not always taken comprehensively in clinical practice, and this important lifestyle data is frequently summarised in statements like, '…functions reasonably well socially, at work and in the home environment'. While this statement might be sufficient to make a judgement on the inclusion/exclusion diagnostic criterion for social/occupational dysfunction in many of the clinical conditions, it does not provide enough information for a nursing formulation and care plan.

A lifestyle functioning assessment considers the current status and potential needs of the person in each of the patterns making up the lifestyle. This is a very useful framework for a lifestyle assessment.

Major aspects of a lifestyle function assessment include (but are not limited to) considering:
- exercise
- nutrition and diet (incorporating food selection and supplements)
- use of nature as source of healing (incorporating media immersion and hyper-reality, evolutionary, existential and clinical concerns; therapeutic benefits of nature)
- relationships
- recreation and enjoyable activities
- relaxation
- stress management (incorporating self-management skills)
- religious and spiritual involvement (incorporating religion, spirituality, psychological development)
- contribution and service to others (Walsh, 2011).

The question is: what type of information, and rationale for the information, should be elicited about each of the major aspects? Nursing has generally built its theory based on holistic needs or the 'whole person' perspective of the person and of health and illness. In this approach, the person's current health status is understood in terms of the actual and potential biopsychosocial needs of the person and their capacity for meeting those needs. Thus, both needs and coping mechanisms are important types of data for a healthy lifestyle assessment.

ASSESSMENT RELATED TO DIFFERENT CONTEXTS

Mental health nursing assessment takes place in different contexts and while the principles of a comprehensive assessment apply, there are times when the nurse may be inclined to focus in on specific aspects of the MHCU's lifestyle functioning, such as a specific symptom or set of symptoms, or a particular behaviour. There are two approaches that may be adopted either individually or in combination:
1. the MHCU's functioning may be assessed as a whole
2. a specific area of functioning may be assessed.

More detailed and comprehensive assessments predominantly occur in inpatient settings and are frequently conducted by members of the multidisciplinary team, individually or as a group. The clinical psychologist, for instance, might pay particular attention to psychodynamic patterns, while the occupational therapist will concentrate mainly on the way in which the MHCU spends work time and free time. Comprehensive assessment is also an important aspect of care in the outpatient context and particularly for new clinic-based MHCUs.

Table 10.6 outlines the different assessment tools and guides covered in this textbook, which might be used in the inpatient and outpatient context as well as with different population groups.

Table 10.6 Assessment tools and guides used in inpatient and outpatient contexts

	Examples of guides	**Examples of contexts**
Overall functioning	Family stages of caregiving	Chapter 5
	Crisis assessment	Chapters 11 and 19
	Case management comprehensive assessment	Chapter 11
	Washington guide for the evaluation of development of young children	Chapter 17

→

	Examples of guides	**Examples of contexts**
	University of Natal Functional Assessment Scale for outpatients and inpatients	Appendix 2
Behaviour	Alcohol problems	Chapter 15
	Assertive behaviour	Chapter 9
	Violence	Chapter 11
	Functional assessment for psychosocial rehabilitation	Chapter 11
	Suicide	Chapter 13
	Trauma counselling and interventions	Chapter 19
	Hamilton Anxiety Rating Scale	Appendix 7
	Stanford Panic Appraisal	Appendix 7
	Fear questionnaire	Appendix 7
Environment	World Health Organisation (WHO) QualityRights tool kit for mental health care, treatment and rehabilitation facilities	Chapter 11

SPECIFIC, FOCUSED MENTAL HEALTH ASSESSMENTS

In certain instances, it is necessary to obtain information about a specific aspect of the MHCU's mental health status. These instances will be determined by the mental health concern(s) presented by the MHCU. Examples of this type of assessment are:
- Assessing the sleeping pattern of an MHCU who complains of an altered sleep pattern
- Assessing the intake of an MHCU with a problem relating to eating habits
- Assessing aggressive outbursts or any other episodic behavioural problems.

This type of assessment is done by means of a specialised assessment instrument or through incident recording. The instrument in Table 10.7 is an example of a specialised assessment instrument.

Table 10.7 Instrument to assess sleep-related problems

Assessment of sleep-related problems
Interview
Background
1. How long have you had this problem?
2. What were your circumstances when the problem started?
3. What measures have already been tried to solve the problem?
4. What activities do you do during the day?
5. What activities do you do in the evening?
6. Are you on any medication?
7. What could have caused the problem?

Sleep pattern
1. For how many nights a week do you suffer from initial insomnia? How long does it take you to fall asleep?
2. For how many nights a week do you suffer from intermittent insomnia? How often during the night does this happen? How often do you have difficulty in falling asleep again? Judge on a scale of 1 to 10 how difficult you find it to fall asleep again.
3. Judge on a scale of 1 to 10 how rested you feel in the morning.
4. How often do you feel tired during the day because you slept badly the previous night?
5. Specify how insomnia affects your daily life.

Contextual factors
1. What time do you go to bed?
2. Do you wake up with or without an alarm clock and when?
3. Do you have your own bedroom or do you share a bedroom?
4. Do you sleep alone in bed or do you sleep with someone?
5. What are the noise and light levels in your surroundings at night?
6. Do you use your bed for other activities like studying, reading, watching TV or listening to music or the radio?
7. Do you sleep during the day? If so, where and how often?

Cognitive–physiological problems
1. Do you have troublesome or recurrent thoughts? If so, specify what they are.
2. Do you have recurrent dreams or nightmares?
3. Do you experience somatic sensations like a rapid heartbeat, restless legs or muscular tension?

Observations	Night	1	2	3	4	5	6	7

1. Bedtime
2. Periodic observations:
   s = sleep
   a = awake
   r = sleeping restlessly
Remarks
	21:00
	22:00
	23:00
	00:00
	01:00
	02:00
	03:00
	04:00
	05:00
	06:00
	07:00
	08:00							

Incident recording as illustrated in noting sleep pattern 'Observations' at the bottom of Table 10.7 means that a particular type of behaviour, which is the target of interest or treatment, is identified and recorded every time that it occurs. The extent of the problem and the improvement of the condition can be accurately evaluated by establishing how often it occurs. In this way a record can be kept, for instance, of the number of times that an MHCU asks for a painkiller or expresses suicidal thoughts. Incident recording can be performed at home by the MHCU or a family member.

Assessment using a time-to-event chart

A time-to-event chart is a visual representation of the MHCU's mental health concern or illness pattern. In essence, it plots the signs and symptoms of the illness, and associated trigger events, over a period of time. In this way, it gives a longitudinal view of the person's relapse and recovery pattern.

This chart can be used in a number of different situations and it can be adapted to suit the specific kind of information the nurse and the MHCU wish to clarify. It can be used to:

- Plot the onset, duration and recovery periods of the mental health concern or illness. The information may for instance help to distinguish between the depressive disorders and their subtypes.
- Plot specific troublesome symptoms that interfere with daily functioning. For example, a person who is troubled by persistent delusions might wish to monitor the symptom in terms of its onset, frequency, trigger and helping factors, on a weekly or daily basis.
- Plot troublesome side effects associated with medication. For example, a person on lithium might be encouraged to monitor side effects in terms of their onset and relationship to such factors as exercise, salt intake and water consumption.

A time-to-event chart activity can be done at home by the MHCU and family together. MHCUs and family members often have different perspectives on the illness. If they use different colours to complete the chart, differences and similarities can be highlighted, and both can be used as a basis for MHCU/family teaching.

Time–event–symptom chart

This method makes it possible to summarise the MHCU's history (see Table 10.8) on a single page which can then be looked over at a glance. One can see that the MHCU's mental health concerns or illness has been present for nine months; that most of the presenting symptoms are active-phase symptoms which have been present for more than two weeks; that the stresses associated with the university seem sufficiently intense to have precipitated a psychotic episode and that the less stimulating environment of home seems to have helped to reduce the intensity of the symptoms for a while; and that symptoms re-emerged with greater intensity prior to his admission to hospital.

The same chart could be used to map the recovery process until the MHCU returns home. The MHCU and family could be taught to use this method to monitor recovery, and to detect early signs of relapse. Trigger events could also be used as the basis for teaching coping skills.

Table 10.8 Time–event–symptom chart

Event	Time	Symptom
Enrolled for mechanical engineering at the university Academic demands stressful Conflict with roommate	January 2010	
Above events persisted	April 2010	Odd beliefs – people looking at him strangely; suspicious of others, particularly roommate
		Persecutory delusions – food being poisoned; authorities 'out to get him'
		Academic performance deteriorated
Left university and returned home	June 2010	Seemed 'calmer' to parents, but was somewhat socially withdrawn
	August & September 2010	Self-care functioning deteriorated and social isolation increased; persecutory delusion returned – food being poisoned and refused to eat
	October & November 2010	Auditory hallucinations of a persecutory type; grandiose delusions with thought insertion; psychomotor restlessness
Admitted to hospital by parents	End November 2010 (present)	Above symptoms present, along with thought blocking and loosening of associations; loss of weight, appears pale and thin

Monitoring specific troublesome symptoms

Similar to the time-to-event chart, a chart could also be used to plot times that the MHCU experiences an increase or decrease of symptoms.

The example in Table 10.9 shows that the person's troublesome symptom (auditory sound) seems to get worse in situations of conflict and where demands are placed on him to 'do something' constructive. The symptom chart shows that the person does attempt to control the symptoms through withdrawal and quietness. This activity helps but it is not necessarily a long-term solution. The MHCU could be taught to deal with conflict, and both the parents and the MHCU could be taught how to communicate with each other in a more constructive way.

A chart completed by the MHCU could give the most accurate information. However, depending on time constraints, nurses could complete the chart themselves in cases where the information would be less reliable if completed by the MHCU. Alternatively, the MHCU can be referred to a specialist mental health nurse.

Table 10.9 Monitoring specific, troublesome symptoms

Event	Time	Symptom
Had an argument with father about not looking for a job	15/2/2011 8:00	Felt anxious, started hearing funny sounds in the right ear; wandered around the house
Went to buy the newspaper to look for work advertisements	10:00	Felt people were looking at him strangely; couldn't turn the pages of the newspaper; sound in right ear got worse
Went to bed and locked bedroom door	11:00	Sounds became softer; felt a bit calmer
Slept so couldn't take lunchtime dose of medication; woke up when mother came home and had tea with her	11:30– 15:00	Felt calmer but a bit anxious; sound in ear hardly troublesome
Father came home and apologised for shouting at him	17:00	Felt a bit anxious but had a nice supper together

CONSTRUCTING CLINICAL MENTAL HEALTH NURSING FORMULATIONS

Although assessment frameworks guide the data collection process, they do not usually provide a way of interpreting or formulating the data and developing a synthesis of the case. A clinical formulation bridges the gap between assessment description and intervention because it provides a way of understanding why the needs have arisen, how they are linked, what the important issues are and what the possible outcomes of intervention might be for the person's mental and health status. It is very difficult to cross from descriptive data into the realm of interpretation without a guide.

An interpretive guide is generally developed from one or more theories about health and health behaviour and then used, like a bridge, to link descriptions with interventions in a way that provides insight into intrapersonal and interpersonal aspects of the case, and gives meaning to nursing work. Working in an interpretive vacuum means the nurse will have difficulty identifying the common thread running through an MHCU's needs, in succinctly hypothesising why these needs might have arisen, and in identifying the important issues for nursing attention and the anticipated outcomes.

There are many different, equally valid and useful interpretative devices for use in mental health assessment in the vast body of nursing and mental health nursing theory. These can also be found in biological health sciences, social health sciences and other human sciences. Nevertheless, for the purposes of this chapter, consider the stress–vulnerability framework as one explanatory device.

Think about a mental health assessment you have completed for an MHCU. However, this time do it through the interpretive lens of the stress–vulnerability model outlined earlier in the chapter. Illustrate each of the dimensions of this model with data you obtained during your assessment. Try to explain how dimensions are linked, what the important issues for intervention are and how interventions might interrupt the 'unhealthy' links to produce healthier links (Figure 10.2).

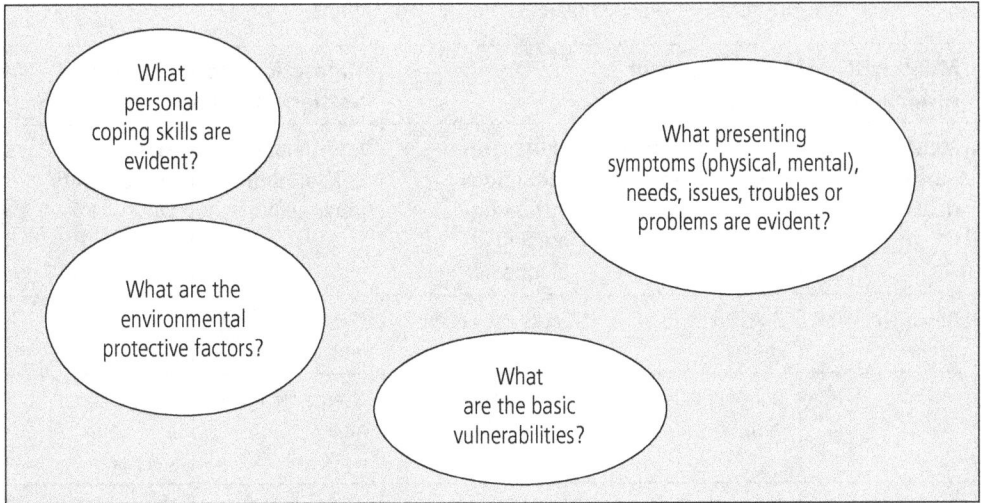

Figure 10.2 Linked dimensions of the stress–vulnerability model

FORMULATING A MENTAL HEALTH NURSING DIAGNOSIS

There is an ongoing debate between researchers in nursing practice and clinical practitioners about the usefulness of a mental health nursing diagnoses. Some argue that the way in which mental health nursing diagnoses are formulated has the potential to fragment, rather than integrate, the nurse's holistic understanding of the client. For example, a list of symptoms and problems, which constitutes a typical biomedical worldview with hypothesised causes, does not paint a holistic picture of the mental health of an MHCU. Neither does this highlight the possible links between the various 'issues' an MHCU is dealing with.

On the other hand, the problem might lie not so much with the concept 'mental health nursing diagnosis' but with the worldview informing the mental health diagnosis.

Mental health nursing diagnoses like, for example, 'overprotected by mother/parents' (see Table 10.10) could be inferred from an interpersonal–behavioural perspective, but also from a psychodynamic viewpoint. Irrespective of the worldview on which a mental health nursing diagnosis is based, actions displayed by the MHCU might be the consequence of overpowering anxiety that renders the person powerless. Bear in mind that separating out mental health nursing diagnoses in this very distinct way (ie, considering the worldview informing the diagnosis) does not identify or nullify the interrelationship between various mental health diagnoses and causes related to these diagnoses. If more than one mental health problem is to be addressed simultaneously their interrelated nature should be the focus of the intervention. Either of the diagnoses (see Table 10.10) is acceptable, provided the interpretation is theoretically sound and does not rely on personal assumptions and opinions.

Table 10.10 An example of a mental health nursing diagnosis of an MHCU with residual schizophrenia who is being treated as an outpatient

MHCU with DSM-5 diagnosis of residual schizophrenia			Theoretical model informing nursing assessment	
Mental health nursing diagnosis	Action informing nursing diagnosis	Explanation for actions informing nursing diagnosis	Interpersonal–behavioural perspective	Stress–vulnerability view
Absence of work behaviour	Does no home chores	Lacks motivation	Overprotected by mother	Environmental stress
	Does not make the bed	Lacks motivation	Overprotected by mother	Personal and environmental stressors
Absence of community involvement	Does not take out own library books	Previous institutionalisation	Overprotected by parents	Neurological/psychological vulnerability
	Does no shopping	Previous institutionalisation	Overprotected by parents	Environmental stress
	Listens to church services on the radio	Previous institutionalisation	Overprotected by parents	Environmental stress

GROUP ASSESSMENT

It may be necessary for a mental health nurse to assess groups of people instead of individuals. In this section special attention is given to three ways in which this can be done.

Genogram for family assessment

A genogram is a diagrammatic, historical 'map' reflecting generations of a family. The preparation of a genogram commences during the first interview with the MHCU. Universally known symbols, typically used by human geneticists and genetic counsellors, are used for the visual representation of facts about the family. The symbols may be viewed as a kind of shorthand understood by all professionals who use genograms as a means of data collection and records of MHCU/family interactions.

A genogram also gives the MHCU and family a visual image of the information that they have already given and information that is still missing. Using a genogram as a method of gathering information enables the mental health nurse to compose a visual image of the MHCU's development, genealogical ('family tree') relationships and present social interaction patterns. It also affords the MHCU the opportunity of giving the nurse further information at a later stage about areas that have already been covered but on which the MHCU wishes to expand. The mental health nurse thus 'draws' the history obtained from the MHCU and keeps the 'map' (visual representation) at hand to obtain more information or to work therapeutically with the MHCU. A genogram can also be used as part of the family assessment (see Figures 10.3a and 10.3b).

Masculine	☐	Death	×
Feminine	○	Divorce	⇥
Marital relationship	—	Separation	⊢
Parent–child relationship	│	Twins (boys)	⬜⬜
Relationship	—	Remote relationship	⊥
Adopted child	△	Intense relationship (over-involved)	∥∥
Pregnancy	⊗		
Abortion	△	Relationship with conflict	∼∼

Figure 10.3a Universal genogram symbols used for people and their relationships (see https://www.edrawsoft.com/genogram/genogram-symbols.php)

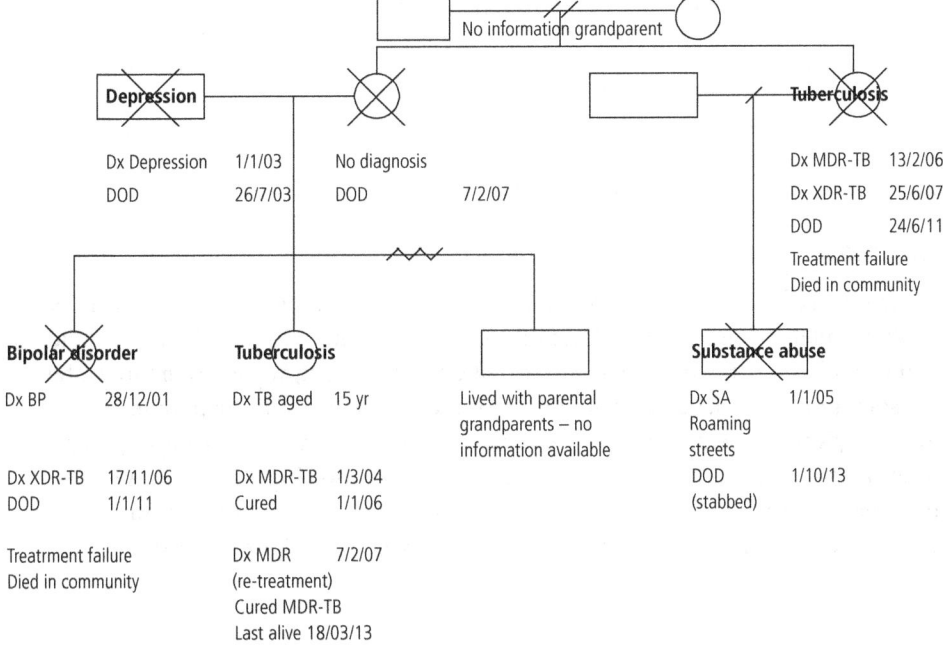

Figure 10.3b Example of genogram

Ecochart

An ecochart (Figure 10.4) is a review of a nuclear family within the context of the world beyond the family, for example in the family's residential area and community. It demonstrates the relationship of the family members with the community and systems outside the structural boundaries of the nuclear family.

An ecochart is particularly useful to a mental health nurse working with a family that has manifold problems. It also serves as a guide for cooperation and the consolidation of services for families. The use of an ecochart alerts a mental health nurse to the possible isolation of a family.

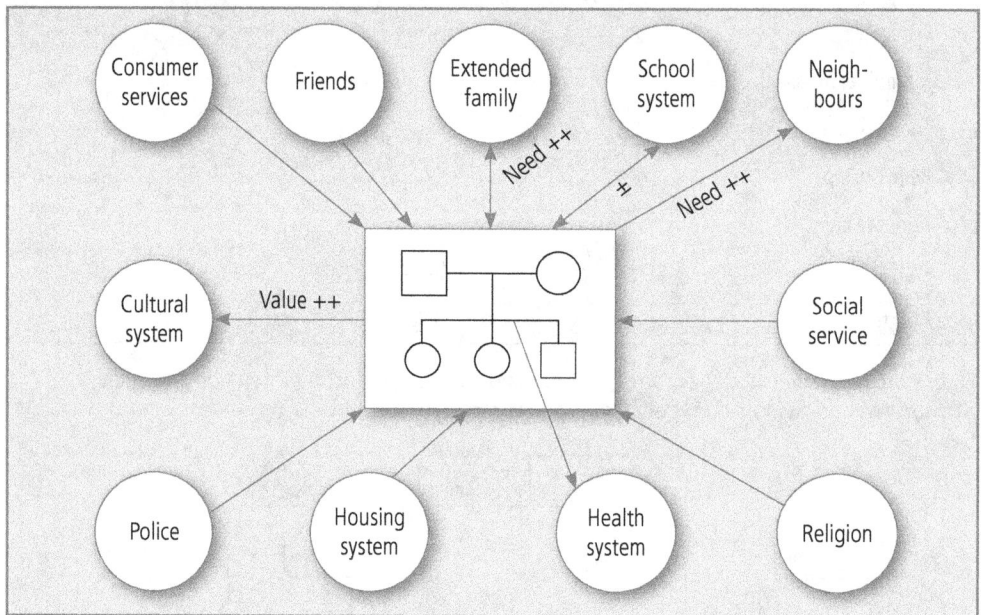

Figure 10.4 An ecochart representing a family

Sociogram

If the members of any one group associate with one another for a period, they will at some stage show interaction patterns. Certain people associate with particular individuals and ignore others. Some people make a great deal of contact, while others make hardly any. A sociogram is a visual representation of the interaction among people.

A sociogram can be drawn up by an observer merely by watching a group of people for a certain period. This is done with the use of the symbols (Figure 10.5a). A sociogram is most useful both in identifying factors that hamper or prevent socialisation and in demonstrating the interaction patterns of specific MHCUs (Figure 10.5b).

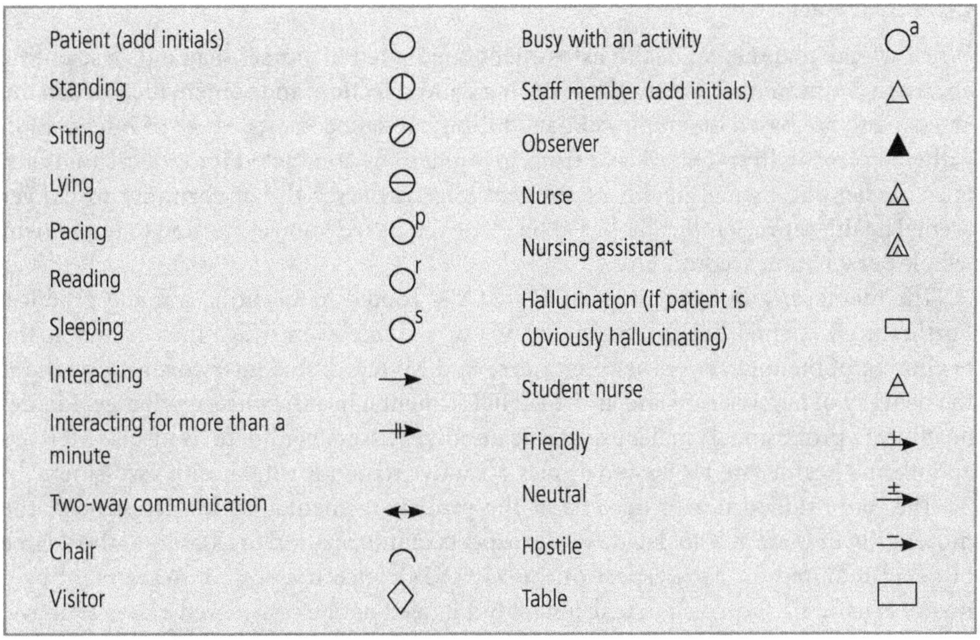

Patient (add initials)	○	Busy with an activity	○ᵃ
Standing	⌽	Staff member (add initials)	△
Sitting	⊘	Observer	▲
Lying	⊖	Nurse	⩙
Pacing	○ᵖ	Nursing assistant	⩙
Reading	○ʳ	Hallucination (if patient is obviously hallucinating)	▢
Sleeping	○ˢ		
Interacting	→	Student nurse	△
Interacting for more than a minute	⇻	Friendly	+→
Two-way communication	↔	Neutral	±→
Chair	⌒	Hostile	−→
Visitor	◇	Table	▭

Figure 10.5a Symbols used in a sociogram

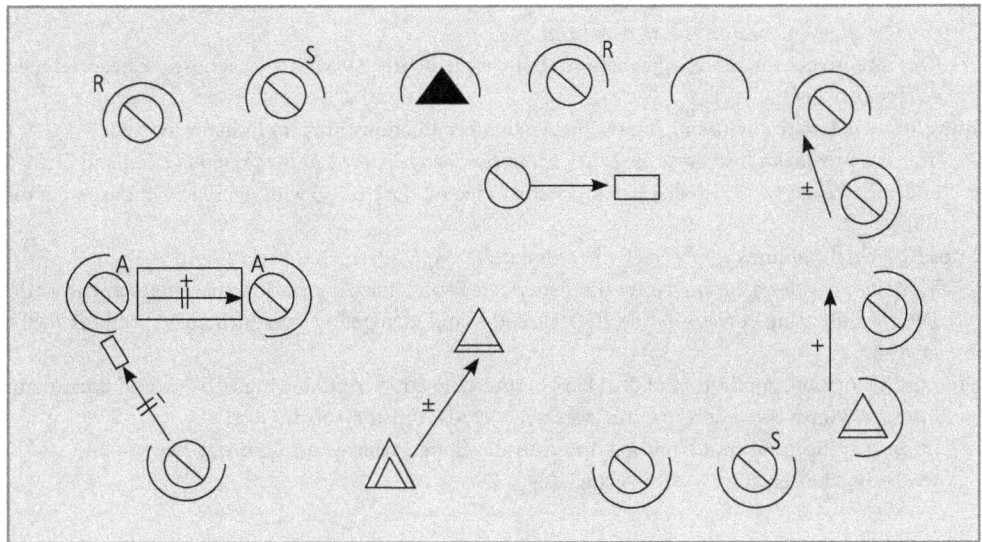

Figure 10.5b Example of a sociogram

CONCLUSION

When we say that mental health assessment conducted by nurses demands a scientific approach, we mean that actions taken during data collection, and content included in the assessment, are based on empirical data. Empirical data consists either of information gathered directly from MHCUs or from investigations conducted into their situations. Such a scientific mental health assessment affords nurses the opportunity to deliver mental health care scientifically, based on evidence-based knowledge, and to implement 'whole person' care accordingly.

The mental health assessment of MHCUs is rooted in scientific nursing practice. Furthermore, mental health assessment is not a single event/stage that occurs at the beginning of the interaction between nurse and MHCU but is interwoven throughout the delivery of nursing care and as the MHCU's mental health concerns change. Mental health care professionals make use of one another's assessment data. Both the MHCUs and mental health care professionals play an active role in mental health assessment.

The more skilled nurses become at the process of mental health assessment, the more easily they are able to decide which aspects of information to assess and the degree of detail required for each aspect of the MHCU's concern assessed. Assessment by a novice is naturally expected to take longer but it need not be considered as less effective.

WEB RESOURCES

http://www.allpsych.com/disorders/dsm.html
> This site gives you more information about each of the DSM-5tm diagnostic categories (see reference below).

https://dhss.delaware.gov/dsamh/files/si2013_dsm5foraddictionsmhandcriminaljustice.pdf
> This site provides a history of the DSM, indicates changes between the previous DSM and DSM-5 and a shortened version of diagnostic criteria based on the DSM-5 with references at the end of the slides.

https://psychiatryonline.org/pb-assets/dsm/update/DSM5Update_October2017.pdf
> This site provides a summary, by the American Psychiatric Association, as a supplement to the DSM-5 indicating corresponding ICD-10 codes and changed versus unchanged sections in the DSM-5.

Find the history and application of the DSM-5, summarised in the following websites and document:
> https://www.psychiatry.org/psychiatrists/practice/dsm/history-of-the-dsm
> https://psychcentral.com/blog/how-the-dsm-developed-what-you-might-not-know/
> ww2.odu.edu/~eneukrug/DSM5/dsm5.doc

REFERENCES

American Psychiatric Association. 2013. *Diagnostic and Statistical Manual of Mental Disorders – DSM-5*. Washington, DC: American Psychiatric Association.

Beckett, J. 2017. 'Evaluating some of the approaches: biomedical versus alternative perspectives in understanding mental health'. *Journal of Psychiatry and Psychiatric Disorders*, 1 (2): 103–107.

City of Toronto. 'Quick Facts. Mental Health in our Workplace'. https://www.toronto.ca/city-government/accessibility-human-rights/mental-health-in-our-workplace/quick-facts/ (Accessed June 2019).

Deacon, B J. 2013. 'The biomedical model of mental disorder: A critical analysis of its validity, utility, and effects on psychotherapy research'. *Clinical Psychology Review*, 33 (7): 846–861.

Morrison, J. 2014. *DSM-5 Made Easy: The Clinician's Guide to Diagnosis*. Guilford Publications.

Seddigh, R, Keshavarz-Akhlaghi, A-A and Azarnik, S. 2016. 'Questionnaires measuring patients' spiritual needs: a narrative literature review'. *Psychiatry Behav Sci*, 10 (1): e4011.

Slide 3/34. 'Chapter 14. Psychological Disorders'. https://slideplayer.com/slide/10425521/ (Accessed June 2019).

Walsh, R. 2011. 'Lifestyle and Mental Health'. *American Psychologist*, 66 (7): 579–592. doi: 10.1037/a0021769.

World Heatlh Organisation (WHO). 2010. *mhGAP intervention guide for mental, neurological and substance use disorder in non-specialized health settings: Mental Health Gap Action Programme (mhGAP)*. ISBN 978 92 4 154806 9.

World Health Organisation (WHO). 2018. *ICD-11 International Classification of Disease for Mortality and Morbidity Statistics (ICD-11 MMS)*. 2018 version. Eleventh Revision. https://icd.who.int/browse11/l-m/en (Accessed June 2019).

World Health Organisation Disability Assessment Schedule 2.0 (WHODAS 2.0). http://www.who.int/classifications/icf/WHODAS2.0_36itemsSELF.pdf (Accessed February 2018).

CHAPTER 11

Mental Health Nursing Interventions

L R Uys and Y Havenga

> **Learning Outcomes**
>
> After studying this chapter, you should be able to:
> - describe the promotive, preventative, curative and rehabilitative nursing interventions applicable to mental health nursing
> - implement all mental health nursing interventions appropriately and evaluate own practice in this regard.

INTRODUCTION

The chapter gives attention to the basic methods that the nurse uses in mental health care, treatment and rehabilitation. This range of methods, once mastered, can be applied to the nursing care of mental health care users (MHCUs) with various psychiatric disorders, or to persons in other health areas, or to life generally. In many ways these methods are not applicable only in a psychiatric setting or only to one diagnostic group.

The previous chapter addressed assessment methods; this chapter addresses intervention methods, commencing with methods related to prevention and promotion of mental health; then care and treatment; and finally, rehabilitation. Interventions for individuals, groups and families will be addressed. As the basic approach is similar, the reader will find the same themes recurring in all the different methods. For instance, the theme of empowering people through teaching is evident throughout the many references to teaching. The methods are not watertight compartments: they flow into one another, and one method is often used with others.

MENTAL HEALTH EDUCATION

Objectives:
- Distinguish between different approaches to and methods of mental health education
- Implement different methods of mental health education to promotive, preventative, curative and rehabilitative mental health nursing.

Education in the promotion of mental health has been recognised as an essential component of nursing care – so much so that Peplau calls mental health nursing an educative and therapeutic process (Peplau, 1952: 9). However, in nursing literature much more is said about the therapeutic role than about the educative role. Mental health education of MHCUs, groups, families and communities to prevent mental illness or to treat and manage their conditions, is one of the most empowering interventions the nurse can implement.

Mental health education has been linked to primary preventative approaches while the concept of psycho-education has been associated with secondary and tertiary preventative approaches. In this section the concepts are used interchangeably, implying that education is provided to MHCUs, groups, families and communities with the goal of preventing mental illness, treating and rehabilitating existing conditions.

Mental health education: primary prevention

Objectives:
- Describe the approaches to primary preventative mental health education
- Describe and implement life skills education.

Promotive and primary preventative mental health education provides individuals, groups and families with knowledge of and insight into all aspects of the promotion of mental health and the prevention of mental illness. The broad aims of mental health education may be set out as follows:
- To enhance the understanding, knowledge and ability of individuals, groups and families so that they are able to manage their daily problems more effectively
- To enhance the understanding, knowledge and ability of the community so that it is able to manage the problem of mental illness effectively and eliminate the stigma of mental illness.

Note: Also read 'Primary prevention' in Chapter 3.

Approaches to primary preventative mental health education

The following are five different approaches to primary preventative mental health education:
1. *Total population approach.* An attempt is made to provide the total population of a particular area with certain information through the mass media. The aim is to bring about a change in the entire community.
2. *Milestone approach.* Individuals are prepared by means of instruction for the maturation crises or the predictable situation crises that await them. They are assisted in finding alternative coping mechanisms and in mastering their feelings.
3. *Gatekeeper approach.* Professional and non-professional groups in a community that have a caring or protective function, such as teachers, community nurses, ministers and police, are taught certain skills. These individuals work with large numbers of people every day and can serve as 'gatekeepers', ensuring early detection and promoting better insight and a positive attitude in the community.
4. *Community or group approach.* A community per se or a group that belongs together geographically (such as factory workers) is the target group for mental health education.

5. *High-risk approach.* The focus is on individuals who run a high risk of succumbing to a particular mental illness. A special teaching programme is prepared for them. For instance, the South African Police Service (SAPS) has been identified as a high-risk group and a teaching programme on stress management has been compiled to help members cope more effectively with stress, thereby maintaining their mental health.

Methods of primary mental health education

Mental health education at the primary level may be given to individuals, groups and communities. Individual and group education can be effective if it is given in an understandable form by means of, for instance, lectures, demonstrations, group discussions, information leaflets, educational videos and even educational theatre programmes. During individual and group education it is important to engage individuals and groups actively rather than following the speech or lecture approach. Behavioural change seldom takes place if people are not given a chance to discuss a matter. The community approach often emphasises the use of the mass media. This approach is more effective when it includes both the high-risk and gatekeeper approaches as well as group tuition.

The life skills approach to mental health education

The teaching of life skills as a way of preventing mental illness has recently received much attention. Of course, this technique is not only useful in terms of primary prevention: enhancing people's competency can also be part of treating them once disorders have already occurred (see 'social skills teaching' in the 'Social skills and learning' section under 'Psycho-education'). However, as a prevention technique it is used in healthy people to enhance their ability to cope with the circumstances and problems of everyday life.

Life skills include all those skills that make it possible for a person to maintain a healthy and well-balanced life. Such a person must be able to:
- recognise and manage their emotions
- identify and acknowledge present and potential difficulties
- recognise the short-term and long-term consequences of their behaviour
- manage stress and negative feelings
- be self-assertive
- solve problems and manage conflict
- make and implement sound decisions
- affirm positive behaviour with self-praise and increased self-regard.

One only needs to think of the many people who come to social services in distress to observe how many of them have a deficiency in one or more of these areas. For example: a young girl comes to the clinic with the symptoms of depression. She tells the story of a series of sexual relations with boys in her school, in search of somebody 'who loves me'. She now has a small baby, and nobody to support her financially or emotionally. She is currently abusing alcohol, both to make her feel better and as a way of seeking a group of friends. Her health is not good and neither is that of the baby, who has been hospitalised for malnutrition. This example shows a series of decisions which are not leading to health and happiness. If she had had more life skills, she might have been able to see the problems more clearly, anticipated the consequences of her behaviour, made different plans for her life, and implemented them. This is the aim of life skills training.

Life skills can be taught through games or educational theatre programmes (ETPs). One such example is the ETP programme for health promotion by Kayser Permanente, one of the USA's largest non-profit health plans. Theatre performances portray scenes about topics relevant to children, such as self-esteem, drug abuse, bullying and sexually transmitted diseases. During these performances by schoolmates or professional actors, questions are asked of the audience regarding, for example, how they would have dealt with a specific problem portrayed in a scene. The principles of active engagement in learning such as using movement, interactive discussion and peer learning are implemented through this ETP (Stevens et al, 2008).

The life skills approach to health education is far removed from what is sometimes called the 'information only' approach. It does not just dish out information, hoping the person will change their behaviour; it focuses on developing skills that will lead to different lifestyles and different life trajectories.

Psycho-education: secondary and tertiary prevention

Objectives:
- Define psycho-education and discuss its importance
- Design and implement an appropriate psycho-educational programme for MHCUs and their family
- Do a functional assessment and facilitate learning of required skills
- Describe the steps in the process of facilitating skills learning and work out a programme for selected social skills.

Psycho-education aimed at MHCUs and their families has been shown to increase their ability to cope with the mental illness and to decrease the possibility of relapse. Sometimes this kind of education is given to an individual patient, often to groups of MHCUs in inpatient settings, and sometimes to MHCUs and their families together on an outpatient basis.

Goals of a psycho-education plan

The goals of a psycho-education plan are to:
- Increase the MHCU and the family's understanding of the condition (for example, schizophrenia), the treatment (for example, medication) and management (for example, symptom management)
- Increase the understanding and cooperation between the MHCU, family and service providers

- Increase the control of the MHCU and the family over the illness and its trajectory
- Decrease the family's feelings of guilt and anxiety, and increase their self-confidence, leading to a more stable family life.

Psycho-education methods

This type of education should include audio-visual material, short presentations, and much discussion and question time. Use could be made of e-learning platforms, social media and other online discussion platforms. Through e-learning platforms MHCUs and families who are far from health services could be reached.

It should be recognised that MHCUs will have a short attention span and may display some side effects, making it difficult for them to sit still for prolonged periods. Anxiety symptoms can also be expected and nurses should accommodate and manage such behaviour.

The nurse providing the education should be a role model to both MHCUs and their families, exhibiting a therapeutic way of dealing with problematic symptoms and behaviour in the group. In this way the process of teaching becomes part of the teaching. A warm, caring and structured environment should be part of every course.

Course content

The following sessions are examples of how a full course in psycho-education could be implemented but should be adapted based on the specific diagnosis and needs of the MHCU and their family:

- *Session 1.* Participants introduce themselves. Provide an explanation of terms used in psychiatry (this gives people a common language to use). Show a DVD or video clip depicting the most common disorder experienced by the participants and discuss this.
- *Session 2.* The adapted psychiatric classification system is explained, together with the main diagnoses in the group and their diagnostic criteria. The MHCUs and their families are encouraged to share experiences of symptoms and diagnosis. Biopsychosocial and stress–vulnerability theories of causality are then discussed.
- *Session 3.* Anxiety, stress and ways of dealing with anxiety are explored. Participants are encouraged to identify their own levels of anxiety and manifestations of these. Families are encouraged to discuss the impact of the MHCU's illness on themselves, and ways of reducing anxiety are explored.
- *Session 4.* Hallucinations and delusions are explained. Participants are encouraged to share their own experiences with hallucinations and delusions, and how they interact with family members during such episodes.
- *Session 5.* Psychotropic medication and the concerns people have regarding their use are discussed. Brain anatomy and physiology are explained and audio-visual material illustrating the work of these medications is presented. Medication categories, side effects and adverse effects are discussed.

- *Session 6.* Symptom management. This is described in the section under 'symptom management and relapse prevention'.

Social skills and learning

Social skills learning is also part of psycho-education. Social skills are learned response components which together comprise a behavioural repertoire that the individual can use in social encounters. Skills are situationally specific, and behaviour which is totally appropriate in one situation, may be inappropriate in another. Those individuals who – as a result of faulty learning experiences or a mental illness – lack particular skills are said to have social skills deficits. These deficits can be identified though a functional assessment and can be remedied by facilitation of social skills learning.

Functional assessments have been used in various contexts such as dealing with challenging behaviour, post injury physical therapy and geriatric care. Functional assessments are done of the physical, psychological and intellectual skills needed by a person to function successfully and be satisfied in his or her unique environment (Cohen et al, 1986a; 1986b). Doing a functional assessment is the first step in the process of rehabilitation and is required as it gives direction to facilitation of social skills learning.

The emphasis of a functional assessment involves an individual being assessed in the context of their environment. A functional assessment is not a general assessment of functioning – in other words, it measures the person's capabilities against the demands of the environment they are in. A functional assessment focuses on tasks a person should be able to perform, such as personal hygiene; the tasks a person would like to perform, like socialising with friends; and the tasks they are required to perform, for example, cleaning and cooking (Rogers & Holm, 2016).

With the development of technology, conducting functional assessments has been enhanced and extended to more persons, even those who cannot readily access health care services. This is through the use of virtual reality, simulators, electronic methods of monitoring (Rogers & Holm, 2016), and even social media platforms.

The process of functional assessment consists of the following steps:
- listing critical skills
- describing skill use
- evaluating skill functioning and
- coaching the MHCU/facilitating learning of the skill (Cohen et al, 1986b).

A social skill is made up of the following components, all of which should get attention in skills teaching:
- *Expressive elements.* These include speech content and paralingual elements such as pace, tone, and pitch.
- *Non-verbal behaviour.* This involves eye contact, facial expression, body proximity/distance and body movements.
- *Social perception.* This has to do with attention and recognising cues.

- *Interactive balance.* This involves response timing, turn taking (waiting your turn and giving others a chance) and social reinforcement (reacting positively to the input of others).

In this context, social skills teaching is discussed with reference to its rehabilitative role. Persons living with mental illnesses such as schizophrenia, bipolar disorder, autistic spectrum disorders and others have impairments of their social skills. This is particularly true of persons who have been treated over long periods by hospitalisation. The person with a mental health disorder is often socially isolated. To reintegrate the person in the social world, it is essential that social skills training be part of the treatment and rehabilitation programme.

In assessing whether an MHCU has a skills deficit, the following questions are helpful:
- Is the MHCU able to initiate and maintain a conversation?
- Can they express feelings?
- Can they get others to respond positively?
- How do they deal with conflict, problems or decisions?

If the answer indicates a deficit, and the MHCU is on optimal treatment for the underlying mental problem, skills teaching is indicated.

The basic steps in the process of facilitating skills learning can be summarised as follows:
- *Identify the skill* to be learned and describe it in behavioural terms. The description must be kept simple; if it is a complex skill, it might have to be broken down into smaller steps. The description of the skill is usually followed by a discussion of why the skill is important or useful. For example: Opening a conversation.
- *Identify essential components.* Ensure that the components of the skill are clear. When skills teaching is done with MHCUs, it is also important to devote attention to the development of correct social perceptions. For instance, an MHCU needs to be able to read non-verbal cues in others accurately. For example: A conversation involves people talking together. People talk about everyday matters, such as what they have been doing, or what others have been doing.
- *Model the skill.* Skills can be modelled in different ways: by role-playing, or by playing a video or audio recording. Such modelling has to be prepared carefully, so that all the correct behaviours are reflected in the example. It is important to give more than one example and to reinforce the important components of the skill. If models are used, they are more effective if they resemble the group members in as many respects as possible, for example: age, gender, status and competence. For example: One group facilitator demonstrates two or three conventional ways of starting a conversation with an MHCU or another professional, for example a greeting and a question about a current event such as soccer results. The different ways of starting the conversation are listed on the board.

- *Rehearse the skill.* Each person in the group should get the opportunity to practise the skill in the group. The person is usually encouraged to choose a situation with which they are familiar and to role play this situation. For example: The person travels by bus to the workshop every day. She is encouraged to turn to the person sitting next to her in the group and to start a conversation as though they are sharing a seat on the bus. She may use any of the ideas listed on the board.
- *Give feedback.* Feedback is given by describing and discussing the behaviour the person displayed during the role play. Other group members are encouraged to identify what was correctly done, and what needs improvement. The role play can be repeated immediately, or a section of it can be repeated. In order to give everyone a chance to practise, the leader might also move to the next person after the feedback. Feedback should always be given in a supportive manner, with clear suggestions for improvement. The feedback should also be specific and focus on not more than one or two aspects of the behaviour at one time. For example:
Leader: What did you think of the conversation Mpo started?
Mary: Well, she looked friendly ...
Precious: She talked too softly. I could not hear her. She should speak up a bit.
- *Give homework.* If participants only practise the skill in the group, they might never transfer the skill to the real-life situation where they need it. They are therefore given a homework task, which requires them to apply the skill in the appropriate environment. This should only follow after reasonably successful rehearsals in the group. For example: The MHCUs are asked to open a conversation with one person each day until the next session.

In setting up a skills teaching and learning group, the group facilitator should remember that the lower the functioning of the MHCUs, the shorter the sessions should be. Short sessions of 30 to 45 minutes each are recommended for MHCUs with serious and long-term illnesses. The group members should be reasonably homogeneous in terms of their social functioning. Preferably, the session should be offered in the language in which group members are comfortable expressing themselves. The optimal number of group members is about four to six members, but this can double with a co-leader. Pace the tempo of the group according to their reaction. They should not feel overwhelmed but must also be kept interested in what is happening.

CRISIS INTERVENTION

Crisis counselling and critical incident stress management (CISM) are important aspects of mental health nursing interventions.

Crisis counselling

Objectives:
- Define and discuss crisis
- Distinguish between the different types and phases of a crisis
- Do a crisis assessment and intervene effectively on the basis of this assessment.

A crisis is characterised by the loss of psychological balance also referred to as disequilibrium. The person's usual coping mechanisms have been unable to re-establish equilibrium, leading to functional distress or impairment (Kneisl & Trigoboff, 2013). A crisis is associated with a 'critical incident' or a turning point which refers to an event outside the person's usual range of experience. A crisis presents both danger and opportunity and does not lead to dysfunction in all cases; every person is unique in their reaction to critical incidents (Hoff, 2009).

All crises are self-restricting and therefore temporary. The emotional discomfort caused by a crisis drives the person to take action to decrease anxiety to an acceptable level as soon as possible. The estimated duration of a crisis is one to six weeks. This is why it should be emphasised that crisis intervention takes place in the short term and is aimed at the solution of the immediate problem. A solution is sought to transform the disturbed state into one of equilibrium. Crisis intervention has been described as a primary preventative measure for post-traumatic stress disorder (Kneisl & Trigoboff, 2013).

A crisis may have one of the following consequences:
- The individual returns to the pre-crisis state. This does not necessarily imply psychological growth, merely a *return to the normal state*.
- The individual not only returns to the pre-crisis state but *grows* as a result of the discovery of new resources and new problem-solving methods. *Lifestyle functioning is better* after the crisis than before.
- The individual diminishes unbearable stress by falling into *personality disorganisation* or *significant impairment of functioning* by presenting for example, with withdrawal, suspicious or depressed mood.

You may wonder why some persons regain their equilibrium and return to a pre-crisis state and others go into crisis. The ability to regain this equilibrium is referred to as resilience. Sources of resilience could be within the person (adaptive personality, problem-solving abilities), relational characteristics (close supporting family relationships) and community characteristics (involved caring people, safety) (Baumgardner & Crothers, 2010). Mental health nurses should assess, uncover and stimulate ways to resilience in individual MHCUs, families and communities (Kneisl & Trigoboff, 2013).

Types of crises

Most sources classify crises into two main groups: situational crises and developmental crises, as described in the following sections.

Situational crises

Situational crises could have a material environmental, personal or interpersonal origin (Kneisl & Trigoboff, 2013). These crises occur as a result of sudden events such as loss of employment or a disaster. These are also known as external crises.

Situational crises can be further subdivided into anticipated, non-anticipated and victim crises, as shown in Table 11.1.

Table 11.1 Situational crises

Type	Description	Examples
Anticipated crisis	The individual experiences a crisis and is partly involved by participation	Starting nursery school, divorce, promotion
Non-anticipated crisis	This is an unexpected crisis; the individual is involved without having been able to predict the situation	Death of a loved one, imprisonment, hospitalisation, diagnosis of terminal cancer, bodily disfigurement
Victim crisis	This is a traumatic event that includes physical aggression and forced action by other individuals or the environment	War, rape, murder, assault, an aircraft disaster, a tornado

Developmental crises

Developmental crises, also referred to as maturational crises, are internal crises and are associated with the normal development stages or life cycle changes, such as the birth of a child, puberty, marriage, retirement and menopause.

Phases in the development of a crisis

One can identify the following four phases in the typical course of a crisis:
1. An individual, confronted with a problem that is threatening, responds with increasing tension. The individual uses the usual problem-solving measures in an attempt to resolve the problem and restore emotional equilibrium.
2. If the usual measures fail and the problem or threat continues, tension and distress increase and the individual feels ineffective. Functioning becomes disorganised and hit-or-miss methods are used to find a solution.
3. If a solution continues to evade the individual, tension rises further and this is viewed as a stimulus to mobilise emergency and new problem-solving methods. The individual may identify with the problem to such an extent that some of the objectives may be abandoned in the process because the individual believes that they are unattainable. The individual may, on the other hand, solve the problem and regain emotional equilibrium.
4. If the individual cannot solve the problem, tension rises above 'breaking point' and the person develops cognitive, emotional and behavioural disturbances (RNAO, 2017).

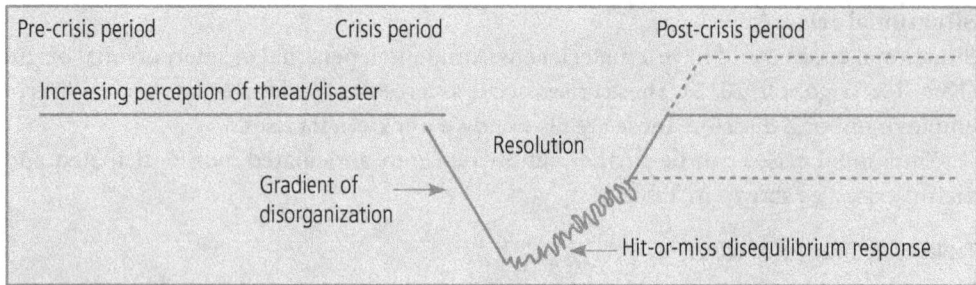

Figure 11.1 Phases in the course of a crisis
Source: Hoff (2009)

Crisis intervention counselling

Crisis intervention is an urgent and short-term acute counselling intervention, close to the event in time and place, and simple and brief to execute. (See also Chapter 19, which deals with people who have suffered trauma.)

Crisis intervention may take place by means of an emergency helpline such as Lifeline or Childline, or by means of counselling from a member of a health service. Special crisis groups may also be established to which individuals or groups in crisis may be referred. Sometimes a natural social group experiences a crisis, in which case the people involved are viewed as a group. Examples are a family in the process of divorce, a group of people who work together and who lose a colleague through suicide, and a community after a natural disaster.

The long-term goal is to facilitate a return to the previous state or improve functioning. Short-term goals are to facilitate emotional release, generate a realistic plan of action, mobilise resources and prevent potential catastrophe, for example suicide or homicide. Crisis intervention follows a formal process of assessment, planning, intervention, referral (Hoff, 2009) and evaluation. Roberts's model for crisis intervention (2005) has been integrated into the approach to crisis intervention described below. It should, however, be noted that crisis intervention is not a linear process and it may be necessary to move back within the steps and tasks mentioned here as needed by the person. There are aspects that are included throughout the crisis intervention namely assessment, safety and support (Myer, Lewis & James, 2013).

Establishment of interpersonal contact
A relationship and rapport should be quickly established. This should be done by demonstrating the interpersonal attributes and competencies discussed in Chapter 9.

Assessment of a crisis
Assessment is a continuous process during the crisis intervention with the focus differing depending on where in the intervention it is used (Myer, Lewis & James, 2013). Initially there should be an assessment of the immediate risks, dangers and most pressing physical and psychosocial needs. For example, a patient may need physical

treatment and pain management after a physical assault or if they are concerned about starting post-exposure prophylaxis after a rape. The person may want to close bank accounts after a robbery or contact a close family member to retrieve a husband's personal belongings should he have died in a motor vehicle accident.

The following aspects should be included in the assessment (Kneisl & Trigoboff, 2013; Myer, Lewis & James, 2013):

- *Precipitating events.* More than one stressful event puts strains on a person's coping skills and makes them more prone to experiencing a crisis.
- *Severity of the crisis.* The signs and symptoms (such as depression, anxiety, rage and disorganisation) and the degree and duration of the crisis should be observed. The more severe the degree of the symptoms and the duration of the crisis, the greater the disorganisation already present in the lifestyle and the more urgent the necessity is of restoring balance.
- *Response to the crisis.* This should be assessed by considering the physical, emotional, social, academic and occupational reactions to the crisis.
- *Perception of the events.* If the individual has a realistic perception of the events, it allows for the recognition of the relationship between the events and the feeling of stress. Problem solving is then directed at reducing stress and successful resolution is probable. If the individual has a distorted perception of the events, it prevents the recognition of the relationship between the events and the feeling of stress. Efforts to solve the problem are unsuccessful and stress is therefore not reduced.
- *Support systems.* This includes people in the individual's environment who are available and who can be depended on to help resolve the problem. Lack of such support when confronted with a stressful situation may lead to disequilibrium and possibly a crisis.
- *Coping mechanisms.* One generally applies one's coping mechanisms when confronted with a problem. Some people think about the problem or discuss it with someone. Others cry or relieve their feelings by swearing, kicking a door or breaking something. Yet others are able to withdraw from the situation temporarily while they consider the problem.
- *Risk of life.* This includes an assessment of suicide and homicide risk.
- *Balancing factors.* This involves an assessment of the risk and balancing factors (see Figure 11.2).

Balancing factors
- Realistic perception of the crisis
- Social support
- Effective coping and problem-solving skills

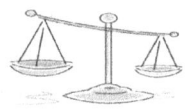

Risk factors
- Intensity of exposure to the situation
- Prior history of traumatic exposure
- Pre-existing psychopathology
- Degree of threat to life
- Coping prior to crisis

Figure 11.2 Balancing and risk factors

Planning and implementation during crisis intervention
Planning and implementation are based on the assessment data and most urgent priorities. Implementation is focused on emotional cognitive and environmental approaches. During the planning and implementation phase of a crisis intervention, dimensions of the problem are explored, feelings and emotions are dealt with, alternatives are generated and explored, and a plan of action is formulated. During this phase the nurse should:
- Listen actively and with empathy to facilitate understanding of what has occurred and the impact of the event and to help identify emotions
- Be direct and supportive and provide hope
- Assist the person to accept reality gradually
- Assist the person to acquire new coping mechanisms
- Assist with decision making and problem solving to encourage self-reliance
- Reinforce newly learned coping mechanisms
- Collaboratively compile a plan of action (RNAO, 2017).

Formal and informal support systems should be mobilised during this phase. These could include family, friends, relevant members of the community, multiprofessional team members and other services, for example the SAPS or relevant legal services.

Evaluation
During the evaluation phase the person in crisis is evaluated in terms of:
- emotional discharge
- perception of the crisis
- connectedness to the support system
- immediate plan of action
- presence of any threat.

Referral is done and a follow-up plan made and agreed on with the person. Table 11.2 provides a summary of tasks during the crisis intervention based on the three phases of a therapeutic relationship.

Table 11.2 Phases and key tasks in crisis intervention

Phases	Key tasks	
Relationship phase	Achieve contact	Establish a rapport and rapidly establish the relationship
	Identify major problem and priority needs	Critical incident assistance is sought for physical, and psychosocial needs
	Assessment*	Assessment is conducted of crisis precipitants, perception of crisis, reaction to crisis, balancing factors, risk factors, risk to life (suicide risk assessment, violence risk assessment)
	Ensure safety*	Physical and psychological safety

Phases	Key tasks	
Work phase	Deal with emotions and provide support*	Facilitate ventilation of feelings Attentive listening Facilitative communication skills
	Address the identified problem	Investigate previous attempts to solve the problem Generate and explore alternatives Collaboratively formulate a plan of action
	Mobilise support system	Formal and informal resources Internal and external resources
Termination phase	Evaluate	Emotional discharge, perception of the crisis, immediate plan of action, connectedness to the support system, threats
	Follow-up and referral	

*Continuous tasks

Source: Adapted from Hoff (2009); Myer et al (2013); RNAO (2017); and Roberts (2005).

Intervention involving CISM

Objectives:
- Define and explain the relevance of CISM
- Describe and implements the components of CISM.

A more comprehensive model has been developed and replaces the term critical stress debriefing. Called CISM, it involves a multitude of crisis intervention techniques that span the crisis continuum from the pre-crisis phase, through the acute phase, to the post-crisis phase, and usually involves more than one session. Critical incident stress debriefing is one component of CISM (Everly & Mitchell, 2000; Kneisl & Trigoboff, 2013).

Debriefing is a form of crisis intervention used with groups of individuals who have experienced a stressful or tragic event and created an opportunity for the ventilation of feelings and sharing of thoughts in a safe and contained environment. It can be used with persons who were raped, or within a school where a learner committed suicide, or in communities where disasters have taken place.

Hospitals are also areas where critical incidents take place and critical incident reactions by staff in hospitals are often overlooked and the management thereof neglected. Sources of critical stress could be managing mass casualties after a motor pileup on the freeway, the brutal assault of a nurse by a psychotic patient, suicide or self-harm of a patient in the ward, the sudden unexpected death of a patient, a patient fall or medication error. One of the authors, who was a student nurse at the time, experienced a psychotic MHCU climbing through a window and falling five stories to his death after she and other nurses desperately attempted to pull him back into the window. After such scenarios the potential for a critical stress reaction is great. Intervention could assist the whole team in debriefing and preventing potentially unhealthy coping mechanisms or decreased functioning in the workplace. Hospitals should have in place critical stress management programmes and teams that are ready to intervene when required (Müller-Leonhardt et al, 2014).

This kind of intervention should take place as soon as possible after the experience. The best time to hold a debriefing session is 24 to 48 hours after the incident. The effectiveness of debriefing diminishes with the passage of time after the event, as the person builds up defences around the memories. Every effort should be made to conduct the debriefing within six weeks of the event.

Debriefing is aimed at allowing the survivors to express their impressions, reactions and feelings in order to reduce their tension. It also allows them to improve their understanding of what happened, and their reactions to it, and to reach closure.

Debriefing goes through the following stages (Mitchell in Blacklock 2012; Mitchell in Pender & Anderton, 2016):

- *The fact stage*. Each person in the group is asked to describe briefly what happened to them during the incident. The sequence of events, and how they came to be where they were, are important elements of this description. The leader can ask a few questions which encourage factual cross-referencing, so that participants get an overall picture of the incident.
- *The thought stage*. Each person is encouraged to describe their first thoughts when the incident happened, and what they saw, heard or felt. These sensory impressions form the basis of the intrusive images and thoughts which may become very disruptive in the post-impact phase. It would seem that verbalising and confronting these memories decrease their power.
- *The reaction phase*. Once thoughts and experiences have been verbalised, the participants are asked to describe their feelings. During this sharing of feelings, the normality of feelings is brought to light. Everyone should be allowed to share their feelings and no one should be interrupted or cut short. No feeling is unimportant or irrelevant. Participants are also encouraged to link their feelings with events earlier in their lives. Questioning participants about the worst part of the experience is important, because post-traumatic reactions are often built up around such events. Feelings of helplessness, frustration, fear or loneliness often surface. The leader should identify people who have suffered a lot, who appear silent or who have extreme symptoms, since they may need additional support later.
- *The symptom phase*. Participants are asked to describe their reactions in more detail. They should identify emotional, cognitive and physical symptoms experienced at the scene and afterwards. Familiar themes are an initial numbness, with feelings only surfacing a day after the event.
- The *educating phase*. In this phase stress is unpacked and effective ways of dealing with stress and a traumatic event.

- *The preparatory and re-entry phase.* In this phase the input of the group is summarised in a way that organises the experience, and normalises it. It is emphasised that reactions are understandable given the abnormal events. It is helpful to outline feelings which participants may experience in the near future, such as being anxious, feeling vulnerable, having difficulty sleeping or concentrating.

Participants should be encouraged to seek further help if their symptoms do not decrease after about six weeks or even increase over time, or if they cannot function at work or at home. It is advisable that a follow-up meeting be planned for the whole group a few weeks later. This follows much the same format as the first meeting, but in less detail.

INDIVIDUAL COUNSELLING

Objectives:
- Distinguish between a counselling and a social interview
- Describe what antecedent and consequent support are, and how these can be shown
- Describe the different phases and tasks of a counselling conversation
- Define and describe constructive confrontation
- Describe how conflict is managed during a discussion.

Counselling is helping a person to analyse interpersonal and intrapersonal patterns in order to understand and improve them. It is an interpersonal process in which one person (the counsellor) facilitates the exploration of a feeling or situation which another person (the counselee) is experiencing.

Characteristics of a counselling interview

A counselling interview has a few characteristics that distinguish it from ordinary social encounters:
- The counselee usually already has a relationship of trust with the counsellor, since people seldom share their concerns with a person they do not know or trust.
- The topic is usually directly related to something the counselee is currently experiencing, and is specific. The counselee provides concrete information and observations. Vague discussions about the past or future rarely lead to change.

To ensure that counselling opportunities will emerge, nurses should build the antecedents of support into relationships; that is, they should make sure that their relationships with people are supportive. This will open the door to counselling should the person need it at a later stage. The *elements of antecedent support* are any action that builds the person's trust in the counsellor, congruence in the counsellor's behaviour over time, availability when the counselee needs the counsellor, and acceptance of the person. Unless these elements are in place, the counselee will probably not choose to talk to the counsellor.

Once the counselling session has commenced, the counsellor should make sure that the *elements of consequent support* are in place, so that the counselee will continue to feel supported and therefore be willing to explore the issues. Consequent support consists of listening carefully so as to understand the person's experiences, recognising the feelings of the counselee and giving accurate empathic responses as soon as these feelings are expressed. The counsellor has to show not only that they are concentrating on what is said, but also that they are beginning to understand; frequent responses will show such understanding. Sometimes it is comforting to touch a person who is expressing such suffering, but this will depend on the person and the context.

There are some responses which are regarded as less effective, since they make the counselee feel *unsupported*. These are the following:

- *The cliché*. A cliché is an automatic response of superficial reassurance, for instance: 'It will be OK', or 'I'm sure he did not mean that!' This comment departs from the counsellor's point of view, could create false hope and the superficiality in this comment will bring to an end the discussion of feelings and interpretations.
- *The 'Band Aid' response*. This is the 'quick fix' response, in which the counsellor reacts to the first mention of the problem by saying 'Why don't you do such and such?' Such a response makes the counselee's problems look trivial, since the counsellor can solve them so easily!
- *The judge*. This is the kind of response, which tells the persons that they are wrong to feel this way or to have done what they did. 'How could you do that!' or 'You should not feel like that!' are typical responses in this category. Once a counsellor has become a judge, it is difficult for the counselee to feel confident that the counsellor respects their feelings.

Phases in a counselling session

A successful counselling session moves through the relationship phase, the work phase and the termination phase.

Relationship phase

The counsellor should establish rapport through a friendly, warm and interested approach. Introductions are done and structure is provided for the session, for example details about the length of the session, frequency and matters of confidentiality.

The counsellor then draws out the counselee and clarifies the presenting problem after which goals for counselling and objectives for the specific session are collaboratively set (Okun & Kantrowitz, 2015).

Work phase

The work phase of the counselling session involves the following:

- The counselee describes the situation and the feelings associated with it, while the counsellor responds in a supportive way.
- The counsellor deals with the feelings first, since the expression of feelings decreases anxiety, which allows for improved problem solving later in the interview. The counsellor deals with feelings by encouraging their expression and description, usually by giving empathic responses for example: 'You are disappointed because you did not pass the subject.'
- The counsellor then encourages a thorough exploration of the situation by focusing on different aspects. The counselee should look again and again at what happened, how it happened, who was involved, what happened before and after, etc. The counsellor tries to help the counselee to see and understand something not understood or seen before. Useful questions may be: 'If you were in her shoes, what would you have thought/done?' or 'What could be another explanation?' or 'What other ways could be used?'
- At this stage of the counselling session it is important to give positive feedback about the strengths the counselee has shown. There should be a focus on what the person did right, or what the strengths were that could build the person up for the challenges that lie ahead. For instance, the following could be said at this time: 'You did not lose your temper, but you rather sought to resolve the issue in a positive way. That is a mature way of handling such conflict situations.' or 'You really have survived enormous hardship. You are clearly a survivor, and that enduring quality is a strength you have.'
- Once the feelings and the situation have been thoroughly explored, it may be appropriate to move into problem solving. The core problem should be distinguished from the peripheral issues, and the counselee should also be encouraged to concentrate on one problem at a time. It is just not feasible to work on a whole series of problems at the same time: one moves mountains by breaking them up into molehills.

The counselee and counsellor then identify which strategies have been tried and they look for different ones that could still be tried. It is not useful to keep on saying things over that clearly have not worked in the past – this just repeats the failure. However, it might be useful to analyse why strategies which looked promising have failed, since that could provide insight into the counselee's own behaviour and may assist with future planning.

One should look at all the options or alternatives, even those which seem impossible. Investigate the implications of each alternative. Does it seem possible to the counselee? If not, do they need additional skills which can be taught, or additional support which can be given? It is important to generate more than one alternative, since that gives the counselee hope. If there seems to be only one option, imagine what the counselee will feel like when that fails.

The counselee is then assisted with choosing an alternative for implementation. A plan is also generated to implement the alternative, and the implementation is encouraged through homework and assignments.

Termination phase

The termination phase is just as important as the first two phases, since poorly managed termination could lead to distress for the counselee. The following tasks are performed in this phase:

- A few minutes before the end of the time the counsellor indicates verbally and non-verbally that the session is coming to an end.
- Time could be spent on summarising and reflecting on the discussion to regain composure, especially if it was a very emotional session (Okun & Kantrowitz, 2015).

In Table 11.3 the phases and key tasks of the individual counselling session are summarised. It is important to note that this is a basic generic structure, which would be adapted based on the theoretical perspectives and strategies used in the counselling session.

Table 11.3 Phases and key tasks for individual counselling

Phases	Key tasks
Relationship phase	Establish rapport Provide structure and promote trust Clarify the problem/main concern Collaboratively set objectives
Work phase	Provide opportunity for ventilation of feelings Make use of therapeutic communication skills* Explore the situation and alternative solutions Establish an action plan Highlight strengths
Termination phase	Indicate approaching termination Engage in summary and reflection Follow-up if agreed or referral if required.

*Continuous tasks

Source: Adapted from Kneisl and Trigoboff (2013); Okun and Kantrowitz (2015)

Throughout individual counselling, the counsellor should maintain a neutral stance, by not including their personal frame of reference. Making suggestions that reflects the counsellor's frame of reference is less effective. Comments such as: 'I am happy you chose to leave your girlfriend' or 'One should forgive and forget' are examples of less effective comments reflecting the counsellor's personal frame of reference.

Counselling interviews with specific goals

There are types of counselling interviews which have specific requirements because their goals are more targeted than those of the generally supportive, problem-solving interview. These are dealt with the following sections.

The constructive confrontation interview

This kind of interview has many uses in the work setting, but in terms of therapeutic settings, it is used mainly in the process of getting a person to change their behaviour to taking responsibility for getting help (for example when abusing a substance). This is done by giving honest feedback. Constructive confrontation is a planned intervention by the confronter (counsellor) where growth is facilitated through drawing attention to inconsistencies. It is always for the benefit of the person being confronted, and the hope is that the person will thus obtain insight into the perceptions of others and that this will result in a better insight into the situation, which will lead to change (Okun & Kantrowitz, 2015).

Confrontation is based on genuineness or inconsistencies (Okun & Kantrowitz, 2015). Examples of confrontative statements based on genuineness are (Okun & Kantrowitz, 2015):

- 'It seems as though you change the topic every time we talk about your relationship with alcohol.'
- 'I notice that you often make excuses for your partner's alcohol misuse.'
- 'It sounds as if you think you need to shout for others to hear your perspective.'

Examples of confrontative statements based on inconsistencies are:

- 'On 15 January you said you would go for help, but it is now 11 February and you have not done so.' (Inconsistencies between what the person says and what the person does.)
- 'You tell students to rub pressure parts with soap and water, but research has shown that friction increases the chances of pressure sores.' (Inconsistencies between theory and practice).
- 'You say that you are a poor communicator, but I have seen you being very effective in the women's group.' (Inconsistencies between what you perceive and what the person says.)

The conflict resolution interview

Conflict is not an uncommon occurrence in life. It often happens between colleagues, between friends, between family members and between MHCUs and nurses. It is important that conflict be dealt with in a way that allows for its resolution. If that is not done, conflict either goes underground, where it festers and undermines the relationship or organisation, or it builds into an explosion which is destructive. The first stage in handling conflict is to recognise that it exists, and that it needs attention. Sometimes little flare-ups between people can be ignored and the tension will pass. At other times, because of the people involved and the intensity or duration of their differences, or because of the importance of the issue, what was once a minor problem becomes a more serious clash, and this must be addressed.

There are six steps to managing conflict in interpersonal relationships. The counsellor must facilitate this process. Usually all the people involved in the conflict should be present for these discussions. If this is not done, individuals may be able to rally support outside the group after the meeting, and undermine the decision reached. Meeting with everybody decreases the chances of disinformation being spread, thus fuelling conflict, and increases the flow of correct information between all concerned. In this way different participants in the conflict are also prevented from manipulating facts and people.

The six steps of conflict management are (Johnson, 2014):

Step 1: Each party describes what they want using 'I messages' while the others listen attentively.
Step 2: Each party describes their feelings about the problem leading to the conflict.
Step 3: Each party explains the reasons for their position.
Step 4: Each party tries to understand the others' perspective.
Step 5: Options are developed where all parties are able to benefit.
Step 6: A beneficial agreement is reached.

THERAPEUTIC GROUPS

Objectives
- Explain the curative factors of group therapy as described by Yalom
- Discuss and effectively facilitate therapeutic groups based on the following phases:
  - preparation for the group
  - relationship phase
  - work phase
  - termination phase
- Explain and enhance interaction of all group members during a therapeutic group
- Manage the following dynamics in the group
  - silent MHCU
  - dominating MHCU.

Group therapy is a structured or semi-structured interpersonal process of therapeutic intervention managed by a trained facilitator. The behaviour and emotional responses of the individual members of a group towards one another and towards the group facilitator are used to improve the mental health and manage the mental illness of the group members. Participation in group therapy provides an experience in re-education. It is a learning and problem-solving process in which each individual is involved with their 'own self' and the group is involved as a 'collective self'. The aim is for group members to assist one another in bringing about meaningful intra- and interpersonal change. The vehicle for these changes is interaction between group members that the skilled facilitator should manage (Yalom & Leszcz, 2005).

Classification of groups

There are a number of group classifications, such as open and closed groups, structured and unstructured groups, and heterogeneous and homogeneous groups. Homogenous groups consist of group members with similar characteristics, concerns and experiences. For example, a group of adolescents who experience difficulties with anger management would be homogeneous. A heterogeneous group have limited characteristics in common. Open groups have 'open borders', implying that members may enter and leave the group, yet the group size remains the same. A closed group does not allow new members until a predetermined number of sessions are complete (Yalom & Leszcz, 2005).

Further groups can also be classified by the methods used, as shown in Table 11.4.

Table 11.4 Classification of groups

Classification	Explanation	Example
Didactic inspirational groups	This type of group emphasises the educational experiences of its members and promotes intellectual and emotional changes while reflecting ethical, religious or societal values.	- Alcoholics Anonymous - Reproductive health education - Hospital discharge planning - Diet group
Conversation groups: exploratory, intervening groups	This type of group emphasises the exploration and verbalisation of its members' emotional and psychological problems within the context of their past and present relationships and their interpersonal relationships in the group.	- Personal growth group - Family therapy - Psychodrama - Intensive psychotherapy - Marriage therapy
Activity groups	This type of group uses a particular activity as the structure around which the interaction of the group members is built, encouraging the development of ego strengths and control.	- Music therapy - Play therapy - Exercise group - Reality orientation

Therapeutic factors

Participation in group therapy has a therapeutic effect on group members, provided the following 11 therapeutic factors are present in the group experience (Yalom & Leszcz 2005):

1. *Instillation of hope*. Observing how members progress and overcome their problems gives the other group members hope. Confidence in the therapeutic process is engendered and group members begin to believe that their condition will improve.
2. *Universality*. Sharing experiences and finding that others respond positively lead to the discovery that problems, feelings and behaviour are not unique but are shared by others. This is part of the wider human experience and confirms that the group member is not an exception or 'different', which is a reassuring realisation.

3. *Shared information.* Group members often share important information because they come from similar backgrounds and have had similar problems.
4. *Altruism.* An opportunity to help a fellow group member acts as an important stimulus to an ego that may feel worthless and useless.
5. *Corrective recapitulation of the primary family group.* Group members learn new ways of dealing with unhealthy family relationships that they consciously or unconsciously project on other group members.
6. *Development of socialising techniques.* In the group process social skills are learned in interaction with other group members.
7. *Imitative behaviour.* Role-modelling by the facilitator and other group members with more effective skills enables group members to imitate this behaviour.
8. *Interpersonal learning.* Group members not only learn from one another's life experiences, but also analyse their own feelings and behaviour in the group.
9. *Group cohesion.* A feeling of belonging and empathy for other group members develops and the group becomes an important source of support.
10. *Catharsis.* Emotional insight is gained and expressed through intense emotions during the group.
11. *Existential factors.* Issues like loss and death can be discussed in a safe and contained environment.

It is important for the group facilitator to give thought to how these therapeutic factors can be brought about and to how the group should be facilitated in such a manner that these factors will be optimally used. The group facilitator should enable optimal interaction between group members. Interaction should ideally not only be through the facilitator. Various factors influence group interaction. These factors include mental health conditions, language barriers, previous experiences, power imbalances between the facilitator and the group members, and the ability of group members to concentrate. The group facilitator should address these factors by establishing trust among group members, making sure the position of the facilitator is collaborative, and asking questions that would facilitate interaction for example:

- I wonder what the rest of the group thinks about what Joe has said about…?
- Mapula discussed her difficulties in relationships. Who has had similar experiences or different experiences?

Group leader's tasks

The various tasks for the group leader will be looked at in the preparation, relationship, work and termination phases of the therapeutic group process.

Preparation phase

Meticulous planning is required before a group is started. The following aspects should be covered:

Objectives
The group facilitator decides on the objectives of the projected series of group sessions or single session. The clearer the formulation of the objectives, the easier the planning and evaluation. Objectives may be set for the group and for each individual member.

Selection of group members
Decisions should be made about the selection criteria for inclusion in the group, the number of members to be included, whether it will be an open or closed group and from where the members will be recruited. These decisions are taken in accordance with the needs of the MHCUs, the objectives of the group and the rest of the therapeutic programme.

Group members should be:
- motivated
- willing to take responsibility for their 'problems'
- experiencing problems in the interpersonal domain, for example loneliness or inability to trust
- able to perform the group task
- having problems compatible with the goals of the group, for example, if the group is about dealing with loss, persons who have experienced the death of a spouse, child, parent or divorce should be appropriate for selection (Yalom & Leszcz, 2005).

Creating the formal structure or group composition
The next decision is choosing the method to be followed in the group. Will it be a didactic group, an activity group or a conversation group? This decision is based on needs of group members, goal of the group and expertise of the facilitator. The facilitator should decide whether it is a homogenous, heterogeneous, open or closed group.

Further decisions should be taken about the duration and frequency of the groups and the number of group members. Generally, group sessions last from 50–90 minutes and could meet one to five times per week. In the outpatient setting sessions are usually further spaced but should be no more than a week apart. In the inpatient setting sessions should be held daily.

The ideal size for a group is seven to eight persons. Groups with three to four group members lack group cohesion while large groups lend themselves to more of a lecture format.

Preparation of the group members
It is important to conduct an interview with each member during which the objectives and process (method) are explained and any misconceptions about the group are clarified.

Once the group has been established, the group facilitator is responsible for its maintenance and the achievement of its objectives. The following aspects in the relationship phase are important in this respect.

Relationship phase

During this phase the leader is responsible for establishing the culture and cohesion of the group.

Setting objectives

The group facilitator should facilitate the process of setting objectives and facilitate the group's acceptance of these objectives. An example would be as follows:

Group leader: Today's group is about managing relationships with families after being discharged from hospital. I wonder what you would like to achieve at the end of this discussion.

Ms X: I would like to get ideas from other members in the group on how they deal with the frustrations of being treated 'differently than before' when going home after being discharged from hospital.

Group leader: It sounds as though you would like to speak about how to fit in again with your family once discharged. I wonder if anyone in the group has a similar or a different objective for today's discussion.

Creation of rapport and group cohesion

Rapport should be established to promote open discussion and facilitate optimal interaction between group members. This is done through the introduction of the group facilitator and group members, an explanation of the role of the group and the basic structure to be followed. This includes the number of sessions, duration of these and what would be expected during the group. Ice breakers could be used if applicable and could be incorporated with the introduction. It is important that the ice breakers are related and relevant to the topic of discussion and contribute meaningfully to group cohesion.

In order to build group cohesion, the group leader should show respect, warmth and empathy to all the members and teach them to do the same by example. This is conducive to a safe and supportive environment. The group facilitator should also, at all times, verbally and non-verbally, emphasise the importance of the group by, for instance, always arriving on time for the meetings. The feeling of hope that the group interaction brings about, and of a safe, warm environment, are important elements in group cohesion.

Creation of therapeutic group norms

All groups should have rules by which they function. In an ideal group, the group facilitator helps the members to formulate their own rules to reach their objectives. The group facilitator should not be the one to make and announce the rules. Rather, the group should discuss each problem as it occurs and then make a sound rule to cope with the issue. Below is an example of how a group facilitator can help a group to accept a group norm:

Ms X: I know I should get help, but I'm afraid to discuss my problem with just anyone. The whole town will know in next to no time.

Group facilitator: It sounds as though you are worried that some of these group members might discuss your personal matters with others?
Ms X: I don't want to accuse anyone. I'm just a private person.
Group facilitator: It sounds as though confidentiality is important to enable you to open up in the group. What do the rest of you think?

After a discussion, the group decides that no one may disclose to outsiders anything they hear in the group.

There are a number of important group norms, which the group facilitator should instil in the group as soon as possible. The first is confidentiality, which was discussed in the example above. Secondly, an equally important norm is that the group should not, as far as possible, be leader dependent – the members should talk directly to one another, not through the group leader; they should decide for themselves what they want to talk about and they should give honest feedback to one another. A third important norm is that the members should talk as frankly as possible about their own experiences and, in the fourth place, they should receive self-disclosures with empathy; they should not be judgemental or aggressive. Building such norms is a sensitive matter that requires wisdom from the group leader. Without group norms the group will not be able to survive or function.

Work phase

During this phase the group facilitator facilitates the process to enable achievement of the objectives of the group. Facilitation is based further on the type of group session being held.

Creation of a focal point

If a group is not helped to focus, the members may chat or work quite happily without ever achieving their objective. There are various ways of focusing a group. In an activity group the activity is usually the focal point, and all the group facilitator has to do is to help the members concentrate on a well-planned activity. In a didactic group there are generally clear learning objectives that the group facilitator can highlight. In a conversation group, however, it is more difficult to maintain a therapeutic focus. In such a case, a here-and-now focus is a valuable aid:
Ms E: I find it difficult to get on with women. I enjoy the company of men far more.
Group facilitator: With which woman in this group do you have the most problems?

After a discussion, Ms E's perceptions of a specific female group member and the latter's response to her are analysed. This makes her problem far more concrete than the vague statement in the 'there-and-then' with which she began.

Enhancing interaction between group members
The group facilitator should encourage group interaction throughout the process. This is done by setting the tone for the group, namely building rapport, and setting appropriate rules, for example that group members will treat each other with respect and keep information in the group confidential. Questioning should not be focused on individual dialogues but should be open and encourage others to participate. Encouraging interaction facilitates optimising the use of the curative factors. Disagreements should not be smoothed over but should be used in a constructive manner. Interaction could be facilitated through the use of therapeutic silence, asking open-ended and follow-up questions for example:
- What do the other group members think about what Mr A said?
- I wonder if anyone else in the group has felt this way?
- Mr J seems to disagree with my point about ... I wonder what the other group members think?

Managing the dynamics of the group
The dynamics of the group are the processes that take place between group members and the group facilitator. Group members often display behaviour that threatens the effectiveness or even the survival of the group. The group facilitator should recognise and cope effectively with such behaviour. Examples are a member who monopolises the group, the very silent group member, people who all talk at the same time or arrive late, a member who loses contact with reality or becomes aggressive.

A general rule for managing problem behaviour involves three strategies:
1. Direct the attention of the group to the behaviour and to help the members to set limits themselves for coping with it.
2. A second strategy is for the group facilitator to use modelling to demonstrate how to cope with unacceptable behaviour. An example is to show the members how to respond when a patient describes hallucinations.
3. The group members are encouraged to describe and discuss their response to the incident.

These three interventions should enable the group to cope with most types of problem behaviour.

Working in the here and now
The focus is moved from discussing content to the process and the relationships between the group members. The facilitator must activate the here and now and then illuminate it (Yalom & Leszcz, 2005).

Termination phase
Group members should be assisted with taking leave of one another from the group experience. Members are often very dependent on the group and are resistant to

termination. Feelings of anger, fear, loss and affection should be verbalised and the members should be encouraged to evaluate the entire group experience. The group facilitator should allow enough time for this phase. Tasks that could be performed in this phase to wrap up a session include summarising of the discussion, discussion of group members' experiences of the group and possible follow-up or referral.

Table 11.5 summarises the phases and tasks during therapeutic groups. However, flexibility should be encouraged based on the type of group being held.

Table 11.5 Phases and tasks in therapeutic groups

Phases	Key tasks
Preparation phase	Recruitment of group members Information sharing and preparation of group members Physical preparation of the group venue
Relationship phase	Introduction States objectives and facilitate group acceptance Ice breaker Sets rules/group norms
Work phase	Facilitates group process towards obtaining objectives Encourages group participation* Effective management of group dynamics* Therapeutic use of communication skills* Works in the here and now
Termination phase	Summary Explores experiences Refers and/or explores follow-up

*Continuous tasks

Source: Adapted from Yalom and Leszcz (2005)

MILIEU THERAPY

When reading this section, also refer to Chapter 1 which describes the international history and development of the therapeutic environment.

Objectives
- Discuss the standards and principles of milieu therapy and of a therapeutic environment
- Evaluate therapeutic environments and develop strategies to promote optimal healing in the therapeutic environment.

What is milieu therapy?

The concept 'milieu therapy' is often used interchangeably with therapeutic community, therapeutic environment, therapeutic milieu, and more recently optimal healing environments. Discussions on the essence of what milieu therapy is and whether its efficacy can be measured have led to criticism and questions as to whether this concept has value for future use (Pearce & Haigh 2017; Smith & Spitzmueller, 2016). In literature it is both referred to as a 'treatment' or 'intervention' (milieu therapy) and a context wherein treatment takes place (therapeutic milieu).

In general, milieu therapy can be defined as a treatment that takes place in a flexible, responsive and therapeutic environment designed purposely to encourage positive change, personal growth and development. This treatment takes place in a physical and interpersonal space where people are busy with daily life activities (Espinosa et al, 2015; Smith & Spitzmueller, 2016).

Inpatient psychiatric hospitals are increasingly challenged with creating and maintaining treatment settings that are therapeutic spaces. The once stable inpatient 'community' is now characterised by MHCUs moving in and out more rapidly due to reduced lengths of stay because of funding pressures, managed care and budget cuts. Private psychiatric hospitals are increasingly required to provide evidence of what therapy takes place in the 23 hours when the MHCU is not on the psychotherapist's so-called 'couch'. Furthermore, dependence on psychopharmacology, focus on managing symptoms, disjointed mental health services and shortages of mental health nurses all challenge the practice of milieu therapy. A number of questions arise that require further development and research, namely:
- Is the inpatient setting we currently manage truly a space where MHCUs can recover from acute episodes of mental illness and return to their optimal level of functioning?
- What should the therapy in the inpatient space and time look like and how can it be optimally developed and maintained?
- What constitutes an environment that would promote or, at the very least, not retract from the MHCUs' optimal level of functioning?
- What is the organising framework of milieu therapy and how can it be measured?

Principles of a therapeutic milieu

All inpatient units and institutions in which large numbers of people live together, such as inpatient psychiatric units old-age homes, children's homes and halfway houses, should apply the principles for creating a therapeutic environment or milieu.

Democratisation of the treatment process

The traditional power structure of the treatment environment was based on a strong hierarchy with the doctor at its head. The milieu therapy approach flattens the hierarchy, giving all the participants a voice in decision making; referred to as shared decision making. Shared decision making is based on the principle of respect for the humanity of the MHCU and of acknowledging the patient's autonomy. Shared decision making in mental health care is a challenge as nurses have a responsibility to ensure safety of the MHCU and also to promote autonomy. Allowing MHCUs to make decisions is especially challenging when they present with impaired communication, questionable insight, and when their ability to act in their own best interest is questionable (Beyene et al, 2018).

The ability to make informed and voluntary decisions, also referred to as the capacity to make decisions, should be assessed considering the MHCU's understanding of that which they are consenting to, their ability to appreciate the consequences, their reasoning about the alternatives and communicating a choice (Applebaum, 2007). The mental health care nurse should be able to give information and in a non-judgemental manner, to assess a mental health care user's capacity to make a decision and then be brave enough to promote autonomy if the MHCU evidences the capacity to do so.

Shared decision making requires active participation and collaboration by MHCUs and their families in:
- Sharing information about the MHCU's illness and treatment so that they are then able to take part in decision making with the necessary insight
- Identification of the problems and treatment options
- Consideration and planning of treatment
- Making or deferring decisions.

Group discussions and meetings are used to ensure that everyone becomes a member of the therapeutic team. The MHCUs share responsibility with the staff for their own treatment and that of other MHCUs. The responsibility that they are given is coupled with authority.

Open communication

An essential element of the democratisation of the treatment process is the establishment of open communication channels between staff and MHCUs; staff and staff; and MHCUs and MHCUs. Each person is considered to be an important source of information and therapy and should therefore be fully informed and involved. Secrets are actively opposed.

Group therapy, group discussions, and staff and ward meetings are freely used to achieve this goal. Information is limited to the extended therapeutic team, which includes other MHCUs and families.

Open communication channels and democracy within the therapeutic framework can be very threatening to the staff. These methods can succeed only if the staff are prepared to run the risk of accepting frank communication and to acknowledge their own faults.

Positive staff attitudes

An emotional climate is created largely by the attitudes of the staff. Negative attitudes lead to antitherapeutic behaviour such as rigidity, teasing, withdrawal and the formation of cliques. Karl Menninger was the pioneer of planned interaction patterns as the basis of therapeutic attitudes. He regarded the following as essential (Menninger Clinic & Menninger Foundation, 1982):

- *Flexibility.* Rules and rituals are viewed as a means to an end and not an end in themselves.
- *Active friendliness.* Staff take the initiative in interaction and show special interest in each patient.
- *Passive friendliness.* The MHCUs take the initiative in interaction and the staff respond positively.
- *Casualness.* This is an element of informal interaction to establish a comfortable interaction pattern.
- *Vigilance.* This means constant observation of and sensitivity to change in the MHCUs or situations.
- *Friendly firmness.* This entails a direct, clear approach indicating self-confidence, which, in turn, gives the patient confidence.

Relationships and connectedness are important components of the therapeutic environment for MHCUs (Thibeault et al, 2010) and the mental health nurse should enhance such positive relational environments.

See also the section on interpersonal competence in mental health care nurse–MHCU relationships in Chapter 9.

Work-related activities

In the early days of custodial care, MHCUs were often forced to take part in occupational activities to the advantage of the institution. Some work did have some therapeutic value, but MHCUs were not paid for their efforts. If there are no work-related activities, idleness, boredom and emotional blunting are experienced.

Milieu therapy programmes reinstated work-related activities as part of the therapeutic process. A number of factors contribute to the effectiveness of occupational therapy programmes. First, MHCUs should be able to choose what they would like to do. This enables them to participate in activities that they find meaningful. Secondly, there should be a variety of activities to enable MHCUs to investigate various work-related areas with a view to possible employment at a later stage. Other types of therapy, such as art, dancing, music and educational therapy, are also used to develop social and expressive skills.

Community and family involvement

In the past, institutions for the mentally ill were far removed from the community. The idea was to protect the community against 'disturbed' MHCUs. The MHCUs could spend their whole lives in an institution without ever going beyond its gates. In the era of the therapeutic milieu, attempts are made to keep MHCUs in their 'normal' environment as much as possible to enable them to continue with most of their usual activities while receiving treatment.

Open visiting times are maintained to keep family and friends involved with the MHCUs. Contact by telephone calls and messages are encouraged and home visits over weekends and holidays often take place. The MHCUs are encouraged to use recreational and commercial services outside the hospital and not to be dependent on the hospital for all their free-time activities. The community is encouraged to become involved with the psychiatric hospital and its residents.

Pleasant and safe physical facilities

The physical facilities should be acceptable to the staff, MHCUs, their families and the community. Physical facilities in psychiatric hospitals often leave much to be desired. Important aspects that demand the attention of nurses are the following:
- adequate privacy
- acceptable standards of hygiene
- facilities for work, recreation, socialisation, therapy and safety.

The physical environment can promote or impede normal, healthy behaviour. For instance, a ward in which the radio blares forth all day may foster withdrawal in a sensitive patient. On the other hand, an attractive sitting room with chairs cosily arranged in groups encourages socialisation.

World Health Organisation (WHO) QualityRights tool kit for mental health care, treatment and rehabilitation facilities

The WHO *QualityRights tool kit* enables assessing and improving the quality and human rights of persons receiving mental health care, treatment and rehabilitation in psychiatric hospitals, psychiatric wards in general hospitals and outpatient mental health care facilities. The toolkit is based on the five themes included in the United Nations Convention on the Rights of Persons with Disabilities (WHO, 2012) summarised in Table 11.6.

Table 11.6 WHO QualityRigths tool kit themes and standards

Theme 1: The right to an adequate standard of living	
Standard 1.1	The building is in good physical condition
Standard 1.2	The sleeping conditions of service users are comfortable and allow sufficient privacy
Standard 1.3	The facility meets hygiene and sanitary requirements

Standard 1.4	Service users are given food, safe drinking water and clothing that meet their needs and preferences
Standard 1.5	Service users can communicate freely, and their right to privacy is respected
Standard 1.6	The facility provides a welcoming, comfortable and stimulating environment
Standard 1.7	People are able to enjoy a fulfilling social life
Theme 2: The right to enjoyment of the highest attainable standard of physical and mental health	
Standard 2.1	Facilities are available to everyone who requires treatment and support
Standard 2.2	The facility has skilled staff and provides good-quality mental health services
Standard 2.3	Treatment, psychosocial rehabilitation and links to support networks and other services are elements of a recovery plan driven by service users and contribute to a service user's ability to live independently in the community
Standard 2.4	Psychotropic medication is available, affordable and used appropriately
Standard 2.5	Adequate services are available for general and reproductive health
Theme 3: The right to exercise legal capacity and the right to personal liberty and the security of person	
Standard 3.1	Service users' preferences regarding the place and form of treatment are always a priority
Standard 3.2	Procedures and safeguards are in place to prevent detention and treatment without free and informed consent
Standard 3.3	Service users can exercise their legal capacity and are given the support they may require to exercise their legal capacity
Standard 3.4	Service users have the right to confidentiality and access to their personal health information
Theme 4: Freedom from torture or cruel, inhuman or degrading treatment or punishment and from exploitation, violence and abuse.	
Standard 4.1	Service users have the right to be free from verbal, mental, physical and sexual abuse and physical and emotional neglect
Standard 4.2	Alternative methods are used in place of seclusion and restraint as means of de-escalating potential crises
Standard 4.3	Electroconvulsive therapy, psychosurgery and other medical procedures that may have permanent or irreversible effects, whether performed at the facility or referred to another facility, must not be abused and can be administered only with the free and informed consent of the service user
Standard 4.4	No service user is subjected to medical or scientific experimentation without their informed consent
Standard 4.5	Safeguards are in place to prevent torture or cruel, unhuman or degrading treatment and other forms of ill-treatment and abuse

Theme 5: The right to live independently and be included in the community	
Standard 5.1	Service users are supported in gaining access to a place to live and have the financial resources necessary to live in the community
Standard 5.2	Service users can access education and employment opportunities
Standard 5.3	The right of service users to participate in political and public life and to exercise freedom of association is supported
Standard 5.4	Service users are supported in taking part in social, cultural, religious and leisure activities

Source: WHO (2012)

The specific criteria for each of the standards are stated in the toolkit and can be accessed online.

Elements of an optimal healing environment

The concept 'healing environment' has been proposed by many in different fields of mental health to replace the much-criticised 'therapeutic milieu' (Mahoney et al, 2009). According to the Samueli Institute, an optimal healing environment focuses on holistic treatment that consists of seven elements summarised in Table 11.7. Note that this approach should still take place within a safe, contained and structured environment.

Table 11.7 Elements of an optimal healing environment

ELEMENTS	EXPLANATION
Building healing spaces	Physical spaces that promote healing by stimulating the senses by using, nature, natural light, colour, fresh air, art, architecture, aroma and music in the physical environment
Creating healing places	Leadership, mission, culture, teamwork, technology, evaluation, and service that is oriented towards intentional healing
Developing awareness and intentions	Mental health care providers who are knowingly committed to being 'healers' Mental health care providers who have knowledge about the biological, psychosocial and spiritual factors related to the MHCU's health A belief in the MHCU's ability to heal
Experiencing personal wholeness	Holistic integration of body, mind and spirit in care, treatment and rehabilitation
Supporting healing relationships	Provision of care, compassion, communication, empathy, and social support for MHCUs and families
Practising healthy lifestyles	Promotion of healthy lifestyles related to diet, exercise, relaxation and work–life balance

ELEMENTS	EXPLANATION
Applying collaborative medicine	Integration of conventional, complementary, traditional, and alternative therapies Interdisciplinary team approach Patient-centred care

Source: Adapted from Jonas and Chez (2004) and Mahoney et al (2009)

Measuring the therapeutic environment

Measures of success in creating and maintaining a therapeutic environment could include (Espinosa et al, 2015):
- patient and staff satisfaction scores
- Ward Atmosphere Scale (WAS) (Rossberg & Friis, 2003)
- number and severity of violent episodes
- number and total time in use of restraint and seclusion
- acuity indicators such as length of stay and numbers of admissions and discharges
- number of psychiatric emergencies
- percentage of staff up to date in training on milieu improvement
- percentage of staff up to date in training on violence prevention and intervention.

Refer also to the section on limit setting, restraint and seclusion in this chapter, which are issues that are related to the therapeutic environment.

HOSPITAL DISCHARGE PLANNING

Objectives
- Define and describe discharge planning
- Outline what hospital discharge planning involves and what the problems are.

Discharge from the hospital is often a crisis for MHCUs and their families. They are confronted with many uncertainties, are deprived of the care team with whom they have become familiar and learned to trust, and they are expected to access a range of care services with which they have not had previous contact.

Discharge planning is an interdisciplinary process that helps MHCUs and families to develop feasible plans for post-hospital care. Although the whole care team is involved, nurses and social workers usually take the lead in the process. Ideally, the outcomes of discharge planning are mutually agreed-upon decisions for the continuation of care.

The foundation of discharge planning is a thorough knowledge of the available resources for care in the community. On this foundation the following elements are built:
- A comprehensive assessment of the care needs of the MHCU, which begins early in the hospitalisation, but is updated as the MHCU's condition changes.

- Involvement of the family or other caregivers. Some MHCUs may not want their families to be involved, but if they are to be involved in aftercare, they have to be involved in the discharge planning.
- The planning has to be interactive and collaborative. The health care team need to bring their input, but enough provision should be made for the voices of MHCUs and their families to be heard.
- Communication is central to the whole process – between team members; the team and the MHCU; the team and the family; and the team and community services.

Usually discharge planning has three stages:
1. *Stage one*. Getting to know the MHCU during the hospitalisation. The information gathering focuses on the functioning of the person, the home environment, the social support and the preferences of the MHCU and family.
2. *Stage two*. Setting a tentative discharge date. Usually a discharge planning conference is held a few days before the MHCU is to be discharged. This conference is attended by the interdisciplinary team in the hospital which has worked with the MHCU, the MHCU and family, as well as central people from the community services who will be involved in future care. With the MHCU's permission, it is important to prepare the caregivers in their support of the MHCU. In a study conducted with MHCUs and their families, preferred preparation for discharge included information about: the MHCU's health status, prevention of readmission to hospital, services for relatives, and signs of relapse (Perreault et al, 2005).
3. *Stage three*. Getting ready for discharge by doing things like arranging for transport, making sure the take-home medications are available, sending the discharge report (DR) out.

The DR is a brief summary of the diagnosis and treatment the MHCU received during hospitalisation, the level of functioning and the discharge plan. It should be sent to the services who referred the MHCU to the hospital for feedback, and to the services to whom the MHCU is being referred for follow-up.

Discharge planning is often not a smooth process; discharge dates get changed, or the decisions are made suddenly without adequate time for stages two and three. Team members might be paternalistic and do not heed the concerns of the MHCU and their families. A major problem in the South African context is often the lack of appropriate accessible community resources, and case management processes so that the family is left to take on too much by default.

SYMPTOM MANAGEMENT AND RELAPSE PREVENTION

Objectives
- Discuss the phenomenon of relapse and the factors related to it
- Describe the process of symptom monitoring and teach it to an MHCU and their family
- Identify and describe strategies to deal with symptoms.

People with severe mental disorders such as schizophrenia and bipolar disorder have an increased potential for relapse. Approximately 40 per cent of MHCUs with schizophrenia relapse within a year after being hospitalised (Csernansky & Schuchart, 2002). These figures seem to be higher in low-income countries. Relapse leads to rehospitalisation with the resultant cost and trauma (Ayano & Duko, 2017).

The risk factors for relapse are listed in Table 11.8. Complete relapse can be prevented if symptoms are identified and managed timeously. Early symptom identification and improvement of functional skills are there for essential in relapse prevention. Families and MHCUs can be taught to identify the symptoms pre-empting relapse.

The process of symptom monitoring and management can be taught to MHCUs and their families by the nurse or another mental health worker. The three steps in symptom management are as follows:
1. Identify the trigger symptoms which are associated with the onset of illness in this particular mental health care user.
2. When the trigger symptoms are present, identify factors which are related to relapse.
3. Develop problem-specific interventions.

These steps will be dealt with in the following sections.

Identifying trigger symptoms

There are different ways in which trigger symptoms can be identified. Professionals sometimes use standardised instruments, such as the Brief Psychiatric Rating Scale, to monitor symptoms at each clinic visit. The findings can then be used to assess the possibility of relapse.

Another way of doing this is to engage with the MHCU and the family about the sequence of symptom increase that preceded a recent relapse, so that warning signs can be identified for future monitoring. The goal is to identify 'marker' or 'trigger' symptoms which are always present when relapse is in progress, but which are not present at other times. For instance, one MHCU reported that he continually hears voices, but he knows that he is relapsing when a particular woman from his past talks to him. Some MHCUs can identify two levels of triggers: the first level consists of symptoms which occur almost weekly, and which they handle through self-regulatory strategies, while the second level occurs only when relapse is imminent and can be dealt with only by getting help. The MHCUs and/or families are asked to monitor their symptoms over time by filling in a rating scale about every two weeks. The rating scale helps the MHCU and/or the family to assess both the presence and severity of symptoms, since some indicators of relapse are the presence of a specific symptom (for example, paranoia) or the increased severity of a symptom that is always present (for example, the voices become too loud to ignore). It has been found that there is a good correspondence between the ratings of MHCUs and those of their families. However, for MHCUs not to see the family's involvement as intrusive, it is important that the process be discussed openly with both the family and the MHCU present, and that agreement be reached regarding what should be done when the 'triggers' are identified.

The nurse should then use the completed rating scales to identify the specific symptom or degree of severity which reliably indicates that the MHCU is in danger of relapse. This decision is crucial.
- The indicator should be sensitive enough to point reliably to all episodes of threatened relapse in time for them to be prevented.
- It should not be too sensitive, so that minor fluctuations lead to increased medication.

The MHCU and their family can then be given a card with the trigger symptoms listed, and asked to check weekly and report to the clinic if any of the symptoms are present at the indicated level.

Identifying factors related to relapse

Generally, relapse is caused by a range of factors, both internal and external to the MHCU. A summary of such factors is given in Table 11.8. It will be noticed that all of these factors describe situations of increased stress, or of decreased support.

Table 11.8 Factors related to relapse

Health	Social/Environment	Attitudes/Behaviour

▪ Poor nutrition
▪ Lack of sleep
▪ Fatigue
▪ Infection
▪ Substance abuse
▪ Lack of exercise
▪ Poor adherence associated with:
  − Medication side effects
  − Complexity of the medication regime
  − Severe lasting psychopathology
	▪ Hostile environment
	▪ Housing difficulties
	▪ Pressure to perform
	▪ Change in life events
	▪ Interpersonal crisis
	▪ Loneliness
	▪ Stigmatisation
	▪ Lack of support
	▪ Financial difficulties
	▪ Transport difficulties
	▪ Weak interpersonal relationships
		▪ Low self-concept
		▪ Feeling hopeless – lack of confidence
		▪ Feeling 'I'm a failure'
		▪ Lack of control
		▪ Feeling overpowered by symptoms
		▪ Poor social skills
		▪ Feeling 'healthy' or recovered
		▪ Limited insight

In each case, the nurse counsels the MHCU and the family to assist them in identifying which factors are playing a role in the increased symptoms. It is important that they identify the factors themselves, and that the nurse does not 'tell them what is wrong'. Autonomy should be encouraged. Honouring the MHCU's self-determination increases their own ability to identify problems and improves their problem-solving ability.

Further therapeutic interventions that have proven to be effective in improving insight, relapse prevention and positive symptom management for MHCUs with schizophrenia are brief cognitive behavioural therapy (Liu et al, 2019) and motivational interviews (Ertem & Duman, 2017). Motivational interviews request MHCUs to change their behaviour based on internal motivation to change ineffective behavioural patterns

(for example taking medication regularly, or abstaining from using harmful substances). An example of such a motivational interviewing process is the intervention by Ertem and Duman (2017) intended to promote treatment adherence by an MHCU with schizophrenia. This motivational interviewing, based on treatment-adherence intervention, was designed with the following goals for each of the six sessions (Ertem and Duman, 2017):
1. Determine and explore the resistance of MHCU's to changing their behaviour.
2. Promote the MHCU's understanding of the symptoms of the disorder, identifying the factors that prevent consistent medication use, evaluating the benefits and side effects of the treatment and addressing the MHCU's indecision in using the medication.
3. Promote the MHCU's understanding of the specific mental illness, evaluating the side effects of the medicines used and weighing the benefits of treatment. By using self-reflection and explorative questions during the interview, awareness by the MHCU is enhanced.
4. Encourage behaviour change by facilitating the MHCU to become aware of the positive and negative effects of past choices and experiences.
5. Enhance MHCU collaboration by evaluating the new choices made by the MHCU towards change and reconfirming and strengthening trust in the therapeutic and professional relationship between the MHCU and nurse.
6. Encourage self-efficiency of an MHCU in maintaining the treatment.

Identifying problem-specific strategies

Early intervention strategies are then necessary to avert the threatened relapse. Usually a temporary increase of medication is needed, coupled with psychosocial strategies to decrease stress and increase support.

The following symptom management categories and strategies are positive promoters of health. They are action-oriented and often involve others:
- Distraction:
  - talking with a friend
  - listening to music
  - prayer
  - dancing
  - meditation
  - watching television
  - working
  - writing
  - going to a nature setting
  - going for a ride or a walk
- Fighting back:
  - positive self-talk
  - positive thinking

- not paying attention to the thoughts
- avoiding situations which increase symptoms
- Help seeking:
  - going to the clinic/hospital/therapist
  - phoning a health care worker
  - seeking the support of a family member
  - contacting a support group
- Attempts to feel better:
  - using medication
  - taking a bath or shower
  - hugging a pillow or stuffed animal
  - using relaxation techniques
  - medication reminders.

The following techniques are not as positive, although they may help the MHCU to remain stable. They do not involve positive action and tend to be passive and reflect the attitude of 'there is nothing I can do'.
- Isolation:
  - going to bed
  - staying at home.

The last category of strategies is negative and should be discouraged at all times. They lead to instability, since the use of self-medication counteracts the positive effects of medication and interferes with positive symptom management.
- Escape oriented:
  - using alcohol
  - using harmful substances.

The nurse and the MHCU and family, if necessary, work out what to do to decrease the symptoms. Many of the strategies are fully under the control of the MHCU, and they can implement them without assistance once they have been taught what to do. However, since decompensation has already started, MHCUs often need support from family, friends and health care providers to implement positive strategies. The longer it takes to identify the potential relapse, the greater the need for support to turn the process around.

The process of symptom management is an essential part of discharge preparation, but the MHCU may not be well enough by the time of discharge to take in the whole process. It might also not be possible to involve the family at that stage, since hospitalisation often takes place far away from where the family lives. This task then falls to the primary health care nurse, who can take a few monthly sessions or a home visit to teach both the family and the MHCU the process of symptom management. This one strategy should make a significant contribution to decreasing relapse and rehospitalisation.

HOME VISITS

Objectives
- Describe the objectives and phases of home visits
- Implement effective home visits and deal successfully with the main problems associated with home visits.

Home visits by a health care provider entail rendering a mental health service to an MHCU and their family in their personal home or within another residential setting such as old-age homes (Canberra Hospital and Health Care Services, 2017). Home visits are mentioned in the nursing literature mainly with regard to preventative health care for new mothers and babies, and for the elderly. In the recent past, it has also become part of the services offered to people living with HIV/AIDS. In the psychiatric literature, home visitation is mainly referred to as part of the assertive community outreach approach to community care. Nevertheless, it is a service approach that has much potential for community mental health care. A study conducted in Iran found that aftercare services, such as home visits, phone calls and psycho-education to family members reduced hospital readmissions for MHCUs with severe mental illnesses, improved general level of functioning and reduced the severity of symptoms related to mental health (Barekatain et al, 2014).

A home visit is usually aimed at gaining an understanding of the MHCU and the family or caregivers as people and their physical, social and emotional context. Having come to such an understanding, the visitor usually assists the MHCU and family to solve problems and access appropriate resources to address their needs. Home visits often also focus on health education to promote the adoption of health-promoting behaviours. Table 11.9 shows the different phases of home visiting.

Table 11.9 Phases of home visiting

Phase of visits	Specific tasks
Relationship phase	Build rapport Complete assessment Set mutual objectives
Working phase	Provide health information Give support Advocate for optimal mental health care and access to health services Engage in mutual problem solving
Termination phase	Make mutual plans for future care Implement referrals and follow-ups.

Source: Adapted from McNaughton (2005)

Because the nurse is visiting the MHCU in a domain where the nurse has no authority, the relationship is more equal than when the MHCU is in the hospital. Byrd (2006) points out that the relationship will only flourish if both the nurse and the MHCU/

caregivers voluntarily provide one another with resources that they each see as valuable. The nurse provides resources such as reassurance, validation, health information, referral and goods like prescribed medication. The MHCU or family provides access to the home, attentiveness, receptivity, the opportunity to interact with the MHCU, and readiness to implement plans or act on advice.

Home visits present a few challenges. First, there may be concerns about the safety of the nurse visiting the home of an MHCU alone where they are subjected to violence (Magin et al, 2008). It is preferable to do home visits with a colleague and to leave when the situation seems unsafe (Kneisl & Trigoboff, 2013). The second major issue is the cost of such a service, especially in a poorly resourced service area like South Africa. A study in Korea (Ryu, 2009) calculated that the average home visit by a nurse costs $US 69.75. In South Africa limited resources such as having no vehicle impacts on the ability to render follow-up services through home visits. To make the service cheaper, non-professionals (community health workers) are often used, but their effectiveness has not been established in the field of mental health.

CASE MANAGEMENT

Objectives
- Define and describe case management
- Distinguish between the different models of case management
- Describe and illustrate the process of case management.

Background

With the reintegration of MHCU's into the community, a need for case management of MHCUs within the community has developed. Case management is relatively underutilised in South Africa and is often used to manage funds of medical aids optimally. Case managers are often found in sub-departments of medical funding companies and those dealing with medical insurance and managed health care services, or they might be found to be working within specific institutions. For example, a private psychiatric hospital may employ a case manager to liaise with funders and to coordinate mental health services within the health institution and among health care providers in the institution.

Case management is necessary because the health and social service systems are fragmented and have limited access, especially for those living in poverty, so that it is extremely difficult for MHCUs to benefit maximally from them. Furthermore, the provision of services is often so expensive that new services cannot continually be created every time a need is identified. It is essential that available services be utilised fully and even be changed to address new needs.

The objectives of case management in its broadest sense are not only to contain costs, but also to ensure that MHCUs with chronic illnesses and complex health needs receive the best quality services available, and that they experience continuity of care and enhanced MHCU and family outcomes (White & Hall, 2006). Case management of MHCUs, if optimally implemented, would imply more than managing services within one institution. It should be implemented across various services, for example in services that have to do with acute inpatient care and long-term community-based care, treatment and rehabilitation. There are various models of case management in psychiatric mental health nursing.

Case management models

The role and workload of the psychiatric nurse as case manager is influenced by the model used. Models are based on the amount of involvement of the case manager. Ernst (2012) describes the following four case management models:

1. *Inpatient model.* This model implies case management from the moment the MHCU enters a casualty or admission ward in a psychiatric hospital. The case manager is a health care practitioner who does the initial assessment, designs the treatment plan and is then responsible for coordinating all services. Typically, such a person would be employed by a hospital.
2. *Continuum of care model.* This model is an integration of individual therapy for the MHCU, assertive community treatment (ACT) and family-centred care. This is done in a process whereby the MHCU family and multiprofessional health team collaboratively design the treatment plan with the main focus of reintegrating the MHCU back into the community.
3. *Broker case management model.* This model requires assessment and referral of MHCUs. The case manager is not directly involved in MHCU care. This model is more often used in a community mental health setting. As the case manager is less directly involved, a caseload of about one case manager to one hundred MHCUs is typical.
4. *Clinical case management model.* In this model the case manager is directly involved in clinical care of an MHCU as the primary health care provider or in a team. This could imply the case manager be available all hours every day of the week. Services could include telephonic helplines and crisis centres. Due to the high level of involvement the ideal caseload is between 12–15 MHCUs per case manager.

Case management models and programmes vary considerably, but they all seem to share the following functions:
- identification of MHCUs and outreach
- individual or family involvement
- assessment of needs, service planning and monitoring
- linking MHCUs to services, health care providers
- multidisciplinary approach
- advocating for service improvement (Ernst, 2012; Kneisl & Trigoboff, 2013).

What constitutes a 'case' can vary from one programme to the next. Although the primary MHCU will be the first responsibility of the professional helper, the 'case' will include the family and significant others when following a family approach. It is impossible to work with the individual separate from their social group in community settings. The case worker will also find families who have multiple problems, of which the identified MHCU is only one. In such instances the whole family becomes the 'case', since the problems and solutions are usually linked.

Various studies have set out to evidence the effectiveness of different case management models. There is some weak to moderate evidence suggesting that case management reduces cost and emergency department visits and that it increases retention of MHCUs in the mental health care system. However, more research is required (Dieterich et al, 2017; Hudon et al, 2016).

The process of case management

The process of case management involves identification and outreach; assessment; service planning; linking of services; monitoring services and advocating for service improvements. These will be expanded on in the following sections.

The identification of MHCUs and outreach

This first step requires that service staff identify the MHCUs to be serviced by the case management programme.
- It might not be possible to give every client a case manager. In this case those clients who have the greatest need of the service must be identified.
- The clients who are in greatest need of the service might not come to the clinic/institution/service. Outreach to where the clients are, and marketing of the programme, are then necessary.

Assessment of MHCUs

This assessment is not the same as an assessment for treatment. In this case the assessment is focused on long-term rehabilitation or support needs and should also follow a holistic approach. The main aspects needing assessment are summarised as follows (Leavitt, 1982):
- ability to perform activities of daily living
- health and medication management skills
- social support and functioning
- financial resources
- residential placement and history
- transportation
- vocational/occupational skills
- service linkages and community resources.

Service planning

Service planning involves devising detailed schemes for meeting an MHCU's needs for assistance.

This includes the following skills:
- clarifying priority areas for services needed
- setting service goals
- choosing service providers
- formulating service plans, which include clear actions to be taken and timeframes for completion.

Linking MHCUs to services

Linking the MHCU to services requires much more than simply referring the MHCU to services such as disability grants, housing facilities and health care services. It includes the marketing of the MHCU to the service, dealing with barriers to service utilisation by the MHCU and negotiating with the service provider to overcome service provider barriers. These barriers might be related to the MHCU's knowledge, emotional function, skills or behaviour. Examples of service provider barriers are limited access for MHCUs (for example, inaccessible service hours), cost, availability of medications, and service provider attitudes.

Monitoring the use and delivery of services

The objectives of the monitoring function are to ensure that the MHCU receives the expected services. If the MHCU is not using this service, or the service is not that which was contracted, the case worker must address these issues.

Monitoring does not involve only telephonic or mail contact but should also include on-site visits while the MHCU is using the service. This allows for first-hand observation, which places the case manager in a stronger position regarding decision making.

Monitoring also includes the aspect of evaluating whether the goals that were set when the MHCU was linked to that service have been achieved, and when the service could be terminated. An added benefit is that it allows the case worker to build up a clearer idea of how the service functions, which is of benefit for future case management.

Advocating for service improvements

It is often not possible to link MHCUs to services because the appropriate services do not exist. In such cases the case manager acts as advocate for an MHCU group in order to improve the level of community services available to them.

Having documented the problem, the case manager has to mobilise action groups, which are core groups of key people committed to solving the problems. These groups should not only include professionals; it is essential that the community at large and consumers of the services or potential services be involved from a very early stage.

Having identified potential action group members, the case worker makes individual plans to involve the groups/individuals. This could be by means of a personal meeting, or a larger group could be brought together, or open invitations could be extended.

The action group then plans the advocacy campaign. Planning a campaign involves the usual steps of setting an overall goal, setting objectives and designing action steps to be taken in order to reach the objectives. Advocacy activities include meetings, writing letters and proposals, building coalitions, demonstrations, petitions, media coverage and investigative research.

LIMIT SETTING

Objectives
- Define limit setting and indicate why it may be used in psychiatric care
- Discuss ways of setting limits as part of a therapeutic environment.

Limit setting can be defined as verbally setting clear limits to behaviour that is acceptable, without relinquishing empathetic, sensitive responsiveness to the cues of the other person. McLean and Nathan (2007) stated that limit setting is authoritative without being forceful or intimidating. The need for something is stated and agreement is sought from the other person (MHCU) that this is indeed essential. It is not just a response to problem behaviour, but is also a means of providing structure and guidance which enhance security and consistent expectation (Sharrock & Rickard, 2002).

Civilisation is characterised by society broadly agreeing on a set of behaviour standards, and usually families, schools and other social institutions are tasked with transmitting these values to the next generation. Society then sanctions the social control necessary to set limits on people's behaviour according to the agreed standards. In health care settings the basic set of behaviours that are enforced through limit setting include the following:
- Staff and MHCUs will be treated with respect.
- The holistic health care needs of MHCUs will be met.
- The MHCUs will comply with reasonable requests from health professionals and vice versa.
- The MHCUs will comply with the usual norms of behaviour, unless their illness makes this impossible.
- The MHCUs will refrain from certain behaviours not considered appropriate for inpatients in a mental health facility, such as using harmful substances or reading pornography.

Setting limits is a strategy used extensively in the therapy of children, but also in other therapy settings. The practice is used for the following reasons (Perez et al, 2007; Vatne & Fagermoen, 2007):
- To maintain or create a safe environment for MHCUs, staff and others

- To make therapy possible, and thus facilitate the MHCU's recovery, rehabilitation, growth and development
- To strengthen self-control
- To allow therapists to maintain attitudes of acceptance, empathy and positive regard
- To prevent waste, such as in the destruction of property.

The following principles should be followed when enforcing selected limits (Sharrock & Rickard, 2002; Department for Health and Ageing, nd):
- Limit setting should be age and context appropriate.
- A friendly, non-emotional tone should be used.
- There should be clarity and simplicity: no mixed messages should be given.
- There should be consistency: no favourites or special exemptions.
- Rationales should be provided: explain why without extensively debating the issue – 'When you … it prevents other MHCUs from resting.'
- Give reasonable choices with consequences.
- With regard to consequences, explain the *natural* consequences of actions. Example: 'If you … then … will happen.'. Enforce *consequences* as soon as possible after the limit has been broken.
- Allow time for responses to happen, especially for the MHCUs who are cognitively challenged and slower in responding.
- Make provision for alternative actions/options/behaviour. Offer more acceptable alternatives to harmful behaviour.

Limit setting is a learned skill and should not be seen as a separate intervention as it is linked to the creation of a therapeutic milieu and is also part of the management of aggression.

DEALING WITH ANGER AND AGGRESSION

Objectives
- Differentiate between anger, agitation, violence, aggression and acting out, and discuss their dynamics
- Discuss factors influencing the potential for violence and assess the potential in an inpatient situation
- Describe and illustrate the process of handling violence
- Discuss the use of seclusion and describe how this can be used in a safe and dignified manner
- Discuss the use of physical and chemical restraint in a safe and dignified manner.

Nurses encounter violence in emergency departments, community health care settings and in inpatient settings. Nurses working in inpatient psychiatric settings and emergency departments are particularly vulnerable to violence (Pekurinen et al, 2017).

Members of the multidisciplinary team working in various health care settings have to be emotionally and physically prepared to deal with violence. Denial is dangerous and under-preparedness can endanger the MHCU, the nurse, other MHCUs, other health care providers, the family and the community.

In this discussion the following definitions apply:
- *Anger* is a common subjective feeling experienced in response to a threat, a feeling of powerlessness or fear (Kneisl & Trigoboff, 2013).
- *Agitation* is a general psychological symptom and is a form of motor hyperactivity that impairs functioning and poses a risk to the safety of self and others (Baumann, 2015).
- *Aggression* is a more general term, referring to behaviour aimed at causing harm. It is a behaviour that leads to the violation of the rights of others. This might be only verbal behaviour, such as an insult, or it might be physical behaviour, in which case it is called violence, regardless whether injury was sustained or if the reason was known (NICE, 2015).
- *Violence* is any physical behaviour which results in injury to self or others or damage to property. It is part of a larger set of behaviours, including acting out and aggression.
- *Acting out* refers to an aggressive type of behaviour which does not include violence, such as verbal threats, cursing, breaking rules, leaving the hospital without permission or self-medicating. It is often seen in inpatients with personality disorders. Acting out relieves the MHCU's feelings of frustration or anger without their actually becoming violent.

In the following discussion, the focus will be on managing aggression and violence. The aim of dealing with violence and aggression in the health care setting, be it the emergency department, inpatient setting or in community settings, should be to prevent violence and to provide safe management of the violence (NICE, 2015). In order to do so, an assessment of various internal and external factors associated with aggression and violence is required.

Factors associated with the risk for aggression and violence

Assessment is part of the management of aggression and violence. It is not possible to predict violence in the long term, that is, to predict whether a particular MHCU will become violent in the future. However, it is quite possible to predict violence in the short term. It is essential that nurses be aware of the risk of violence presented by a specific MHCU at a specific time and within a specific space. Aggression and violence are multifaceted phenomena with internal and external risk factors (NICE, 2015). It is this unique combination of internal and external factors that should be assessed and managed.

Internal factors

The internal factors associated with the risk for violence have to do with causes of violence that are intrinsic to the person; in this case the MHCU.

Internal factors could be history, a medical condition, substance intoxication or withdrawal, a mental health condition or a combination of these factors (NICE, 2015; Rintoul et al, 2009). These factors increase the risk of violence and, should they be present, the MHCU should be regarded as possessing a potential risk for violence.

History

A history of recent violent fights and previous violent convictions is a risk factor for violence (Dack et al, 2013; NICE, 2015). A further factor is associated with childhood history of trauma (Bevilacqua et al, 2012).

Medical conditions

Medical conditions associated with violence include brain injuries, -infections, -lesions, -tumours; seizures, toxic levels of medication, adverse drug reactions, thyroid disease, metabolic imbalances, infection or pain (Garriga et al, 2016; Rintoul, 2009).

Mental conditions

Some mental conditions are associated with a higher risk for aggression and violence due to the person's impaired impulse control, cognitive functioning, perceptual disturbances, social skills and associated agitation. These disorders include personality disorders, psychotic disorders, anxiety disorder, cognitive disorders, bipolar disorder (manic and mixed states), schizophrenia, substance-related disorders, intellectual disability and autistic spectrum disorder (Dack et al, 2013; Garrigaa et al, 2016; Kneisl & Trigoboff, 2013; Lozzino et al, 2015; Petit, 2005; Sadock et al, 2015). The nurse should not use this as an exclusive list as aggression can present in a person, with or without a mental disorder and sometimes the reason might be planned and goal directed for personal gain (Rintoul et al, 2009).

Factors that contribute to violence are, however, not only internal (related to an individual MHCU's characteristics) but are also external and related to the immediate environment of the MHCU.

External factors related to the environment

The external factors are environmental factors that increase the risk for violence. These include staff variables (attitudes and behaviours), unit and hospital structures (physical space rules and procedures) and restriction of freedom (Bowers et al, 2014; NICE, 2015).

Physical environment

A physical environment that restricts freedom and autonomy, such as involuntary admission (Cornaggia et al, 2011; Lozzino et al, 2015), longer hospital stay (Cornaggia et al, 2011), locked doors, inability to go out of the hospital grounds and restriction of relationships with, and contact with, the opposite sex (same sex wards) are contributing factors to violence (Greenwood & Braham, 2018). Furthermore, in these restricted spaces there is limited personal space and privacy (Greenwood & Braham, 2018) and these are triggers for violence. Emergency departments further compound the internal triggers for violence as they are busy, often overpopulated and noisy environments (Rintoul et al, 2009).

Nurse–MHCU relationships
The difficult dual role that nurses fulfil, which involves controlling and caring at the same time, is a trigger for conflict. An example would be a nurse being empathic but also denying certain requests. Nurses' attitudes and their manner of interaction are important factors associated with aggression and violence (Greenwood & Braham, 2018).

Safe management of aggression and violence

Aggression and violence do not occur in isolation, but are part of a process that involves the MHCU, the environment and the staff. The management of aggression and violence requires a graded, multipronged and multidisciplinary approach. Three steps in management of aggression and violence involve (1) anticipation and risk reduction, (2) prevention; and (3) implementation of restrictive interventions (NICE, 2015). These steps are expanded on as follows (NICE, 2018):

1. *Anticipation and risk reduction* require the removal of triggers for violence, violence risk assessment, ensuring a safe environment and optimising the therapeutic milieu.
2. *Prevention of* aggression and violence requires de-escalation and environmental manipulation.
3. *Restrictive interventions* imply physical and chemical restraint, and seclusion.

The process of aggression and violence management is represented in Figure 11.3 with the main focus being risk reduction. Thereafter, prevention methods are applied and as a last resort, restrictive measures are used.

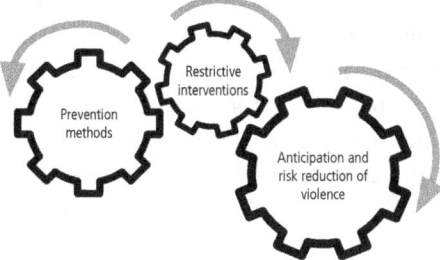

Figure 11.3 The process of aggression and violence management

Source: Adapted from NICE (2015) and Petit (2005).

The process of managing aggression and violence will be applied to the four stages of progression from heightened emotions to violence.

Stage 1: Heightened emotions

During this stage the MHCU shows signs of increased anxiety, anger or irritation. Prevention of further escalation of these emotions is required. The first step in the prevention is early identifications of agitation and aggression.

During this stage the nurse should be on the lookout for the following behavioural cues of heightened emotions shown by the MHCU (Garriga et al, 2016; Kneisl & Trigoboff, 2013; Petit, 2005):

- tension or nervousness
- a hostile mood
- aggressive facial expression
- increased restlessness
- threatening posture and gestures (clenched fists and jaw, staring)
- increased volume in speaking (yelling, swearing, screaming)
- sudden movements
- decreased body distance
- flushed face and neck.

A physical and mental status examination should be done to determine the presence of any internal and external risk factors that require immediate intervention (Rintoul, 2009). Sometimes there is limited time to do such an assessment and at other times a more comprehensive assessment is possible. If possible, in addition to clinical judgement, valid violence risk-assessment tools such as the Broset Violence Checklist (BVC) or the Dynamic Appraisal of Situational Aggression – inpatient version (DASA-IV) could be used (NICE, 2015).

After assessment, de-escalation and environmental manipulation are indicated. De-escalation is the frontline management of aggression and violence, occurring at the inpatient, emergency unit or community clinic. During de-escalation the nurse uses verbal and non-verbal communication to reduce or remove aggression and violence that occurred during the escalation phase (Lavelle et al, 2016). There are many tips regarding how to approach angry MHCUs. These are summarised below. However, it is important to use your own knowledge of the MHCU, the other staff and the ward situation to de-escalate the crisis. The MHCU should usually be given five to ten minutes to calm down. Table 11.10 summarises the approach that should be used in de-escalation.

Table 11.10 How to approach the angry MHCU

Approach Be calm, controlled and unprovocative Be concise Treat with dignity Listen attentively
Posture Present with a supportive posture which speaks of support and not of assault Do not approach the MHCU from the front or behind Stay a little to the side, with arms and hands relaxed and open
Space Do not crowd the MHCU but do not stay so far away that a normal tone of voice is impossible Do not touch the MHCU
Speaking Establish verbal contact The voice should be low and calm, but clear. Do not use profanities and do not shout. Do not challenge the MHCU. Avoid the use of stop words such as 'Okay?' at the end of sentences Use open-ended questions which are more specific, rather than direct questions: 'Do you feel that people have been unfair to you?' rather than 'What is the matter?' Give choices
Safety Ensure that you have enough staff as back-up before approaching the MHCU Do not take the MHCU to a secluded area far away from help Do not wear dangling earrings or other jewellery which may cause grave injury Remove dangerous furniture or equipment from the environment

The nurse should be supportive and to allow verbalisation of feelings. Empathic responses and any other intervention that will reduce anxiety are appropriate, for example: 'You feel angry because your family did not visit today. What is it that you need right now? Let's talk about what you are feeling.' Other techniques are the use of distraction and calming, for example deep breathing and progressive relaxation techniques. During de-escalation, the use of *pro re nata* (as needed) medication may be indicated and should be used safely and with caution (NICE, 2015).

Environmental manipulation should involve identifying anything that agitates or angers the MHCU and addressing these, for example allowing for a decrease in stimuli (loud radios and TV, busy and noisy ward environment), ensuring appropriate staff attitudes or identifying MHCU discomfort. Provide a safe, quiet room with comfortable seating and offer something to drink. Furthermore, any dangerous objects should be removed from the ward. When in a closed space, such as an office, staff should position themselves so that they are able to find an escape route, for example near the door (Petit, 2005). De-escalation is also implemented during the challenge level.

Stage 2: Challenge level

At this stage there are clear signs of aggression. The MHCU challenges the staff and their authority. Verbal aggression is evident, the MHCU looks angry and violates other rights. The MHCU is easily irritated and resists or refuses to follow directions.

At this stage the appropriate staff intervention is directive limit setting. The staff takes control in a situation where the MHCU is losing control, by firmly setting limits to behaviour. This should not be done in a threatening way, but by showing concern and empathy. For example, if the MHCU is becoming too loud, the first step is to let them know why such behaviour must cease. A simple explanation of the fact that the noise is disturbing others is often enough to calm the MHCU down. If not, there is no need to threaten the MHCU into compliance. Instead, point out the fact that they can remain in the area if they quieten down. If not, they will have to be escorted out. In this way the MHCU feels that there is a choice, and the consequences are determined by their own choices.

Limit setting means that the boundaries for permissible behaviour are set out. Limits should be clear, concise and above all enforceable: 'You seem very angry and we cannot allow you to harm other people. Please come to the office so that we can talk about what made you angry.'

It would seem that people need to have their basic needs met when in a crisis. It is therefore a good idea to offer a safe place, something to eat or drink, and acceptance. If de-escalation does not occur and there is a risk of safety for the MHCU and others, physical intervention may be required.

Stage 3: Crisis level

During this phase there is a loss of control, and resultant physical violence on the part of the MHCU. The MHCU may be breaking windows or furniture, attacking staff or MHCUs, or injuring themselves.

At this stage, verbal intervention from staff is inadequate and restrictive measures may be necessary. Attempts to de-escalate the situation and attain trust should, however, continue (Rintoul et al, 2009). The MHCU may have to be physically controlled by staff and either placed in seclusion or chemically restrained. Pharmacological interventions include the use of benzodiazepines or antipsychotics. It is preferable that the MHCU be given a choice of the type and route of medication; choice provides a sense of regaining control and de-escalating the violence (Petit, 2005).

Non-violent physical intervention is a safe, non-harmful behaviour management system designed to aid staff members by maintaining the best possible care for individuals who are agitated or out of control, even during their most violent moments. Restrictive practices may be indicated in the crisis level if the MHCU is a danger to themselves and others.

Restrictive practices

Restrictive practice in nursing care is a broad concept which implies any action that 'limits a person's movement, day to day activity or functioning' (Royal College of

Nursing, 2016: 7). There are several nursing practices that are seen to be preventative of potential harm. These include controlling visitation times or restricting certain visitors, controlling and managing MHCUs' finances and valuables, preventing MHCUs from entering certain places in the ward like the kitchen, implementing seclusion and administering sedation.

The Royal College of Nursing (2016) has proposed a rights-based approach to the use of restrictive practices that should also be read with the relevant legislative framework in South Africa (see Chapter 6). Restrictive measures should not be used as a hit and miss method when a crisis ensues in the ward but should be part of a carefully considered, multidisciplinary approach to the MHCU's care treatment and rehabilitation. Furthermore, restrictive measures should never be used as a form of punishment or to establish dominance (NICE, 2015). When considering any restrictive measure, the nurse should ensure that it is:

- in the MHCU's best interest
- considerate of the person's human rights
- within the legal framework wherein the nurse practises mental health care, treatment and rehabilitation
- the least restrictive measure to ensure safety of the MHCU and others
- therapeutic in nature based on evidenced-based practice
- part of a multidisciplinary treatment plan
- regularly and timeously reviewed; reduced and removed as soon as possible
- ethical.

(Royal College of Nursing, 2016)

Physical restraint

When physical restraint is essential, it is important that the staff ensure that they and others remain safe, while at the same time ensuring that the MHCU remains safe. This intervention should be the last resort after all other measures have failed to defuse the situation and should be implemented by a team with a team leader (Rintoul, 2009). Minimum force should be used with the intention only of containing the violent MHCU.

Figures 11.4 to 11.12 on the following pages illustrate some non-violent, self-defence and MHCU-control strategies – that is, avoiding a reaction to MHCU violence in the form of staff violence. These strategies should be practised by nurses and security staff so that they can be performed smoothly and efficiently.

The principles behind the self-defence and MHCU-control techniques are the following:

- *Do the unexpected.* For example, when the MHCU pulls your hair and expects you to pull away, move your head quickly towards the MHCU. This kind of action unbalances the MHCU and often induces them to let go.
- *Do it fast.* This kind of strategy only works if it is done fast, since it often relies on unbalancing the MHCU. If it is done slowly, the person has time to adapt their stance.
- *Use your whole body.* In the MHCU-control techniques, for example, staff should place the entire length of their legs against those of the MHCU in order to improve control, rather than standing far away from them.

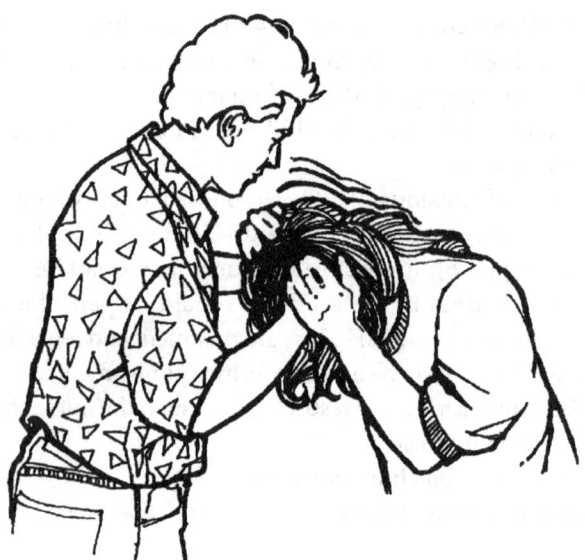

Figure 11.4 Two-handed hair-pull release

Clasp the MHCU's hands and immobilise these against your head to prevent injury. Move your head towards the MHCU's body at a 45° angle. The grip of the hair-pull is levered backwards, which reduces its strength. Move out of the way.

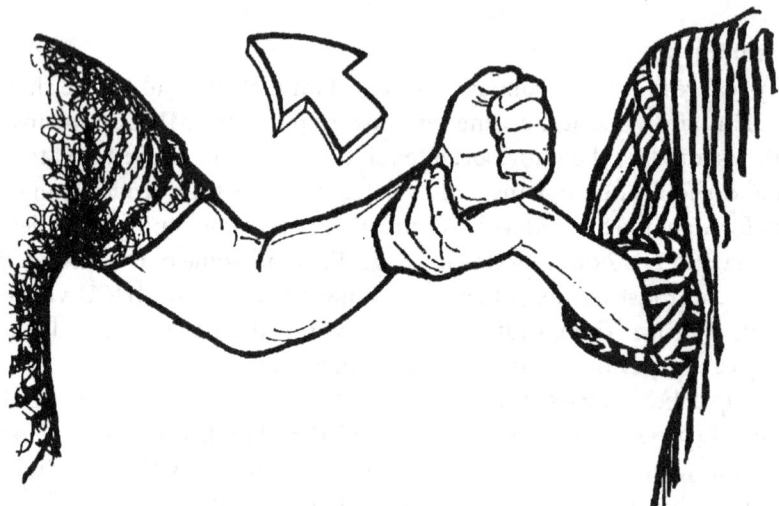

Figure 11.5 One-handed wrist-grab release

Use the laws of physics – momentum and leverage. Pull away from the weak link between thumb and fingers. Increase momentum and leverage by using both hands. Move out of the way.

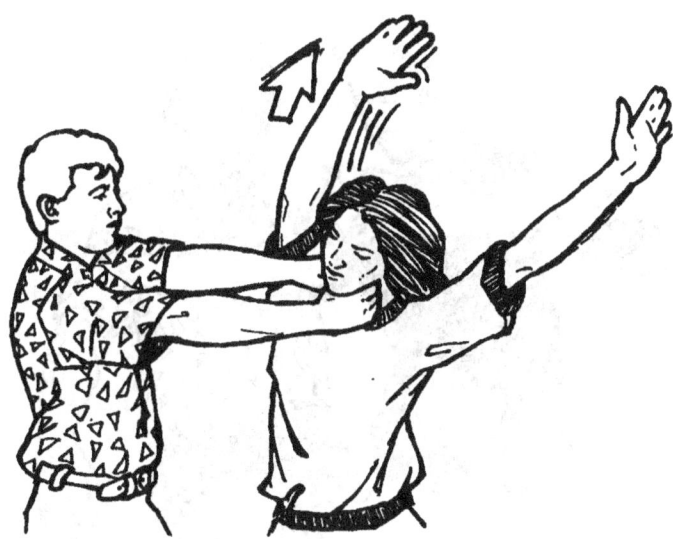

Figure 11.6 Front choke release

Throw the arms straight up for momentum and leverage; this will also cause a distraction. Lean away from the MHCU so as to extend their arm, which weakens the hold. Your shoulders will supply leverage as you turn away from the hold. Move out of the way.

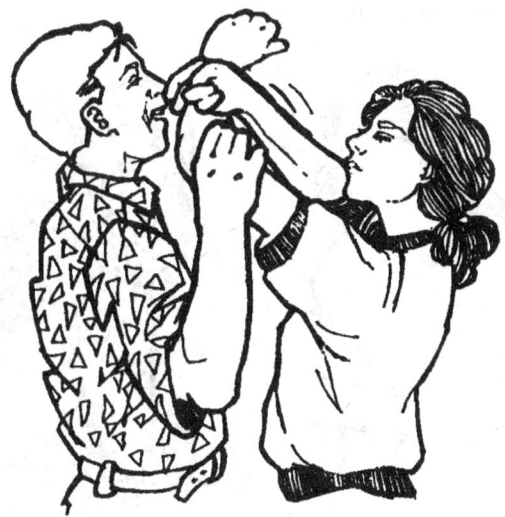

Figure 11.7 Bite release

Lean into the bite and use a vibrating motion above the MHCU's upper lip to induce them to open their jaws. The vibrating motion causes a parasympathetic response. Use the minimum force necessary to effect a release. Avoid pulling away from the bite. Move out of the way.

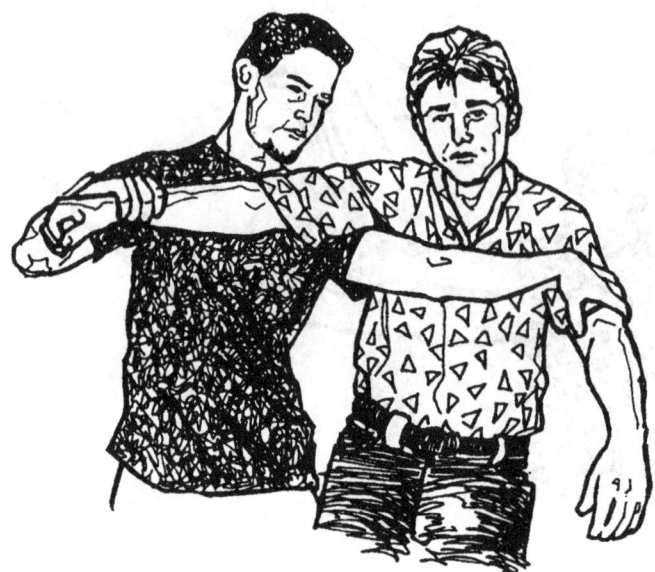

Figure 11.8 Interim control position

This is a temporary control position. The staff member who is with the acting-out person should always maintain control of one of the arms (do not let go of the wrist) and move their (staff's) hand under the acting-out person's arm to possibly gain control of the acting-out person's free arm.

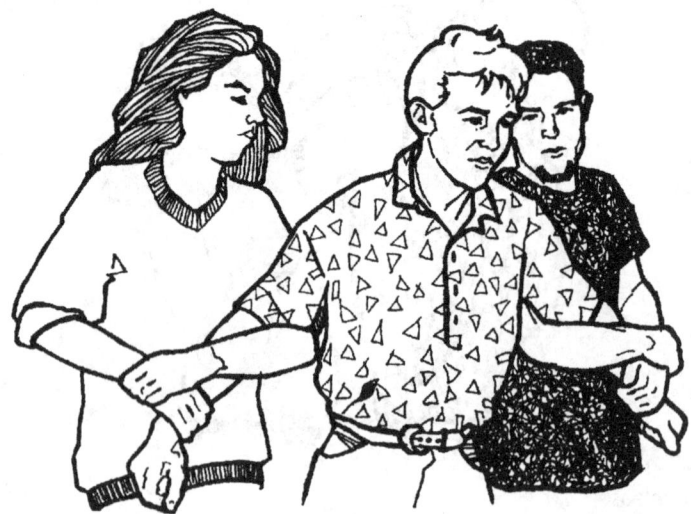

Figure 11.9 Transport technique

Staff remove their hands from the MHCU's shoulders, move them under the MHCU's hands and clasp their own wrists. This forms a cross-grained grip which secures the MHCU. Remain close to the MHCU.

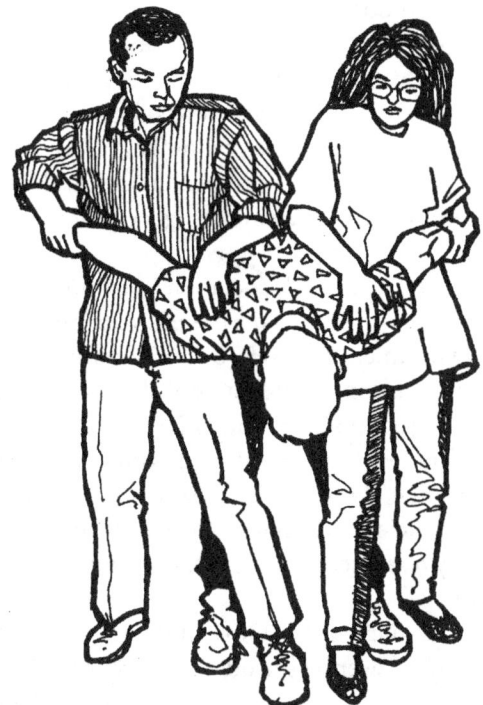

Figure 11.10 Team control position

Staff face in the same direction with the inside legs placed in front of the MHCU and outside hands holding the MHCU's wrists. Staff's inside hands form a C on the MHCU's shoulders.

It is advisable to approach an aggressive or violent MHCU as a team. The leader will communicate with the MHCU to request cooperation, for example to lie down or accompany the team to a quiet and safer space. If the team needs to hold down the MHCU, it should preferably be in a seated or kneeling position. Laying an MHCU in a prone position and/or sitting on the MHCU could lead to airway obstruction and restriction of breathing. Care should be taken not to cause physical injury to the MHCU (Harwood, 2017).

Seclusion and restraint
Seclusion means the containment of an MHCU in a room or other enclosed area from which the MHCU cannot exit for a specific time without the freedom to leave as they choose. Restraint could be by holding down a person or by using some mechanical or chemical method to prevent free movement of another person (Goulet & Larue, 2016). Seclusion and restraint are emergency interventions with the potential for abuse and cause of harm if not implemented according the guidelines discussed above for restrictive measures. Seclusion and restraint should, however, be actively managed and reduced on an institutional level by changing staff cultures about the use thereof, regular

training in de-escalation methods, implementation of de-escalation techniques and the use of aggression management protocols (Knox & Holloman, 2012).

Seclusion has psychological and physical consequences for MHCUs and nurses. There are multiple physical risks during seclusion, such as injury and death of MHCUs. Psychological consequences could include feeling degraded, dehumanised, frightened and lonely. Nurses could also experience physical injury in the process of secluding or restraining an MHCU and could have psychological reactions to secluding MHCUs (Goulet & Larue, 2016).

The American Psychiatric Nurses Association's position statement (APNA, 2018) supports the reduction and elimination of the use of seclusion and restraint yet maintains there should be a safe environment for MHCUs and nurses. Reduction and elimination are supported by position statements that focus on all levels of health care. These include levels of health care relating to individual nurses (attitudes, competencies), professional standards (standards of practice), organisational issues (philosophy, culture, policies, procedures, therapeutic milieu, staffing ratios, resources, training), and at the provincial/national level (laws and policies). Reducing and eliminating the use of seclusion and restraint is also affirmed by research that supports evidence-based practice in preventing and managing aggression.

Self-harming MHCUs, suicidal MHCUs, children under 12, medically ill and unconscious MHCUs should never be secluded. Elderly MHCUs, cognitively impaired MHCUs or those with a history of physical, sexual or psychological trauma and abuse are at increased risk for further trauma and adverse events when secluded or restrained. Note that this list is not exclusive and the nurse's accurate assessment and clinical judgement should be applied in all cases where restrictive measures are implemented (Department of Health, 2012). Under no circumstances may a person be restrained and then left alone in a locked room (APNA, 2014).

In the Mental Health Care Act 17 of 2002, regulations 36 and 37 deal with the use of seclusion and restraint. They stipulate that seclusion shall not be used for punishment, but only to contain severely disturbed behaviour, which is likely to harm to self, others, or property and where other treatment techniques have failed. Furthermore, the act indicates that the least restrictive measures should be used.

According to the Department of Health, Republic of South Africa (2012) the following principles regarding seclusion and restraint should be applied:

1. Seclusion and restraint should be prescribed by a registered medical practitioner. The prescription must be renewed every 24 hours after a face-to-face consultation has been conducted.
2. Seclusion and restraint should be prescribed for not more than four hours for adults and less than two hours for adolescents (12–18 years). The minimum time should be used and measures to expedite release should be implemented.
3. Ongoing comprehensive assessment of the MHCU should be done. According to APNA (2014), a registered medical practitioner or competent professional nurse should do a face-to-face evaluation within an hour of initiating seclusion or restraint with special attention to their cardiac and respiratory condition.

4. Seclusion and restraint should be implemented in a safe environment that ensures human dignity. Objects of risk and potential harm must be removed from the MHCU and the environment. Observation of all areas of the room must be possible. A toilet and basin should be present. Ways of attracting the nurse's attention, such as an intercom and a fire detector must be in place. The room should be of a comfortable temperature and have adequate lighting.
5. Optimal monitoring (observation), care and record-keeping should be ensured. The MHCU must be observed at least every 30 minutes, and a register must be kept, signed by a medical practitioner, which documents the period and the reasons for seclusion or restraint. Monitoring, care and record-keeping must include (Department of Health, 2012):
    (a) behaviour of the MHCU
    (b) medication administered and reaction to medication
    (c) physical and psychological needs and care provided (for example, fluids provided, support and assurance of safety)
    (d) interventions to promote comfort and safety
    (e) assessment of mental status and physical condition of the MHCU
    (f) vital signs (including saturation).
6. The head of the institution should receive these reports daily.
7. The head of the institution should report to the review board on a quarterly basis or when there are injuries or MHCU deaths.

Nursing notes should, in addition to the half hourly observation and care, include a description of (Department of Health, 2012):
- the behaviour leading to the seclusion and restraint
- alternative nonphysical measures that were used to prevent seclusion and restraint
- all persons contacted and notified
- therapeutic goals of seclusion or restraint
- the therapeutic response to the seclusion or restraint
- the measures implemented to expedite release from seclusion or restraint
- the post-seclusion debriefing that was conducted.

Mechanical restraint means the use of any instrument or appliance whereby the movements of the body or any of the limbs of a user are restrained or impeded (Mental Health Care Act 17 of 2002). Mechanical restraint (for example lap belts, hand restraints) should very seldomly be necessary if chemical restraint is used effectively and efficiently. In the Mental Health Care Act, article 38 deals with this form of restraint. It stipulates that it should only be used if chemical restraint is inadequate to ensure that the person does not harm self or others, or where it is done for a short period to administer the chemical restraint.

Stage 4: Tension reduction level

In the aftermath of violence there is a reduction of tension in the MHCU, both physically and emotionally. The MHCU is often drained emotionally and physically. They may be quiet, remorseful and apologetic. They may also not remember everything that occurred before. They may be afraid, confused and/or ashamed. This is the start of regaining control.

The appropriate staff response is to establish therapeutic rapport and communication with the MHCU. The nurse can assist the MHCU with gaining control by assisting with physical grooming, for example combing mussed hair, offering a drink of water, etc. It is advisable also to discuss the events and the MHCU's feelings about them, opening the way for in-depth counselling at a later date.

The physical and psychological well-being of other MHCUs and staff who were involved in the violent incident should be assessed with physical treatment and debriefing provided. Reporting of the incident according to hospital policy and procedures should be done (NICE, 2015).

Post-violent incident debriefing and review

After incidents of violence a team consisting of internal and external members to the unit or ward should conduct an evaluation and make recommendations regarding (NICE, 2015):

- The physical and emotional effect on all involved
- Cause of the violence and less restrictive alternatives in the future
- Challenges in the environment that may negatively influence a situation and if changed, could prevent the same incident in the future
- Recommendations that should address the unit or ward philosophy, policies, therapeutic environment, treatment approach and staff education.

CONCLUSION

This chapter demonstrates the centrality of mental health education and psycho-education as tools for empowering MHCUs and their families. Skills teaching, mental health education, social skills teaching, psycho-education and symptom management are the foundations of this important function. Another important aspect is the way that MHCUs and their families can be helped to deal with the mental health problems they face. This is the core focus of therapeutic groups, counselling, crisis intervention, case management, discharge planning and home visiting strategies. There is also a discussion on using the therapeutic environment in mental health nursing, as seen in milieu therapy and the management of violence. These functions are interrelated, and together they form the rich fabric of mental health nursing.

WEB RESOURCES

http://www.crisisprevention.com
   The Crisis Prevention Institute gives very useful information on this site. One can order the following brochures, for example: 'How to stay safe during home visits,' and 'The art of setting limits'.

http://rnao.ca/bpg/guidelines/crisis-intervention
   This website by the Ontario Nursing Association provides a free download of an evidence-based guideline on crisis intervention.

https://www.who.int/mental_health/publications/QualityRights_toolkit/en/
   This is the WHO QualityRights tool kit for assessing and improving quality and human rights in mental health and social care facilities.

https://www.rcn.org.uk/professional-development/publications/pub-006075
   This website by the Royal College of Nursing describes the three Steps to Positive Practice: A rights-based approach when considering and reviewing the use of restrictive interventions.

https://www.nice.org.uk/guidance/ng10
   This is the National Institute for Health and Care Excellence's web resource with information about violence and aggression: short-term management in mental health, health and community settings.

REFERENCES

American Psychiatric Nurses Association (APNA). 2014. 'Seclusion and restraint standards of practice'. https://www.apna.org/i4a/pages/index.cfm?pageID=3730#Standards (Accessed 11 July 2018).

American Psychiatric Nurses Association (APNA). 2018. 'Position statement on the use of seclusion and restraint'. https://www.apna.org/i4a/pages/index.cfm?pageid=3728#PositionStatement (Accessed 11 July 2018).

Applebaum, P S. 2007. 'Assessment of Patients' Competence to Consent to Treatment'. *New England Journal of Medicine*, 357: 1834–1840.

Ayano, G and Duko, B. 2017. 'Relapse and hospitalisation in patients with schizophrenia and bipolar disorder at the St Amanuel Mental Specialized Hospital, Addis Ababa, Ethiopia: a comparative quantitative cross-sectional study'. *Neuropsychiatric Disease and Treatment*, 13: 1527–1531.

Barekatain, M, Maracy, M R, Rajabi, F and Baratian, H. 2014. 'Aftercare services for patients with severe mental disorder: A randomized controlled trial'. *Journal of Research in Medical Science*, 19 (3): 240–242.

Baumann, S E. 2015. 'The agitated or violent patient'. In: Baumann, S E (ed). *Primary Care Psychiatry A practical guide for southern Africa*. 2nd edition. Cape Town: Juta & Company.

Baumgardner, S R and Crothers, M K. 2010. *Positive Psychology*. London: Pearson.

Bevilacqua, L, Carli, V, Sarchiapone, M, George, D K, Goldman, D, Roy, A and Enoch, M A. 2012. 'Interaction between FKBP5 and childhood trauma and risk of aggressive behavior'. *Archives of General Psychiatry*, 69 (1): 62–70. doi: 10.1001/archgenpsychiatry.2011.152.

Beyene, L S, Severinsson, E, Hansen, B S and Rørtveit, K. 2018. 'Shared Decision-Making – Balancing Between Power and Responsibility as Mental Health-Care Professionals in a Therapeutic Milieu'. *SAGE Ope Nursing*, 4: 1–10.

Blacklock, E. 2012. 'Interventions Following a Critical Incident: Developing a Critical Incident Stress Management Team'. *Archives of Psychiatric Nursing*, 26 (1): 2–8.

Bowers, L, Alexander, J, Bilgin, H, Botha, M, Dack, C, James, K, Jarrett, M, Jeffery, D, Nijman, H, Owiti, J A, Papadopoulos, C, Ross, J, Wright, S and Stewart, D. 2014. Safewards: evidence and appraisal. Journal of Psychiatric and Mental Health Nursing, 21: 354–364. doi: 10.1111/jpm.12085.

Byrd, M E. 2006. 'Social exchange as a framework for client-nurse interaction during public health nursing maternal-child home visits'. Public Health Nursing, 23 (3): 271–276.

Canberra Hospital and Health Care Services. 2017. 'Canberra Hospital and Health Services Operational Procedure: Home Visiting'. ACT Government Health & Canberra Hospital Health Care Services.

Cohen, M, Farkas, M and Cohen, B. 1986a. *Functional Assessment: Reference Handbook* 6. Boston: Boston University.

Cohen, M, Farkas, M and Cohen, B. 1986b. *Direct Skills Teaching: Reference Handbook* 6. Boston: Boston University.

Cornaggia, C M, Beghi, M, Pavone, F, Barale, F. 2011. 'Aggression in psychiatry wards: A systematic review'. *Psychiatry Research*, 189: 10–20. doi: 10.1016/j.psychres.2010.12.024 PMID: 21236497.

Csernansky, J G and Schuchart, E K. 2002. Relapse and rehospitalisation rates in patients with schizophrenia: effects of second-generation antipsychotics. *Central Nervous System Drugs*, 16 (7): 473–484.

Dack, C, Ross, J, Papadopoulos, C, Stewart, D and Bowers, L A. 2013. 'Review and meta-analysis of the patient factors associated with psychiatric in-patient aggression'. *Acta Psychiatrica Scandanavia*, 127: 255–268. doi: 10.1111/acps.12053 PMID: 23289890.

Department for Health and Ageing, Government of South Australia. nd. *Mental Health Restraint and Seclusion Toolkit Fact Sheet 3*. Government of Australia.

Department of Health, Republic of South Africa. 2012. *Policy Guidelines on Seclusion and Restraint of Mental Health Care Users*. Pretoria: Department of Health.

Dieterich, M, Irving, C B, Bergman, H, Khokhar, M A, Park, B and Marshall, M. 2017. 'Intensive case management for severe mental illness'. *Cochrane Database Systematic Review*, 1: CD007906.

Ernst, E J. 2012. 'Chapter 7: Psychiatric Case Management'. In: Rogers, V L, Fitzpatrick, J J and Jones, J S. *Psychiatric-Mental Health Nursing: An Interpersonal Approach*. New York: Springer Publishing Company.

Ertem, M Y and Duman, Z Ç. 2017. 'The effect of motivational interviews on treatment adherence and insight levels of patients with schizophrenia: A randomized controlled study'. *Perspectives in Psychiatric Care*, 55: 75–86. doi: 10.1111/ppc.12301.

Espinosa, L, Harris, B, Frank, J, Armstrong-Muth, J, Brous, E, Moran, J and Giorgi-Cipriano, J. 2015. 'Milieu Improvement in Psychiatry Using Evidence-Based Practices: The Long and Winding Road of Culture Change'. *Archives of Psychiatric Nursing*, 29: 202–207.

Everly, G S and Mitchell, J T. 2000. 'The Debriefing "Controversy" and Crisis Intervention: A Review of Lexical and Substantive Issues'. *International Journal of Emergency Mental Health*, 2 (4): 211–225.

Garriga, M T, Pacchiarotti, I, Kasper, S, Zeller, S L, Allen, M H, Vázquez, G A, Baldaçara, L, San, L, McAllister-Williams, R H, Fountoulakis, K N, Courtet, P, Naber, D, Chan, E W, Fagiolini, A, Moeller, H J, Grunze, H, Llorca, P M, Jaffe, R L, Yatham, L N, Hidalgo-Mazzei, D, Passamar, M, Messer, T C, Bernardo, M and Vieta, E. 2016. Assessment and management of agitation in psychiatry: Expert consensus. *The world journal of biological psychiatry: the official journal of the World Federation of Societies of Biological Psychiatry*, 17(2): 86–128.

Goulet, M and Larue, C. 2016. 'Post-Seclusion and/or Restraint Review in Psychiatry: A Scoping Review'. *Archives of Psychiatric Nursing*, 30: 120–128.

Greenwood, A. and Braham, L. 2018. Violence and aggression toward staff in secure settings. *Journal of Forensic Practice*, 20 (2): 122–133.

Harwood, J H. 2017. 'How to deal with violent and aggressive patients in acute medical settings'. *Journal of the Royal College of Physicians of Edinburgh*, 47: 176–182.

Hoff, J A. 2009. *People in Crisis: Clinical and diversity perspectives*. 6th edition. New York: Routledge.

Hudon, C, Chouinard, M, Lambert, M, Dufour, I and Krieg, C. 2016. Effectiveness of case management interventions for frequent users of healthcare services: a scoping review. *British Medical Journal Open*, 6 (9): e012353. doi: 10.1136/bmjopen-2016-012353.

Johnson, D H. 2014. *Reaching Out Interpersonal Effectiveness and Self-Actualization*. 11th edition. New York: Pearson.

Jonas, W B and Chez, R A. 2004. 'Toward optimal healing environments in health care.' *The Journal of Alternative and Complementary Medicine*, 10 (Suppl 1): S-1-S-6.

Kneisl, C R and Trigoboff, E. 2013. *Contemporary Psychiatric-Mental Health Nursing*. 3rd edition. New York: Pearson.

Knox, D K and Holloman, G H. 2012. 'Use and Avoidance of Seclusion and Restraint: Consensus Statement of the American Association for Emergency Psychiatry Project BETA Seclusion and Restraint Work'. *Western Journal of Emergency Medicine*, 8 (1): 35–40.

Lavelle, M, Stewart, D, James, K, Richardson, M, Renwick, L, Brennan, G and Bowers, L. 2016. 'Predictors of effective de-escalation in acute inpatient psychiatric settings'. *Journal of Clinical Nursing*, 25: 2180-2188. doi: 10.1111/jocn.13239.

Lozzino, L, Ferrari C, Large, M, Nielssen, O, de Girolamo, G. 2015. 'Prevalence and Risk Factors of Violence by Psychiatric Acute Inpatients: A Systematic Review and Meta-Analysis'. *PLoS ONE*, 10(6): e0128536. doi: 10.1371/journal.pone.0128536.

Leavitt, S S. 1982. 'Case management: a remedy for problems of community care'. In: Sanborn, C, ed. *Case Management in Mental Health Services*. New York: Haworth Press.

Liu, Y, Yang, X, Gillespie, A, Guo, Z, Ma, Y, Chen, R and Li, Z. 2019. 'Targeting relapse prevention and positive symptoms in first-episode schizophrenia using brief cognitive behavioural therapy: A pilot randomized controlled study'. *Psychiatry research*, 272: 275–283.

Magin, P J, Adams, J, Sibbritt, D W, Joy, E and Ireland, M C. 2008. 'Effects of occupational violence on Australian general practitioners' provision of home visits and after-hours care: a cross-sectional study'. *Journal of Evaluation in Clinical Practice*, 14 (2): 336–42

Mahoney, J S, Palyo, N, Napier, G and Giordano, J. 2009. 'The Therapeutic Milieu Reconceptualized for the 21st Century'. *Archives of Psychiatric Nursing* 23 (6): 423–429.

Mclean, D and Nathan, J. 2007. 'Treatment of Personality Disorder: Limit Setting and The Use of Benign Authority'. *British Journal of Psychotherapy*, 23 (2): 231–246.

McNaughton, D B. 2005. 'A naturalistic test of Peplau's theory in home visiting'. *Public Health Nursing*, 22 (5): 429–438.

Menninger Clinic and Menninger Foundation. 1982. *Bulletin of the Menninger Clinic*. Topeka Kansas: Menninger Foundation.

Müller-Leonhardt, A, Mitchell, S G, Vogth, J and Schürmann, T. 2014. 'Critical Incident Stress Management (CISM) in complex systems: Cultural adaptation and safety impacts in healthcare'. *Accident Analysis and Prevention*, 68: 172–180.

Myer, R, Lewis, J and James, R. 2013. 'The introduction of a task model for crisis intervention'. *Journal of Mental Health Counselling*, 35 (2): 95–107.

National Institute for Health and Care Excellence (NICE). 2015. 'Violence and Aggression: Short-Term Management in Mental Health, Health and Community Settings'. *NICE Guideline, NG10*. https://www.nice.org.uk/guidance/ng10 (Accessed 20 April 2019).

Okun, B F and Kantrowitz, R E. 2015. *Effective Helping: Interviewing and Counseling Techniques*. 8th edition. Stamford, USA: Cengage learning.

Pearce, S and Haigh, R. 2017. 'Milieu approaches and other adaptations of therapeutic community method: past and future'. *Therapeutic Communities: The International Journal of Therapeutic Communities*, 38 (3): 136–146.

Pender, D A and Anderton, C. 2016. 'Exploring the Process: A Narrative Analysis of Group Facilitators' Reports on Critical Incident Stress Debriefing'. *The Journal for Specialists in Group Work*, 41 (1): 19–43. doi: 10.1080/01933922.2015.1111485.

Peplau, H E. 1952. *Interpersonal Relations in Nursing*. New York: G P Putnam's Sons.

Perez, R, Ramirez, S Z and Kranz, P L. 2007. 'Adjusting limit setting in play therapy with first-generation Mexican-American children'. *Journal of Instructional Psychology*, 34 (1): 22–27.

Pekurinen, V, Willman, L, Virtanen, M, Kivimäki, M, Vahtera, J, Välimäki, M. 2017. 'Patient Aggression and the Wellbeing of Nurses: A Cross-Sectional Survey Study in Psychiatric and Non-Psychiatric Settings'. *International Journal of Environmental Research and Public Health*, 14: 1245.

Perreault, M, Tardif, H, Provencher, H, Paquin, G, Desmarais, J and Pawliuk, N. 2005. The role of relatives in discharge planning from psychiatric hospitals: the perspective of patients and their relatives. *Psychiatric Quarterly*, 76 (4): 297–315. doi: 10.1007/s11126-005-4964-z.

Petit, J R. 2005. 'Management of the Acutely Violent Patient'. *Psychiatric Clinics of North America*, 28: 701–711.

Registered Nurses' Association of Ontario (RNAO). 2017. *Crisis intervention for adults using a trauma-informed approach: Initial four weeks of management*. 3rd edition. Toronto, Ontario

Rintoul, Y, Wynaden, D and McGowan, S. 2009. 'Managing aggression in the emergency department: Promoting an interdisciplinary approach'. *International Emergency Nursing*, 17: 122–127.

Roberts, A R, ed. 2005. *Crisis intervention handbook: Assessment, treatment and research*. 3rd edition. New York: Oxford University Press.

Rogers, J C and Holm, M B. 2016. 'Functional assessment in mental health: lessons from occupational therapy'. *Dialogues in Clinical Neuroscience*, 18 (2): 145–154.

Rossberg J I and Friis S. 2003. 'A suggested revision of the Ward Atmosphere Scale'. *Acta Psychiatrica Scandinavica*, 108 (5): 374–80.

Royal College of Nursing. 2016. *Three Steps to Positive Practice: A rights-based approach when considering and reviewing the use of restrictive intervention*. London: Royal College of Nursing. https://www.rcn.org.uk/professional-development/publications/pub-006075#detailTab (Accessed 9 July 2018).

Ryu, H. 2009. 'An estimation of the cost per visit of home care nursing services'. *Nursing Economics*, 27 (2): 111–118.

Sadock, B J, Sadock, V A and Ruiz, P R. 2015. *Kaplan & Sadock's synopsis of psychiatry*. 11th edition. Philadelphia: Wolters Kluwer.

Sharrock, J and Rickard, N. 2002. 'Limit Setting: A Useful Strategy In Rehabilitation'. *Australian Journal of Advanced Nursing*, 19 (4): 21–26.

Smith, Y and Spitzmueller, M C. 2016. 'Worker Perspectives on Contemporary Milieu Therapy: A Cross-Site Ethnographic Study'. *Social Work Research*, 40 (2): 105–116.

Stevens, N H, Foote, S and Wu, P W. 2008. 'Educational Theatre Programme: Promoting Health'. *The Permanente Journal*, 12 (3): 90–92.

Thibeault, C A, Trudeau, K, d'Entremont, M and Brown, T. 2010. 'Understanding the Milieu Experiences of Patients on an Acute Inpatient Psychiatric Unit'. *Archives of Psychiatric Nursing*, 24 (4): 216–226.

Vatne, S and Fagermoen, M S. 2007. 'To correct and to acknowledge: two simultaneous and conflicting perspectives of limit-setting in mental health nursing'. *Journal of Psychiatric and Mental Health Nursing,* 14: 41–48.

White and Hall, 2006. 'Mapping the literature of case management nursing'. *Journal of the Medical Library Association,* 94 (2) Supplement: 99–106.

World Health Organisation (WHO). 2012. *QualityRights tool kit to assess and improve quality and human rights in mental health and social care facilities.* Geneva, World Health Organisation. https://www.who.int/mental_health/publications/QualityRights toolkit/en/ (Accessed 1 June 2019).

Yalom, I D and Leszcz, M. 2005. *The theory and practice of Group Psychotherapy.* 5th edition. New York: Basic Books.

SECTION 3
Psychopathology and Nursing Interventions

CHAPTER 12

Nursing the Mental Health Care User with an Anxiety Disorder

L Middleton and G E Pietersen

> **Learning Outcomes**
>
> After studying this chapter, you should be able to:
> - differentiate between variations of anxiety (stress, anxiousness, pathological anxiety)
> - describe the concept of anxiety from a cognitive behavioural perspective and describe the multidimensional responses associated with anxiety
> - diagnose anxiety disorders and obsessive-compulsive disorders, and manage these disorders in a primary health care setting
> - apply the strategies in each phase of the scientific process of nursing which are related to the care of mental health care users (MHCUs) with anxiety
> - explore the sources of the nurse's own feelings of anxiety in dealing with MHCUs and implement a plan for change.

INTRODUCTION

Many theorists have devoted a great deal of time and energy to unravelling the mysteries that surround anxiety. Developing a valid conceptualisation of anxiety has been a goal since the advent of Freud's pioneering work. Since anxiety is considered to be at the very root of what it means to be human, this is not surprising.

There is a common belief that the prevalence of anxiety has increased in the 21st century as a result of political, social, economic or environmental changes. However, efforts to quantify the prevalence of anxiety disorders are hampered by the ubiquitous nature of stress and anxiety which does not always result in pathological anxiety.

It is known that different anxiety disorders often occur together and also have a high comorbidity with other mental health disorders. Major depression occurs in almost two-thirds of MHCUs with generalised anxiety disorder, panic disorder in a quarter, and alcohol abuse in more than one-third of MHCUs with generalised anxiety disorder (Bandelow & Michaelis, 2015: 327–335). Anxiety disorders are the most prevalent class of lifetime disorders. Furthermore, among mental disorders the range of anxiety disorders is most common. The MHCUs with anxiety disorders are, however, mostly not hospitalised as most are treated in community-based and general medical settings, followed by complementary and alternative medicine practitioners (usually traditional healers) and then by other mental health professionals.

The idea that anxiety shapes and directs human behaviour, and disease, has important implications for mental health nursing practice, especially when the care is delivered in the community or at a community-based health facility. These implications lie in the impact anxiety has on healthy lifestyle functioning in that the greater the anxiety, the greater the degree of disorganised lifestyle functioning. To the extent that anxiety can be perceived as the pulse of lifestyle functioning, it can also be seen as one of the vital signals for action or intervention in mental health nursing.

THE ANXIETY RESPONSE

Clinical anxiety can be experienced and/or observed in the cognitive, affective/subjective and behavioural dimensions (see Figure 12.1). These responses are often interpreted as further sources of threat and this leads to an increase in the intensity of the anxiety experienced.

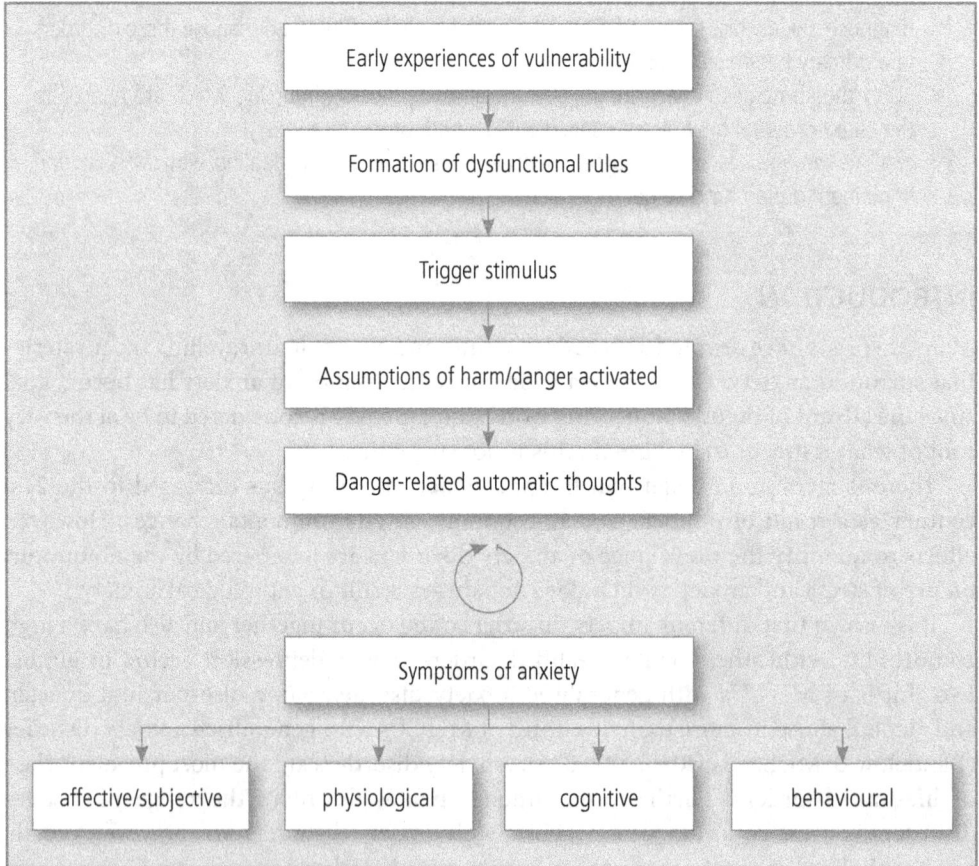

Figure 12.1 The cognitive model of anxiety

The effects of anxiety are diffuse and uneven; although all aspects of lifestyle functioning are affected, the effects are unlikely to manifest uniformly in each dimension. An MHCU may, for example, show signs of cognitive disorganisation, yet appear calm and controlled.

Subjective responses associated with anxiety

This refers to the MHCU's descriptions and interpretations of symptoms. The MHCUs sometimes present with anxiety as their chief complaint. More commonly, they present a range of physiological symptoms, such as heart palpitations, and cognitive symptoms like not being able to concentrate, or a fear of dying.

Typical terms used to describe the subjective experience of anxiety are listed below. Some people, especially those presenting at general medical facilities, will use the term 'stressed' when describing these experiences.

- tense
- shaky
- worried
- terrified
- wound-up
- highly strung
- nervous
- on edge
- panicky
- anxious
- scared
- jittery
- apprehensive
- fearful

Physiological responses associated with anxiety

These responses are primarily mediated through the autonomic nervous system. When the MHCU appraises a situation as dangerous, a number of physiological changes occur. These responses serve a useful function in the face of realistic dangers, because they help to prepare the person concerned for flight, fight or fainting. However, when the threat arises from a misperception, the responses activated are inappropriate for the situation. Instead of serving a useful function, these responses are often interpreted as further sources of danger. This interpretation sets up a series of vicious circles that tend to maintain and increase the intensity of the anxiety. In some cases, these physiological responses are at first understood as general medical conditions. Table 12.1 lists the symptoms associated with physiological responses to anxiety.

Table 12.1 Symptoms associated with physiological responses to anxiety

System	Symptoms
Musculoskeletal	Pains and aches, twitching, myoclonic jerks, grinding of teeth, unsteady voice, increased muscle tone, spasms, tremors, restlessness, wobbling legs, clumsiness

Sensory	Tinnitus, blurring of vision, hot and cold flushes, feelings of weakness, prickling sensations, flushed face, pale face, sweating, itching
Cardiovascular	Tachycardia, palpitations, pain in chest, throbbing of vessels, feeling faint, skipped heartbeat
Respiratory	Pressure or constriction in chest, choking feeling, sighing
Gastrointestinal	Difficulty in swallowing, flatulence, abdominal pain, burning sensations, abdominal discomfort, nausea, vomiting, looseness of bowels, loss of weight, loss of appetite, constipation
Genitourinary	Frequency of urination, amenorrhoea, menorrhagia, premature ejaculation, loss of libido
Autonomic	Dry mouth, flushing, pallor, tendency to sweat, giddiness, tension headache, raising of hair

Cognitive responses associated with anxiety

A number of diffuse changes in cognitive functioning take place in response to anxiety. These are listed in Table 12.2.

Table 12.2 Symptoms associated with changes in cognitive functions

Cognitive functions	Symptoms associated with changes in cognitive functions
Sensory-perceptual	<ul><li>Hazy, cloudy, foggy, dazed</li><li>Objects seem blurred/distant</li><li>Environment seems different/unreal</li><li>Feeling of unreality</li><li>Self-conscious</li><li>Hypervigilant</li></ul>
Thought impairment	<ul><li>Cannot recall important things</li><li>Confused</li><li>Unable to control thinking</li><li>Difficulty in concentrating</li><li>Distractibility</li><li>Blocking</li><li>Difficulty in reasoning</li><li>Loss of objectivity/perspective</li></ul>
Content of thought	<ul><li>Cognitive distortion</li><li>Fear of losing control</li><li>Fear of not being able to cope</li><li>Fear of physical injury/death</li><li>Fear of going crazy</li><li>Fear of negative evaluations</li><li>Frightening visual images</li><li>Repetitive fearful ideation</li><li>Obsessive thoughts</li></ul>

Behavioural responses associated with anxiety

Several coping strategies may be evident in the MHCU's behaviour. These represent the person's conscious and unconscious attempts to manage the problem situation and to deal with the affective consequences of the problem, namely anxiety.

Conscious coping behaviours

There are two types of conscious coping behaviours:
1. *Problem-focused* coping involves taking direct action to modify or eliminate the source of threat. This includes behaviour such as physical and interpersonal withdrawal, aggression and external blaming.
2. *Emotion-focused* coping includes responses with the primary function of managing the affect aroused by stressful situations. Behaviour such as crying, eating or smoking more, the use of alcohol and drugs, excessive sleeping, immobility, hyperactivity, talking about the experience and seeking help are examples of this type of coping.

Unconscious coping behaviours

These unconscious manoeuvres include denial, projection, rationalisation, intellectualisation and suppression. Although these mechanisms are useful in protecting the person from feelings of worthlessness and inadequacy, they can, if used in the extreme, limit the person's functioning in all lifestyle dimensions.

UNDERSTANDING ANXIETY AS A PHENOMENON (AN EXPERIENCE/HAPPENING/EVENT)

Anxiety is a universal human emotion. It is experienced by everyone in mild form at some time or another; in a more extreme form it leads to fears of impending death or catastrophe:

> *It comes over me all at once. First of all it is like something pressing only on my eyes. My head gets so heavy, there's a dreadful buzzing and I feel so giddy that I almost fall over. Then there's something crushing my chest so I can't get my breath ... My throat's closed together as though I were going to choke ... I always think I'm going to die. I'm brave as a rule and go about everything by myself – into the cellar and all over the mountain. But on a day when this happens, I don't dare go anywhere ...* (Freud's description of Katharina in Meissner, 1979)

Stress, in contrast to anxiety, is described as a feeling of strain and pressure. Stress may be considered to be a healthy aspect of life, as desired and beneficial, especially when experienced to a limited degree, and as a motivating or energising force. This can be experienced in situations like an athlete drawing upon internal tension to perform, or when someone uses the feeling of internal pressure when completing a task or leaning to adapt to a new work environment or an unfamiliar situation. Excessive and ongoing stress, however, could impact a person's physical health, putting them at an increased risk of stroke, cardiac arrest and ulcers, or their mental health, resulting in depression. Stress is mostly experienced when the person does not have the emotional, social or physical coping resources to deal with the demands of these life experiences. Experiencing these demands as exceeding their ability to deal with them is then described and perceived as stress.

Although stress is mostly considered to be external, related to a person's circumstances or environment, stress may in fact also be created by internal processes and perceptions the person may have. These perceptions ultimately cause the person to experience anxiety which could spill over to become pathological anxiety.

Anxiety defined

An appropriate description of anxiety is (Taylor & Arnow, 1988):

> *... a feeling of uneasiness and apprehension about some undefined threat. The threat is often physical with intimations of bodily harm or death, or psychological with threats to self-esteem and well-being. The feeling is diffuse and ineffable, and the indefinable nature of the feeling gives it its peculiarly unpleasant and intolerable quality.*

When reading most definitions there is an agreement that anxiety occurs in response to a stimulus (event, experience, object, person) which individuals perceive as threatening to their physical, social or psychological integrity. There is as yet little theoretical consensus about what constitutes a 'threat' and the nature of the relationship between the threat and the experience of anxiety.
This is partly because anxiety can be observed or experienced in several dimensions – subjective, cognitive, behavioural, physiological – and these dimensions largely determine 'how' the problem is defined. For example, behavioural theorists believe that anxiety is a learned response to a painful stimulus. The focus of treatment is therefore on helping the person to learn adaptive behavioural responses to anxiety-provoking stimuli.

Physiological theorists emphasise the biological basis of anxiety and describe four neuro-anatomical structures and three neuro-transmitter systems implicated in anxiety. Treatment in this instance is medical, and could take the form of psychotropic medications with the emphasis on symptom control.

Common to most definitions of anxiety are the following six characteristics:
1. It is an emotional state characterised by the subjectively experienced quality of fear or a closely related emotion.
2. The emotion is unpleasant.
3. It is directed towards the future.
4. Either there is no recognisable threat or the threat is, by reasonable standards, quite out of proportion to the emotion it seemingly evokes.
5. There are subjective bodily discomforts during the period of anxiety.
6. There are manifest bodily disturbances.

Levels of anxiety

Four levels of anxiety are generally observed. These are:
1. *Mild.* Here, the ability to cope increases. Alertness is increased and sensory input seems heightened, enabling the person to achieve and succeed in specific tasks, like studying productively for an examination or completing an assignment on time.
2. *Moderate.* At this level, the ability to perceive and to communicate is reduced and a sensation of increased nervousness and tension occurs. Some coping skills are still functional, and the person can follow directions. Therefore, with some help, the anxiety can be dealt with successfully.
3. *Severe.* In this form, a person's perceptual field becomes quite narrow and focused on the short term. The attention span is shortened and the ability to attend to other things is impaired. An accompanying physical discomfort may add to a sense of emotional discomfort.
4. *Panic.* At this level, a person's ability to cope is severely impaired. Perception is distorted. There is a feeling of terror and thoughts may be unfocused, random, fleeting and irrational. A person cannot function at this level for long.

UNDERSTANDING ANXIETY FROM A COGNITIVE BEHAVIOURAL PERSPECTIVE

Although no single theory can comprehensively explain the phenomenon of anxiety, it is still useful to examine in detail a particular approach to addressing anxiety. A working knowledge of one approach is more useful to the practitioner than scanty knowledge of a variety of theories.

The cognitive behavioural approach provides a useful framework for understanding and intervening in anxiety, because it closely parallels the principles of mental health nursing practice. A great deal of emphasis is placed on expressing concepts in descriptive, concrete terms; problem solving is an integral part of treatment; much of the treatment is based on the here-and-now and requires that the MHCU, where possible, be an active participant in the process of care.

Cognitive model of anxiety

This model attributes anxiety to a disorder related to thinking. The central thesis of this approach is that the special meaning that an individual attaches to an event will determine their emotional and behavioural response. The meaning is encased in cognition, namely, a thought or image. In anxiety, the thinking of the anxious person is dominated by cognitions of danger to their personal domain.

Threats to physical integrity include the possibility of physical harm, serious illness or environmental hazards. Threats to the psychosocial well-being of the person encompass anticipated loss of interpersonal support, anticipation of criticism, humiliation or desertion. In addition, the possibility of losing some important object (person, financial security, material possessions) is another common threat to the personal domain.

The cognitive model describes three specific concepts to explain how this process operates in anxiety. This is known as the *cognitive triad* (see Figure 12.2). The cognitive triad consists of three major cognitive patterns that influence the way in which MHCUs view themselves, the future and life experiences.

The first aspect of the triad centres on the MHCU's negative view of self. Anxious MHCUs see themselves as vulnerable in the face of potentially harmful situations.

Because of this, they believe that they do not possess the necessary resources to cope with untoward events and therefore live in a constant state of anticipation of physical and/or psychological harm.

The second aspect of the triad involves the tendency of anxious MHCUs to consistently misinterpret their ongoing experience in a threatening way.

The third component of the cognitive triad consists of a fearful view of the future. Fear of the future generally revolves around the theme of suffering. This may be experienced in response to the anticipation of physical harm or to the anticipation of a painful emotional state resulting from psychosocial hurt. Fear of loss of control leading to feelings of humiliation, embarrassment and sadness is common. This may include fear of losing control of one's faculties, for instance 'going crazy', not being able to function, or harming others. Fear of death is also common, especially in MHCUs who experience panic attacks.

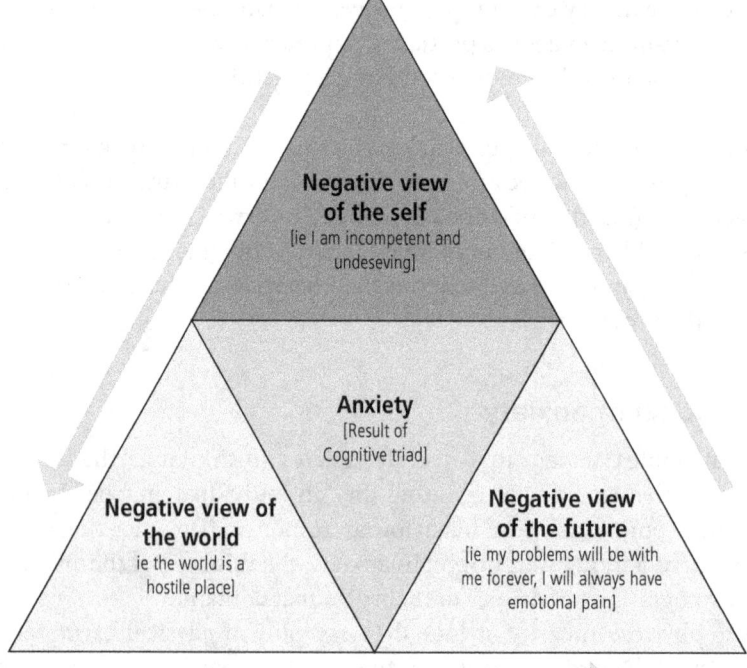

Figure 12.2 Cognitive triad

All people have, embedded in their self-concept, a set of general rules that guide behaviour and form the basis for specific interpretations. For MHCUs experiencing anxiety these are mostly dysfunctional rules or beliefs. Furthermore, these rules are thought to arise from memories of early experiences that were never fully processed or accepted by the individual. Beliefs are overcompensation for painful emotional memories. A person's emotional memory of being inferior to others may have a corresponding belief, such as 'I have to be loved at all times'. Since this is an impossibility, the overcompensating beliefs often create precisely the experience the person is trying to avoid, namely anxiety.

Although the rules involved in anxiety are varied, they are generally concerned with the concept of danger and MHCUs' assessment of their capacity for coping with it. Most revolve around themes of acceptance, competence, control, responsibility and the symptoms of anxiety themselves. Table 12.3 shows the beliefs an MHCU might hold about themselves.

Table 12.3 Common beliefs held by MHCUs

Themes	Examples of belief
Acceptance	I am nothing unless I am loved I always have to please others Criticism means rejection I should always like others
Responsibility	I am responsible for what others feel or think when they are with me If something goes wrong, it is my fault
Competence	I must never make a mistake If I make a mistake, I will fail I cannot cope I am not strong or capable Strong people don't ask for help
Control	I must be in control at all times If I let someone get too close, they will control me Any strange situation should be regarded as dangerous My security and safety depend on anticipating and preparing myself at all times for any possible danger
Symptoms of anxiety	I must be calm at all times I am having a heart attack I am dying/going mad

When people encounter novel situations, their perception of the situation is coloured by past emotional experiences, namely, a belief system. In the case of anxiety, beliefs about one's vulnerability are activated at an unconscious level but manifest themselves at a conscious level in the form of negative, automatic thoughts.

Beck's (1976) classic description of these thoughts as automatic, since they arise as if by reflex and are unsolicited by the person, is still relevant. Because these thoughts tend to spring to mind easily, people regard them as plausible and worthy of belief. Negative, automatic thoughts of vulnerability or threats to one's personal domain are triggered by one's perception of the situation as dangerous and, in turn, trigger the experience of anxiety. People about to enter a social situation might automatically think 'I'd better keep my mouth shut or people will think I'm stupid' or 'I will not be able to cope with this situation'. At the same time, pictorial images of looking foolish, saying the wrong thing and having people laughing at them may flash through their minds.

Cognitive errors (faulty information processing)

Negative thoughts are a product of errors in processing, through which perceptions and interpretations of experience are distorted. These include the following:

- *Selective abstraction.* A person who is concerned about social evaluation may conclude that they are socially boring because they notice one person in the group yawning.
- *Stimulus generalisation.* The same person may hear other people in the room laughing and conclude that these people are laughing at them because they are boring.
- *Catastrophising.* The same person will dwell on the most negative extreme consequences imaginable, such as being alone for ever in the world because they are boring.
- *Dichotomous thinking.* On the basis of selective abstraction, stimulus generalisation and catastrophising, the person may classify all social situations as unsafe, rather than arrange them in gradations of safety.

In summary, the individual's interactions with self, others and the environment are guided by a set of dysfunctional or irrational rules and/or thoughts that predispose the individual to misinterpreting a wide range of situations and experiences in a threatening fashion. This process of faulty information processing gives rise to a stream of negative thoughts and images that set the anxiety response in motion.

NORMAL VERSUS PATHOLOGICAL ANXIETY

It is often difficult to draw a line between everyday 'normal' and clinical or pathological anxiety. Anxiety can be considered pathological if any one of the five questions appearing below is answered in the affirmative. Furthermore, the levels of anxiety mentioned earlier might help to decide whether the anxiety is 'working for' or 'working against' the person.

1. Is the degree of anxiety out of proportion to the danger?
2. Is anxiety present in the absence of objective danger?
3. Has the person sought treatment for anxiety?
4. Does the person engage in self-destructive behaviour to control the anxiety?
5. Is the intensity/frequency/duration of the anxiety experience such that it interferes with adaptive functioning?

Diagnostic criteria of anxiety disorders based on the DSM-5

All the diagnostic criteria for anxiety disorders are characterised by excessive fear and anxiety and related behavioural disturbances, which are not normative based on their persistence and the extent of their presentation. Anxiety disorders may also be seen in children, but they present differently (see Chapter 22). All the diagnostic criteria for obsessive-compulsive disorders are characterised by the presence of obsessions (recurrent and persistent intrusive thoughts and urges) and/or compulsions (repetitive behaviours or mental acts that the MHCU is driven to perform because of obsessions or rigid mental rules). In all the diagnoses related to trauma and stressors, exposure to a traumatic or stressful event is an explicit part of the diagnostic criteria.

Mental health nurses, although not expected to have advanced psychiatric diagnostic background knowledge, should be aware of the range of pathological anxieties described in the DSM-5, including their specific diagnostic criteria. Table 12.4 shows the DSM-5's three categories of anxiety disorders (APA, 2013).

Table 12.4 The three separate categories of anxiety disorders specified by the DSM-5

DSM-5 categories of anxiety disorders	Examples of disorders
Anxiety disorders	Separation anxiety disorder, selective mutism, specific phobia, social phobia, panic disorder, agoraphobia, social anxiety disorder, generalised anxiety disorder
Obsessive-compulsive disorders	Obsessive-compulsive disorder, body dysmorphic disorder, hoarding disorder, trichotillomania, and excoriation disorder
Trauma and stressor-related disorders	Reactive attachment disorder, disinhibited social engagement disorder, PTSD, acute stress disorder, and adjustment disorder

Anxiety disorders

This section briefly describes the key features of selected anxiety disorders, followed by a summary of the DSM-5 diagnostic criteria.

Specific phobias

Phobias are relatively common, with a prevalence in the general population of 7–9 per cent. They are more common in females than in men (2:1) and they occur at a slightly lower rate in children. Although the rate is also lower in the elderly, they remain a common condition in this age group. Phobias are often related to a traumatic event, either by experiencing it personally, witnessing it or viewing it on television (for example, watching the reporting of a tsunami). They might also be related to an unexpected panic attack in a situation that then becomes a phobic one, such as having a panic attack in a lift and then becoming phobic about enclosed spaces. However, in many people the trigger cannot be identified. The condition is usually lifelong, although it waxes and wanes over the lifetime.

DSM-5 criteria for specific phobias
The DSM-5 criteria for specific phobias are as follows (APA, 2013):
A. Marked and persistent fear that is excessive or unreasonable, cued by the presence or anticipation of a specific object or situation (for example, flying, heights, animals, receiving an injection, seeing blood).
B. Exposure to the phobic stimulus almost invariably provokes an immediate anxiety response, which may take the form of a situationally bound or situationally predisposed panic attack.
Note: In children, the anxiety may be expressed by crying, tantrums, freezing, or clinging.
C. The person recognises that the fear is excessive or unreasonable.
Note: In children, this feature may be absent.
D. The phobic situation(s) is avoided or else is endured with intense anxiety or distress.
E. The avoidance, anxious anticipation, or distress in the feared situation(s) interferes significantly with the person's normal routine, occupational (or academic) functioning, or social activities or relationships, or there is marked distress about having the phobia.
F. In individuals under age 18 years, the duration is at least six months.
G. The anxiety, panic attacks, or phobic avoidance associated with the specific object or situation are not better accounted for by another mental disorder, such as obsessive-compulsive disorder (for example, fear of dirt in someone with an obsession about contamination), post-traumatic stress disorder (PTSD) (for example, avoidance of stimuli associated with a severe stressor), separation anxiety disorder (for example, avoidance of school), social phobia (for example, avoidance of social situations because of fear of embarrassment), panic disorder with agoraphobia, or agoraphobia without history of panic disorder.

Specify phobia type:
Animal type
- Natural environment type (for example heights, storms, water)
- Blood-injection-injury type
- Situational type (for example airplanes, elevators, enclosed places)
- other type (for example phobic avoidance of situations that may lead to choking, vomiting, or contracting an illness).

Note: In children, avoidance of loud sounds or costumed characters.

Social anxiety disorder

Intense fear or anxiety about situations in which the person may be under scrutiny of others is characteristic of this condition. The person fears negative evaluation by others. This anxiety sometimes develops without the person being very shy before and may be related to a stressful social event such as bullying. It often develops during adolescence and if it is not treated, may last for many years. It is more common in females and the prevalence decreases with age.

DSM-5 criteria for social anxiety disorder
The DSM-5 criteria for social anxiety disorder are as follows (APA, 2013):
A. Marked fear or anxiety about one or more social situations in which the individual is exposed to possible scrutiny by others. Examples include social interactions such as having a conversation, meeting unfamiliar people, being observed eating or drinking, and performing in front of others such as giving a speech.
B. Individual fears that they will act in a way or show anxiety symptoms that will be negatively evaluated such as feeling humiliated or embarrassed or will lead to rejection or offend others.
C. The social situations almost always provoke fear or anxiety.
   Note: In children, the fear or anxiety may be expressed by crying, tantrums, freezing, clinging, shrinking, or failing to speak in social situations.
D. The social situations are avoided or endured with intense fear or anxiety.
E. The fear or anxiety is out of proportion to the actual threat posed by the social situation and to the sociocultural context.
F. The fear, anxiety, or avoidance is persistent, typically lasting for six months or more.
G. The fear, anxiety, or avoidance causes clinically significant distress or impairment in social, occupational, or other important areas of functioning.
H. The fear, anxiety, or avoidance is not attributable to the physiological effects of a substance such as drug of abuse, a medication or another medical condition.
I. The fear, anxiety, or avoidance is not better explained by the symptoms of another mental disorder, such as panic disorder, body dysmorphic disorder, or autism spectrum disorder.
J. If another medical condition such as Parkinson's disease, obesity, disfigurement from burns or injury is present, the fear, anxiety, or avoidance is clearly unrelated or is excessive.

Specify if:
Performance only: If the fear is restricted to speaking or performing in public.

Panic disorders

A panic attack is a sudden episode of intense fear that triggers, in most instances, severe physical reactions when there is no real danger or evident cause. Panic attacks are more frightening than life-threatening but could significantly affect the quality of life of a person. Panic attacks in themselves are not a mental disorder. They may occur with a range of other mental disorders, and also in the absence of a mental disorder.

A panic disorder, characterised by reoccurring unexpected panic attacks, is an anxiety disorder and meets the diagnostic criteria as discussed below. Panic disorders affect about 2–3 per cent of the population and affect females more than males on a 2:1 ratio. They usually affect children after the age of 14 and decline with age. Panic attacks may occur from a calm or anxious state and escalate within minutes.

Sometimes a person may expect the attack due to a specific cue or trigger, while other attacks are unexpected. It is important to realise that the symptoms of panic attacks can mimic serious physical disorders such as myocardial infarction, cardiac arrhythmias, hyperthyroidism and different types of epilepsy. If not properly diagnosed, panic disorders can therefore result in repeated unnecessary physical investigations and even treatment.

To differentiate panic disorders from medical disorders, it is important to do a thorough physical evaluation. It is also important to explore the emotional component of the attack, since MHCUs often concentrate on only a few physical symptoms, and do not talk about their fears and symptoms of depression. Panic attacks may be triggered by large doses of caffeine, some cold medications and dagga.

Panic disorders are eminently treatable conditions. The usual treatments involve cognitive behavioural or pharmacological therapies or a combination of the two. The cognitive behavioural therapy usually involves weekly sessions for eight to 12 weeks, and the MHCU should show improvement by the third week. Pharmacological treatment includes tricyclic or monoamine oxidase inhibitor (MAOI) antidepressants and high-potency benzodiazepines.

DSM-5 criteria for a panic disorder
The DSM-5 criteria for a panic disorder are as follows (APA, 2013):
A. Recurrent unexpected panic attacks. A panic attack is an abrupt surge of intense fear or intense discomfort that reaches a peak within minutes, and during which time four (or more) of the following symptoms occur;
   Note: The abrupt surge can occur from a calm state or an anxious state.
   1. Palpitations, pounding heart, or accelerated heart rate.
   2. Sweating.
   3. Trembling or shaking.
   4. Sensations of shortness of breath or smothering.
   5. Feelings of choking.
   6. Chest pain or discomfort.
   7. Nausea or abdominal distress.
   8. Feeling dizzy, unsteady, light-headed, or faint.
   9. Chills or heat sensations.
   10. Paresthesias (numbness or tingling sensations).
   11. Derealization (feelings of unreality) or depersonalization (being detached from oneself).

12. Fear of losing control or "going crazy."
13. Fear of dying.

Note: Culture-specific symptoms (e.g., tinnitus, neck soreness, headache, uncontrollable screaming or crying) may be seen. Such symptoms should not count as one of the four required symptoms.

B. At least one of the attacks has been followed by 1 month (or more) of one or both of the following:
   1. Persistent concern or worry about additional panic attacks or their consequences (e.g., losing control, having a heart attack, "going crazy").
   2. A significant maladaptive change in behavior related to the attacks (e.g., behaviors designed to avoid having panic attacks, such as avoidance of exercise or unfamiliar situations).
C. The disturbance is not attributable to the physiological effects of a substance (e.g., a drug of abuse, a medication) or another medical condition (e.g., hyperthyroidism, cardiopulmonary disorders).
D. The disturbance is not better explained by another mental disorder (e.g., the panic attacks do not occur only in response to feared social situations, as in social anxiety disorder: in response to circumscribed phobic objects or situations, as in specific phobia: in response to obsessions, as in obsessive-compulsive disorder: in response to reminders of traumatic events, as in posttraumatic stress disorder: or in response to separation from attachment figures, as in separation anxiety disorder).

Agoraphobia

Agoraphobia is the fear of being in places or situations from which escape from the phobic stimulus might be difficult (or embarrassing) or in which help might not be available in the event of an emergency. This type of phobia involves a cluster of situations, of which the most common are fear of confined spaces (for example, supermarkets, hair salons and cinemas), of public transportation and of being far from home. These situations are then avoided. These people generally feel safest at home or in the company of a trusted person; the further they venture from home and safety, the more fearful they become. If escape from the phobic situation seems impossible, they may experience panic. Agoraphobia seems to start either in late adolescence, when particularly women are expected to become more independent, or around the age of 30.

The adolescent's skill at describing and expressing their feelings and internal experiences are generally more sophisticated than in young children. This could lead to the phenomenon that teens may be better at describing anxiety than younger children. However, in western societies, 'panic attack', is a term commonly used. Youth may already be familiar with this and other anxiety-related expressions and thus easily state, 'I have a panic attack.' Even though adolescents might be more able to express their anxiety they would still require gentle support to have the courage to share what is happening with them.

Generalised anxiety disorder

Generalised anxiety disorder (together with social phobia) is one of the more common anxiety disorders. More than half the people suffering from this disorder have had high anxiety levels since childhood, when the anxiety often centred around school performance or catastrophic events such as nuclear war. It is not common in people older than 20.

DSM-5 criteria for generalised anxiety disorder
The DSM-5 criteria for generalised anxiety disorder are as follows (APA, 2013):
A. Excessive anxiety and worry (apprehensive expectation), occurring more days than not for at least 6 months, about a number of events or activities (such as work or school performance).
B. The individual finds it difficult to control the worry.
C. The anxiety and worry are associated with three (or more) of the following six symptoms (with at least some symptoms having been present for more days than not for the past 6 months):
   Note: Only one item required in children.
   1. Restlessness, feeling keyed up or on edge
   2. Being easily fatigued
   3. Difficulty concentrating or mind going blank
   4. Irritability
   5. Muscle tension
   6. Sleep disturbance (difficulty falling or staying asleep, or restless, unsatisfying sleep).
D. The anxiety, worry, or physical symptoms cause clinically significant distress or impairment in social, occupational, or other important areas of functioning.
E. The disturbance is not attributable to the physiological effects of a substance (for example, a drug of abuse, a medication) or another medical condition (for example, hyperthyroidism).
F. The disturbance is not better explained by another medical disorder (for example, anxiety or worry about having panic attacks in panic disorder, negative evaluation in social anxiety disorder [social phobia], contamination or other obsessions in obsessive-compulsive disorder, separation from attachment figures in separation anxiety disorder, reminders of traumatic events in PTSD, gaining weight in anorexia nervosa, physical complaints in somatic symptom disorder, perceived appearance flaws in body dysmorphic disorder, having a serious illness in illness anxiety disorder, or the content of delusional beliefs in schizophrenia or delusional disorder).

Obsessive-compulsive disorders

This category includes obsessive-compulsive disorder, body dysmorphic disorder, hoarding disorder, trichotillomania, and excoriation disorder.

Obsessive-compulsive disorder

Obsessions are unwanted and intrusive thoughts and urges or impulses that are involuntary. They generally concern topics that are distasteful to the person and difficult to dismiss. Once the thought occurs, it is accompanied by anxiety or by feelings of discomfort and the urge to neutralise the thought. Neutralising generally takes the form of overt and covert compulsive behaviour.

Overt behaviour might include avoiding situations that trigger obsessional thoughts or performing a particular activity, for example checking repeatedly that all the doors are locked for fear of being physically harmed. Covert behaviour involves changes in mental activity, such as thinking a different thought in response to the obsessional thought or thinking the same thought an even number of times in order to feel better.

These behaviours are usually carried out in a stereotyped way or according to personally defined 'rules' or rituals. They are coupled with temporary relief from anxiety as well as with the belief that, if the behaviour is not carried out, the anxiety will increase. Anxiety relief thus reinforces compulsive behaviour. As obsessions persist and rituals become extensive, MHCUs sometimes prevent obsessional thoughts from occurring by performing neutralising behaviour. Someone may wash their hands 100 times a day to prevent the original obsessional thought of contamination by germs from occurring. The disorder usually manifests itself in adolescence or early adulthood. Table 12.6 identifies examples of obsessions and related compulsive behaviours.

Table 12.6 Obsession and compulsive behaviour

Content and examples of obsession	Examples of compulsive behaviour
Contamination (ideas of being harmed by contact with substances believed to be dangerous, for example dirt, germs, urine, faeces, blood, radiation, poison) ▪ The hairdresser's comb has the HIV/AIDS virus on it	Rings doctor; checks body for symptoms of AIDS; washes hands and hair; sterilises all things that others may touch
Physical violence to self or others by self or others ▪ I will harm my baby	Will not be alone with the baby; seeks reassurance; hides knives, plastic bags
Accidental harm (not due to contamination or physical violence, for example accident, illness) ▪ I may have hit someone with my car	Telephones hospitals, police; retraces route driven; checks car for marks
Socially unacceptable behaviour (for example, shouting, swearing, losing control of behaviour) ▪ I am going to shout an obscenity	Tries to 'control' behaviour; avoids social situations; asks others whether behaviour was acceptable in a particular situation
Sex (preoccupation with sexual organs, unacceptable sexual acts) ▪ I am going to commit rape	Avoids being alone with women; tries to keep mind off sexual thoughts
Religion (for example, blasphemous thoughts, religious doubts) ▪ I am going to offer my food to the devil	Prays; seeks religious help/makes confession; offers other things to God

→

Content and examples of obsession	Examples of compulsive behaviour
Orderliness (things being in the right place, actions done in the right way, according to a particular pattern or number) ■ If I don't clean my teeth in the right way, I'll have to do it again until I get it right	Repeats action a 'good' number of times; repeats until it 'feels right'
Nonsense (meaningless phrases, images, tunes, words, strings of numbers) ■ Hears (in the head) the tune of a TV sports programme while reading	Repeats action until managing to read the same passage without tune occurring

Source: Adapted from Hawton et al (1989)

DSM-5 diagnostic criteria for obsessive-compulsive disorder

The DSM-5 diagnostic criteria for obsessive-compulsive disorder are as follows (APA, 2013):

A. Presence of obsessions, compulsions, or both:

Obsessions are defined by (1) and (2):
1. Recurrent and persistent thoughts, urges, or impulses that are experienced, at some time during the disturbance, as intrusive and unwanted, and that in most individuals cause marked anxiety or distress.
2. The individual attempts to ignore or suppress such thoughts, urges, or images, or to neutralise them with some other thought or action (ie by performing a compulsion).

Compulsions are defined by (1) and (2):
1. Repetitive behaviours (for example, hand washing, ordering, checking) or mental acts (for example, praying, counting, repeating words silently) that the individual feels driven to perform in response to an obsession or according to rules that must be applied rigidly.
2. The behaviours or mental acts are aimed at preventing or reducing anxiety or distress, or preventing some dreaded event or situation; however, these behaviours or mental acts are not connected in a realistic way with what they are designed to neutralise or prevent, or are clearly excessive.

Note: Young children may not be able to articulate the aims of these behaviours or mental acts.

B. The obsessions or compulsions are time-consuming (for example, take more than one hour per day) or cause clinically significant distress or impairment in social, occupational, or other important areas of functioning.
C. The obsessive-compulsive symptoms are not attributable to the physiological effects of a substance (for example, a drug of abuse, a medication) or another medical condition.
D. The disturbance is not better explained by the symptoms of another mental disorder. These include excessive worries, as in generalised anxiety disorder; preoccupation

with appearance, as in body dysmorphic disorder; difficulty discarding or parting with possessions, as in hoarding disorder; hair pulling, as in trichotillomania (hair-pulling disorder); skin picking, as in excoriation (skin-picking disorder); stereotypies, as in stereotypic movement disorder; ritualised eating behaviour, as in eating disorders; preoccupation with substances or gambling, as in substance-related and addictive disorders; preoccupation with having an illness, as in illness anxiety disorder; sexual urges or fantasies, as in paraphilic disorders; impulses, as in disruptive, impulse-control, and conduct disorders; guilty ruminations, as in major depressive disorder; thought insertion or delusional preoccupations, as in schizophrenia spectrum and other psychotic disorders; or repetitive patterns of behaviour, as in autism spectrum disorder.

Specify if:
- *With good or fair insight.* The individual recognises that obsessive-compulsive disorder beliefs are definitely or probably not true or that they may or may not be true.
- *With poor insight.* The individual thinks obsessive-compulsive disorder beliefs are probably true.
- *With absent insight/delusional beliefs.* The individual is completely convinced that obsessive-compulsive disorder beliefs are true.
- *Tic-related.* The individual has a current or past history of a tic disorder.

Trauma and stressor-related disorders

These disorders are outlined in Chapter 19 on trauma.

THE EXPERIENCE OF INTERACTING WITH AN ANXIOUS MHCU

Health care of anxious MHCUs can be particularly stressful. This is partly because of the helplessness mental health care workers may experience in the face of the person's obvious distress and discomfort, and partly because anxiety itself is communicated interpersonally. In addition to the anxiety-reducing techniques mentioned later in the chapter, there are a number of other strategies the nurse can use to maintain personal and professional efficiency when delivering care to an anxious MHCU.

Recognising one's own feelings of anxiety

The first strategy centres on recognising one's own anxiety and the thoughts, events and feelings that may be responsible for provoking it. Many students enter the clinical situation beset by a range of fears about their own competencies and resources for coping: 'What if I say something wrong?'; 'What if the MHCU doesn't like me?'; 'What if I get hurt or hurt the person?'; 'Will I be able to cope with mentally ill health care users?' These responses are quite normal considering that one is entering a novel situation, and often not voluntarily. No amount of preparation for the clinical experience can allay anxiety in students. What can be of help is to explore the beliefs that give rise to these negative thoughts and to work actively to reframe them as reasonable statements of intent.

The nursing socialisation process is to some extent responsible for the beliefs that nurses develop about themselves. Explicit images of the responsible, independent practitioner abound in nursing. Thus, the mismatch between what we think we should be thinking, feeling and doing when delivering health care and what we are actually thinking, feeling and doing often leads to the development of a belief system that is at best confusing and at worst the source of much anxiety and distress.

Hence, when thoughts of incompetence arise, it is important to question their validity:
- Is it reasonable to expect that one should be able to cope with all situations all the time?
- Is it reasonable to expect that all people should like us all the time?
- Is it reasonable to expect that nurses should never make mistakes?
- Is it unreasonable to expect that nurses are capable of directing and controlling their own profession?

The nurse should work at challenging these and other unfavourable thoughts that pop up and at restating them in ways that allow for your own humanness. Thoughts such as 'What if I do something to hurt the MHCU?' can be rationally restated as 'I will use what skill and knowledge I have at this point to care for MHCUs'. With persistence and practice, nurses can contribute towards challenging the values and beliefs that cause anxiety and work towards developing a realistic belief system that enhances their natural abilities and talents.

Skills that can be used in interacting with the highly anxious MHCUs

The second strategy involves developing a set of verbal, non-verbal and environmental management skills that can be used in dealing with anxious MHCUs, especially those with a high level of anxiety.

Verbal communication

The mental health care nurse should follow these principles when using verbal communication skills:
- Communicate with the person simply and directly, without being patronising.
- Avoid lengthy, in-depth discussions with the extremely anxious MHCU since their ability to process information is likely to be impaired.
- Speak in a calm, even tone of voice.
- Avoid criticising or making judgements about what the person does to curtail their anxiety, even if these coping behaviours are maladaptive, for instance neutralisation of behaviour or avoidance.
- If the MHCU is talking fast and breathlessly, suggest they slow down and draw a breath between words to decrease cardiovascular arousal.

Non-verbal communication

The mental health care nurse can also use non-verbal communication when dealing with a highly anxious MHCU and should follow these guidelines:

- Allow the person sufficient body space; being too close to the MHCU can increase the anxiety response.
- Make sure that physical gestures convey an intention to help, not harm; move slowly towards the person and reach out with the palms of the hand facing up so that the gesture is not misinterpreted by the person as an attempt to 'attack'.
- When moving towards the person, inform them verbally of what your actions mean, for example: 'I'm going to sit down on the bench with you for a few minutes.'
- Sometimes restless and panicky MHCUs need reassurance about the availability of support and nurture; provide this by holding the person gently while making verbal statements about the desire to help the MHCU feel in control, for example: 'I'm here to help you cope with the distress and tension you seem to be feeling.'

Environmental management

Managing the environment is another way in which the mental health care nurse can assist the highly anxious MHCU. This can be done in the following ways:

- Decrease environmental stimulation by limiting the MHCU's interactions with others; by monitoring the noise level in the ward/home/clinic and by intervening to decrease the level of noise, if possible.
- Identify and modify situations that provoke anxiety for the person until they are able to participate in this process; for example, ask the family to visit or not to visit if this is a source of anxiety for the person.
- Offer supportive physical measures, for example, a warm bath or shower, or massages if the MHCU is able to tolerate physical touch.
- Administer prescribed medications to provide relief of symptoms.

MENTAL HEALTH NURSING AND ASSESSMENT OF ANXIETY

Health care workers who are aware of their own feelings of anxiety, who have prepared themselves to be competent in managing MHCUs experiencing anxiety, and who have developed a comprehensive skill set (verbal, non-verbal and environment management) for interacting with anxious MHCUs, are prepared for conducting mental health assessments of such persons.

Mental health assessments have three aims, which involve:
1. determining the precise nature of the problem
2. defining the goals of possible nursing interventions
3. identifying appropriate nursing interventions.

The precise nature of the problem

Determining the precise nature of the problem involves identifying:
- what the problems are and which are most distressing to the MHCU
- when the problems started and how they have developed over time
- what behavioural, cognitive, physiological and affective responses are associated with the problems
- in what situations and contexts the problems occur
- what factors serve to maintain the problems and
- what coping strategies and resources the person employs to manage the problems and their emotional consequences.

The examination of a person's state of mental health and the identification of lifestyle patterns are the basic assessment tools of the nurse. There are a variety of assessment strategies that can aid the systematic and accurate collecting of information. These include: the behavioural interview; self-monitoring; self-reporting (for example, questionnaires); information from others (for example, interviews with key individuals); direct observation of behaviour in clinical settings; and physiological measures.

The behavioural interview

Chapter 10, 'Mental Health Assessment of Hospitalised or Community-based Individuals', deals in detail with this method of assessment.

A time–event chart can be used to plot the course of the problem. Variations in severity of the problem are recorded down one side of the timeline, and life changes or stressful events down the other side (see Appendix 6 for an example of such a chart).

Self-monitoring

This can be used as an adjunct to behavioural interviewing. Self-monitoring is flexible and can be applied to a wide range of problems or symptoms. There are two stages in self-monitoring. The MHCU first has to recognise that the behaviour, thought, emotion or event has occurred and then has to record that it has happened. The behaviour to be monitored should be clearly defined; 'feels anxious' is too vague a concept to measure. Criteria that indicate the person is anxious should rather be used. These criteria can include self-critical thoughts when in the company of others, palpitations, breathlessness, etc. Alternatively, self-monitoring can be used to help specify what the problems are.

A number of aspects of the problem can be monitored:
- How often the target behaviour occurs (frequency)
- How long the target behaviour lasts (duration)
- The situation in which the target behaviour occurs (context)
- Emotions associated with the target behaviour
- Thoughts associated with the target behaviour.

Rating scales can be used to establish the intensity of the various aspects of the problem and the extent to which the MHCU believes their negative thoughts. A scale of 0 to 100 can be used, where 0 = the absence of emotion, sensation or belief, 50 = a moderate degree, and 100 = as strong as it could be.

To ensure the relative accuracy of self-monitoring, the MHCU should be instructed to record the information as soon as it is noted and not to delay doing so until later.

Example
Ms B reported that she felt 'terrified' all the time. She was unable to be any more specific than this, so the nurse asked her to keep the following record for one day. The purpose of this exercise was to reinforce the need for concrete as opposed to global thinking, as well as to determine specific problem areas.

From Ms B's log, it seems that she feels most anxious in the company of others and is concerned about how other people perceive her. The same method could be used to clarify further in what specific social situations she feels anxious and with whom, and the nature and intensity of the anxiety response. Table 12.7 shows how her emotions can be recorded and rated.

Table 12.7 Assessing emotion

Date & time	Emotion	Situation	Negative thoughts
	What is it? How bad is it? 0–100	Where were you; what were you doing at the time and with whom?	What were your thoughts? To what extent do you believe each of them? 0–100
22.8 07:00	Nervous: 80 Angry: 80	Lying awake in bed; person next to me snored all night	I can't stand this: 80 I would have slept if I was at home alone: 50
08:00	Flustered: 90 Racing heart: 60 Muddled thoughts: 70	Sitting with other MHCUs in the lounge; ward sister came to speak to me	What have I done wrong: 80 Fellow MHCUs don't like me, the ward sister has to talk to me: 90
09:00	Relaxed: 50 Lonely: 70	Sitting outside alone, knitting	If I avoid people, I feel better: 90 Other people are much happier without me around: 90

Note how the MHCU's self-rating gives an indication of her cognitive thought patterns. Ms B concludes that, because she is alone and feeling relaxed, her anxiety must have something to do with being with other people (selective abstraction). This cognitive error might prevent her from considering the possibility that other factors, such as focusing on a distracting task (knitting), might also be partly responsible for her feeling relaxed.

Direct observation of behaviour

The nurse can gather information about naturally occurring behaviours that indicate anxiety by using time sampling, interval recording and continuous recording methods. If specific target behaviour is to be observed, that which is to be observed should be clearly defined. For example, if MHCUs deals with their fear of social ridicule by withdrawing, the focus of observation could be on trying to establish the frequency of the person's interactions, how long they last and with whom they interact.

It is insufficient to state simply 'socially withdrawn'; it is the degree to which MHCUs isolate themselves that determines what intervention strategies are appropriate.

Physiological measures

Physiological processes can be monitored indirectly. An MHCU can be asked to monitor the frequency, duration and contexts. Physiological symptoms such as sweating, headaches, nausea, respiration and blood pressure can be monitored regularly to determine the extent of physiological arousal and the extent to which intervention strategies have helped decrease physiological arousal. Sometimes, especially with MHCUs who deny feeling anxious, yet obviously appear to be so, tangible evidence of physiological arousal can help them to develop an awareness of the possibility that they might be feeling anxious.

Analysing the data for the purpose of goal setting and nursing diagnosis/intervention

Once the exact nature of the anxiety symptoms or disorder has been determined, the mental health nurse identifies goals that are relevant to the nursing diagnoses. This will illuminate the nature and intensity of the problem, the frequency and duration of the verbal and non-verbal behaviours that describe the problem; the specific stressors associated with the problem, and the range of nursing interventions required for the particular person's needs.

Characteristics of 'anxiety' as a nursing diagnosis

Anxiety is most frequently cited as a *nursing* diagnosis in a wide variety of practice settings. Nurse researchers attempt to develop a workable formulation or diagnosis of anxiety that has universal meaning for nurse practitioners. The extent of the research done in this area and the apparent lack of consensus as to what the critical defining characteristics of anxiety are, reflect the elusive nature of anxiety.

Common alternative nursing diagnoses applicable to MHCUs with anxiety (as meeting the DSM-5 diagnostic criteria) are the following:
- Anxiety *related* to threat to self-concept *evidenced* by feelings of unreality and insomnia.
- Panic *related* to being exposed to phobic stimulus (name the MHCU's phobic stimulus), *evidenced* by palpitations, fear of dying, fainting, trembling and shaking.

Defining the precise nature of the problem sets the stage for identifying treatment goals and nursing intervention strategies.

NURSING INTERVENTIONS RELATED TO STRESS/ANXIOUSNESS AND/OR PATHOLOGICAL ANXIETY

Nursing intervention takes place within the context of the supportive, collaborative relationship initiated between the nurse and the MHCU during the assessment phase.

The three broad, interrelated goals of intervention are to:
1. Help relieve the MHCU's immediate distress associated with anxiety
2. Help the person to gain an understanding of their experience of anxiety and
3. Help the person to identify and cope with the source of their anxiety.

Cognitive behavioural therapy

Cognitive behavioural therapy has already been mentioned as a mode of intervention a mental health nurse can apply when dealing with an MHCU, irrespective of the variations of anxiety experienced. The following strategies are used in cognitive behavioural therapy to help people to develop new constructions of themselves at specific points.

Cognitive distraction techniques

These strategies can be used for managing the consequences (emotional and behavioural) of anxiety – in other words, for immediate symptom management and to help MHCUs realise that they can exercise some measure of control over their anxiety. These strategies aim to shift the person's awareness from their anxiety to neutral things beyond self. The choice of strategy depends on the MHCU's degree of distress and cognitive ability: a highly anxious person with marked cognitive impairment would not be asked to participate in mental exercises; this would serve to increase their level of anxiety; absorbing physical exercise or activities would be more appropriate. The nurse should also ensure that these techniques are not perceived as competitive; this is a potential source of danger for the person. The way in which the strategy works, and its potential benefits, should be explained to the MHCU.

Focusing on an object
The MHCU can be taught to focus their attention on a neutral object, such as a bowl of flowers, chair, carpet or piece of furniture and to describe it in as much detail as possible when they feel anxious. As an example, an MHCU, Pete, was interested in woodwork. When he felt anxious, he focused his attention on a piece of furniture and asked himself a series of questions: 'What is it made of?', 'How big is it?', 'What colour is it?', 'What could it be used for?' This technique helped to reduce his level of anxiety in the situation and he was able to use his knowledge in conversation with others.

Sensory awareness
This involves teaching the MHCU to focus on their surroundings, using all their senses. In this instance, Pete learned a series of cue questions to stimulate awareness: 'What can I see if I look around me?', 'What sounds can I hear?', 'What is the texture of this wood/leaf/tree trunk?'

Mental exercises
Any absorbing mental activity can serve as a distraction from feelings of distress. An example would be counting backwards from 50, doing jigsaw or crossword puzzles, or playing general knowledge games.

Absorbing activities
Physical activities can help to distract the MHCU and reduce physical tension associated with anxiety. Activities such as playing tennis, setting the table, table-tennis, swimming, brisk walks, stretching exercises, yoga, arranging flowers, making beds, or serving meals are useful.

Visualisation techniques
Therapeutic visualisation is similar to the process of 'reframing'. Reframing is based on the idea that, because people choose to interpret or frame their experience in a particular way, it is possible for them to learn other, more positive ways of interpreting their experiences.

This technique has been used successfully for problem solving. In one study, 15 respondents were instructed in the technique and then asked to apply it daily, for one week, to an interpersonal problem. Of the seven respondents who practised the technique on a daily basis, five reported significant, measurable outcomes. What follows is an example of the technique:

Instructions:
- Imagine a blue picture frame.
- Try to imagine your problem of ... inside the frame.
- Stand back from the picture and look at all the elements in it. Who is in it? What are they doing? What colours are in the picture?
- Look at the picture for two minutes, then let the picture fade.
- Now imagine a white picture frame.
- Inside the frame, see the problem of ... resolved.
- Stand back again and look at the elements in the picture. Who is in it? What are they doing? How do they feel about each other?
- Try to hold the picture for two minutes, then let the picture fade.

This technique should be practised twice daily for five minutes. Initially, the MHCU will experience some difficulty in imagining and holding the picture frames. This is to be expected, but it should improve with practice.

Behavioural strategies of self-monitoring and rating

This has been discussed in the section dealing with assessment. This strategy can be used at any time during treatment, as it is especially useful as a method of monitoring and charting progress.

Cognitive behavioural strategies

The aims of these strategies are to reduce anxiety by teaching MHCUs how to identify, evaluate, control and alter their negative, danger-related thoughts and associated behaviours.

Identifying unhelpful beliefs underlying negative thoughts and the specific situations in which they occur

This may take some time. Negative thoughts may be so habitual and believable that the MHCU frequently fails to notice them. In addition, the visual images may be so brief that the person might not notice or remember them. These images, especially those associated with high anxiety, are often so bizarre (for example, lying on a shop floor screaming) that MHCUs are many a time reluctant to discuss them. In this case, it would be helpful to reassure the person that such images are normal in the face of high anxiety. Again, thoughts concerned with danger can provoke anxiety; MHCUs may then engage in a variety of obvious and not-so-obvious avoidance behaviour, such as talking about experiences in general terms, removing themselves from the situation or giving diluted versions of their anxious thoughts.

A useful principle for the nurse to use when helping the MHCU to identify negative thoughts or images is to ask: 'Would I be as anxious as the MHCU if I had this thought and believed it?' If the answer is 'no', the identified thought is possibly inaccurate or requires further exploration.

Exploring a recent emotional experience

Ask the MHCU to recall and describe in detail a recent event or situation in which they felt anxious. Questions such as 'When were you in the situation?', 'What thoughts were going through your mind?', 'What is the worst thing you think could happen to you?' and 'What image did you have of yourself at that moment?' will help to identify some of the thoughts associated with the onset and maintenance of the emotional reaction.

Using imagery to elicit automatic thoughts

If questioning fails to draw out automatic thoughts, the nurse may ask the MHCU to relive the experience using imagery. Instructions such as 'Imagine yourself back in the situation we were talking about, at the point just before you noticed yourself becoming anxious. Briefly describe to me what you see, whom you are with, what is going on around you, how you are feeling, what thoughts are going through your mind, what do you see now? At the time your anxiety increased, what was going through your mind?'.

Picking up on shifts in the mental health care user's mood

Picking up on shifts in the person's mood while talking to them can also be a useful source of automatic thoughts. For example, while talking to an MHCU (Pete) about an approaching birthday celebration party, the nurse noticed that he suddenly became quiet when dancing was mentioned.

Nurse: What went through your mind when I mentioned dancing?
Pete: I was thinking about dancing.
Nurse: What were you thinking?
Pete: About not being able to dance.
Nurse: Did you have a picture in your head of yourself?
Pete: Yes.
Nurse: Describe the picture to me.
Pete: I was standing alone watching all the people.
Nurse: How did you feel?
Pete: Horrible ... all tense ... I wanted to dance but I felt too embarrassed to ask anyone.

The nurse then went on to help Pete to describe the picture in more detail and to clarify what he meant by 'tense', where he felt the tension in his body and what he meant by 'horrible'.

Finally, the nurse helped Pete to 'put it all together' by writing a list of the anxiety-provoking situations, corresponding thoughts or images and anxiety response. Table 12.8 shows how this list could be written.

Table 12.8 Anxiety responses to different situations

Situations	Thoughts or images	Anxiety response
Being at a party with people I don't know	Picture of myself standing all alone, looking foolish and awkward; thinking 'I can't cope with this'; other people thinking I am boring, an idiot; everyone looking at me	Feels tense and awkward; chest is tight; heart is beating fast; on edge, jittery, nervous
	I am going to trip and fall if I move; I am going to make a fool of myself; I am going to suffocate; there is something badly wrong with my heart	Tachycardia; breathlessness; hypervigilance; feels faint, out of control, terrified

Modifying thoughts and associated behaviours

Help the client to recognise that thoughts influence behaviour and emotions. Ask the MHCU what they make of the idea that their responses came after the identified negative thoughts. In other words, it is possible that the person's interpretation of the situation (as revealed in their thoughts) may have led to the feelings of anxiety in the situation. Use each of the instances written down by the MHCU to reinforce this idea.

It is important at this point not to lecture the MHCU on the relationship between thoughts, feelings and behaviour. Statements such as 'If you had more positive thoughts about yourself you would feel and think differently and wouldn't be so anxious' are not helpful. The person must be brought to this realisation slowly, at a pace they able to deal with. Again, many people confuse this technique with positive thinking; the goal here is to help the person develop more rational ways of thinking that include a realistic awareness of the positive as well as the negative aspects of the situation.

For example, the nurse's interaction with Pete may continue like this:

Nurse: Did you feel anxious before you had that image of yourself?
Pete: No, I felt okay before.
Nurse: What do you make of that? You had a picture of yourself looking, as you say, foolish, and then you started feeling tense?
Pete: (*sceptical*) Well, maybe the two are related, but I don't really see how. I mean, I feel tense whenever there are people around, not just when I have to go to a party.

Picking up on Pete's message, 'I feel tense whenever there are people around', the nurse helped Pete to be specific about describing the situations in which he felt anxious (in what situations, with whom, when, where).

It turned out that Pete was generalising (this is known as stimulus generalisation). In reality, he felt more anxious in situations involving people he did not know. Pete felt a certain sense of relief when the nurse pointed this out to him; the problem seemed more manageable.

Other strategies in nursing interventions
The following strategies can also be used when nursing an MHCU with anxiety.

Give information about anxiety (or depression)
Giving information about the symptoms of anxiety, their possible origins and functions, the lack of relationship between anxiety and insanity and the fact that the automatic changes that occur are not dangerous, may help the MHCU to see that a series of seemingly unconnected problems such as insomnia or difficulty in concentrating are aspects of an anxiety state and not a huge array of insurmountable problems. This information might also help to correct any misconceptions about anxiety.

Whatever information is given should be tailored to suit the MHCU's needs and mental state.

Test automatic thoughts of threat
Because the MHCU's first interpretation of the event is usually the worst, the goal here is to help them find more realistic and helpful alternatives to these thoughts.

Verbal challenging
This technique is used to teach MHCUs how to re-evaluate their thinking for themselves.

A series of questions, as outlined below, can be asked to stimulate this process.

Question: What evidence do you have for that thought?
The evidence used to support a negative thought is likely to be distorted because the MHCU's thinking is dominated by themes of danger and because non-threatening information (contrary evidence) is less easily recalled than threatening information. This means that conclusions are reached on the basis of faulty information.

Nurse: Pete, you mentioned that you think people find you boring – what makes you think this?
Pete: Well, when I'm in a group and they are all talking, no one talks directly to me.
Nurse: Are you the only one they don't talk directly to?
Pete: No.
Nurse: Is there anything that people do when you are at a party that goes against this idea?
Pete: Some friends do come over and talk to me.
Nurse: How do you think that fits in with the idea that people don't talk directly to you because they find you boring?
Pete: I suppose it's not entirely true.

Question: What alternative views are there?
Nurse: Can you think of any other reasons for people not talking directly to you?
Pete: Not really.

Question: When explanations are not easily available, supplementary questions can be asked.

Nurse: What would you say to another person who came to you with the same problem?

Pete: Something like 'Sometimes you give the impression that you are not interested in what's being said because when people try to involve you, you withdraw and don't talk'.

Nurse: So another reason for people not looking directly at you might be that they don't think that you are interested because you withdraw?

The nurse then went on to help Pete make a list of at least four different but equally plausible interpretations for each event.

It is not necessary for the different interpretations to be absolutely accurate. It is more important for the MHCU to realise that different interpretations are possible and that the first interpretations are not automatically correct simply because they are the first. Finding alternatives helps to weaken the plausibility of the first thought.

Question: Are your judgements based on how you felt rather than on what you did?

Sometimes anxious MHCUs evaluate their behaviour in particular situations as inappropriate simply because they feel anxious. Often their actual behaviour is appropriate.

Nurse: You say that you were feeling uptight when your friend's girlfriend came over to talk to you and that you couldn't cope. What did you do?

Pete: I offered her a drink and listened while she told me about her job.

Nurse: That sounds like coping.

Question: Are you thinking in all-or-nothing terms?

When anxious, people tend to evaluate themselves and their experiences in extremes.

Pete: If people don't show an interest in me, then that means that they don't like me.

Nurse: I'm going to draw a line and mark the one end 'strongly hate', the middle 'neither like nor dislike' and the other end 'strongly like'. Think of all the people you know and mark how you think each person feels about you on the scale.

Pete was able to see that people cover the whole range of the scale and not just the two extremes.

Question: Are you concentrating on the things that frighten you and forgetting about positive experiences? (selective abstraction)

Nurse: Let's try to divide each of your experiences at the party into good and bad. What was good about the time you spent with your friend's girlfriend?

Pete: It all seemed bad ... but okay, I felt a little more relaxed while she was talking to me; I didn't feel as if I was so boring.

Exploring each experience in this way, Pete was able to realise that his tendency to select and focus on the threatening aspects of situations clouded his perception of the entire experience.

Question: Are you overestimating how responsible you are for the way things turn out?/Are you overestimating how much control you have over how things work out? (personalisation)
Anxious MHCUs tend to believe that they are responsible for what other people think and feel, and for the way events proceed. A friend told Pete he didn't enjoy the party. Pete believed that this was because he was anxious. The nurse helped Pete to make a list of all the causes that might have contributed to his friend's not enjoying the party and which were out of Pete's control. Pete was then asked to draw a pie chart (see Figure 12.3), allocating a section of the circle to each cause. It became clear to Pete that there were other factors involved.

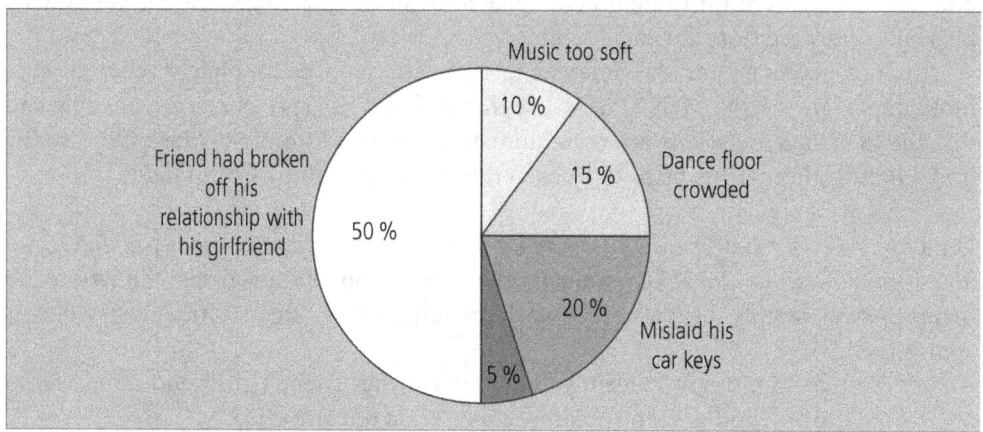

Figure 12.3 Pete's pie chart

Question: What if it happens? What would be so bad about that? (catastrophising)
Anticipating harm is often more distressing that the event itself. Using this question may help the MHCU to realise this.

Nurse: If you went to the ward party, what do you think is the worst thing that could happen?
Pete: No one would talk to me.
Nurse: Has this ever happened before?
Pete: Not really.
Nurse: Imagine that no one came to talk to you, what do you think would happen to you?
Pete: Well, I'd feel really bad.
Nurse: How bad, on a scale from 0 to 100?
Pete: I suppose 40.
Nurse: So you would feel moderately bad?
Pete: It's not so terrible, but not pleasant.

The nurse then went on to point out that Pete had already learned a number of distraction techniques that he could use in the situation, thus reducing the intensity of the feeling even further.

Questioning negative thoughts encourages MHCUs to evaluate realistically the costs and advantages of thinking differently and opens the way for changes in behaviour.

Take action to test negative thoughts
Arguing against negative thoughts is often not enough to convince MHCUs that they are incorrect. The person needs to build up a body of experience that contradicts the thoughts. Testing predictions (negative thoughts) helps to break old patterns of thinking and pave the way for new ones.

There are five steps in this process:
1. *State the negative thought (prediction) clearly in concrete terms, using 'who', 'what', 'when', 'where' and 'how' questions.*
   Pete predicted that, if he went to the party, he would not be able to talk to anyone and that he would have a terrible time.
2. *Help the MHCU to review the existing evidence for and against it.*
   'Before I became so anxious, I used to enjoy parties. It's true that since I've been so anxious I have been avoiding going to parties. Still, I have gone to one or two and not felt anxious. This one will be with people I know in the ward; they know how I am, so maybe they won't expect too much from me. If I don't go, I might miss an opportunity to feel better; I am sure it will take me out of myself.'
3. *Help the MHCU to work out an action plan.*
   'Go and see what happens. Use distraction beforehand to stop anxiety building up, for example visualisation exercises, a brisk walk. Walk there with people I know, sit with them and talk to them first. Focus my attention on what they are saying, listen to them.'
4. *Teach the MHCU how to make a note of the results.*
   There are two main possibilities: the prediction is borne out or it is not. If the prediction is verified, reassure the person that this is valuable information and not a sign of their incompetence. Work with the person to develop a new action plan based on their experience.
   'Did not enjoy it, left early. Spent the whole evening thinking that people were wondering why I wasn't dancing; felt uncomfortable, foolish. I couldn't concentrate on what was going on.'
   New action plan: 'Next time, practise distraction techniques for a longer period and practise them while I am at the party; see if I can get to know one of my fellow MHCUs on the ward a bit better; start by asking Ms B to play cards with me; practise visualising myself coping at the party; practise progressive relaxation before the party.'
5. *Help the MHCU to draw conclusions on the basis of the results.*
   What do the conclusions tell the MHCU about the way they feel about themselves or the way anxiety affects them? What general rules can the person draw up to help them deal better with similar situations in the future?
   'My original prediction was correct, mainly because I was so concerned with how

I was feeling that I couldn't look outwards. Even so, two people did sit with me for a while, so I suppose one bad evening does not mean that everyone thinks I'm boring.'

As with any new skill, it takes time to learn how to test the validity of negative thoughts in real-life situations. In the beginning, the MHCU should be encouraged to test negative thoughts in situations that are least threatening, namely, in situations where they are likely to experience some measure of success. As the person becomes more adept at testing negative thoughts in practice, this new learning can be generalised to apply to more difficult situations. Setbacks are not uncommon, and the MHCU should be helped to see them as valuable sources of information that can themselves be tested in the same way.

Nursing strategies when dealing with panic

The nurse can educate or assist the MHCU with various strategies for coping with panic, by making these types of statements:

- Remember that, although your feelings and symptoms are very frightening, they are not dangerous or harmful.
- Understand that what you are experiencing is just an exaggeration of your normal bodily reactions to stress.
- Do not fight your feelings or try to wish them away. The more you are willing to face them, the less intense they will become.
- Do not add to your panic by thinking about what 'might' happen. If you find yourself asking 'What if ...?', tell yourself 'So what!'.
- Stay in the present. Notice what is really happening to you as opposed to what you think might happen.
- Label your fear level from 0 to 10 and watch it go up and down. Notice that it does not stay at a very high level for more than a few seconds.
- When you find yourself thinking about the fear, change your 'what if' thinking. Focus on and carry out a simple and manageable task such as counting backwards from 100 in 3s, or snapping a rubber band on your wrist.
- Notice that when you stop adding frightening thoughts to your fear, it begins to fade.
- When the fear comes, expect and accept it. Wait and give it time to pass without running away from it.
- Be proud of yourself for your progress thus far and think about how good you will feel when you succeed this time.

Relaxation training

The relaxation response is the physiological opposite of the anxiety response; increased physiological–affective–behavioural–cognitive arousal is associated with anxiety, whereas a decrease in autonomic arousal is associated with relaxation. Because of this, relaxation training forms an important part of the MHCU's treatment.

Learning to relax takes time and the person should be made aware of this. Any relaxation technique, if it is to be ultimately effective, should be practised daily. There are a number of techniques. Those that require the MHCU to withdraw their consciousness and engage in fantasy are not suitable for MHCUs with a high level of anxiety, neither for persons who are psychotic.

Nursing strategies when dealing with families of MHCUs

Nurses can help families who have an MHCU with an anxiety disorder by giving them the following advice:

- Don't make assumptions about what the affected person needs; ask them.
- Be predictable; don't surprise them.
- Let the person with the disorder set the pace for recovery.
- Find something positive in every experience. If the affected person is only able to go part of the way to a particular goal, such as a movie theatre or party, consider that an achievement rather than a failure.
- Do not enable avoidance; negotiate with the person with panic disorder to take one step forward when they want to avoid something.
- Do not sacrifice your own life and build resentments.
- Do not panic when the person with the disorder panics.
- Remember that it is all right to be anxious yourself; it is natural for you to be concerned and even worried about the person with the panic disorder.
- Be patient and accepting, but do not settle for the affected person being permanently disabled.
- Say: 'You can do it no matter how you feel. I am proud of you. Tell me what you need now. Breathe slowly and low. Stay in the present. It's not the place that's bothering you, it's the thought. I know that what you are feeling is painful, but it's not dangerous. You are courageous.'
- Do not say: 'Relax. Calm down. Don't be anxious. Let's see if you can do this (ie setting up a test for the affected person). You can fight this. What should we do next? Don't be ridiculous. You have to stay. Don't be a coward.'

PSYCHOPHARMACOLOGY RELATED TO TREATMENT OF ANXIETY DISORDERS

The psychotropic medications used in the treatment of anxiety can be regarded as a 'window of opportunity' for the nurse and the MHCU. This is because the most helpful outcome of these medications is rapid symptom relief, which allows the nurse to move closer to MHCUs and to work with them on changing unhealthy lifestyle patterns.

Because some of the anxiety disorders (phobias, obsessive-compulsive disorders, panic disorders) are more responsive to antidepressant medication, it has been suggested that these might be more closely related biochemically to depression than to generalised anxiety.

At present, medication for anxiety states is prescribed according to the specific anxiety disorder from which the MHCU suffers. Table 12.9 lists medications used in the treatment of anxiety.

Table 12.9 Psychopharmacological management of anxiety and related disorders

Disorder	Clinical presentation	Emergency medication	First-line medication	Second-line medication options
Generalised anxiety disorder	■ Excessive anxiety and worry (apprehensive expectation) ■ Somatic symptoms eg restlessness, fatigue, difficulty concentrating, irritability, muscle tension, sleep disturbance	Benzodiazepines eg oxazepam, lorazepam (short-term use ie maximum 2–4 weeks)	■ SSRIs eg fluoxetine or sertraline (transient exacerbation of symptoms may occur; low starting doses usually required)	■ Other antidepressants eg mirtazapine, venlafaxine, duloxetine, agomelatine, imipramine, clomipramine ■ Beta-blockers eg propranolol, atenolol ■ Atypical antipsychotics eg quetiapine
Panic disorder	■ Sudden, abrupt and unpredictable episodes of intense fear or discomfort (usually reaches a peak within minutes and lasts less than one hour) ■ Somatic symptoms eg palpitations, tachycardia, sweating, trembling, shortness	Benzodiazepines eg alprazolam (have rapid effect but transient ie symptoms often return quickly if medication withdrawn)	■ SSRIs eg fluoxetine (transient exacerbation of symptoms may occur; therapeutic response may be delayed)	■ Other antidepressants eg imipramine ■ Beta-blockers eg propranolol

→

Disorder	Clinical presentation	Emergency medication	First-line medication	Second-line medication options
	of breath, choking, chest pain, nausea, dizziness, numbness or tingling, fear of losing control/ dying			
Social anxiety disorder (social phobia)	▪ Marked fear of social situations eg eating in public, having a conversation or meeting unfamiliar people ▪ Fear of humiliation, embarrassment or rejection ▪ Avoidant social behaviour ▪ Anxious anticipation of social situations ▪ Exposure to extreme traumatic event eg actual or threatened death, serious injury or sexual violence, followed by: – Intrusive symptoms eg recurrent and distressing memories, dreams, flashbacks	Benzodiazepines (have rapid effect; may be useful to use as needed in anticipation of social situations that may cause distress)	▪ SSRIs eg fluoxetine or citalopram (transient exacerbation of symptoms may occur; therapeutic response may be delayed)	▪ Other antidepressants eg venlafaxine ▪ Anticonvulsants eg gabapentin, sodium valproate ▪ Benzodiazepine augmentation eg clonazepam ▪ Beta-blockers eg propranolol, atenolol ▪ Atypical antipsychotics eg quetiapine, olanzapine

Disorder	Clinical presentation	Emergency medication	First-line medication	Second-line medication options
Post-traumatic stress disorder	– Persistent avoidance of stimuli eg avoidance of similar situations or reminders – Negative cognitions or mood symptoms eg fear, horror, shame, guilt, depression, detachment – Altered arousal and reactivity eg irritability, hyper-vigilance, sleep disturbances	Not usually appropriate	■ SSRIs eg fluoxetine or citalopram (therapeutic response may be delayed; high doses may be necessary)	■ Other antidepressants eg mirtazapine, venlafaxine, duloxetine, clomipramine ■ Alpha-blocker augmentation eg prazosin ■ Atypical antipsychotic augmentation eg risperidone, olanzapine
Obsessive compulsive disorder	■ Obsessional thinking (recurrent, persistent, intrusive thoughts eg constantly thinking the door has been left unlocked) and attempts to ignore, supress or neutralise such thoughts	Not usually appropriate	■ SSRIs eg fluoxetine, paroxetine or citalopram (therapeutic response may be delayed; high doses may be necessary)	■ Other antidepressants eg clomipramine, mirtazepine ■ Atypical antipsychotic augmentation eg risperidone ■ Benzodiazepine augmentation eg clonazepam

→

Disorder	Clinical presentation	Emergency medication	First-line medication	Second-line medication options
	• Compulsive behaviour (repetitive acts in response to obsessions eg constantly and repeatedly checking that the door is locked) • Obsessions and compulsions are time-consuming and distressing			

Best psychopharmacology nursing practice involves being cognisant of the risk of treatment-related adverse events. This information informs what nursing precautions to take, implications to consider and educating to provide regarding the MHCU's treatment.

A summary of the more typical adverse events related to Benzodiazepines, selective serotonin reuptake inhibitors (SSRI) and Beta-blockers are listed in Table 12.10. It is evident that when an MHCU has drug-related complaints, in most instances, it is not possible to identify which drug caused the adverse event. Furthermore, it is necessary to be knowledgeable of current evidence-based related adverse event information by keeping up to date with printed material or the use of electronic applications (app). Depending on the severity of an adverse event treatment might need to be discontinued before a therapeutic level is reached. As some adverse events could impair decision making and reflexive responses the nurse should caution and educate the MHCU to therefore avoid activities such as driving, working with heavy, dangerous machinery and being unprotected at dangerous heights until drowsy or dizziness related to medication has been ruled out. Furthermore caution the MHCU about the interaction of alcohol, CNS depressants and benzodiazepines. Be aware that most medications should be slowly withdrawn to reduce the intensity of possible withdrawal symptoms. Ultimately, despite treatment being prescribed, the nurse has a duty to constantly review whether the need for the treatment continues.

Table 12.10 Common adverse events ascribed to psychopharmacological management of anxiety and related disorders

Adverse event	Psychopharmacological management*		
	Benzodiazepam	SSRI	Beta-blockers
Bradycardia	–	–	Yes
Confusion	Yes	–	Yes
Constipation	–	–	Yes
Diarrhoea	–	Yes	Yes
Dizziness	Yes	Yes	Yes
Drowsiness	Yes	Yes	–
Dry mouth	–	Yes	Yes
Dry skin and eyes	–	–	Yes
Fatigue	–	–	Yes
Feelings of depression	Yes	–	–
Headache	Yes	Yes	–
Impaired coordination	Yes	–	–
Insomnia	–	Yes	–
Memory loss	–	–	Yes
Nausea	–	Yes	Yes
Nervousness and agitation	–	Yes	–
Oedema (hands and feet)	–	–	Yes
Sexual problems	–	Yes	Yes
Sleep disturbance	–	–	Yes
Trembling	Yes	–	–
Visual problems	Yes	Yes	–
Weakness	–	–	Yes
Weight gain	–	–	Yes

*Adverse events related to antidepressants, anticonvulsants and antipsychotic drug is discussed in Chapters 14, 17 and 18.

Another aspect of best psychopharmacology nursing practice is being cognisant of the risk of an MHCH becoming dependent on, or abusing, prescribed treatment. Both could lead to withdrawal symptoms when treatment is terminated. This implies that a thorough nursing assessment is necessary to identify possible abuse patterns (the potential for abuse is increased if there is a history of abuse of other substances) and tolerance (the MHCU requires increased dosing or frequency for the medication to achieve the same effect). If abuse of treatment is suspected, follow policy guidelines as specified by the health care service provider.

An additional consideration regarding psychopharmacological treatment relates to dietary intake. Some foods enhance the absorption of medication. Dietary guidelines, meaning prescriptions or restrictions, related to specific treatment need to be kept in mind. Lastly, the nurse should skilfully enquire whether an MHCU is pregnant as this would determine whether the prescribed treatment should be started or continued.

General education related to psychopharmacological treatment is to caution the MHCU that the effects of the treatment might not be felt immediately and alternative anxiety management strategies might thus be necessary to explore concurrently. It is vital to educate the MHCU to use treatment as prescribed, in terms of dose, frequency and whether to take medication with food or not. Support the MHCU to develop a routine related to taking treatment that is compatible with their lifestyle and demands related to the medication.

CONCLUSION

Anxiety is, to a greater or lesser degree, a component of both 'normal' and pathological functioning. Reasonable levels of anxiety are necessary for healthy functioning, whereas intense anxiety contributes to disorganised functioning. Anxiety should not be seen as a discrete entity; it is pervasive and infiltrates almost every facet of human experience. Because of this, the presence of anxiety, its manifestations and its level of intensity constitute an important aspect of any mental health assessment and intervention.

WEB RESOURCES

http://www.who.int/medicines/publications/essentialmedicines/en/index.html

    The latest version of the WHO Model List of Essential Medicines can be found on the website.

http://www.sadag.org/

    This address leads to the South African Depression and Anxiety Group (SADAG). It provides information on depression, panic disorder, social phobia, generalised anxiety disorder, PTSD, bipolar disorder, and specific information regarding children and the elderly, electroconvulsive therapy (ECT) and suicidal behaviour. It also has a telephone helpline with trained counsellors and lists support groups in various areas.

REFERENCES

American Psychiatric Association (APA). 2013. *Diagnostic and Statistical Manual of Mental Disorders – DSM-5.* 5th edition. Washington, DC: American Psychiatric Association.

Bandelow, B and Michaelis, S. 2015. Epidemiology of anxiety disorders in the 21st century. *Dialogues in Clinical Neuroscience,* 17: 327–335.

Beck, A T. 1976. *Cognitive Therapy and the Emotional Disorders.* New York: International Universities Press, Inc

Hawton, K, Salkovskis, P, Kirk, J and Clark, D. 1989. *Cognitive Behaviour Therapy for Psychiatric Problems: Practical Guide.* USA: Oxford University Press.

Meissner, W W. 1979. 'Studies on hysteria – Katharina'. *Psychoanalytic Quarterly,* Oct 48 (4): 587–600.

Republic of South Africa. *Essential Drugs Programme. Hospital level (Adults) Standard Treatment Guidelines and Essential Medicines List.* 4th edition. Republic of South Africa: National Department of Health; 2015.

Roy-Byrne, P, Sherbourne, C, Miranda, J, Stein, M, Craske, M, Golinelli, D and Sullivan, G. 2006. 'Poverty and response to treatment among panic disorder patients in primary care'. *American Journal of Psychiatry,* 163: 1419–1425.

Taylor, C B and Arnow, B. 1988. *The Nature and Treatment of Anxiety Disorder.* New York: Free Press.

Whitley, G G. 1989. Anxiety: defining the diagnosis. *Journal of Psychosocial Nursing,* 27: 7–12

Wood, S D, Kitchiner, N J and Bisson, J I. 2005. 'Experience of implementing an adult educational approach to treating anxiety disorders'. *Journal of Psychiatric and Mental Health Nursing,* 12: 95–99.

RESOURCES NOT REFERRED TO IN THE TEXT

Beck, J and Reilly, C. 2006. 'Nurses integrate cognitive therapy treatment into primary care: Description and clinical application of a pilot program'. *Topics in Advanced Practice Nursing e-journal,* 6 (3).

Benson, H. 1975. *The Relaxation Response.* USA: William Morrow & Co.

Chiang, Y-H, Beckstead, J W, Lo, S-C and Yang, C-Y. 2018. 'Association of Auditory Hallucination and Anxiety Symptoms with Depressive Symptoms in Patients with Schizophrenia: A Three-month Follow-up'. *Archives of Psychiatric Nursing.* doi: 10.1016/j.apnu.2018.03.014.

Conn, M K, Shafer, S and Cline, T. 2017. 'Anxiety Management in Primary Care: Implementing the National Institute of Clinical Excellence Guidelines'. *Archives of Psychiatric Nursing,* 31 (2): 205–210. doi: 10.1016/j.apnu.2016.09.016.

Duhoux, A, Menear, M, Charron, M, Lavoie-Tremblay, M and Alderson, M. 2017. 'Interventions to promote or improve the mental health of primary care nurses: a systematic review'. *JONM Journal of Nursing Management,* 25 (8): 597–607.

Goette, L, Bendahan, S, Thoresen, J, Hollis, F and Sandi, C. 2015. Stress pulls us apart: Anxiety leads to differences in competitive confidence under stress. *Psychoneuroendocrinology,* 54: 115–123.

Jacobson, E. 1938. *Progressive Relaxation.* Chicago: University of Chicago Press.

Lam, D and Gale, J. 2000. 'Cognitive behaviour therapy: teaching a client the ABC model – the first step towards the process of change'. *Journal of Advanced Nursing,* 31 (2): 444–451.

Musey, P I, Lee, J A, Hall, C A and Kline, J A. 2018. 'Anxiety about anxiety: a survey of emergency department provider beliefs and practices regarding anxiety-associated low risk chest pain'. *BMC Emerg Med BMC Emergency Medicine,* 18 (1).

Sasaki, N, Somemura, H, Nakamura, S, Yamamoto, M, Isojima, M, Shinmei, I, … Tanaka, K. 2017. 'Effects of Brief Communication Skills Training for Workers Based on the Principles of Cognitive Behavioral Therapy: A Randomized Controlled Trial'. *Journal of Occupational and Environmental Medicine*, 59 (1): 61–66.

Shah, L B I, Klainin-Yobas, P, Torres, S and Kannusamy, P. 2014. 'Efficacy of Psychoeducation and Relaxation Interventions on Stress-Related Variables in People with Mental Disorders: A Literature Review'. *Archives of Psychiatric Nursing*, 28 (2): 94–101. doi: 10.1016/j.apnu.2013.11.004.

CHAPTER 13

Nursing a Person with a Mood Disorder

M A Jarvis and L Middleton

Learning Outcomes

After studying this chapter, you should be able to:
- undertake a comprehensive physical, mental, and social assessment on a mental health care user (MHCU) presenting with symptoms indicative of a mood disorder and reach an accurate nursing diagnosis
- use assessment scales/screening tools as an adjunct to assess for depression, including suicide and mania
- present findings, inclusive of a nursing diagnosis post-assessment framed within a social model
- explore with the MHCU and/or support structure(s) treatment options and implement specific evidence-based nursing care to ensure the MHCU is supported in their recovery
- apply relevant legislation to care delivery, in particular the Mental Health Care Act 17 of 2002, and debate ethical implications
- reflect on personal and professional ability to deal with suicidal tendencies in people with mood disorders
- conduct risk–benefit counselling, involving antidepressants and mood stabilisers with the MHCU and/or support structures
- identify various cultural manifestations and the influences these have on management plans
- record physical, mental, and social condition, risk assessment and precautions taken on an ongoing basis
- discuss electroconvulsive therapy as a treatment method.

INTRODUCTION

Caring for people with mood disorders makes up a large proportion of the work of mental health care nurses. Although the DSM-5 separates bipolar-related disorders from depressive disorders, this chapter recognises that mood disorders encompass both diagnostic classes. For each of these two groups there are three main categories: the major illness (either depression or bipolar) which can be a single episode or recurrent; the low-grade type of illness (low-grade depression, called dysthymia and low-grade bipolar disorder, called cyclothymia); and then a group of disorders, which does not fit into either of these categories. Comorbidity often exists with anxiety, substance abuse, and depression; however, this chapter focuses on mood disorders. The median age of onset of mood disorders in South Africa is 37 years (Stein et al, 2008). Mood disorders are important not only because of their prevalence but also because of the related challenges, the risk-taking behaviours and suicidal tendencies associated with these disorders.

DEFINITIONS

The World Health Organisation (WHO, 2017: 7) defines *depressive disorders* as:

Characterised by sadness, loss of interest or pleasure, feelings of guilt or low self-worth, disturbed sleep or appetite, feelings of tiredness, and poor concentration. Depression can be long lasting or recurrent, substantially impairing a MHCU's ability to function at work or school or cope with daily life. At its most severe, depression can lead to suicide. Depressive disorders include eight main sub-categories but here we shall focus on two:

1. *Major depressive disorder (MDD), which involves symptoms such as depressed mood, loss of interest and enjoyment, and decreased energy; depending on the number and severity of symptoms, a depressive episode can be categorised as mild, moderate, or severe*
2. *Persistent depressive disorder (Dysthymia), a persistent or chronic form of mild depression; the symptoms of dysthymia are similar to depressive episodes but tend to be less intense and last longer.*

In summary, depression is a state of low mood and aversion to activity that can affect an MHCU's thoughts, behaviour, feelings and sense of well-being.

Bipolar disorders are defined by the WHO (2010: 24) as follows:

Bipolar disorder is characterised by episodes in which the MHCU's mood and activity level are significantly disturbed. This disturbance consists on some occasions of an elevation of mood and increased energy and activity (mania), and on others of a lowering of mood and decreased energy and activity (depression). Characteristically, recovery is complete between episodes. People who experience only manic episodes are also classified as having bipolar disorder.

DEPRESSIVE AND BIPOLAR DISORDERS
Introduction to depressive and bipolar disorders

The WHO (2017: 5) reported depression as 'the single largest contributor to global disability', and a principal contributor to suicide deaths, estimated at 788 000 globally in 2015 (WHO, 2017: 5). Depression affects 4.4 per cent of the world's population, which equates to 322 million MHCUs of whom 9 per cent are in the African region (WHO, 2017: 8). Bipolar disorders affect a smaller percentage of the population compared to depressive disorders; 0.5–0.8 per cent of the world's population and 0.5–0.9 per cent of South Africa's population. Although bipolar disorders have a lower prevalence rate, the burden estimates of the two groups of disorders are similar because of the high disability weighting for a manic episode in a bipolar disorder. Bipolar disorders fall into the top 30 leading causes of disability globally and are one of the top five causes of the burden relating to mental and substance-abuse disorders (Vos et al, 2016).

The possibility exists for under-reporting of figures for Africa. This is in light of the existence of a large gap between mental health needs and access to mental health care (WHO, 2016); low mental health literacy (Chipps et al, 2015); and with depression three times greater, the possibility of consultation with a traditional or spiritual leader rather than a western medicine mental health practitioner (Tomlinson et al, 2009: 371). In South Africa, second to alcohol abuse, depression is the most prevalent lifetime psychiatric disorder with the age of onset ranging between 23 and 53 years (Stein et al, 2008).

Note that the WHO (2017: 17) presents South Africa's prevalence of depressive disorders as 4.6 per cent. However, in some South African contexts, despite the variance in age the prevalence is high, with evidence of 50.3 per cent in postnatal mothers in a rural setting (Stellenberg & Abrahams, 2015: 7), 57.9 per cent in women 18–30 years, living in an informal urban settlement in Durban (Gibbs et al, 2018) and 49.3 per cent in elderly persons in an urban residential care setting (Chipps & Jarvis, 2016: 1266). Ardington and Case (2010: 70) confirm that older South Africans are at greater risk of depression. Depression is likened to the 'common cold' of psychiatry as it occurs so frequently in the general population.

In recognition of the fundamental role of mental well-being in overall health, the WHO set global targets through the Mental Health Action Plan (2013–2020), one of which is that the rate of suicide will be reduced in countries by 10 per cent in 2020 (WHO, 2013). Health care professionals, in particular mental health care nurses, have a significant role in the attainment of global targets, starting in South Africa.

Aetiology of depression

Depression is not typical in its presentation or cause, but it is complex in nature with many studies recognising the relevance of resilience as a protective factor.

There are multiple causes of depression that 'the result of a chemical imbalance' cannot explain away. Factors such as genetic vulnerability, socio-determinates of depression like life stressors, substance/alcohol misuse, bipolar disorder, certain medications, and physical conditions can all act as contributory factors or presenting features of depression. Recent studies show a link between depression and excessive amounts of proinflammatory cytokines, in particular C-reactive protein (CRP), that result in the reduction of serotonin production and increase neurodegenerative products (Komori, 2017: 58).

In addition, the presence of physical symptomatology can exacerbate the MHCU's vulnerability to depression, resulting in the emergence of symptoms. Hence, a thorough initial assessment is vital. Furthermore, physical symptomology can present with features similar to depressive disorders. It is imperative in the assessment process to eliminate physical conditions. A discussion of some of these follows.

Depression is a symptom of hypothyroidism. There is a link between the thyroid stimulating hormone (TSH) and lowered serotonin levels. A function of the thyroid gland is to regulate serotonin levels. Further, there is increased cortisol release during stress. Cortisol contributes to serotonin depletion. Cortisol inhibits the D2 enzyme, which is responsible for the conversion of the thyroid hormone, T4, into T3 (Hage & Azar, 2012). TSH changes are evidenced in weight change, dry skin, constipation, intolerance of cold or heat, menstrual changes, fatigue, anxiety, tachycardia, tremor or thyroid enlargement.

Certain medications may have depression as a side effect. Examples are Accutane (isotretinoin) used for acne; long term use of benzodiazepines such as Valium (Diazepam); cholesterol-lowering drugs such as Lipitor; Premarin for menopausal symptoms; Atenolol used in ischaemic heart disease, Efavirenz, an antiretroviral, and oral contraceptives.

Assessment and diagnosis of depression

Common presentations of depression are multiple persistent physical symptoms with no clear cause, low energy, fatigue nearly every day (anergia), sleep problems nearly every day, significant appetite or weight change, reduced concentration, psychomotor retardation, psychomotor agitation, thoughts of worthlessness, guilt or suicide attempts or thoughts (WHO, 2016: 17). The following unhealthy cognitive patterns (cognitive distortions) most commonly occur in an MHCU presenting with depressive features, which if consistently present lead to and maintain a feeling of depression:

- *Selective abstraction.* Because of the MHCU's negative mindset, the tendency is to pick out the negative in most situations and ignore the positive.
- *Overgeneralisation.* From one negative aspect, there is generalisation to all situations and people most of the time.
- *Catastrophising.* Having generalised the negative freely, the resulting conclusion is that the worst will happen.

Linked to these cognitive distortions, the MHCU's sense of mastery becomes undermined because they do not account for the fact that in depression the simplest of tasks requires tremendous effort. The MHCU might be plagued with thoughts such as: 'I'm not doing anything', 'I'll never get anything done', 'I can't do anything', 'Nothing I do is worthwhile', 'I should be able to do that anyway'. Because MHCUs presenting with depression tend to think in global, negative ways about themselves, what they do and what they do not do, it is important to establish the 'hard facts'. Is the MHCU inactive, withdrawn, incapable of solving problems, beset by negative thoughts and unpleasant emotions all day and in every situation they encounter? Or, are there in fact some situations in which they feel less withdrawn, more active and more capable? This is important information in the

> 'Hope is being able to see that there is light despite all of the darkness.' Desmond Tutu

assessment that will be valuable when collaborating a path with the MHCU out of the depression. If the MHCU finds it difficult to provide this information, make enquires from the family/friend.

The mentioned list of features needs to be accompanied by at least one of the core symptoms of a loss of interest or pleasure in activities that were normally pleasurable (anhedonia) and/or a persistent sadness/depressed mood (dysphoria) *for at least two weeks* (WHO, 2016: 19).

A number of other observations could be made. Screen for alcohol/substance abuse. Consider alcohol or substance abuse if the MHCU consumes more than 21 standard drinks per week (male); or more than 14 standard drinks per week (female); and/or five standard drinks per session; or misuses illicit or prescription drugs (Department of Health, 2016). In South Africa a standard drink contains 12 grams of pure alcohol which equates, for example, to 30 ml spirits or 100ml wine.

The mental health care nurse is to ensure the physical status is not overlooked in the assessment. Check TSH if there are signs of changes in thyroid function and monitor the management of chronic diseases. Identify the use of medication that might have depression as a side effect. Identify whether the MHCU is pregnant and what the period of gestation is.

Another consideration in a diagnosis of depression is whether daily functioning is affected in the realms of personal, family, educational, social, or family functioning. Assess if there are home, occupational, or social stressors. In addition, other mental health conditions such as a depressive episode in bipolar disorder need identification and management (WHO, 2016: 19), or if mania develops while taking antidepressants (Department of Health, 2016).

> *Suicide eliminates the possibility of life getting better.*

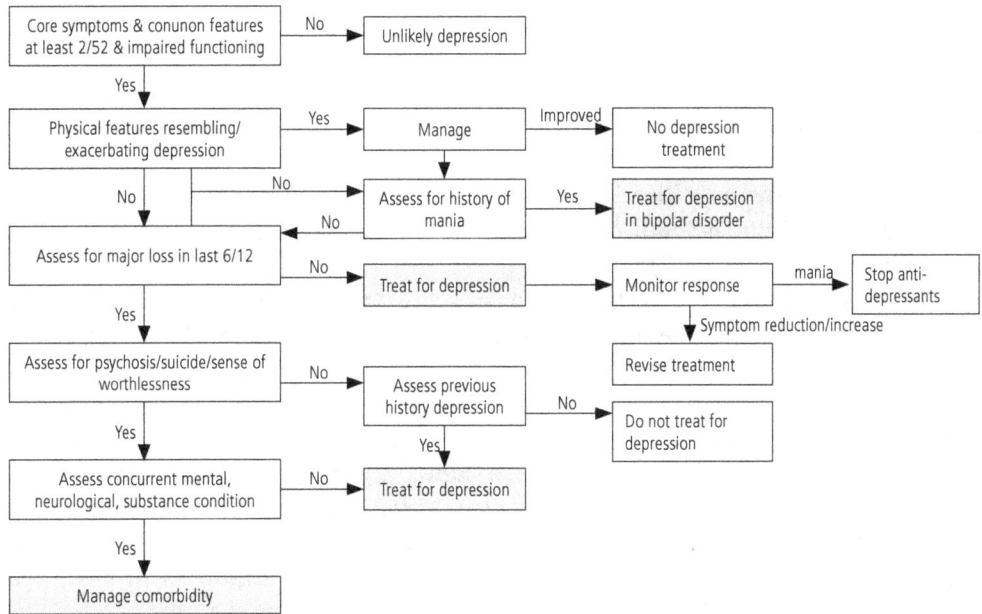

Figure 13.1: Flow diagram representing the diagnostic pathway for depression (Adapted from WHO, 2017)

Screening tools

The use of screening tools is an adjunct to the general assessment and confirms the level of depression providing a baseline score, which serves as a comparative, as the MHCU engages with treatment modalities, inclusive of psychotropic medication.

Examples of such depression scales are: self-rating inventories used by the MHCU, for example the Hamilton Depression Rating Scale (HDRS), Hudson's Generalised Contentment Scale, the Beck Depression Inventory (BDI-II), Zung's Self-rating Depression Scale (SDS), Centre for Epidemiologic Studies Depression Scale (CES-D), CES-D-10, Geriatric Depression Scale (GDS) and the WHO-five Well-being Index (WHO-5). Discussion follows below of a few assessment scales.

The BDI-II is widely used with persons over 13 years by either the practitioners or the MHCU to self-rate depressive features in the areas of negative attitude, performance difficulty, somatic complaints and depression (Makhubela & Debusho, 2016: 522). The BDI-II has been used in South African studies and contains 21 questions, assessing feelings over the previous two weeks and scores on a scale from 0–3, range 0–63, with scores of 17 and above indicating clinical depression (Makhubela & Debusho, 2016: 523).

> *Depression is not being able to talk about your problems, while taking on everyone else's problem just to hide your own.*

The 20-item Centre for Epidemiological Studies on Depression (CES-D) Scale uses a four-point Likert Scale, which asks questions about depressive symptoms in the previous week, and has been applied in a variety of South African studies (Gibbs et al, 2018; Nduna & Jewkes, 2012). Studies have used ≥ 16 and other studies have used ≥ 21 as cut-off scores on the CES-D for symptoms of depression (Gibbs et al, 2018). Refer to the Annexure for the scale. In addition, the CES-D-10, a shortened version, has shown reliability and validity in South African settings as a tool to identify persons at risk for depression (Baron et al, 2017).

The five questions in the WHO-5 are positively formulated but at the same time the tool is able to measure for the characterising symptoms of depression (Heun et al, 2001). It encompasses the three primary items of depression, namely mood, energy and interests, as positive constructs. The WHO-5 assesses for emotional well-being over 14 days using a six-point Likert Scale (range 0–5) with a cut-off score of ≥13 showing mental well-being (WHO, 1998). In a Danish study, the WHO-5 was compared (n=9542) against the psychometrics of the Short Form-36 (SF-36) questionnaire which has a mental health subscale (Bech et al, 2003). The unidimensionality of the WHO-5 was recognised, and the acknowledgement that positive well-being is more easily measured (Bech et al, 2003). The WHO-5 takes about two minutes to complete and can be self-administered.

Student activity: Carefully read the scenario below and thereafter record the mental state examination for Monica. Choose a scale and assess the level of depression.

Monica, a 30-year-old registered nurse, is in charge of the diabetic clinic of the local district hospital where you work. She realised that she was not well and today she referred herself to the employee assistance programme (EAP). The EAP referred her to your unit for further consultation. On arrival, she looks uncomfortable about being seen, but after your reassurance, she settles into the chair and appears more relaxed. You comment on how smart she looks in the new unit manager uniform and while tugging at her skirt, she admits that it takes a lot of her energy every day to get to work. You inquire into her work setting to which she openly admits, 'Diabetes used to be my passion and it gave me such joy to run workshops, but now the clinic is a drudge. I find myself avoiding the patients and yesterday I realised it was bad when I caught myself thinking that if a patient's glucose level goes out of control its their own fault, as I have given "my all" to teaching them.' You respond to her level of apathy, by asking for how long this has been going on. She says that she once had similar feelings at the age of 15, after her first boyfriend broke up with her. You ask if the scars on her wrists are linked to that event; she looks at you with eyes surrounded by dark rings and says, 'Yes, but after therapy, I have been well and managed to deal with loss and change, until three weeks ago.' She goes on to tell you that three weeks prior to admission her boyfriend of two years, David, had ended their relationship as he had fallen in love with someone else. Monica states: 'I don't know why you are bothering with me, I am of no importance, and even David fell out of love with me and found someone else. Look at how thin I have got!' She begins to weep silently and states, 'I'll never find anyone else; he was the one and now I'm going to be alone forever. I feel so low and have done so for the last three weeks.' Monica goes on to tell you all the plans and dreams she had for herself and David. She is so devastated and hopeless about her future that you find yourself feeling great empathy for her.

→

You invite her mother in, as she had been sitting outside. Her mother who has come from Cape Town tells you that she is very worried about Monica as David was her only friend and she went everywhere with him. Her mother tells you that she thinks that since the breakup Monica has not left her flat except to go to work and that Monica seems to spend the entire weekend alone in her flat, not bothering to cook or clean the place. Monica confirms this and states, '*What is the point of going out, alone? I don't know anyone to go out with.*' Further probing reveals that Monica spends the evenings and weekends reading David's letters and listening to songs they both enjoyed. She tells you that when she wakes up at 3am she feels like she is the only person in the world. No one is up and she can see from her veranda all over Durban and imagines that everyone is asleep with their families and she is all alone. She wonders what David and his new girlfriend are doing and finds herself hating him so much and imagining all kinds of ways to get back at him. The only thing that helps her get back to sleep is a strong alcoholic drink. While she waits for the alcohol to send her to sleep, she wonders why she goes on.

Mental status examination of Monica

General description
- *Care for self.* In areas where she has the possibility of being critiqued, such as in a work setting, she is paying attention to self-care, but it is requiring effort; however, there are signs of neglect through her weight loss and dark rings under her eyes
- *Care for others.* Although not enduring there is evidence of loss of care for her clients, a previous source of concern
- *Care of the environment.* Declined interest in her care for environment, not giving her home attention
- *Psychomotor activity.* Calm disposition
- *Attitude to examiner.* Initially embarrassed and possibly conscious of being in the unit. However, her need for care overrides this awareness and soon she is demonstrating a high level of trust regarding disclosure to the examiner, opening up and being honest

Mood and Affect
- *Mood.* Describes a dysphoric mood (lost, alone, and hopeless)
- *Affect.* Blunted
- *Congruency.* Affective expression is congruent with the mood
- *Appropriateness.* Mood is appropriate to the content of conversation focused on loss

Perceptual disturbances. Nil evident

Thought processes
- *Flow and form.* Sentence structure is intact; answers are appropriate to questions; preoccupied with thoughts of her loss and has a fatalistic view of her future
- *Thought content.*
    - Suicidal risk in her ability to access potentially lethal medication for diabetics and has a working knowledge of the medication
    - Cognitive distortions
    - Evidence of rumination of past relationship
    - Decreased sense of self-worth based not on her senior position, but on failed relationship

→

Cognition
- *Cognition.* Not impaired
- *Concentration.* Able to concentrate for the entire interview
- *Memory.* Long-term memory appears intact – recounts teenage suicide attempt; short-term memory appears intact – can remember break up of relationship
- *Alert* and attentive
- *Orientation.* Oriented to place and person, time – arriving correct place, when EAP was open and responding to person

Judgement
- *Occupational and social judgement.* Impaired in relation to fatalism, hopelessness, and evidenced by her using self-medication a few hours before needing to be at a demanding job.

Insight
- *Intellectual insight.* Despite being a professional nurse and having had therapy before, she uses less effective measures to sleep; yet knows there is a problem and accesses EAP.

Vegetative shift
- Decreased energy, anhedonia; impaired eating patterns and loss of weight; initial insomnia; uses alcohol to self-medicate.

NURSING INTERVENTIONS WITH MHCUs PRESENTING WITH DEPRESSIVE FEATURES

It is important to be aware of the multideterminants of depression and where relevant, attempt to prevent its occurrence or be alert to depression as a side effect of medication, alcohol abuse or social determinants. Social determinants (for example, gender or socioeconomic status) of depression might need a variety of social, economic, political or educational counter measures. There are a number of different interventions for addressing depression.

Collaborative MHCU and family-centred care

MHCUs with depression may have attached themselves to many people in their search for help, often with either overt or covert suicidal threats due to their use of passive dependence as a coping mechanism. Relating in this way leads to a great deal of anxiety, helplessness and guilt in the other person and very little pleasure or fulfilment, with the result that they gradually withdraw from the MHCU. It may also be that the MHCU uses passive withdrawal as a coping mechanism – not contacting friends or family, never accepting invitations, not talking or sharing – thereby making it difficult for the maintenance of relationships.

The presenting symptomatology of depression might result in the emergence of power discourses in the relationship between health care professionals, family members and the MHCU with the diagnostic label of depression. Language use might reflect power discourses with statements like 'you must', 'you ought to', 'comply with your treatment', or 'the doctor says you must take your medication'. However, this is counter to collaborative patient-centred care.

The elements that are to be visible in collaboration involve:
- Mutual respect for skills and knowledge, focusing on the multideterminants of mental health
- Engaging the lived experiences of the MHCU with depression and the family as 'experts by experience'
- Honest, clear communication regarding the value of all parties and arriving together at mutually agreed-on goals
- Creating an environment that allows for a more hospitable space for the MHCU to examine, reflect and creatively look at options for their mental health care
- Allowing for an awakening within the MHCU of the power they have in their treatment plan and the ability they have to reason and weigh up their treatment options
- Acknowledging cultural differences
- Bracketing by health care professionals of their own agendas
- Re-evaluating at mutually agreed intervals of progress
- Absence of power differentials, stigmatisation and blaming.

Interventions for cognitive distortions

Peter Block said, 'The shift in the world begins with a shift in our thinking. Shifting our thinking does not change the world, but it creates a condition where the shift in the world becomes possible.' (AZ Quotes).

The nursing interventions for destructive cognitive patterns/distortions are as follows:
- Identify the cognitive pattern.
- Encourage the MHCU to be self-aware regarding the cognitive patterns they utilise, and their effect on how they perceive situations and the consequences on their mental health.
- Assist the MHCU in learning how to test the truth of the belief or thought and to correct it. For example:
  - Selective abstraction: to identify positive aspects of their circumstances.
  - Overgeneralisation: to confine a negative aspect to where it belongs.
  - Catastrophising: to identify different scenarios, not just the one that is most negative.

The following transcript of a conversation between the mental health care nurse and Monica illustrates how these principles work.

Nurse: At our interview yesterday when talking about David you said that you would never find anyone else, and that David was the one and you felt you would be alone forever. You strongly feel that there is no chance of meeting anyone again.

Monica: Yes, there is literally no chance at all. David was an exception, but it did not last. I guess I should have realised that it would not have lasted. It is the story of my life. I will go back to being unnoticed. I was only noticed in the clinic because the patients needed something from me, but they did not notice ME.

Nurse: It is important that you get noticed for who you are.
Monica: Yes, it is. Yesterday was another example. I went down to the hospital café and it was terrible. The person at the till didn't notice me standing there and I had to wait while he served others who arrived at the counter after me … he did apologise but as I said to you – it's the story of my life – no one notices me or cares about me.
Nurse: It sounds as if how others see you is really important to you. (*Reflecting feeling*). You have mentioned that with David and you no longer in a relationship, you feel you are at risk of being alone forever. This was followed by yesterday's example at the café. Those are two examples; I would like it if you could give me an example of another situation where you also felt unnoticed? (*Collecting information to identify the cognitive pattern*)
Monica: Well, as I said, it's the story of my life … but okay, this morning this other patient promised to keep me a seat in front of the TV. I got there, and she had forgotten. She offered to fetch me a chair but that's not the point.
Nurse: From the stories you've told me, it seems as if two things happen to you when you feel other people aren't noticing you. First, you think that it must mean that you are a totally worthless person all the time, and secondly, you forget to look at the positive part of each situation; for example, David and you were in a relationship for two years, the shop assistant apologised to you and the other patient offered to fetch you a chair. Does that sound familiar to you? (*Summarising, identifying cognitive patterns of overgeneralisation and selective abstraction; checking this out with her*)
Monica: A bit … but still, that's what happens to me all the time. If people noticed me, for me and not for what I can offer I would not feel so bad and then it wouldn't happen.
Nurse: So if people noticed you, you wouldn't feel so bad … let's look at it in another way and see what you think. I'd like you to think back to a time before you became depressed. How did you feel about yourself then? (*Helping her to see that faulty thoughts are the problem, not the situation itself*)
Monica: I remember feeling good and strong, a few ups and downs, but mostly well.
Nurse: Imagine yourself feeling good … you're in the café you were in yesterday and the shop assistant serves people who came after you before he serves you. If you had to rate your feelings of worthlessness on a scale from 0 to10, where 0 meant not feeling worthless at all and 10 meant feeling totally worthless, what rating would you give yourself? (*Helping her to see the relationship between thoughts, feelings and behaviour*)
Monica: Maybe one or two at the most.
Nurse: So, what do you make of the idea that because you saw yourself as a strong, capable person, what happened in the shop didn't really bother you so much? (*Pointing out the influence thoughts have on feelings and behaviour without 'lecturing' her*)

Monica: Maybe it works like that … but right now it's hard to even imagine feeling good …

Nurse: It sounds as if you're fed up with feeling bad all the time. Let's try to get a good idea of how things really are. What I'd like you to do is to keep a diary for the next week about the specific situations where you felt useless and worthless. (*Helping her to get a baseline for negative thinking and teaching her to 'diagnose' patterns and the relationship between patterns, feelings and behaviours*) I have written an example of how you can lay it out, but you might choose another format.

> Date: _____
>
> Situation (who was involved, what happened, who said what and did what):
>
> _____
>
> Thoughts about myself: _____
>
> How I felt and behaved: _____

Monica: Okay … I probably won't be able to do it properly.

Nurse: That's one of the good things about this exercise. There aren't any 'proper' ways of doing it.

The following meeting (after social niceties):

Nurse: How did your homework go?

Monica: Well, I tried, but it's probably not much good.

Nurse: Let's look at it together. On Sunday you felt bad about yourself after the nurse forgot to call you for lunch … the same on Monday and Tuesday when the social worker asked to postpone her appointment. I see that after each incident you felt 'awful' for the rest of the day.

Monica: Yes, well, more evidence that I'm a nobody.

Nurse: Let's think of a few other reasons why the nurse forgot to call you, and why the social worker had to postpone her appointments. (*Helping the her to test the thought and correct it through learning more rational ways of interpreting the situation*)

Monica: The nurse was busy, I'll admit that. She was working on her own and there was a new admission. The social worker was called away to some special meeting at head office, but still …

Nurse: Okay, it seems that there are fairly good reasons why the nurse and the social worker behaved as they did, and that it's not just because you are so 'forgettable'. Maybe what's happening here is that you're forgetting about the more positive, realistic aspects of the situation and focusing on the negative. (*Reinforcing the relationship between patterns, feelings and behaviours*)

Monica: Maybe.

Nurse: It takes time to change the way we think about things. Keep your diary for another week and add an extra column, 'New ways of thinking, feeling and behaving'. (*Teaching her to find alternative and more rational ways of seeing things, so that eventually new thought patterns become as entrenched as the old, thus leading to a change in the way she feels about self, and subsequently behaves.*)

Interventions for social withdrawal

Coping mechanisms used by the MHCUs who present with depressive features are usually passive in character and often involve dependence behaviour and social withdrawal. A definition of *social withdrawal* is: the physical and psychological removal of the self from an environment, thus resulting in detachment and isolation. This is not always a passive process but may be very active and strongly enforced by the MHCU.

Heath care users who display social withdrawal have retreated from both external and internal stimuli. Involvement with others and with their own feelings is seen as a source of overwhelming threat and they do not have the resources to cope with this.

The following are some guidelines or principles which may be useful when intervening with MHCUs who are socially withdrawn:

1. Establish and maintain a trusting relationship.
   Health care practitioners need to be aware that this may be a lengthy process that requires patience and perseverance and that the MHCU may initially reject them. Health care practitioners often think that they have 'failed' if, after one or two interactions, the MHCU does not seem willing to express their feelings and talk about their problems. The practitioner who measures their own therapeutic ability against how much the MHCU talks and shares will possibly identify such behaviour as difficult to deal with.
2. The greater the pressure and/or the absence of pressure on the withdrawn MHCU to interact, the more likely they are to retreat physically and emotionally.
   - Make contact or link with the MHCU. Therapeutic use of family or close friends may be helpful, discussing the family or friends' approach individually and as part of the multisectoral team.
   - Respect the need for physical distance and emotional and social privacy, while at the same time ensuring that the MHCU knows the health care practitioner is available.
   - Respect the MHCU's need for silence and inform them that the health care practitioners are available when there is a need to communicate.
   - Keep the MHCU informed of what is happening in the ward – for example, new admissions, discharges (without disclosing confidential information) and ward activities (without pressurising participation).
   - Adjust the demand for interaction according to their non-verbal behaviour, while at the same time following a programme of graded social involvement that starts with the least threatening social activities.

3. Therapeutic use of touch may be used by staff who feel comfortable with touch and according to the MHCU's reception of touch.
   Touch needs careful consideration and the mental health care nurse's overwhelming need to 'get the MHCU to talk' might result in it being used inappropriately.
4. The more consistent and reinforcing the withdrawn MHCU perceives the environment to be, the greater the likelihood of their engaging with the environment.
   - Provide an environment that is consistent and reliable in its demands on the MHCU and one that realistically reinforces the MHCU's attempts to engage with it.
   - Keep promises of returning to spend time with them. Maintain consistency regarding appointment times and keep all other promises or commitments made to the MHCU.
   - Realistically reinforce attempts to engage with the environment. Use friends and family as a link with the community.
   - Assist the family in their understanding of the condition by inviting the family and the MHCU to a 'family session' where the focus is on all members developing insight about all the aspects of depression. The MHCU with depression will often be told by family to 'pull yourself together'. This indicates the void between the family's perception of depression and the MHCU's feelings. Teach family and friends how to cope with both dependent and withdrawal behaviour.
   - Give positive feedback to both verbal and non-verbal responses.
   - Teach the MHCU to identify the kinds of behaviour that scare people off and assist in behaviour and change; offer interpersonal skills training, if necessary.
5. Gradually increase the demand for interaction, first at a physical level and later at an emotional and social level (the amount and type of demand at any given moment is determined by the MHCU's level of anxiety evident in verbal and non-verbal behaviour).
   - Gradually introduce and involve the MHCU in lifestyle activities.
   - Provide for safety in the ward setting with regard to other MHCUs, but gradually introduce the MHCU to other people and then explore their feelings regarding the contact made with others.
   - Identify the family and friendship network of the MHCU prior to the illness and gradually reactivate these contacts.
   - Set up a plan of graded activity.

Read the following scenario about Cathy who presents with social withdrawal.

Cathy is a 24-year-old woman who is exhibiting severe social withdrawal. She spends the large part of each day sitting on the floor in her room, facing the corner. She avoids eye contact with the staff and turns away her face when they enter the room. She refuses to eat in the dining room but eats if the mental health care nurse brings the food to her. Her only form of communication with others is through non-verbal gestures and even then, these are designed to isolate herself from others. Mental health care nurse

Zuma and mental health care nurse Mkhize (on opposite shifts) are assigned to care for Cathy.

Mental health care nurse Zuma enters the room, moves close to Cathy and puts her arm around her, saying: 'Hello, Cathy, I'm Nurse Zuma … look at me … look at me, please, I'd like to talk to you. You'll feel better if you talk about what's bothering you.' Cathy turns away and curls up into a ball. At the same time, she tries to shrug off mental health care nurse Zuma's arm from her shoulder. Mental health care nurse Zuma hugs Cathy tighter and tries to turn her head to face her while saying, 'I can see you are upset about something. I'm here to help you, please talk to me.' Cathy tries to retreat further; her body becomes rigid and she buries her head in her lap. After a minute or so mental health care nurse Zuma gets up and quietly leaves the room. Over the course of the day she repeats her approach to Cathy, who continues to resist her.

Mental health care nurse Zuma's entry in the nursing notes reads as follows: 'The MHCU very withdrawn and reluctant to engage in any form of communication and becomes very anxious when approached, for example, shrinks away from contact, body tense. To continue trying to interact with Cathy.'

The following day mental health care nurse Mkhize approaches Cathy. She enters the room and squats down on the floor a good few metres from Cathy, saying, 'Hello, Cathy, I'm Nurse Mkhize … (*few moments of silence*) … I can see from the way you are sitting curled up in a ball that you'd really like to be by yourself … (*few moments of silence*) …. That's okay … I'd like to sit quietly with you for a few minutes … (*few moments of silence*) … (*Cathy peeks at mental health care nurse Mkhize from under one arm and then looks away. Her body relaxes slightly*). If you'd like to sit more comfortably, that's all right. I'm not coming any closer … (*Cathy shifts her position slightly but is still turned away from the mental health care nurse*). I've brought you a magazine I thought you might like to look at – I'll leave it here for you. I'm going back to the ward now, but I'll come back in an hour's time and sit with you for a short while.' Over the course of the day, mental health care nurse Mkhize makes regular contact with Cathy. Before her shift ends, she notices that the magazine has been moved and assumes that Cathy has looked at the front cover.

Mental health care nurse Mkhize's entry in the nursing notes reads as follows: 'The MHCU is showing some non-verbal evidence of communication, for example fleeting eye contact and relaxing of body posture. To continue programme of graded interaction based on her non-verbal responses.'

Mental health care nurse Zuma and mental health care nurse Mkhize discussed their approaches to Cathy and decided to be consistent in their approach and follow the principles discussed above as they graded Cathy's social activity. With regard to their professional interaction they agreed to avoid comments to each other as health care practitioners like 'Seeing you aren't busy …' if either is sitting in silence with Cathy.

Table 13.1 is a detailed example of Cathy's programme of graded social activity. The mental health care nurse might not write such detail, but the table shows the possible contact, the grading and the possible outcome. The amount of detail will depend on the context.

Table 13.1 Cathy's programme of graded social activity

_____			
Example of Cathy's programme of graded social activity			
Day	Time	Activity	Outcome
Monday	07:30	Greet Cathy while putting the table in her room. Place her food on the table and invite her to eat at the table.	Cathy moved the table to the corner of the room and stood while eating her food.
	09:30	Identify from Cathy's family her choice of radio channel. Place a radio (playing softly) in her room, notifying Cathy of the reason for the channel.	Volume on the radio was turned up slightly.
	10:30	Return to talk to Cathy about how she feels about having the table in her room and hearing news about the outside world on the radio. Acknowledge any attempt at communication.	Shrugged her shoulders.
	12:30	Place Cathy's food on the table and invite her to eat.	Ate at the table but got up immediately when nurse entered the room.
	14:30	Cathy's sister to visit for 10 minutes.	Withdrawn after the visit, sitting hunched up in the corner. Staff reported hearing sister say, 'Pull yourself together.' Discuss with sister alternate approach and explanation of the condition.
	16:30	Mental health care nurse Zuma to spend five minutes with Cathy, in silence if necessary.	Seemed more relaxed, made eye contact with the mental health care nurse and 'grunted' in response to a question.
	17:00	Place Cathy's food on the table and invite her to eat.	Sat at the table, did not get up until the mental health care nurse asked her how she felt sitting at the table.
Tuesday	07:00	Invite Cathy to wash once the other MHCUs have finished.	Checked she was alone but carried out ablutions.
	07:30	Ask Cathy to join mental health care nurse at table for coffee after breakfast.	Came after all mental health care nurses had left the dining room. Drank coffee in silence. Responded with a thin smile when thanked for joining mental health care nurse.
	09:30	Ask Cathy if she would like the radio turned on and to indicate yes or no with a nod or shake of her head. Respect her decision and acknowledge her communication.	Nodded affirmatively. Body posture seemed to relax when non-verbal attempt acknowledged.

Interventions for physical inactivity

As the MHCU presenting with depression tends towards social withdrawal, physical inactivity can also be a concern. Inactivity occurs in all spheres of life, for example at home, at work, in community involvement and in relationships. The strategies of monitoring, scheduling and grading task assignments can be adapted to the specific situations in which the MHCU is inactive.

Involvement and choice are important to the sense of self-efficacy that is often low. Exercise patience and understanding, as the health care practitioner awaits a response. The process starts with the MHCU recording their activities in a 24-hour period.

Using the case study involving Cathy as a point of reference (see Table 13.1), start by finding out what Cathy does on an hour-by-hour basis over a specified period of time, and encourage her to rate each activity out of 10 for how much they enjoyed it (10 = most pleasurable) and the sense of achievement the task gave them (10 = greatest sense of mastery).

Because people with depression tend to have unrealistically high expectations of themselves, it is important to stress that Cathy should rate her sense of mastery in terms of how she felt at the time and not in terms of how well she thinks she should have performed the activity. Table 13.2 shows Cathy's self-monitoring record of her activities.

Table 13.2 Self-monitoring of activities

Example of Cathy's self-monitoring record of her activities P= Pleasure M = Mastery		
Time	Monday	Tuesday
07:00–08:00	Got out of bed (P0, M5), got dressed (P1, M3), had breakfast at the table in the room (P3, M4).	Got out of bed (P1, M4), got dressed (P1, M5), had breakfast at the table in the room with Ms King (MHCU) (P0, M6).
08:00–09:00	Sat at the table, looked at a magazine (P2, M5). Nurse came to see me (P3, M5).	Went to have a bath (P4, M6). Nurse came to see me (P4, M5).
09:00–10:00	Ms King brought me tea (P3, M4), listened to youtube clips (P4, M6).	Asked Ms King to have tea with me (P4, M7), took my cup back to the kitchen (P1, M8).
10:00–11:00	Nurse came to see me, went to have a bath (P3, M7).	Walked down the corridor (P1, M8) but turned back when I saw all the other MHCUs (P0, M0).
12:00–13:00	Had lunch with the nurse (P4, M6).	Ms King and nurse had lunch with me at the table (P4, M9).
13:00–14:00	Rested in bed (P8, M3).	Rested for half an hour (P6, M3) and then got up (M9) and listened to the radio (P7).

The schedule of Cathy's programme also reflects her increasing involvement in social activities, which were a part of her graded social involvement programme worked out by the mental health care nurses.

The information from the self-monitoring is used to plan a schedule of activities for each day in advance, aimed at slowly increasing the activity and optimising mastery and pleasure. The schedule of activities should be realistic, clearly itemised and achievable. The amount of activity expected from Cathy should be consistent with how she is feeling, and with the level of activity identified during the self-monitoring phase. An MHCU who feels severely depressed might be able to accomplish one activity in a day, whereas another MHCU might be able to accomplish more.

Cathy's self-monitoring chart shows that spending time with the mental health care nurse and Ms King, and listening to youtube clips, gave her the greatest pleasure, while leaving her room gave her the greatest sense of mastery. Activity scheduling for Cathy would focus on providing similar activities – that is, socialising with a limited number of familiar people outside the setting of her room. The level of demand for social interaction outside Cathy's room would be graded (broken down into small steps) to maximise the chances of success with the task, thus increasing pleasure and mastery. A graded task assignment details the steps to be taken to achieve each task, as well as personalised rewards for achieving each task. Rewards help to maximise pleasure and mastery, and to reinforce activity. Rewards can be anything Cathy regards as worthwhile. Pleasurable activities identified in the self-monitoring can be used as personalised rewards. Rewards can increase Cathy's interaction with the environment, like having lunch with a select person.

A graded task assignment can also be used to determine mastery and pleasure levels. The therapist can ask Cathy to rate each step achieved in terms of these two concepts. This gives important evaluation information about how successful the MHCU perceived the task assignment to be in improving activity levels.

A graded task assignment

What follows is an example of Cathy's graded task assignment.

Goal. Within seven days, Cathy should be able to spend 10 minutes a day outside her room with Ms King and one other MHCU with whom she feels comfortable. Table 13.3 shows the small steps needed to achieve the goal and Cathy would then select the personalised rewards linked to each step.

Table 13.3 Steps to be taken for achieving Cathy's goals

Day	Small steps to achieve goal
Monday	Identify the second MHCU with whom she would feel comfortable List the MHCUs she knows Rate her feelings about each MHCU on a 'comfort' scale of 0–10 Select the MHCU by name
Tuesday	Invite Ms Dlamini and Ms King to have afternoon tea with Cathy in her room Mental health care nurse will approach Ms Dlamini Cathy will approach Ms King
Wednesday	Identify an area outside her room in which she would feel comfortable spending time Walk around the ward with mental health care nurse while other MHCUs are having lunch Identify an area by name Imagine being in that area and discuss feelings and thoughts about it Invite Ms King and Ms Dlamini to try to join Cathy for tea in her room
Thursday	Become familiar with the area Spend five minutes sitting in the area with mental health care nurse, listening to the radio while other MHCUs are having morning tea Discuss feelings and thoughts about being outside her room Invite Ms King and Ms Dlamini to watch TV with her in her room
Friday	Invite Ms King to sit with her in the area for 10 minutes on Friday morning Invite mental health care nurse and Ms King to join her for afternoon tea in the area
Saturday	Invite Ms King, Ms Dlamini and mental health care nurse to join her for morning tea in the area

Narrative approach as an intervention

The narrative approach can also be used as a method of intervening with an MHCU. According to the Dulwich Centre (nd): 'narrative therapy seeks to be a respectful, non-blaming approach to counselling and community work, which centres people as the experts in their own lives. It views problems as separate from people and assumes people have many skills, competencies, beliefs, values, commitments and abilities that will assist them to reduce the influence of problems in their lives.'

It might be easier for MHCUs to describe depression and its influence on their lives using metaphors and moving the problem into a space outside of themselves where they can take action against it, and be able to answer the questions: 'Does depression define me?' or 'Do I define depression?' Often MHCUs can have a 'spoiled identity', which is a limited definition of themselves according to which they have come to live their lives. Winston Churchill referred to depression as 'The Black Dog' (see http://www.who.int/campaigns/world-health-day/2017/videos/en/).

These are some principles to consider in a narrative interview:
- The therapist never presumes to 'know' how the problem works, as the therapist is asking questions, of an expert in their own lives, to which the therapist does

- not know the answer. The therapist declines the invitation to be the expert in the MHCU's life.
- The therapist recognises their role as a conversational architect and that the MHCU is the primary author of their story (Wallis et al, 2010).
- Central to the conversation are the MHCU's views, preferences, hopes and purposes. The therapist is decentred, meaning they are not the expert. The therapist works alongside the MHCU, yet is influential through scaffolding questions and reflections that make it possible for descriptions of alternate stories, and explorations of neglected areas (Morgan, 2002).
- Narrative therapy recognises that there are many possibilities for conversations with the MHCU as lives are multistoried, and no story is free of ambiguity or contradiction, nor can a single story encapsulate all the contingencies of the MHCU's life. However, the MHCUs themselves choose the story they wish to tell and the direction of the story. The therapist offers to the MHCU a range of options regarding the directions that can be taken and the MHCU makes the decision that the therapist follows, facilitating the conversation, and opening spaces for dialogue (Morgan, 2002). Narrative therapy understands that lives are shaped by stories created by the person and seeks to re-author conversations for rich story development (Hibbel et al, 2010; Morgan, 2002).
- The therapist will assist the MHCU to find the alternate story and to 'thicken the story' (develop the alternate preferred story) that does not sustain the problem-saturated story, which is part of the depression (Dulwich Centre, nd). Initially stories are often thin descriptions with thin conclusions about the MHCU's identity, drawn from problem-saturated stories, possibly of failure and worthlessness.
- The therapist encourages externalising (renaming) the conversation by using 'it' or 'the' to separate the problem from the MHCU. When writing it down they are encouraged to use a capital letter, for example, 'Does this inadequate feeling only visit when Mr Fear is at home? Are there times when it is more likely for The Inadequate to come as an uninvited visitor?' The therapist is to use only language that separates and keeps the separation between the problem and the MHCU.
- The therapist is to remember that problems are socially constructed and created over time, and that all stories have a context. Although the therapist may have encountered a similar problem before, such as depression, they would never before have encountered this MHCU, with their particular context. Hence, the therapist is to raise questions about everything that would be routinely accepted and to 'keep questioning those taken for granted ideas of self', avoiding seeing people as ill, but rather as having problems that have come into their lives (Hibbel et al, 2010).
- The therapist is to create the context, showing genuine interest in everything about the MHCU with whom they are talking, showing curiosity, respect, and collaboration regarding the values, beliefs and preferences that are fundamental to this process. Thus, the therapist is attempting to understand the MHCU's telling their story and using the story to understand the problem – it is not about problem solving (Hibbel et al, 2010).

- The narrative therapist aims to use words accurately, sensitively and with delicacy.
- The therapist is to assist the MHCU in examining the effect of the problem, the discourses sustaining it and collaborate on an outcome. Together with the MHCU, the therapist looks for the structures of power and questions these. This involves questioning discourses (particular ways of thinking/talking about a person/activity with meanings located in particular cultures or groups of people) and challenging dominant discourses (created by persons in power and accepted as the way to perceive people/events, often associated with conflict). Collaboratively they re-author their story with possibility (Hibbel et al, 2010). Reconstruction helps the MHCU to search for unique outcomes outside of the dominant, thin story and for the MHCU to revise their relationship with the problem. In such a way, the MHCU builds personal agency, experiencing moments when they defeat the problem (O'Connor et al, 2004: 28).

Intervening with participation in group and community life

Owing to the dependence/withdrawal coping patterns used by the MHCU with depression, there is a possibility that participation in recreational, religious and cultural groups has diminished, while involvement with groups that reinforce the sick role has increased. For many there appears to be a lack of interest in the political climate, such that political issues are too far removed and not of importance.

There is often ambivalence in the MHCU's approach to religion. Some MHCUs who are depressed tend to use religion as a support system – religious practices may increase, prayers may become more intense, with a fervent plea for God to help them. On the other hand, there may be anger towards God, accompanied by such statements as 'Where's God – doesn't He know I exist?'. From here, the MHCU may distance themselves from God, making such statements as 'even God doesn't want me any more'. This is an indication of the intensity of the MHCU's sense of hopelessness and impending doom. This is a very vulnerable period for the MHCU, requiring respect for their religious beliefs, without imposition of other religious on them. It is often necessary to arrange for sensitive spiritual counselling by an appropriate person.

The MHCU may find it very difficult to participate in group activities and this limits their resocialisation and rehabilitation. Involve the MHCU in group therapy to prepare for re-entry into community life.

Intervening with participation in work

The MHCU's work becomes a means to an end and is often only of extrinsic value. The MHCU alienates themselves from their product, their peers, and ultimately themselves. They often have a temporary blind spot that prevents them from recognising themselves as a capable, productive, confident, and creative worker. The results are decreased work performance, participation, and productivity and, perhaps, ultimately the loss of their job.

The following aspects of work habits may become affected:
- *Personal presentation.* A decrease in punctuality and an unkempt appearance
- *Social presentation.* Difficulty in accepting feedback, an increase in negativism and complaining, and difficulty in relating to peers
- *Work competence.* Impaired concentration and forgetfulness, a low frustration tolerance and an inability to organise and plan
- *Work tolerance.* An inability to tolerate a full day's work and its stress and pressures, and difficulty in completing a job in the required time and producing quality work

The health care provider can assist the MHCU's reintegration into the work environment by making use of simulation techniques, such as role playing a job interview, or supported employment (assistance in obtaining and maintaining employment). Referrals can be made for job sampling, job trials and job placement through members of the multidisciplinary team like the social worker or occupational therapist.

Intervening with motivation to access available resources

An MHCU with depression may deny the availability of accessible resources such as community or faith-based activities, the internet, the library, social media, parks, museums, the beach and the mountains or may have reasons for not using them, like issues relating to distance or transportation. This pattern is strongly influenced by changes in other patterns, for example the MHCU who presents with insomnia may be fatigued and lethargic, which reinforces social isolation and ultimately the motivation to use available resources. As MCHUs improve, they become more inclined to use these resources.

The principles of graded task assignment, pleasure mastery or the narrative approach can be used to encourage the use of free time for positive, rewarding engagement such as volunteering, as opposed to spending free time in ways that increase or maintain the depression. Activities should be identified that the MHCU finds enjoyable and interesting or that give a sense of accomplishment; the activities during which the MHCU feels either least depressed or most depressed should be monitored. The MHCU can be assisted in scheduling positive activities during emotionally low times, for example, a widow who feels very depressed in the evening when missing her late husband and who enjoys talking to friends can be scheduled to make two phone calls to friends every evening, or to chat on a social media group. The MHCU is taught to reward themselves for every prescheduled task performed or to involve people on social networks to do the reinforcement. The widow in the above example could have a bubble bath after her two calls.

Interventions with fulfilling biological needs

In order to fulfil the biological needs of the MHCU, identify biological problems or changes in areas like sleep, libido, exercise and eating patterns.

Sleep health

The effects of sleep deprivation are deleterious and influence mood, cognition, quality of life, cortisol production, glucose metabolism, energy levels, stress response, weight regulation and cardiovascular health (Nedeltcheva & Scheer, 2014; Passos et al, 2014), spotlighting the importance of sleep health. Insomnia is a 24-hour problem, which needs examination for the total amount of time slept. Mastery of sleep health occurs through measures such as managing underlying physical pathologies, addressing psychological problems and developing and maintaining a structured sleep–wake cycle. In addition, the nutritional input to sleep of essential amino acids needs to be recognised. These amino acids include tryptophan, a precursor of serotonin, melatonin, and nicotinamide, which play a part in the sleep–wake rhythm (Kokturk & Kanbay, 2015). Melatonin has a strategic role in the induction of spontaneous sleep. Assessment of sleep patterns begins with self-monitoring by means of a sleep–wake diary or a sleep–wake clock for each 24-hour cycle. If the clock is used the time spacing will vary according to the MHCU's lifestyle. The following patterns regarding the sleep patterns of MHCUs should be monitored:

- The ease with falling asleep initially and if awake how easily they return to sleep, ie sleep efficiency (Buysse, 2014: 11)
- The estimated time they fell asleep
- Sleep fragmentation – the time they awaken, how frequently they awake and for how long they are awake, monitoring sleep duration and continuity (Buysee, 2014: 11)
- The average number of hours they sleep in 24 hours, divided into sleep in the day and sleep in the night
- Factors that might precipitate awakening and falling asleep, for example, bad dreams, noise, preoccupation with specific thoughts
- What they do when awake, for example, lie in bed, read a novel, get up and do an activity
- Subjective assessment of the quality of the sleep (Buysee, 2014: 13)
- Subjective assessment of sense of alertness during waking hours (Buysee, 2014: 13)
- Measures used to self-medicate in order to return to sleep, such as alcohol, over-counter medication. Alternatively, there might be increasing reliance on benzodiazepines.

Instead of the universal goal of eight hours sleep per night it is more applicable to develop a structured programme around actual sleep time. This could involve the following suggestions to the MHCUs:

- Get into bed six hours before they due to wake up and set the alarm if they have one, for example, into bed at 00:00 and wake at 06:00.
- Darken the room before sleep, open the curtains, and turn on lights/light a candle at rising time.
- If awake and relaxed during sleep time, stay in bed.
- If awake and anxious during sleep time, do relaxation exercises and stay in bed. If anxiety persists, get out of bed.

- If out of bed, become involved in an activity without disturbing others in the dwelling and return to bed if feeling sleepy. Get up at the designated time even if they returned to bed only an hour before.
- Avoid caffeine (tea, coffee), alcohol, and cigarettes (if possible) within five hours of scheduled bedtime.
- Avoid exercise and spicy, heavy meals within two hours of bedtime.
- If plagued by worrying thoughts before bedtime, set aside a 20-minute 'worry time' after supper in which to worry as much as possible. Keep a 'worry' diary with possible solutions to the problems. When entering the sleep area, leave 'worries' (the diary as well) outside the door.
- Avoid naps during the day – rather do something else, for example, household or gardening tasks.
- Be involved in exercise during the day to improve sleep quality (Passos et al, 2014).

Note: Initially eliminate any underlying physiological cause of insomnia.

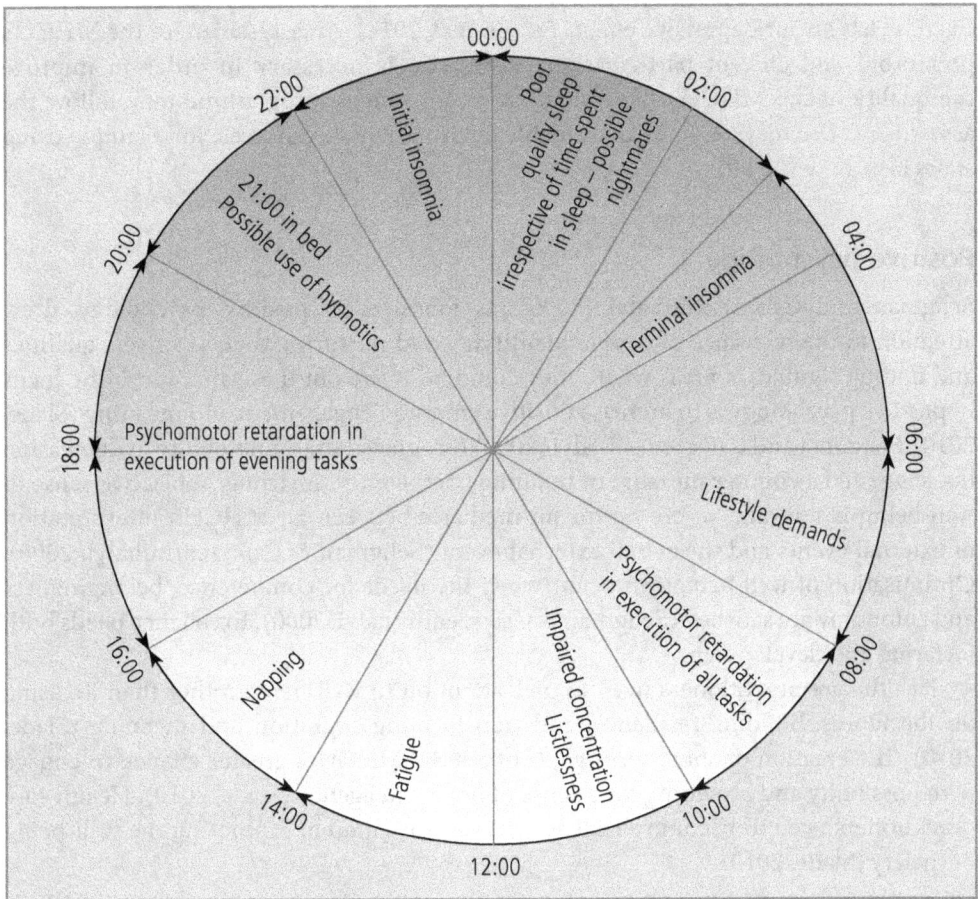

Figure 13.2 An MHCU's sleep–wake clock

Healthy eating patterns

Eating patterns have physiological, social, and psychological links, which underline the need to address these in totality. Eating patterns may vary from MHCU to MHCU, with some presenting with an increase in appetite and subsequent weight gain that can spiral to lowering the self-esteem and possible social withdrawal. The phenomenon of gaining weight for some MHCUs, despite no increase in eating patterns, may indicate a link between hypothyroidism and depression or decreased sleep duration and the link to type 2 diabetes (Nedeltcheva & Scheer, 2014), alternatively hormonal changes. On the other hand, some MHCUs may have a decreased desire to eat and for some, even preparing a meal is an effort. This results in marked weight loss and the resultant deprivation of nutrients, especially the vitamin B group, which perpetuates the existing listlessness and fatigue. Constipation is often an unwanted outcome of decreased intake.

Healthy exercise patterns

Exercise has an antidepressive effect (Passos et al, 2014). An assessment of the MHCU's premorbid and current participation in exercise is necessary in order to improve the quality of the MHCU's life. Initiation of an exercise programme may follow the assessment. Use may be made of available environmental resources, for example using stairs instead of the lift.

Positive psychology

Seligman and Csikszentmihalyi (2000), as founders of positive psychology, drew attention to the relevance of people identifying and nurturing their strongest qualities and finding significant areas where they could best 'live out these strengths'. The focus in positive psychology is to increase positive emotion, engagement and meaning (Slade, 2010). Seligman and Csikszentmihalyi (2000) recognised the vulnerability to depression but suggested a counter measure of building competency. A strong, subjective sense of well-being is relevant, where optimism mediates between an MHCU's interpretation of external events and the actual external event (Seligman & Csikszentmihalyi, 2000). Optimisation of well-being can occur when the needs for competence, belongingness and autonomy are satisfied (Seligman & Csikszentmihalyi, 2000). Excellence needs both fostering and development.

Health care practitioners need to give attention to well-being rather than focusing on the illness, building resilience, and transforming cognition and meaning (Slade, 2010). The creation of short-term goals offers the MHCU a greater chance to engage with possibility and providing for a sense of hope and agency (Slade, 2010). Health care practitioners need to become social activists against stigma, promoting the well-being of society (Slade, 2010).

OTHER INTERVENTIONS

In this section, other therapies used for treating depression are discussed. These include repetitive Transcranial Magnetic Stimulation (rTMS) and electroconvulsive therapy (ECT).

Intervening with rTMS

Transcranial magnetic stimulation is a non-invasive and non-convulsive treatment modality that utilises the principle of electromagnetic induction. It makes use of a high current pulse generator which produces a current that flows through a stimulating coil. This is placed on the MHCU's scalp at the site of the left dorsolateral prefrontal cortex, inducing an electrical field and a magnetic pulse of approximately 1.5 Tesla that activates neural networks in the cortex (Lefaucheur et al, 2014: 2152). Literature suggests that there is an asymmetry of cortical activities in depression. This explains the placement of coil over the left prefrontal cortex, which is considered hypoactive in depression (Lefaucheur et al, 2014: 2178). This treatment option is effective in MHCUs who are unable to tolerate antidepressants or anaesthetics, or who require a non-systemic treatment for the depression, as the MHCU is awake during the procedure (Bernard et al, 2009). To enable therapeutic effects, 20–30 sessions of 37 minutes daily over four to six weeks are required.

The initial contact requires a detailed explanation and discussion with the MHCU about their preferences regarding the milieu during the treatment. This could be their preferences regarding sleeping or watching a DVD or having the company of support of a person of their choice, as well as assessment of the use of caffeine-containing substances, alcohol or benzodiazepine use (Bernard et al, 2009: 328). The mental health care nurse is to assess the level of depression using, for example, Becks Depression Inventory. The MHCU should be asked to wash hair using only shampoo the night before and at the start of the treatment to remove reading glasses and hearing aids; mobile phones must be switched off (Bernard et al, 2009: 331). Ideally, the same mental health care nurse should be present throughout the treatment offerings. The mental health care nurse is to remain with the MHCU for the treatments and monitor for focal motor movements indicating a spread to the trigeminal nerve, which causes discomfort or the rare occurrence of a seizure (Bernard et al, 2009: 328). The MHCU can pre-medicate an hour before with Tylenol or ibuprofen as prescribed for the side effect of headaches and apply topical lidocaine cream to alleviate site pain (Bernard et al, 2009: 328).

Intervening with electroconvulsive therapy (ECT)

This treatment involves the administration of a short-duration general anaesthetic and a muscle relaxant to the MHCU, and then the application of a weak electrical current of (70–130 V) by briefly placing electrodes unilaterally or bilaterally on the temples in order to produce a generalised seizure. Non-dominant hemisphere (usually right) unilateral ECT causes less cognitive impairment compared to bilateral ECT but is considered less effective.

The mechanism of ECT is complex. No unified theory exists on how ECT works or how the cognitive adverse effects are explained, but what is known is that ECT affects multiple components of the central nervous system (Shah et al, 2013; Sienaert, 2014: 85).

When the therapist is racing against time for the MHCU's life, ECT has strong clinical significance. Generally, ECT is considered effective when the MHCU begins to socialise with others, is no longer preoccupied with suicidal thoughts, and verbalises a sense of well-being.

Guidelines for administering ECT

The following section details the indications, contraindications and the number and frequency of treatments.

Indications
- No improvement in MDD after a full trial of antidepressants
- Mood stabilisers fail to control the acute manic phase in bipolar disorder
- Catatonic disorder
- Emergency treatment of active suicide where life is endangered (while waiting for effect of antidepressants)
- Intolerance of side effects of antidepressants with MDD.

Contraindications
Very high risk
- Increased intracranial pressure
- Space-occupying brain lesion
- Intracerebral bleeding
- Myocardial infarction within the last three months
- Conditions presenting as high anaesthetic risk
- Pregnancy

Moderate risk
- Severe osteoarthritis, osteoporosis or a recent fracture
- Cardiovascular disease
- Major infections, recent stroke, chronic respiratory difficulty or an acute peptic ulcer.

Number and frequency of treatments
Each MHCU is assessed individually; thus, the frequency and number of treatments vary. On average, ECT administration is twice a week as opposed to three times a week (three times a week is associated with greater memory impairment). The number of treatments ranges from six to twelve.

Nursing care
Nursing care should take place pre-treatment, during treatment and post-treatment.

Pre-treatment

Assess the attitudes, fears and beliefs of the MHCU about ECT and intervene as indicated.

- Work with the MHCU and family towards an informed decision about ECT, through identification of knowledge, fears and beliefs about ECT. Identify the influence of the media on fear and belief structures.
- Assist in alleviating fears and reducing anxiety. Anxiety is present in up to 75 per cent of MHCUs receiving ECT, with fears of memory impairment or brain damage being the greatest and fear range moving from a little fear to terror (Obbels et al, 2017: 230). In the identification of fears, allow direct and open expression of feelings about the forthcoming treatment, correcting misconceptions and clarifying existing information. Psycho-education with a leaflet or a DVD needs careful consideration, as the source material should be matched with the MHCU at the service centre. Consideration should be given to levels of literacy and education. Discuss the concerns that both the MHCU and the family see as important. Use a positive approach to the treatment, avoiding the use of words like 'shocks' and other negative terms. Talk about the treatment, emphasising its therapeutic value.
- Teach the MHCU and the family what to expect in the treatment – the nature of ECT, reason for recommendation of ECT, number and frequency of treatments, potential side effects and their management, alternatives to ECT inclusive of no treatment and its implications. Provide information to the MHCU and the family about amnesia for autobiographical information as it is a critical adverse cognitive effect of ECT.
- Obtain informed consent, but if one is unable to do this due to the MHCU's condition then a legal guardian, parent, or spouse may provide consent, or in the absence of the aforementioned, the head of the health care establishment may provide authorisation.
- Invite family members to be with the MHCU during the treatment in an attempt to allay anxiety, provide support and later to testify to the MHCU about the safety of the treatment. This is also a measure for countering stigmatisation (Obbels et al, 2017: 235).
- In the event of family not accompanying the MHCU to the treatment, obtain mobile numbers of whom to contact post-treatment.
- Provide reassurance that members of the team will be with the MHCU during each of the treatments.
- Allow the MHCU to discuss ECT with another MHCU who has undergone the treatment.
- Prepare the MHCU as for any other anaesthetic procedure:
  - take a thorough medical history
  - carry out baseline investigations (full blood count, urea and electrolytes, blood sugar levels; chest X-ray, electrocardiogram (ECG) and computed tomography (CT) scan if first psychiatric presentation, vital signs, and test for pregnancy)
  - doctor to review medication and to make recommendations prior to the course

of ECT or prior to each treatment (medication that may interfere with ECT are benzodiazepines, lithium, clozapine, risperidone, anticonvulsants)
- obtain consent after the MHCU has received the above information
- keep nil per month for eight hours, administer pre-medication inclusive of anxiolytic
- Monitor and record pre-treatment cognition as a baseline measure.

During treatment
Provide supportive care during the treatment:
- The mental health care nurse who has established the relationship with the MHCU is to accompany the MHCU to the operating theatre/treatment centre.
- The mental health care nurse is to stay with the MHCU throughout the treatment, talking the MHCU through every aspect of the treatment. In the event of a family member accompanying the MHCU, the family member is included in all explanations and talked through the procedure.
- It might be the MHCU/family member's first time in such a setting. Hence, it is vital to allay fears and to provide an explanation about all equipment.
- Carry out relaxation exercises, especially if there is a delay in commencing the treatment.
- Immediately before the ECT verify the MHCU's identity through asking the MHCU to state their name and date of birth, crosschecked against the information in the file. Ask the MHCU what procedure they are having. Check that consent is signed. The doctor will confirm the electrode placement and electrical dosing (Watts, 2016).
- The MHCU is pre-oxygenated, ECG monitor is connected and an intravenous line is inserted for administration of a short-acting muscle relaxant. The ECT is delivered through electrodes to generate a generalised seizure of at least 25 seconds. The clonic phase is usually only visible through the twitching of the toes.
- Thereafter the MHCU is placed in the semi-prone position, oxygen maintained, and vital signs monitored before being transported back to the unit.
- The doctor is to complete the ECT register and submit form MHCA 47 to the Mental Health Review Board on a quarterly basis.

Post-treatment
Monitor and evaluate the MHCU post-treatment for the course of the side effects.

Monitor for negative cognitive side effects
- Be sensitive to the possible short-term postictal confusion immediately post-ECT, characterised by anxiety, restlessness and disorientation (Andrade et al, 2016).
- Nurse in a safe environment and provide orientation.
- Monitor carefully, noting the course for anterograde amnesia (three months after treatment) and retrograde amnesia (prior to treatment) and the anxiety attached to the feeling. Retrograde amnesia involves difficulty in remembering facts or autobiographical information, particularly related to events; both forms of amnesia

appear more lasting compared to amnesia on how to operate certain devices (Verwijk et al, 2017). Enquire about events linked to hospitalisation, weddings, jobs, and events that took place in the past year, and monitor responses at subsequent times. Use family for collateral input. Notify the doctor about the course of the amnesia.
- Pre-empt possible amnesia and provide orientation aids. Place a piece of paper on the locker stating what procedure they received, their name, where they are and the date. Offer to place a call to a significant other to prevent embarrassment of having forgotten how to use a mobile phone.
- Reintroduce primary caregivers.
- Prior to discharge, educate the MHCU and their family about the possibility of amnesia and its management.

Monitor for other adverse effects: headaches, myalgia, nausea and dizziness
- Monitor vital signs.
- Headaches vary from mild to severe, but they are usually mild and self-limiting after 24 hours and need differentiation from headaches linked to depression (Andrade et al, 2016).
- Do not wait for the MHCU to complain about a headache but enquire about the presence of a headache.
- The MHCU may be confused about whom to ask for an analgesic.
- Treating headaches diminishes the headache-related nausea (Andrade et al, 2016).
- Enquire about the presence of myalgia, nausea and dizziness.
- Monitor for postural hypotension.
- Intervene accordingly.

Provide support post-treatment
- Recognise the fear linked to a deprivation of memory and orientation.
- Allay anxiety post-treatment. Talk through what has occurred in the treatment.
- Notify the family that treatment was carried out. Notify the MHCU that the family have been informed.
- Encourage resumption of normal activities. Reinforce the concept of ECT as a therapeutic treatment rather than an incapacitating procedure.

SUICIDE
Background

Suicide occurs throughout the lifespan, and in 2015 was among the top 20 leading causes of death globally, and the second leading cause of death among persons 15–29 years old (WHO, 2017). Globally about 10.7 persons per 100 000 successfully commit

> 'To write a prescription is easy: but to come to an understanding with people is hard.'
> *Franz Kafka*

suicide, with nearly 800 000 deaths due to suicide in 2016 (WHO, 2018). In 2016 South Africa reported suicide mortality rates of 11.6, Swaziland 13.3 and Lesotho 21.2 persons per 100 000 (WHO, 2018: 32). The reasons for the high suicide rates in Africa are many and include suicide being an escape from legal systems with brutal punishments for crimes; a solution to problems linked to poverty and to health issues especially human immunodeficiency virus (HIV)/acquired immunodeficiency syndrome (AIDS); displacement; homelessness and war. Globally, the success rate is greater for males, particularly in the age group 25–34 years (WHO, 2018).

Survivors of suicide have described the experience as something that has links to oppression and to relief, in expressions such as: 'body and mind crushed by life's demands'; 'invisible agony'; and 'death offers a sweet smell'.

Definitions

Suicide behaviour includes thinking about suicide, planning for suicide, attempting the suicide and the suicide itself (WHO, 2014). The various terms are defined as follows:

- *Suicide.* Self-inflicted death with evidence (either explicit or implicit) that the MHCU intended to die
- *Suicidal ideation.* Thoughts of engaging in behaviour intended to end one's life
- *Suicide plan.* Formulation of a specific method through which one intends to die
- *Suicide attempt.* Engagement in potentially self-injurious behaviour in which there is at least some intent to die
- *Suicidal intent.* Subjective expectation and desire for a self-destructive act to end in death
- *Deliberate self-harm.* Wilful self-inflicting of painful, destructive, or injurious acts without intent to die.

Suicide profile

Suicide profiles differ per geographical setting and between the general population of the specific community . The adoption of a public health model will allow for a structured approach to suicide. It is relevant that each clinical area should develop a profile of suicide, identifying what the problem is, and the population-specific risk, while at the same time not ignoring the outliers to the profile. This should be accompanied by the implementation of specific protective factors to buffer against the risk, followed by evaluation and development of policies and programmes (WHO, 2014). In particular, consideration needs to be given to the fact that MHCUs more frequently use medication as a means for suicide due to its accessibility, and to comorbidities such as chronic pain and substance abuse (Bhatt et al, 2018). However, suicide is prevalent in MHCUs with diagnostic labels of mood disorders, psychotic disorders, substance use disorders (Bhatt et al, 2018) and where impulsivity is evident such as in personality disorders.

Global profile and risk factors

The risk factors need identification for specific regions and encompass biological, psychological, social and economic factors. The risk factors cannot be seen in isolation, but in conjunction with the MHCU's bio-psychological vulnerability, stressors and the strength of protective factors like the availability of social and professional support, willingness to seek support and personal resources to deal with challenges. Below are some risk factors (Dumon, & Portzky, 2014; WHO, 2014):

- In lower middle-income countries, (LMICs), suicide is 57 per cent higher in men (WHO, 2014)
- Age in LMIC: young adults (15–29 years) and elderly women (>70 years) have higher risk and middle-aged males (WHO, 2014)
- In LMICs, 44 per cent violent deaths in males and 70 per cent violent deaths in females are due to suicide (WHO, 2014)
- In LMICs, pesticide ingestion is most common (WHO, 2014)
- Ethnicity depending on geographical location
- Unemployment
- Relationship steeped in gender-based violence
- Lack of social support
- High-risk profession, eg police
- Minority group, for example, lesbian, gay, bisexual, transgender persons
- Social isolation, for example, living alone
- Recent criminal offence
- Substance or alcohol abuse
- Medical conditions causing chronic pain
- Recent loss of a significant person.

Suicide prevention

Suicide prevention programmes should incorporate national measures as well as those to be implemented in health care settings.

National measures

National measures that should be put in place include:
- Limiting access to lethal means:
    - changing pack sizes of dispensed medication
    - introducing legislation to limit over-counter purchases of analgesics
    - creating blister packs for medication
    - limiting carbon monoxide emissions from cars
    - implementing firearm laws controlling access
    - restricting pedestrian access to bridges, railways or barricade areas of high-rise buildings
    - creating legislation to limit access to alcohol

- Increasing and supporting national surveillance of suicide for a composite data registry
- Raising awareness through education about warning signs for suicide, alcohol and substance-use disorders and bullying (especially cyber-bullying and sexting)
- Recognising World Suicide Prevention Day on 10 September
- Scaling up treatment of MHCUs attempting suicide
- Providing for national emergency call centres like suicide crisis help-lines
- Providing for accessible 24/7 treatment for crises, relationship issues and mental health disorders
- Controlling insensitive media reporting relating to suicide
- Instituting measures to decrease stigma for health seeking behaviours
- Instituting measures to support MHCUs affected by suicide, inclusive of bereavement
- Providing continued support post-discharge not only for mental health care disorders
- Implementing a national strategy on suicide prevention.

Institutional measures to prevent harm
Allow the MHCU to feel safe in the setting and limit the opportunities for suicide:
- Remove potentially harmful items such as sharp instruments, cleaning agents, matches, medication and electrical cords and ensure medication is always locked away.
- Monitor the therapeutic environment regularly. Be aware of possible means of committing suicide such as large windows.
- Be aware of articles brought into the unit by both MHCUs and visitors.
- Place the MHCU near the nurses' station.

It should be remembered, however, that no unit is suicide-proof and that MHCUs constantly test the environment.

In cases of extreme risk of suicide, short-term chemical restraint might initially be necessary.

Ward policies for preventing suicide
It is important to develop ward policies and to identify plans for the prevention of suicide:
- Maintain a 24-hour observation period, recording accurately and specifically the MHCU's behaviour, with particular attention to changes in mood, energy levels, and ability to concentrate as signs of shifts in depression. The antidepressants might have energised the MHCU prior to the mood changes and the risk is that the energy is mobilised into a suicide attempt.
- Identify a time corresponding to ward activities when the MHCU may be at greater risk of committing suicide.

- Identify and plan for times of low staff/MHCU ratio such as staff changes and night duty. At such times, there is a need for special awareness of the MHCUs' behavioural patterns.

Initiating positive interventions to decrease the risk of suicide
These positive interventions include the following:
- Staff attitudes should be therapeutic:
    - avoid non-therapeutic responses such as indifference, sarcasm, and hostility
    - avoid arguing with or confronting the MHCU about their decisions; rather opt for a therapeutic exploration of the outcome of the decisions and recognise the seriousness of suicidal behaviour
- Reassure the MHCU of staff availability at all times and establish a relationship of trust.
- Explore the MHCU's belief about life after death and how the MHCU would like to be remembered by family and significant others.
- Avoid being drawn into confidential alliances with the MHCU asking not to share with other team members. However, acknowledge the MHCU's distress.
- Avoid the use of pre-printed 'no suicide' contracts, which have no empirical support, and rather opt for an agreement that is individualised per MHCU that targets their motivation towards recovery (Rudd et al, 2006). An example of this has been provided at the end of this section.
- Reinforce positive responses and activities, such as grooming. Encourage the development of a positive self-concept, with mastery and control over their own life.
- Offer the MHCU intensive psychotherapy after the immediate crisis of attempted suicide, with particular emphasis on effective coping strategies and challenging maladaptive cognitions.
- Encourage the MHCU to participate in activities.
- Identify support groups in the community and refer the MHCU on discharge.

Monitoring of risk prevention activities

Audit clinic/hospital files regularly, assessing:
- Highlighted risk indicators per person
- Individual risk management plans for at-risk persons
- Evidence of prompt follow-up for person discharged from hospital with serious mental illness/history recent suicide
- Critical incident review when person attempted suicide to establish what might have been done differently
- Post-discharge follow-up and continued linking with the person.

Suicide warning signs

The warning signs listed below are general and need to be seen in context with other behaviours and not in isolation. For example, it might be appropriate for an older person to be writing a will, but this could be questionable for a 10-year-old child. Warning signs can be grouped under the following pointers:

- *Focus of conversation.* Focuses on death; shows despair and openly talks about unbearable pain or hopelessness; verbal suicide threats; enquiring about lethality; talking about being burdensome; guilt statements like 'It's all my fault'; helplessness. 'I can't do anything that makes a difference'; escape. 'I just have to get out of this mess'.
- *Preparation for death.* Updating/writing a will; giving away possessions; saying good-bye to others; cleaning up room/house; writing a suicide note; stockpiling of tablets; buying a firearm; cancelling social arrangements; taking out extra insurance policies or funeral policy; checking suicide clauses in policies.
- *Signs of depression.* See earlier in this chapter, under 'Assessment and diagnosis of depression'.
- *Social withdrawal.* Choosing to be alone and avoiding friends and social activities.
- *Mood change.* Shifting from hopelessness/agitation to sudden calm.
- *Uncharacteristic reckless behaviour.* Driving dangerously or increased substance abuse evidencing decreased value for life.
- *Electronic search history.* Showing ways to commit suicide.
- *Display status on social media.* Evidencing death cue statements like 'What's the point?'
- *Self-medication.* Using over-counter medication or substances like alcohol or increasing use of prescribed medication in an attempt to ameliorate the feelings of despair/depression.

Suicide risk assessment

People often shy away from asking the MHCU directly about suicide, even if they believe there might be a risk. A common but incorrect statement is, 'What if I put ideas of suicide into his head?' or the mental health care nurse might navigate the MHCU's fear by using vague questions to address the topic. This level of silence or vagueness on the part of the health care provider detracts from an opportunity for the MHCU to receive support, counselling and could even end in a fatality. It also runs the risk of the MHCU answering inappropriately. The mental health care nurses need to reflect on their attitude and where necessary seek counselling regarding their opinions and levels of fear about suicide.

How and what to assess for in suicide risk

The mental health care practitioner, in assessing the suicide risk of an MHCU, should:
- Ensure that at the start of the interaction the MHCU is aware of the limits of confidentiality that absolute confidentiality is not possible, and it might be necessary to include other members of the multidisciplinary team as well as support structures such as family.
- If the MHCU is in the trauma/casualty department following a suicide attempt identify the time and method(s), including the name and dose of medication, and administer emergency measures accordingly. These emergency measures will depend on the time lapse and the method and could include treating the injuries;

administering activated charcoal for oral overdose within two hours; administering naloxone 0.4 mg IV for an opioid overdose (respiration <12 bpm); and supplying oxygen 100 per cent via face mask or 100 per cent oxygen via face mask for carbon monoxide poisoning (Department of Health, 2016).
- Deal with own prejudices and levels of discomfort before engaging in suicide risk assessment. Be prepared to enquire about suicide risk.
- Carry out the risk assessment in conjunction with a detailed history and a mental state examination.
- Carry out risk assessment jointly with the MHCU where possible, working through the risk assessment tool together.
- Listen carefully for suicide risk cues in the conversation.
- Be alert to suicide being a possibility across a range of health care delivery situations.
- Avoid being surprised when it becomes evident in a less expected clinical situation.
- Know that it is a myth that 'people, who talk about suicide, do not mean it'.
- Understand that direct references or cues to suicide often result in contexts of strong trust, hope and rapport. This might be the mental health care nurse's only opportunity to intervene and should not be lost because of the mental health care nurse's personal issues prohibiting engagement in the topic.
- Avoid being apologetic about asking the questions linked to suicide enquiry.
- Enquire about suicide risk in a non-judgemental manner, without interjections of personal opinions and values.
- Avoid pressurising the MHCU into an answer, realising that such disclosure requires a setting steeped in empathy, evidence of genuine concern and letting the MHCU feel they are in charge.
- Avoid guilt-producing statements or statements laden with blame.
- Never hesitate to call on support if the mental health care nurse is feeling they need further professional support in any of the phases of interaction, explaining to the MHCU the reason.
- Do not rely solely on the outcome of suicide risk assessment tools. Sound clinical judgement regarding the path most suited for the MHCU must incorporate a structured clinical interview inclusive of a thorough history linked to the surrounding events. As much as scales give outcome scores, these are only guides and at times it is difficult to quantify suicide. The Adult Primary Care Guidelines use one criterion to assess high suicide risk: 'Does the patient have current thoughts or plans to commit suicide?' (Department of Health, 2016: 52).
- Include family history of suicide when taking the history of the MHCU. Also to be included are attempts at suicide and reasons for these, and mental health history inclusive of current medication, substance use and abuse, chronic illness or new diagnoses, as well as cognitive patterns (see 'Assessment and diagnosis of depression'). Identify maladjusted cognitive patterns. When assessing psychiatric history, enquire about hallucinations, especially command hallucinations. What is the MHCU's history of communication patterns – do they hold grudges, fail to verbalise feelings, frequently misinterpret conversations.

- Enquire about the current attempt or ideation and ask details about the perceived lethality of the plan or attempt, the access to the means, the reason for choosing the time of day, the time taken to plan the attempt, the availability of support and spiritual beliefs.
- Assess for personality characteristics such as manipulation, impulsivity versus self-control, and aggression.
- Allow the unit/hospital to select from the large variety of suicide rating scales and what best suits the setting and the profile of the MHCU profile. In addition, a scale with high specificity and sensitivity will be used. It is important that the mental health care nurse is familiar with its content and scoring system. Date all assessments and repeat these, plotting the outcome in relation to events occurring in the MHCU's life, personal characteristics and current symptoms so that a personalised overview is obtained. This can be used as a reflective tool in relapse management discussions with the MHCU thereby allowing them to become aware of their response patterns and growth points. (See the section for 'Examples of suicide rating scales'.)

It requires clinical expertise to strike the balance between underestimating and overestimating the suicide risk of the health care user. Underestimation can result in injury or a fatality, while overestimation can result in unnecessary hospitalisation and time away from work or support structures.

- Do not leave the MHCU, who is at risk for suicide, alone.
- Develop trust so that the MHCU hands over dangerous items like a firearm. Ask for removal of ammunition.

Record keeping throughout the process is imperative with clear justification of decisions reached and evidence of collaboration with the support structures and consultation with the multidisciplinary team.

> **Clinical practice**
> Use the scenario about Monica described earlier in the chapter. Identify a relevant suicide rating scale. Assess Monica's risk for committing suicide. Justify your choice. Identify additional information you would need to ask Monica.

Examples of suicide rating scales

There are various examples of suicide rating scales. A scale that measures the severity of the suicide is the Columbia Suicide Severity Rating Scale (Posner et al, 2008). The Suicidal Ideation Attributes Scale (SIDAS) is a short scale that offers validity and reliability as an internet assessment scale (Van Spijker et al, 2014). The SAD PERSONS Scale (SPS) is widely used and is effective in identifying a large number of risk factors. However, there are questions relating to its ability to predict suicide risk (Warden et al, 2014).

Bantjes and Ommen (2008) also provide a suicide risk assessment interview schedule, which highlights the following important items: demographic information,

DSM diagnosis, cognitions, history, psychometric tests and assessment interviews, suicidal ideation and intent, collateral information, details of previous psychological assessments and details of consultations and supervision sought by the clinician.

(See Annexure for Beck's Suicide Intent Scale used to assess the intent and perceptions of the MHCU regarding the suicide attempt. This scale is suitable for an MHCU who has made a suicide attempt.)

Care of the MHCU with suicidal ideations or who attempts suicide

A highly suicidal MHCU cannot be cared for at home and should be hospitalised. The decision about whether hospitalisation should occur is dependent on the MHCU's level of suicide risk, the level of support available at home and in the community, as well as the requests from the MHCU and their support structure. However, safety is priority and should be the first consideration.

The discussion of nursing care is from a hospital perspective, but the principles are applicable to the community setting. A nursing goal is to maximise the chances of survival. Efficient and effective nursing care can have a positive influence on the MHCU and shift them into the domain of life with hope. It is significant that all of these nursing actions are therapeutic interpersonal skills, which are regarded by mental health care nurses as the cornerstone of the mental health care nurse–MHCU relationship.

Note: There is legislation that is relevant to suicide interventions, in particular the Mental Health Care Act 17 of 2002. As suicide seldom stands as alone, contributory factors with linked legislation should be considered, for example the Criminal Procedure Act 51 of 1977, and the Prevention of, and Treatment for Substance Abuse Act 70 of 2008. See also Chapter 6 on legislation.

Care of the MHCU with suicidal ideations or who attempts suicide involves the following:

1. *Attend to the MHCU's basic needs*
    - touch and comfort them appropriately, for example, touch to the hand
    - walk and talk with the MHCU outside in the fresh air as safety allows
    - maintain nutritional needs
    - ensure sufficient sleep and rest
    - provide assistance with personal hygiene needs
2. *Create a secure, therapeutic environment that allows for healing*
    - ensure structure and stability in the setting
    - build a trusting relationship with the MHCU
    - ensure that the staff are friendly, welcoming and accommodating
    - communicate acceptance
    - encourage and ensure regular contact with support structures like family
    - create opportunities for community and faith-based organisations to visit and offer support
3. *Make time for the MHCU*
    - seek them out to enquire with genuineness about how they are feeling

- ensure a disturbance-free environment while talking together
- ensure the MHCU feels comfortable to approach staff at any time of the day
- appeal to the desire to live, as the MHCU might feel ambivalent about wanting to die:
  - What are the reasons for living?
  - What are the reasons for wanting to die?
  - When did these feelings start?
- teach techniques in cognitive behavioural therapy.

4. *Interact with the MHCU without prejudice*
   - recognise that they are still emotionally fragile
   - show unconditional positive warmth and respect for their needs and feelings
   - try to understand their experience from their point of view
   - avoid changing the topic when they raise their problems
   - avoid the use of guilt tactics involving significant others or religion in an attempt to convince them that suicide is 'wrong'. An example would be: 'How can you think of killing yourself? What about your child/husband/family?' or 'It is a sin to kill yourself; do you want to go to hell?'

5. *Allow the MHCU to express their feelings*
   - allow them to cry as much as needed and stay with them in silence
   - allow them to talk about suicidal feelings; do not discount the fact that they exist
   - avoid patronising or belittling their experience, for example: 'Don't worry so much, your husband does still love you.'; 'Now you must calm down and act like an adult.'
   - communicate hope through the above therapeutic interactions

6. *Assessment*
   - utilise assessment tools to assess progress or deterioration in mental health status
   - engage the MHCU in risk assessment, emphasising a strengths-based risk management approach.

An example of a treatment agreement

I, _____, agree to make a commitment to the recovery process. I understand that this means that I have agreed to be actively involved in all aspects of my recovery including:

i. attending all nurse-led groups (or letting the nurse leader know when and the reason I can't make it)
ii. setting recovery-based goals
iii. when attending all nurse-led sessions I will be actively involved, expressing my feelings honestly
iv. seeking out the nurse assigned to me for the day when I am feeling emotionally fragile
v. taking prescribed medication
vi. experimenting with newly learned skills
vii. verbalising to my assigned nurse if I feel that I am not progressing as I feel I would like to.

I acknowledge that to a large part, the successful outcome of my stay in hospital is dependent on my involvement. I agree to make a commitment to living.

- Embrace the situation to build shared visions about an enabling environment and discuss challenges. Use the opportunity to review and update existing unit policies or create a new policy document.

> **Practice plan**
> - Learn to be reflective of your practice.
> - Review documentation and reflect on practice outcomes, legislation and the meeting of ethical requirements. In the process, revise protocols and procedures to ensure practice improvement.
> - Critically analyse each situation, looking for evidence of opportunities for improved care to help prevent fatalities.
> - These are the types of questions you can ask in reflective practice:
>   - What was I aiming for when I carried out that specific action?
>   - How successful was I?
>   - What criteria am I using to measure success? Are the criteria based on what I want or what clinical guidelines suggest or what the MHCU would prefer?
>   - How would I do it differently next time?
>   - What do I feel about the whole experience?
>   - In what specific area of the interaction was I unsure?
>   - How did I deal with my lack of surety?
>   - Did I compromise care delivery because of my lack of knowledge/skill?
>   - How helpful do I feel the consultation with the resource person(s) was post-event?
>   - How helpful was the consultant with literature resources?
>   - Have I identified a clinical research gap?
>   - Do I feel competent to tackle the learning suggested?
>   - Have I noticed a progressive improvement in my clinical skills in this area? What evidence is there of scaffolding of my skills?
>   - Have I received feedback this week that contradicts what I initially thought about my performance?

BIPOLAR MOOD DISORDERS

This section covers bipolar mood disorders, nursing interventions and medication for these disorders.

Bipolar disorders: manic episodes

The essential features of a manic episode are a distinct period in which the predominant mood is either elevated, expansive or irritable and the disturbance is sufficiently severe to cause marked impairment in occupational functioning or usual social activities/relationships with others.

The following characteristics can be noted:
- *Appearance.* Colourful and flamboyant with very high energy levels
- *Speech.* Loud, rapid and rumbustious, with the use of puns. Pressure of speech and flight of ideas accompany this disorder
- *Mood.* Labile and the MHCU is easily susceptible to distracting stimuli
- *Social judgement.* The MHCU is intrusive, domineering and demanding. They are typically grandiose and very often sexually inappropriate – promiscuous and hypersexual.

The agreement will apply for the next week at which time it will be reviewed and modified.
Signed: _____
Date: _____
Witness: _____

Adapted from Rudd et al, 2006

Critical thinking about ethical issues and suicide
Debate
The MHCU has a right to commit suicide regardless of their psychiatric diagnosis.
versus
The MHCU has no right to commit suicide regardless of their psychiatric diagnosis.

Care of the survivors of suicide

The involvement of family or significant others may vary on a continuum from detachment to enmeshment. This may be influenced by various factors such as guilt, anger, denial, exhaustion or even shame which might be linked to the previous attempts made by the MHCU or events leading up to the suicide. Regardless of the circumstances, the health care professional needs to be available to the survivor(s) of the suicide who too often are forgotten or ignored. The survivor(s) might not actively reach out for help and the health care professional might need to take the initiative.

It is important to remember that survivors can include health care professionals or other persons working in the unit/clinic and other caregivers who too will experience a myriad of feelings, inclusive of professional failure. The following principles apply:

- The immediate care offered may vary from supportive counselling to crisis intervention. As indicated, offer further counselling at the health care centre or an agency of their choice. The following areas may be explored:
- When sharing feelings about the suicide and feelings preceding the suicide:
  - deal with current feelings and explain that the type of feelings will change as will the intensity. It may be confusing for the survivor to be feeling guilt, anger, and sadness at one time or in close succession
  - manage questions posed by friends and other community members about the suicide
  - cope with grief, the intensity of which will vary, as may its cause, from the physical death of a significant other to the loss of a self-imposed expectation of the significant other.
- When interacting with personnel avoid an atmosphere of unpleasantness that includes naming, blaming, and shaming surrounding the incident.
- Create both support and an opportunity to learn from the incident.
- Create a setting for personnel to discuss and explore their feelings surrounding the incident. Build group cohesion as opposed to division.
- Organise follow up support group meetings.
- Identify personnel who need individual counselling and intervene accordingly.

DSM-5 diagnostic criteria: manic episodes

A. A distinct period of abnormally and persistently elevated, expansive, or irritable mood and abnormally and persistently increased goal-directed activity or energy, lasting at least 1 week and present most of the day, nearly every day (or any duration if hospitalization is necessary).
B. During the period of mood disturbance and increased energy or activity, three (or more) of the following symptoms (four if the mood is only irritable) are present to a significant degree and represent a noticeable change from usual behavior:
   1. Inflated self-esteem or grandiosity.
   2. Decreased need for sleep (e.g., feels rested after only 3 hours of sleep).
   3. More talkative than usual or pressure to keep talking.
   4. Flight of ideas or subjective experience that thoughts are racing.
   5. Distractibility (i.e., attention too easily drawn to unimportant or irrelevant external stimuli), as reported or observed.
   6. Increase in goal-directed activity (either socially, at work or school, or sexually) or psychomotor agitation (i.e., purposeless non-goal-directed activity).
   7. Excessive involvement in activities that have a high potential for painful consequences (e.g., engaging in unrestrained buying sprees, sexual indiscretions, or foolish business investments).
C. The mood disturbance is sufficiently severe to cause marked impairment in social or occupational functioning or to necessitate hospitalization to prevent harm to self or others, or there are psychotic features.
D. The episode is not attributable to the physiological effects of a substance (e.g., a drug of abuse, a medication, other treatment) or to another medical condition.
   Note: A full manic episode that emerges during antidepressant treatment (e.g., medication, electroconvulsive therapy) but persists at a fully syndromal level beyond the physiological effect of that treatment is sufficient evidence for a manic episode and, therefore, a bipolar I diagnosis.

Note: Criteria A-D constitute a manic episode. At least one lifetime manic episode is required for the diagnosis of bipolar I disorder.

Hypomanie Episode

A. A distinct period of abnormally and persistently elevated, expansive, or irritable mood and abnormally and persistently increased activity or energy, lasting at least 4 consecutive days and present most of the day, nearly every day.
B. During the period of mood disturbance and increased energy and activity, three (or more) of the following symptoms (four if the mood is only irritable) have persisted, represent a noticeable change from usual behavior, and have been present to a significant degree:
   1. Inflated self-esteem or grandiosity.
   2. Decreased need for sleep (e.g., feels rested after only 3 hours of sleep).
   3. More talkative than usual or pressure to keep talking.

4. Flight of ideas or subjective experience that thoughts are racing.
5. Distractibility (i.e., attention too easily drawn to unimportant or irrelevant external stimuli), as reported or observed.
6. Increase in goal-directed activity (either socially, at work or school, or sexually) or psychomotor agitation.
7. Excessive involvement in activities that have a high potential for painful consequences (e.g., engaging in unrestrained buying sprees, sexual indiscretions, or foolish business investments).

C. The episode is associated with an unequivocal change in functioning that is uncharacteristic of the individual when not symptomatic.
D. The disturbance in mood and the change in functioning are observable by others.
E. The episode is not severe enough to cause marked impairment in social or occupational functioning or to necessitate hospitalization. If there are psychotic features, the episode is, by definition, manic.
F. The episode is not attributable to the physiological effects of a substance (e.g., a drug of abuse, a medication, other treatment).

Note: A full hypomanic episode that emerges during antidepressant treatment (e.g., medication, electroconvulsive therapy) but persists at a fully syndromal level beyond the physiological effect of that treatment is sufficient evidence for a hypomanic episode diagnosis. However, caution is indicated so that one or two symptoms (particularly increased irritability, edginess, or agitation following antidepressant use) are not taken as sufficient for diagnosis of a hypomanic episode, nor necessarily indicative of a bipolar diathesis.

Note: Criteria A–F constitute a hypomanic episode. Hypomanic episodes are common in bipolar I disorder but are not required for the diagnosis of bipolar I disorder.

Recognising bipolar disorders

Recognition of the disorder is essential for adequate treatment. The early signs of bipolar disorder may be hypomania – a state of high energy, excessive moodiness or irritability, and impulsive or reckless behaviour. Hypomania might feel good to the MHCU who is experiencing it, and family and friends may be the first to recognise that the mood swings are abnormal. In the beginning, bipolar disorder may also present as drug or alcohol abuse or poor school or work performance. If untreated, it worsens into a full episode of mania or depression. The MHCU might need a lot of encouragement from their social circle to seek help.

Nursing assessment and intervention

The patterns of lifestyle functioning will be used to describe the phenomena of mania and hypomania with corresponding psychiatric nursing interventions. Examples of nursing diagnoses which could be used to give substance to the intervention process are also given below.

Psychodynamic patterns

An MHCU's psychodynamic pattern features are strong evidence of high energy levels. This affects pattern maintenance, which in turn affects lifestyle functioning.

Patterns of fulfilling biological needs

Subjectively it seems as if the manic MHCU does not have the need to eat, sleep or rest, although it does seem as if they have an increased sexual need. The MHCU user appears rested with a maximum of two to three hours of sleep. This need to be perpetually active can lead to serious complications like exhaustion and collapse. The decreased need to sit down to a meal can be overcome by making finger food, snacks, fruit and high-calorie drinks available to the MHCU, as these can be eaten while the MHCU is in motion.

Personal hygiene requires supervision; the MHCU has to be instructed with regard to bathing and the use of toiletries, cosmetics and jewellery.

Essential drug list: PHC

For acute management of psychotic MHCUs (including mania), see Chapter 14, 'Nursing the MHCU with schizophrenia, schizophrenia spectrum and other psychotic disorders'.

Patterns of building and maintaining relationships

The MHCU with a manic episode can be either the 'happy' manic, who seems to be loved by all, or the 'irritable' manic, who becomes annoyed easily and has a low frustration tolerance. Both situations create problems for the MHCU, as responses from the people around them may ultimately be negative. They are often intrusive and have poor social judgement. This can lead to them being physically, emotionally and sexually abused. Relationships become strained as people cannot keep up with the MHCU with a manic episode. This may be verbalised or they may be avoided. Family, friends and staff are usually exhausted by their talkativeness, mood changes and increased energy. They seem to be at the mercy of the stimuli in the environment and cannot help themselves. They are hyper alert to everything that they see, hear or touch – even a subdued environment seems to provide a challenge for the MHCU with a manic episode to 'liven' it up. The MHCU also manifests manipulative behaviour, which staff and family have to recognise.

There is evidence to show that group psycho-education and family psycho-education reduced the length of time of manic episodes and improved the quality of life and family relationships (Crowe, et al, 2016; Crowe et al, 2010; Perlick et al, 2018; Van der Voort et al, 2015).

Limit setting is defined as a process through which a person in authority sets temporary and artificial boundaries for another person. Effective limit setting is directed towards the MHCU's physical and emotional safety and the technique creates a therapeutic boundary for the MHCU that can decrease MHCU's feelings of anxiety and uncertainty, minimise disruptive behaviour that is used to manage overt and covert sexual behaviour, and support adaptation to ward rules and routines. Limit setting should only be applied in the presence of an already established caring mental health care nurse–MHCU relationship that respects the rights and dignity of the MHCU and the mental health care nurse. Elements of trust, empathy and unconditional positive regard must be present for limit setting to be applied and to be effective. Limit setting is a therapeutic intervention and not a punishment. Everybody working with the MHCU, such as family and staff, therefore has to be aware of the problems and how they are to be handled. Some guiding principles are:

- As a team, and where possible with the MHCU, determine what types of behaviours need limits and why.
- Work out in advance how the limit will be set, the various types of alternate behaviour suggestions for the MHCU, and the consequences.
- Limits must be explained simply and briefly to the MHCU and they should be included in the setting of these limits where possible.
- Provide the MHCU with various types of acceptable behaviours they should follow.
- The consequences of not adhering to these limits must also be explained. Consequences must be direct and simple and, if possible, must have a bearing on the limits.
- If the MHCU exceeds the limits, the consequences must follow immediately. The rewards for adhering to the limits must be appropriate.
- Consistency in setting limits is of the utmost importance, as mixed messages render the exercise a failure and prevent the MHCU from understanding and assuming responsibility for their behaviour.
- Limit setting must not be taken as an opportunity to be punitive towards the MHCU.
- Unacceptable behaviour must be handled firmly in a non-judgemental manner, with no show of anger or disgust.
- Feedback must be given regarding unacceptable behaviour. Acceptance of the MHCU as an MHCU must be reinforced.
- Positive feedback must be given about acceptable behaviour.

Patterns of participation in group and community life

The MHCU with a manic episode seems to have a need to take over in group settings: they often interrupt discussion and usually want all the attention. While the MHCU may be regarded as 'funny', they may actually disrupt and stunt group progress. They may embarrass group members or ask very personal questions, or they may be manipulative. They are usually flamboyant and convincing and can embark on major projects like making large purchases of furniture and vehicles successfully. They tend to spend money indiscriminately and become extremely extravagant. The MHCU may also be viewed as the community clown due to their expansive mood, their constant change of clothes at short intervals and their over-familiarity. The MHCU relates briefly and superficially to religious and political issues and can be very disruptive in such settings.

Patterns of participation in work

The work environment may be extremely stimulating to an MHCU with a manic episode, which may result in severe distraction and poor concentration. This in turn may result in poor work output. The MHCU may also be either extremely irritable or extremely euphoric, thus creating difficulties with fellow workers and supervisors. This may be aggravated by the MHCU's need to be in control of a situation due to their grandiosity and expansive mood. The MHCU may also be a danger to themselves and others because of their excessive energy, the need to try something different and the speed at which they perform tasks. Fellow workers may be irritated by them or be exhausted by their energy, mood, talkativeness and tendency to manipulate.

In a ward situation, activities such as jogging, painting large areas – all large motor activities – may be suitable for an MHCU with a manic episode.

CONCLUSION

Nursing an MHCU with a mood disorder can be both challenging and rewarding. It provides an opportunity for the mental health care nurse, the MHCU and significant others to work together to restore the equilibrium of the MHCU's lifestyle patterns and to develop a recovery plan. It is important that mental health care nurses look after their own mental health, engage in a healthy work–life balance, and access their support structures and resources to promote their mental health. The mental health care nurses will need a good support system of their own and they are encouraged to be involved in activities that promote their own mental health. They will periodically need to re-examine their feelings and management skills, on the one hand regarding hopelessness, despair, negativism, low energy levels and, on the other hand, exuberance and hyperactivity. Reflection inaction, allowing for ongoing critical thinking about clinical practice, is an important skill and involves constantly reviewing personal and clinical strategies to ensure best practice.

REFERENCES

American Psychiatric Association (APA). 2013. *Diagnostic and Statistical Sanual of Sental Disorders: DSM-5,* doi: 10.1176/appi.books.9780890425596.744053.

AZ Quotes. 'Peter Block quotes'. http://www.azquotes.com/author/38092-Peter_Block (Accessed 15 September 2017).

Andrade, C, Arumugham, S S and Thirthalli, J. 2016. 'Adverse effects of electroconvulsive therapy'. *Psychiatric Clinics,* 39 (3), 513–530.

Ardington, C and Case, A. 2010. 'Interactions between mental health and socioeconomic status in the South African National Income Dynamics Study'. *Studies in Economics and Econometrics,* 34, 3: 69–85.

Bantjes, J and Van Ommen, C. 2008. 'The development and utilisation of a suicide risk assessment interview schedule'. *South African Journal of Psychology,* 38 (2): 391–411.

Baron, E C, Davies, T and Lund, C. 2017. 'Validation of the 10-item centre for epidemiological studies depression scale (CES-D-10) in Zulu, Xhosa and Afrikaans populations in South Africa'. *BMC Psychiatry,* 17 (1): 6.

Bech, P, Olsen, L R, Kjoller, M and Rasmussen, N K. 2003. 'Denmark Measuring well-being rather than the absence of distress symptoms: a comparison of the SF-36 Mental Health subscale and the WHO-Five Well-Being Scale'. *Psychiatric Research*, 12 (2): 85–91. doi: 10.1002/mpr.145.

Bernard, S, Westman, G, Dutton, P R and Lanocha, K. 2009. 'A Psychiatric Nurse's Perspective: Helping Patients Undergo Repetitive Transcranial Magnetic Stimulation (rTMS) for Depression'. *Journal of the American Psychiatric Nurses Association*, 15 (5): 325–332.

Bhatt, M, Perera, S, Zielinski, L, Eisen, R B, Yeung, S, El-Sheikh, W, DeJesus, J, Rangarajan, S., Sholer, H., Iordan, E and Mackie, P. 2018. 'Profile of suicide attempts and risk factors among psychiatric patients: a case-control study'. *PloS one*, 13 (2): p.e0192998.

Buysse, D J. 2014. 'Sleep health: can we define it? Does it matter?'. *Sleep*, 37 (1): 9–17.

Chipps, J and Jarvis, M A. 2016. 'Social capital and mental well-being of older people residing in a residential care facility in Durban, South Africa'. *Aging & Mental Health*, 20 (12): 1264–1270.

Chipps, J, Oosthuizen, F, Buthelezi, M B, Buthelezi, M M, Buthelezi, P F, Jeewa, S, Munsami, S, ... Ramlall, S. 2015. 'Knowledge, beliefs and mental treatment seeking practices of Black African and Indian outs in Durban, South Africa: Mental health'. *African Journal for Physical Health Education, Recreation and Dance*, 21: 186–196.

Crowe, M, Whitehead, L, Wilson, L, Carlyle, D, O'Brien, A, Inder, M, ... Joyce, P. 2010. 'Disorder-specific psychosocial interventions for bipolar disorder – A systematic review of the evidence for mental health nursing practice'. *International Journal of Nursing Studies*, 47 (7): 896–908. doi: 10.1016/j.ijnurstu.2010.02.012.

Department of Health. 2016. 'Adult Primary Care' (APC0 Guide 2016/2017). Pretoria. https://www.knowledgehub.org.za/system/files/Adult%20Primary%20Care%20guide%202016_2017%20%20Final%20for%20sign%20off%2012%20August%202016%20%28002%29_0.pdf (Accessed June 2019).

Dulwich Centre. nd. 'What is narrative therapy'. https://dulwichcentre.com.au/what-is-narrative-therapy/ (Accessed 3 February 2018).

Dumon, E and Portzky, G. 2014. 'General Guidelines on Suicide Prevention' (EUREGENAS project). https://www.academia.edu/15134909/General_Guidelines_on_Suicide_Prevention_EUREGENAS_project. (Accessed 10 October 2017).

Gibbs, A, Govender, K and Jewkes, R. 2017. 'An exploratory analysis of factors associated with depression in a vulnerable group of young people living in informal settlements in South Africa'. *Global Public Health*, 13 (7): 788–803.

Hage, M P and Azar, S T. 2012. 'The Link between Thyroid Function and Depression'. *Journal of Thyroid Research*, 2012, 590648. doi: 10.1155/2012/590648.

Heun, R, Bonsignore, M, Barkow, K and Jessen, F. 2001. 'Validity of the five-item WHO Well-Being Index (WHO-5) in an elderly population'. *European archives of psychiatry and clinical neuroscience*, 251 (2): 27–31.

Hibbel, J, Gallant, P, Polanco, M, Manley, M, Scholtz, C and Schlapper-Colmer, O. 2010. 'Keeping faith with keeping faith: Conversations about a conversation with Michael White'. *Journal of Systemic Therapies*, 29 (3): 1–22.

Kokturk, O and Kanbay, A. 2015. 'Tryptophan Metabolism and Sleep'. In: Engin A, Engin A (eds). *Tryptophan Metabolism: Implications for Biological Processes, Health and Disease. Molecular and Integrative Toxicology*. Humana Press: Cham.

Komori, T. 2017. 'The significance of proinflammatory cytokines and Th1/Th2 balance in depression and action of antidepressants'. *Neuropsychiatry*, 7 (1): 57–60.

Lefaucheur, J P, André-Obadia, N, Antal, A, Ayache, S S, Baeken, C, Benninger, D H, Cantello, R M, Cincotta, M, de Carvalho, M, De Ridder, D and Devanne, H. 2014. 'Evidence-based guidelines on the therapeutic use of repetitive transcranial magnetic stimulation (rTMS)'. *Clinical Neurophysiology*, 125 (11): 2150–2206.

Makhubela, M and Debusho, L K. 2016. 'Factorial invariance and latent mean differences of the Beck Depression Inventory–second edition (BDI-II) across gender in South African university students'. *Journal of Psychology in Africa*, 26 (6): 522–526.

Morgan, A. 2002. 'Beginning to use a narrative approach in therapy'. *International Journal of Narrative Therapy & Community Work*, 2002 (1): 85–90.

Nduna, M and Jewkes, R. 2012. 'Disempowerment and psychological distress in the lives of young people in Eastern Cape, South Africa'. *Journal of Child and Family Studies*, 21 (6): 1018–1027.

Nedeltcheva, A V and Scheer, F A. 2014. 'Metabolic effects of sleep disruption, links to obesity and diabetes'. *Current Opinion in Endocrinology, Diabetes, and Obesity*, 21 (4): 293.

Obbels, J, Verwijk, E, Bouckaert, F and Sienaert, P. 2017. 'ECT-related anxiety: a systematic review'. *The Journal of ECT*, 33 (4): 229-236.

O'Connor, T S, Davis, A, Meakes E, Pickering, R and Schuman, M. 2004. 'Narrative therapy using a reflecting team: An ethnographic study of therapists' experiences'. *Contemporary Family Therapy*, 26 (1): 21–39.

Perlick, D A, Jackson, C, Grier, S, Huntington, B, Aronson, A, Luo, X and Miklowitz, D J. 2018. Randomized trial comparing caregiver-only family-focused treatment to standard health education on the 6-month outcome of bipolar disorder. *BDI Bipolar Disorders*, 20 (7): 622–633.

Passos, G S, Poyares, D, Santana, M G, Teixeira, A A D S, Lira, F S, Youngstedt, S D, ... and De Mello, M T. 2014. 'Exercise improves immune function, antidepressive response, and sleep quality in patients with chronic primary insomnia'. *BioMed Research International*, Volume 2014.

Posner, K, Brent, D, Lucas, C, Gould, M, Stanley, B, Brown, G, Fisher, P, Zelazny, J, Burke, A, Oquendo, M and Mann, J. 2008. 'Columbia-Suicide Severity Rating Scale (C-SSRS)'. *The Research Foundation for Mental Hygiene*, Inc. http://cssrs.columbia.edu/wp-content/uploads/C-SSRS_Pediatric-SLC_11.14.16.pdf (Accessed 17 October 2017).

Rudd, M D, Mandrusiak, M and Joiner Jr, T E. 2006. 'The case against no-suicide contracts: The commitment to treatment statement as a practice alternative'. *Journal of Clinical Psychology*, 62 (2): 243–251.

Seligman, E P and Csikszentmihalyi, M. 2000. 'Positive psychology. An introduction'. *American Psychologist*, 55 (1): 5–14. doi: 10.1037//0003-066X.55.1.5.

Shah, A J, Wadoo, O and Latoo, J. 2013. 'Electroconvulsive therapy (ECT): important parameters which influence its effectiveness'. *British Journal of Medical Practitioners*, 6 (4): a634.

Sienaert, P. 2014. 'Mechanisms of ECT: reviewing the science and dismissing the myths'. *The Journal of ECT*, 30 (2): 85–86.

Slade, M. 2010. 'Mental illness and well-being: the central importance of positive psychology and recovery approaches'. *BMC Health Services Research*, 10 (1): 26.

Stein, D J, Seedat, S, Herman, A, Moomal, H, Heeringa, S G, Kessler, R C and Williams, D R. 2008. 'Lifetime prevalence of psychiatric disorders in South Africa'. *The British Journal of Psychiatry: The Journal of Mental Science*, 192, 2: 112–7.

Stellenberg, E L and Abrahams, J M. 2015. 'Prevalence of and factors influencing postnatal depression in a rural community in South Africa'. *African Journal of Primary Health Care & Family Medicine*, 7 (1): 874. doi: 10.4102/phcfm.v7i1.874.

Tomlinson, M, Grimsrud, A T, Stein, D J, Williams, D R and Myer, L. 2009. 'The epidemiology of major depression in South Africa: Results from the South African stress and health study'. *South African Medical Journal*, 99 (5).

Van der Voort, T Y G, van Meijel, B. Hoogendoorn, A W, Goossens, P J J, Beekman, A T F and Kupka, R W. 2015. 'Collaborative care for patients with bipolar disorder: Effects on functioning and quality of life'. *Journal of Affective Disorders*, 179: 14–22, doi:https://doi.org/10.1016/j.jad.2015.03.005.

Van Spijker, B A, Batterham, P J, Calear, A L, Farrer, L, Christensen, H, Reynolds, J and Kerkhof, A J. 2014. 'The suicidal ideation attributes scale (SIDAS): community-based validation study of a new scale for the measurement of suicidal ideation'. *Suicide and Life-Threatening Behavior*, 44 (4): 408–419.

Verwijk, E, Obbels, J, Spaans, H P and Sienaert, P. 2017. 'Doctor, will I get my memory back? Electroconvulsive therapy and cognitive side-effects in daily practice'. *Tijdschrift voor Psychiatrie*, 59 (10): 632–637.

Vos, T, Allen, C, Arora, M, Barber, R M, Bhutta, Z A, Brown, A, Carter, A, Casey, D C, Charlson, F J, Chen, A Z and Coggeshall, M, 2016. 'Global, regional, and national incidence, prevalence, and years lived with disability for 310 diseases and injuries, 1990–2015: a systematic analysis for the Global Burden of Disease Study 2015'. *The Lancet*, 388 (10053): 1545–1602.

Wallis, J, Burns, J and Capdevila, R. 2010. 'What Is Narrative Therapy and what is it not? The usefulness of Q methodology to explore accounts of White and Epston's (1990) approach to narrative therapy'. *Clinical Psychology & Psychotherapy*, 18 (6): 486–497.

Warden, S, Spiwak, R, Sareen, J and Bolton, J M. 2014. 'The SAD PERSONS Scale for Suicide Risk Assessment: A Systematic Review'. *Archives of Suicide Research*. doi: 10.1080/13811118.2013.824829.

Watts, B V. 2016. 'A time-out before every ECT treatment'. *The Journal of ECT*, 32 (4): 224.

World Health Organisation (WHO). 1998. 'WHO (five) Wellbeing Index (1998 version)'. http://www.who-5.org/ (Accessed 6 April 2013).

World Health Organisation (WHO). 2010. 'mhGAP intervention guide for mental, neurological and substance use disorders in non-specialized health settings: Mental Health Gap Action Programme (mhGAP): 24. https://apps.who.int/iris/bitstream/handle/10665/44406/9789241548069_eng.pdf?sequence=1; http://www.who.int/mental_health/mhgap (Accessed October 2017).

World Health Organisation (WHO). 2013. 'Mental health action plan 2013–2020'. http://www.who.int/mental_health/publications/action_plan/en/ (Accessed 20 January 2016).

World Health Organisation (WHO) (2014). 'Preventing suicide. A global imperative'. Luxembourg. http://www.who.int/mental_health/suicide-prevention/world_report_2014/en/ (Accessed 15 October 2017).

World Health Organisation (WHO). 2016. 'mhGAP Intervention Guide for mental, neurological and substance use disorders in non-specialised health settings'. Version 2.0. http://www.who.int/mental_health/mhgap/mhGAP_intervention_guide_02/en/. (Accessed 15 April 2017).

World Health Organisation (WHO). 2017. 'Depression and Other Common Mental Disorders: Global Health Estimates'. Geneva. Licence: CC BY-NC-SA 3.0 IGO. http://www.who.int/mental_health/management/depression/prevalence_global_health_estimates/en/ (Accessed October 2017).

World Health Organisation (WHO). 2018. 'World health statistics 2018: monitoring health for the SDGs, sustainable development goals. Geneva: World Health Organization; 2018. Licence: CC BY-NC-SA 3.0 IGO. https://apps.who.int/iris/bitstream/handle/10665/272596/9789241565585-eng.pdf?ua=1 (Accessed 24 May 2019).

RESOURCES NOT REFERRED TO IN THE TEXT

Baruch, E, Pistrang, N and Barker, C. 2018. 'Between a rock and a hard place: family members experiences of supporting a relative with bipolar disorder'. *Social Psychiatry and Psychiatric Epidemiology: The International Journal for Research in Social and Genetic Epidemiology and Mental Health Services*, 53 (10): 1123–1131.

Bernardo, M, de Dios, C, Pérez, V, Ignacio, E, Serrano, M, Vieta, E, … Roca, M. 2018. 'Quality indicators in the treatment of patients with depression, bipolar disorder or schizophrenia. Consensus study'. *Revista de Psiquiatria y Salud Mental*. doi: 10.1016/j.rpsm.2017.09.002.

Daggenvoorde, T, Geerling, B and Goossens, P J J. 2015. 'A Qualitative Study of Nursing Care for Hospitalized Patients with Acute Mania'. *Archives of Psychiatric Nursing*, 29 (3): 186–191. doi: 10.1016/j.apnu.2015.02.003

Esan, O, and Esan, A. 2016. 'Epidemiology and burden of bipolar disorder in Africa: a systematic review of data from Africa'. *The International Journal for Research in Social and Genetic Epidemiology and Mental Health Services*, 51 (1): 93–100. doi: 10.1007/s00127-015-1091-5.

Fernandes, F, Rocca, C, Lafer, B, and Nery, F. 2018. 'The association between social skills deficits and family history of mood disorder in bipolar I disorder'. *Rev. Bras. Psiquiatr. Revista Brasileira de Psiquiatria*, 40 (3): 244–248.

Gumus, F, Buzlu, S, and Cakir, S. 2015. 'Effectiveness of Individual Psychoeducation on Recurrence in Bipolar Disorder; A Controlled Study'. *Archives of Psychiatric Nursing*, 29 (3): 174–179. doi: 10.1016/j.apnu.2015.01.005.

Hofer, A, Mizuno, Y, Wartelsteiner, F, Wolfgang Fleischhacker, W, Frajo-Apor, B, Kemmler, G, … Uchida, H. 2017. 'Quality of life in schizophrenia and bipolar disorder: The impact of symptomatic remission and resilience'. *European Psychiatry*, 46: 42–47. doi: 10.1016/j.eurpsy.2017.08.005.

Stegink, E E, van der Voort, T Y G N, van der Hooft, T, Kupka, R W, Goossens, P J J, Beekman, A T F and van Meijel, B. 2015. 'The Working Alliance Between Patients with Bipolar Disorder and the Nurse: Helpful and Obstructive Elements During a Depressive Episode From the Patients' Perspective'. *Archives of Psychiatric Nursing*, 29 (5), 290–296. doi: 10.1016/j.apnu.2015.05.005.

The Effect of Group Psychoeducation Program on Medication Adherence in Patients with Bipolar Mood Disorders: A Randomized Controlled Trial. 2016. *Journal of Caring Sciences*, 5 (4): 287–297.

Salcedo, S, Gold, A K, Sheikh, S, Marcus, P H, Nierenberg, A A, Deckersbach, T and Sylvia, L G. 2016. 'Empirically supported psychosocial interventions for bipolar disorder: Current state of the research'. *Journal of Affective Disorders*. doi: 10.1016/j.jad.2016.05.018.

Van der Watt, A S J J, Roos, T, Beyer, C and Seedat, S. 2018. 'Participants perspectives of weekly telephonic mood monitoring in South Africa: a feasibility study'. *Pilot Feasibility Stud Pilot and Feasibility Studies*, 4 (1) 1–11. doi: 10.1186/s40814-018-0245-0.

ANNEXURE

Centre for Epidemiological Studies Depression Scale (CES-D)

Instructions: Below is a list of the ways you might have felt or behaved. Please tell me how often you have felt this way during the past week.

During the past week	Rarely or none of the time (less than 1 day)	Some or a little of the time (1–2 days)	Occasionally or a moderate amount of the time (3–4 days)	Most or all of the time (5–7 days)
1. I was bothered by things that usually don't bother me.				
2. I did not feel like eating; my appetite was poor.				
3. I felt that I could not shake off the blues even with help from my family or friends.				
*4. I felt that I was just as good as other people.				
5. I had trouble keeping my mind on what I was doing.				
6. I felt depressed.				
7. I felt that everything I did was an effort.				
*8. I felt hopeful about the future.				
9. I thought my life had been a failure.				
10. I felt fearful.				
11. My sleep was restless.				
*12. I was happy.				
13. I talked less than usual.				
14. I felt lonely.				
15. People were unfriendly.				
*16. I enjoyed life.				

→

During the past week	Rarely or none of the time (less than 1 day)	Some or a little of the time (1–2 days)	Occasionally or a moderate amount of the time (3–4 days)	Most or all of the time (5–7 days)
17. I had crying spells.				
18. I felt sad.				
19. I felt that people disliked me.				
20. I could not get 'going'.				
Total score				

Scoring: 0 = column 1; 1 = column 2; 2 = column 3; 3 = column 4; * = reverse score.
Possible range = 0–60, with higher scores showing more depressive symptoms
(http://www.chcr.brown.edu/pcoc/cesdscale.pdf)

WHO (FIVE) WELL-BEING INDEX (WHO-5)

There are five (5) statements. Please indicate for each of the five statements, which is the closest to how you have been feeling over the *last two weeks*.

		All of the time	Most of the time	More than half of the time	Less than half of the time	Some of the time	At no time
(a)	I have felt cheerful and in good spirits	5	4	3	2	1	0
(b)	I have felt calm and relaxed	5	4	3	2	1	0
(c)	I have felt active and vigorous	5	4	3	2	1	0
(d)	I woke up feeling fresh and rested	5	4	3	2	1	0
(e)	My daily life has been filled with things that interest me	5	4	3	2	1	0

Scoring of WHO-5

- If the person has scored a 1 or 0 on any of the items, counselling is recommended.
- A summation score ≤13 requires further investigation for depression.
- Complete at regular intervals monitoring for change.

BECK'S SUICIDE INTENT SCALE

Use this scale for MHCUs who have attempted suicide and survived to obtain an understanding of the desire to die. Carefully consider the context of the attempt, in particular in rural settings where access to emergency help might be lower than urban setting. Interview the MHCU about the *most recent* suicide attempt. Add scores of items 1–15. Mark 'not applicable' as indicated.

Objective Circumstances Related to Suicide Attempt

1. *Isolation*
    1. Somebody present (0)
    2. Somebody nearby, or in visual or vocal contact (1)
    3. No one nearby or in visual or vocal contact (2)
2. *Timing*
    1. Intervention is probable (0)
    2. Intervention is not likely (1)
    3. Intervention is highly unlikely (2)
3. *Precautions against discovery intervention*
    1. No precautions (0)
    2. Passive precautions (as avoiding other but doing nothing to prevent their intervention; alone in room with unlocked door) (1)
    3. Active precautions (as locked door) (2)
4. *Acting to get help during/after attempt*
    1. Notified potential helper regarding attempt (0)
    2. Contacted but did not specifically notify potential helper regarding attempt (1)
    3. Did not contact or notify potential helper (2)
5. *Final acts in anticipation of death* (will, gifts, insurance)
    1. None (0)
    2. Thought about or made some arrangements (1)
    3. Made definite plans or completed arrangements (2)
6. *Active preparation for attempt*
    1. None (0)
    2. Minimal to moderate (1)
    3. Extensive (2)
7. *Suicide note*
    1. Absence of note (0)
    2. Note written, but torn up; note thought about (1)
    3. Presence of note (2)
8. *Overt communication of intent before the attempt*
    1. None (0)
    2. Equivocal communication (1)
    3. Unequivocal communication (2)

Self-report

9. *Alleged purpose of attempt*
    1. To manipulate environment, get attention, get revenge (0)
    2. Components of above and below (1)
    3. To escape, surcease, solve problems (2)
10. *Expectations of fatality*
    1. Thought that death was unlikely (0)
    2. Thought that death was possible but not probable (1)
    3. Thought that death was probable or certain (2)
11. *Conception of method's lethality*
    1. Did less to self than they thought would be lethal (0)
    2. Was not sure if what they did would be lethal (1)
    3. Equalled or exceeded what s/he thought would be lethal (2)
12. *Seriousness of attempt*
    1. Did not seriously attempt to end life (0)
    2. Uncertain about seriousness to end life (1)
    3. Seriously attempted to end life (2)
13. *Attitude towards living/dying*
    1. Did not want to die (0)
    2. Components of above and below (1)
    3. Wanted to die (2)
14. *Conception of medical rescuability*
    1. Thought that death would be unlikely if he received medical attention (0)
    2. Was uncertain whether death could be averted by medical attention (1)
    3. Was certain of death even if he received medical attention (2)
15. *Degree of premeditation*
    1. None; impulsive (0)
    2. Suicide contemplated for three hours or less prior to attempt (1)
    3. Suicide contemplated for more than three hours prior to attempt (2)

Other Aspects (Not included in total score)

16. *Reaction to attempt*
    1. Sorry it was made; feels foolish; ashamed (0)
    2. Accepts both attempt and failure (1)
    3. Regrets failure of attempt (2)
17. *Visualisation of death*
    1. Life after death, reunion with descendants (0)
    2. Never-ending sleep, darkness, end of things (1)
    3. No conceptions of or thoughts about death (2)
18. *Number of previous attempts*
    1. None (0)
    2. One or two (1)
    3. Three or more (2)

19. *Relationship between alcohol intake and attempt*
    1. Some alcohol intake prior to but not related to attempt; reportedly not enough to impair judgement, reality testing (0)
    2. Enough alcohol intake to impair judgement; reality testing and diminish responsibility (1)
    3. Intentional intake of alcohol in order to facilitate implementation of attempt (2)
20. *Relationship between drug intake and attempt*
    1. Some drug intake prior to but not related to attempt; reportedly not enough to impair judgement, reality testing (0)
    2. Enough drug intake to impair judgement; reality testing and diminish responsibility (1)
    3. Intentional intake of drug in order to facilitate implementation of attempt (2)

Note: There is a greater risk of repeated attempts the higher the intent rating.

15–19 Low intent	20–28 Medium intent	29+ High intent
Date: ___/___/20___	Outcome	Assessor name & signature

(https://www.phenxtoolkit.org/toolkit_content/PDF/PX640301.pdf))

SUICIDE RISK ASSESSMENT
Modified SAD PERSONS Scale of Hockbeyer and Rothstein

Parameter	Finding	Points	MHCU score
Sex/Gender of MHCU	Male	1	
	Female	0	
Age	< 19	1	
	19–45	0	
	> 45	1	
Depression or hopelessness	Present	2	
	Absent	0	
Previous suicide attempts or psychiatric care	Present	1	
	Absent	0	
Excessive alcohol or drug use	Excessive	1	
	Not excessive or more	0	

→

Parameter	Finding	Points	MHCU score
Rational thinking loss	Loss due to organic brain syndrome or psychosis	2	
	Intact	0	
Separated, divorced or widowed	Separated, divorced or widowed	1	
	Married or always single	0	
Organised or serious attempt	Organised, well thought out or serious	2	
	Neither	0	
No social support	None (no close family, friends, job or active religious affiliation)	1	
	Present	0	
Stated future intent	Determined to repeat attempt or ambivalent about the prospect	2	
	No intent	0	

Interpretation

Minimum score: 0
Maximum score: 14

The higher the score, the greater the risk of suicide.

Score	Management
0–5	May be safe to discharge, depending on circumstances, rarely requires hospitalisation
6–8	Emergency psychiatric consultation
9–14	Probably requires hospitalisation

Note: This scale is a guide only to the contributing risk factors and must be used in conjunction with history and other assessment.

CHAPTER 14

Nursing the Mental Health Care User with Schizophrenia, Schizophrenia Spectrum and Other Psychotic Disorders

L R Uys and Y Havenga

> **Learning Outcomes**
>
> After studying this chapter, you should be able to:
> - describe the major characteristics of schizophrenia
> - formulate a diagnosis for schizophrenic spectrum and other psychotic disorders based on DSM-5 diagnostic criteria
> - identify the manner in which schizophrenia affects the lifestyle and functioning of the mental health care user (MHCU) and their families
> - apply the nursing process and implement major nursing interventions when caring for the individual and family living with schizophrenia to optimise independent living
> - implement methods to minimise relapse of mental health care users with schizophrenia.

INTRODUCTION

Schizophrenia is a term used to describe a group of complex, severe conditions that are the most chronic and disabling of the mental illnesses. The conditions are characterised by MHCUs experiencing a different reality from that of the people around them. This break with reality is why it is called a 'psychotic' condition. The reality of these MHCUs is distorted, changeable and often frightening. Their sensory perceptions may be distorted by hallucinations, of which auditory voices are the most common. Their thought processes are often confused so that they find it difficult to 'think straight' or to focus on or engage in problem solving. The thought content is often also abnormal, delusions being common. Emotional expression is usually very limited or inappropriate. The symptoms of these MHCUs are grouped into positive symptoms, negative symptoms and cognitive symptoms which are discussed further in this chapter.

Schizophrenia is a major illness for a number of reasons. It affects people in the prime of their lives, often leads to multiple admissions and in many cases it is not possible for an MHCU to fully return to their pre-illness level of functioning. The disorder therefore has a long-term course. The disorder is the most common of the serious mental disorders (Sadock et al, 2015) and therefore forms a large portion of the work of psychiatric nurses.

Some seven in one thousand people (0.7 per cent) of the world's population could be affected by schizophrenia in their lifetime (McGrath et al, 2008). A study conducted by McGrath et al (2008) confirms that men and women are affected equally. Statistics on the prevalence of schizophrenia in South Africa are not available. A study conducted in one general hospital in Gauteng within an acute psychiatric ward, with a total of 2 143 mental health admissions from 2004–2007, indicated that on average 20 per cent were diagnosed with schizophrenia (Janse van Rensburg & Olorunju, 2010).

Schizophrenia is often confused with a 'split personality' by the general public because the word 'schizophrenia' means split. The split of schizophrenia, however, refers to a split between the affect (feelings) and the thoughts and behaviour of the MHCU, and not a split into multiple personalities. Multiple personality is a rare dissociative disorder. Schizophrenia is also confused with substance-induced psychotic disorders that are brought on by the use of alcohol, cannabis, cocaine, sedatives, stimulants and hallucinogens (see the DSM-5 diagnostic criteria). It is, however, true that substance-abuse disorders occur very often among persons with schizophrenia (Drake & Mueser, 2002; Patel et al, 2014).

It is still not clear what causes schizophrenia, with biological and psychosocial theories being suggested. It seems that genetic factors produce vulnerability, with environmental factors precipitating the acute episodes of the disorder. The environmental factors are stressors such as tension in the family or demands at work/school or social problems. Children of parents with schizophrenia have a 10 per cent chance of developing schizophrenia, compared to the 0.7 per cent risk of persons in the general population. Even in the presence of a genetic risk it is not possible to predict who may develop schizophrenia (Roos & Burns, 2016). Similar to many other mental illnesses, schizophrenia is not 'just all in the head', as there are indications of physical causes involving abnormalities in the neurotransmitters, immunology and endocrinology of these MHCUs. Dopamine D2 receptor sites have been linked to a number of the symptoms experienced. Certain structural features of the brain and neural circuits also show abnormalities (Patel et al, 2014). An association between cannabis use and schizophrenia has been shown. People who are genetically at risk of developing a psychotic syndrome have higher psychotic responses to the main psycho-active ingredient in cannabis, delta-9-tetrahydrocannabinol (THC). Cannabis and psychosis are associated in different ways. Persons who are susceptible to psychosis may use cannabis as a form of self-medicating; however, cannabis induces susceptibility to psychosis. Due to the effect of cannabis on neurodevelopment the continued use thereof from adolescence into early adulthood could increase the risk of developing longstanding psychotic disorders (Roos & Burns, 2016).

The prognosis of MHCUs with schizophrenia has always been viewed with great pessimism, but the long-term course and prognosis varies from person to person. Sadock et al (2015) report that 10–20 per cent of MHCUs with schizophrenia have good outcomes five to ten years after the first hospitalisation. However, 50 per cent of first-time admissions will have repeated hospitalisations with poor outcomes. What is concerning, however, are the findings that people with schizophrenia have a two to three times greater risk of dying compared to the expected deaths in the general population. This difference has been increasing over years (McGrath et al, 2008). This increased risk of death has been attributed to suicide and comorbid physical conditions like diabetes and ischaemic heart disease (McGrath et al, 2008), which is addressed further in this chapter.

DIAGNOSIS OF SCHIZOPHRENIA SPECTRUM AND OTHER PSYCHOTIC DISORDERS

Schizophrenia spectrum disorders are complex and present in different ways affecting cognition, emotions, perceptions and behaviour. The schizophrenia spectrum disorders, as included in the DSM-5 (APA, 2013) are summarised in Table 14.1.

Table 14.1 DSM-5 Diagnostic criteria and specifiers: schizophrenia spectrum and other psychotic disorders

Schizophrenia

A. Two or more of the following symptoms present for a significant portion of the previous month:
  1. Delusions
  2. Hallucinations
  3. Disorganised speech
  4. Grossly disorganised behaviour
  5. Negative symptoms

B. Marked impairment of functioning compared to before the disorder.
C. Continuous signs of disturbance for at least six months, even if only negative symptoms.
D. Other mental disorders have been ruled out (eg schizoaffective disorder or bipolar disorder).
E. Not attributable to a substance or medical condition.
F. If there is a history of autism spectrum disorder or communication disorder, the additional diagnosis of schizophrenia is only made if delusions and hallucinations are prominent.
Specifiers: ■ Course: first episode, multiple episodes, continuous ■ With catatonia ■ Severity: according to the severity of symptoms
Schizoaffective disorder: The disorder has features of both schizophrenia and mood disorders (manic or depressive episode). There is a period of two or more weeks where delusions and hallucinations are present in the absence of a mood disorder but symptoms of a mood disorder are present most of the time over the duration of the disorder.
Schizophreniform disorder: The condition looks like schizophrenia, but the episode lasts less than six months without the criteria for other mental disorders being met.

Schizophrenia
Delusional disorder: The person has one major delusional theme (related to real-life situations) but usually without major impairment and disorganisation. Symptoms should be present for at least a month. Delusions could be erotomanic, grandiose, prosecutor, somatic, mixed or unspecified in nature.
Shared psychotic disorder: This disorder presents as delusions being transferred by a primary more dominant person to a more submissive person. They are often closely related and reside together.
Brief psychotic episode: A person has psychotic symptoms for a minimum of one day and a maximum of a month that are not attributed to a mood disorder, a medical condition or substances. The subtypes are (1) with a stressor; (2) without a stressor; and (3) onset during the postpartum period.
Psychotic disorder not otherwise specified: These disorders present with psychotic symptoms without adequate information and do not fit the diagnostic criteria of other psychotic disorders.
Psychotic disorder due to another medical condition: The person has prominent hallucinations and delusions, but these are associated with a medical condition such as an untreated endocrine, metabolic or autoimmune condition.
Substance of medication-induced psychotic disorder: The person presents with psychosis and loss of contact with reality as a result of a substance or medication. The onset could be during intoxication or withdrawal and should be specified.
Catatonia: This condition can be a specifier for other mental disorders or can be linked to medical conditions. It is characterised by psychomotor features such as stupor, catalepsy, waxy flexibility, mutism, posturing, mannerisms, stereotypy, echolalia and echopraxia.

Source: APA (2013); Sadock et al (2015)

Symptoms of schizophrenia

Schizophrenia is characterised by positive symptoms, negative symptoms, cognitive symptoms and mood symptoms.

Positive symptoms

Positive symptoms are unwanted symptoms 'added' to who the person is and are associated with acute episodes. Positive symptoms include hallucinations, delusions, disorganised speech, disorganised behaviour and catatonia (Roos & Burns, 2016; Sadock et al, 2015).

Hallucinations are sensory experiences that are subjective and related to one of the five senses without the external stimuli for such a sensation (Kneisl & Trigoboff, 2013). There are various types of hallucinations, namely auditory (the most common), visual, olfactory, somatic, tactile and gustatory (Sadock et al, 2015; Roos & Burns, 2016)

Different types of hallucinations are associated with different diseases and should therefore be carefully considered during the assessment of the MHCU in order to plan further investigations and treatment interventions. For example, olfactory, tactile, somatic and gustatory hallucinations have been associated with seizure disorders, infections, heavy metal poisoning, vitamin and mineral toxicities and tumours (Sadock et al, 2015; Kneisl & Trigoboff, 2013).

Delusions are fixed false beliefs about self and the environment despite evidence that they are not true (Sadock et al, 2015). There are various types of delusions such as persecutory, jealous, guilt, grandiose, religious, somatic, delusions of reference, delusions of being controlled, delusions of mind reading, thought broadcasting, thought insertion and thought withdrawal (Sadock et al, 2015).

Disorganised speech and form of thought present with symptoms such as tangentiality, incoherence, circumstantiality, thought blocking and neologisms (Roos & Burns, 2016).

Disorganised behaviour could be seen in the MHCU's clothing, appearance, social behaviour and sexual behaviour. It could present as being aggressive–agitated or being repetitive–stereotyped.

Negative symptoms

Negative symptoms 'subtract' from who a person is and reduce existing abilities. Negative symptoms include flatness of affect, social withdrawal, poverty of speech, decreased motivation and the inability to set and follow through on goals (Roos & Burns, 2016; Sadock et al, 2015). Negative symptoms are common and are associated with unfavourable health outcomes (Patel et al, 2014).

Cognitive symptoms

Cognitive symptoms influence a person's ability to understand and process information, understand and interpret social cues and then respond appropriately. Cognitive symptoms involve the thinking of a person and include problems with attention and concentration, memory and learning, and executive functioning (abstract thinking and problem solving). These cognitive symptoms are often noticed when they are severe, but they are present even in the absence of an acute episode (Baumann, 2015; Patel et al, 2014; Roos & Burns, 2016).

Mood symptoms

Mood symptoms include depression, anxiety, agitation and suicidality and could be present during acute illness or develop thereafter (Roos & Burns, 2016).

APPLICATION OF NURSING PROCESS TO ASSESSMENT AND DIAGNOSIS OF MHCUs WITH SCHIZOPHRENIA

This section deals with the mental health nurse's involvement in the assessment and diagnosis of the MHCU with schizophrenia.

Assessment

There is no single test for diagnosing schizophrenia. The mental health nurse should consider various means of assessment such as a physical assessment and other medical assessments, psychiatric history, mental status examination and psychiatric rating scales. It is important to obtain a comprehensive MHCU history as the signs and symptoms of schizophrenia are also present in a number of other psychiatric and neurological disorders, symptoms change over time and could present within the context of culture and religion (Sadock et al, 2015). It is therefore important that both the cultural understanding of mental illness and spiritual assessment are integrated in the assessment process as this understanding of the cause and treatment of schizophrenia is important in deciding on the overall goal and individual treatment plan (Chidarikire et al, 2018).

It has been noted in the literature that MHCUs are often inappropriately given a diagnosis of schizophrenia due to the misunderstanding of indigenous cultural and religious beliefs by western-trained health care professionals. The misunderstanding may also be the result of communication problems and the process of translation or inadequate attention being given to eliminating other physical conditions that cause psychosis:

- Many physical conditions produce symptoms that are similar to those of schizophrenia. Examples of these conditions are: epilepsy, neurosyphilis, herpes simplex encephalitis, degenerative disorders, human immunodeficiency virus (HIV)/acquired immunodeficiency syndrome (AIDS), head injuries, strokes, epilepsy, systemic lupus erythematosus, electrolyte imbalance, Vitamin B12 deficiency, hyper- or hypothyroidism, Cushing syndrome, Addison's disease; Huntington's disease, Parkinson's disease and toxins (Bauman, 2015; Sadock et al, 2015; Roos & Burns, 2016). A thorough examination is therefore essential. Special care and referral should be done if there are unusual or rare symptoms.
- The psychosis could be substance-induced, occurring during substance intoxication or withdrawal. The possibility has to be investigated and excluded (Sadock et al, 2015).
- Psychotic symptoms could also be related to commonly used medications such as antimalarial medications, corticosteroids, ephedrine/pseudoephedrine, antiretroviral therapy (efavirenz), antituberculosis drugs (isoniazid) or some of the anticonvulsants (Bauman, 2015).
- It can be quite difficult to distinguish between schizophrenia and mood disorders, especially when MHCUs present with psychosis in depression or a manic episode. To effectively treat both disorders, it is essential to get the diagnosis right. The DSM-5 stipulates that the delusions experienced during a depressive and a manic episode are mood congruent (Sadock et al, 2015).

Rating scales are available for assessing disorders. These include (Sadock et al, 2015):
- the Brief Psychiatric Rating Scale (BPS): psychotic disorders
- the Positive and Negative Syndrome Scale (PANSS): positive and negative symptoms of schizophrenia

- the Scale for the Assessment of Positive Symptoms (SAPS)
- the Scale for the Assessment of Negative Symptoms (SANS).

Because MHCUs with schizophrenia are at a greater risk of death in comparison with the general population (Mc Grath et al, 2008; Ward, 2017) mental health nurses must ensure that comprehensive physical assessments are done and that physical complaints receive the attention required. Nurses should provide and advocate for improved chronic and specialist medical services in mental health facilities. Suicide risk assessment should form part of the ongoing general assessment of persons with schizophrenia.

Diagnosis

Nursing diagnoses of MHCUs with schizophrenia often include changes in thought content, thought process, communication, emotion, perception and behaviour. Common symptoms in nursing diagnoses are listed in Table 14.2.

Table 14.2 Symptoms in nursing diagnoses of schizophrenia

- Potential for violence, self-directed or directed at others RELATED TO lack of trust, panic level anxiety, hallucinations of delusions EVIDENCED BY increased pacing, tense body posture, overt aggressive acts or threats.
- Social isolation RELATED TO lack of trust, hallucinations or delusions EVIDENCED BY social withdrawal, dull affect, preoccupation with own thoughts and meaningless actions.
- Ineffective coping RELATED TO personal vulnerability, inadequate support systems EVIDENCED BY inability to meet basic needs and alteration in social participation.
- Sensory-perceptual alternation: auditory/visual/tactile RELATED TO chemical imbalance EVIDENCED BY poor concentration, disordered thought, inappropriate responses.
- Risk of suicide RELATED TO command hallucinations EVIDENCED BY suicidal ideations.
- Alteration in thought processes RELATED TO chemical imbalance EVIDENCED BY distractibility, impaired and concrete thinking, abnormal content of speech.
- Impaired verbal communication RELATED TO impaired thinking and sensations EVIDENCED BY loose associations, neologisms, nonsensical talk, echolalia.
- Self-care deficit RELATED TO perceptual and cognitive impairment EVIDENCED BY not eating, deficits in personal hygiene, poor grooming.
- Sleep pattern disturbances RELATED TO anxiety levels, delusions and hallucinations EVIDENCED BY restlessness, insomnia.
- Activity intolerance RELATED TO cognitive and emotional disturbances AS EVIDENCED BY limited interaction, apathy, anxiety about making choices.

Source: Townsend (2011); Kneisl and Trigoboff (2013)

APPLYING THE NURSING PROCESS TO THE CARE, TREATMENT AND REHABILITATION OF MHCUs WITH SCHIZOPHRENIA

A holistic approach to treating schizophrenia has been proven most effective due to the multiple causes and complex nature of the disorder. Antipsychotic medications are the backbone for treating schizophrenia (Roos & Burns, 2016) but are not effective without treating the complex social, economic and health needs of MHCUs and their families affected by schizophrenia. Baumann (2015) proposes the following factors be addressed in the comprehensive and integrated management of an MHCU with schizophrenia:

- Predisposing factors – such as unsympathetic and conflictual family relationships – with family therapy, social skills training
- Precipitating factors – like substance abuse; non-adherence – with counselling like motivational interviewing for behaviour change (Ertem & Duman, 2017), mental health education and methods to improve medication adherence.
- Perpetuating factors – for example, non-adherence to treatment, social and economic challenges – with home visitations, mental health education, brief cognitive behavioural therapy (Liu et al, 2019) social-environmental interventions, and occupational therapy.
- Protective factors – such as a supportive family – with caregiver and family support, education, MHCU support groups, supportive housing and appropriate employment and employment support.

Community-based, psychosocial interventions should be provided in augmenting hospital-based care (Asher et al, 2017). The broader treatment goals for persons with schizophrenia are managing symptoms, enhancing skills needed to function optimally within a family and community, and relapse prevention (Crimson et al, 2014). A schizophrenia outreach team based in the United States proposes eight evidence-based interventions in addition to pharmacological management of schizophrenia, namely: assertive community treatment, supported employment, cognitive behavioural therapy, family-based services, reinforcement using tokens, skills training, psychosocial interventions for alcohol, management of other substances and weight (Dixon et al, 2010).

The following section addresses facilitation of a healthy lifestyle, symptom management, support of family and caregivers, participation in community life, medication management and relapse prevention and management.

Facilitation of a healthy lifestyle

The appropriate type of nursing care is determined by the degree of disorganisation and disintegration of functioning exhibited by the MHCU. In the acute phase of the disease, all life patterns are disorganised, but in the long term the greatest problems are self-care patterns, work patterns and the use of free time. A treatment programme geared towards encouraging MHCUs to take maximum responsibility for their own health is developed in consultation with the MHCUs, families and/or caregivers.

MHCUs living with schizophrenia should be empowered and supported to engage with treatment for both their mental and physical illnesses (Ward, 2017).

In addition to mental health care, treatment, and rehabilitation, a healthy physical lifestyle should be promoted as there is a greater risk of early death in people with schizophrenia. The reasons for the shorter life expectancy of MHCUs with schizophrenia is often due to comorbid physical conditions such as weight gain and the development of metabolic syndrome related to the use of second-generation antipsychotic medications (McGrath et al, 2008). Other contributing factors are high-risk behaviours and lifestyle factors such as unprotected sex, smoking and reduced adherence to medical treatments like oral hypoglycaemic therapy and antiretroviral treatment (Prince et al, 2007). Changeable cardiac risk factors such as tobacco use, minimal physical activity, poor diet and a tendency to weight gain when on antipsychotic treatment should be actively managed. Healthy lifestyle interventions like smoking termination, diet and exercise interventions, and programmes to prevent weight gain when antipsychotic medications are initiated, should be promoted (Ward, 2017).

Symptom management

This section addresses dealing with social withdrawal, managing delusions and hallucinations and dealing with thought disorders.

Dealing with social withdrawal

An MHCU with schizophrenia exhibits a wide variety of coping mechanisms. One of the first to be noticed is withdrawal. Withdrawal occurs mainly in the passive form: an MHCU with schizophrenia avoids contact with others and contributes little to conversations. Sometimes, however, withdrawal becomes more active, for example when word salad – a mixture of words and phrases that cannot be understood (Sadock et al, 2015) – or bizarre behaviour drives people away.

Withdrawal in an MHCU with schizophrenia is probably the result of interaction between three factors:
1. The MHCU might have had limited social skills to begin with, so that they developed few relationships even before they became ill.
2. During the process of treatment, the MHCU might have suffered long periods of hospitalisation in units where social stimulation was limited, which caused withdrawal as a secondary symptom.
3. Withdrawal is also a coping mechanism used by the MHCU to defend themselves against intrusive, critical and over stimulatory interaction.

In addressing withdrawal in an MHCU with schizophrenia, it is important that the problem be correctly identified. A withdrawn MHCU does not generally draw attention to themselves; they are quiet and unobtrusive. Unless nurses in large wards make an effort to identify and approach a withdrawn MHCU, they will simply fade into the background. By spending time with an MHCU, getting to know them and having them participate fully in their own care, treatment and rehabilitation will assist in reducing such social withdrawal.

In an outpatient setting it is more difficult to identify the withdrawn MHCU. One useful technique is to assess the non-verbal behaviour of the MHCU in the interview setting, since this will give an indication of the level of social skills. Although the MHCU might be able to give an accurate indication of whether this is a problem in their life, the family should also be interviewed to deepen and confirm the assessment data.

The treatment of withdrawal would probably need long-term strategies. First, the treatment staff should establish a trusting relationship with the MHCU in which they are willing to become involved in therapy. Unless this trusting and personal relationship is established, it is doubtful whether the MHCU will be susceptible to other treatment methods. Secondly, the nurse should be supportive by showing unconditional acceptance, making frequent brief contacts with the MHCU and supporting them during group-related activities (Townsend, 2011). The third treatment approach is to teach the MHCU the social skills needed to establish and maintain social relationships. The MHCU should be assisted to use these skills by placing them in groups and social settings where the skills can be practised and utilised. When an MHCU initiates interaction with others, the nurse should acknowledge and support this behaviour (Townsend, 2011). Hospital treatment should use the least restrictive measures, and create continued opportunity for individualised care, appropriate level of independence and decision making. See also Chapter 11 for more detail in supporting an MHCU in this regard.

Managing hallucinations and delusions

Hallucinations are one of the most significant problems in both the acute and chronic stages of schizophrenia. Hallucinations are a distressing experience in themselves, but they also depress social functioning. The exact cause is not known; however, multiple theories that attempt to explain the phenomenon of hallucinations have been suggested. These include theories relating to psychodynamics, neuropathology, neural circuits, neurotransmitters, psycho-neuroendocrinology, psycho-immunology, electrophysiological changes and cognitive perceptual theories (Sadock et al, 2015; Kumar et al, 2001).

Specific nursing care is required for MHCUs who *hallucinate*. This situation requires nurses to:
- Assess the risk: for example, whether there are command hallucinations to hurt themselves or another person (Sadock et al, 2015)
- Maintain an understanding and supportive approach
- Diminish the reality of the hallucinations by:
    - touching the MHCU if the MHCU allows this
    - making eye contact
    - maintaining an open posture

- speaking in a calm tone of voice
- not arguing about the hallucinations
- showing scepticism about the hallucinations, for example: 'I don't see them'
- using direct responses, for example: 'Look at me; don't pay attention to the voices'
- making one's voice dominate the hallucinations in cases of auditory hallucinations
- investigating the MHCU's present interests, activities and emotions.
- involving the MHCU individually or in groups in ward activities like walks or any other constructive activities
- encouraging the MHCU to drive away the voices
- identifying the subjects that distress the MHCU and avoid them

- Limit free and unstructured time by:
  - setting up a day programme
  - involving the MHCU in activities
  - providing regular physical activities that require the use of the large muscles and demand concentration

- Involve the MHCU in concrete reality through:
  - discussing everyday subjects
  - asking simple questions
  - giving concrete instructions
  - discouraging discussion of hallucinations

- Reduce anxiety by:
  - encouraging acknowledgement of feelings of being threatened
  - encouraging discussion relating to emotions and anxiety
  - explaining possible causes of hallucinations, for example loneliness or anxiety
  - enhancing the MHCU's ability to test reality by encouraging questions
  - teaching the MHCU alternative coping mechanisms for more appropriate management of identified reasons for hallucinations
  - setting reasonable expectations for the MHCU
  - gradually increasing the MHCU's responsibilities in relation to the level of anxiety

- Block auditory hallucinations by:
  - teaching MHCUs to whistle or sing when they hear voices
  - determining whether hallucinations harm others or the MHCU and, if so, provide protection
  - identifying and evaluating the content of hallucinations and hospitalising if necessary

- Promote the family's understanding and management of hallucinations by:
  - explaining the causes of and the behaviour that may be expected with hallucinations
  - encouraging family members to discuss their emotions about the MHCU's hallucinations.

Specific nursing care is required for MHCUs who have *delusions*. This situation requires nurses to:
- Reduce the reality of the delusions by:
  - avoiding all efforts to convince MHCUs that their views are wrong or unreal
  - saying only that you do not share their views or express your scepticism thereof, for example: 'I hear you believe … but I find it difficult to believe'
  - focusing on facts and reality
  - encouraging the discussion of present feelings
  - changing the subject and giving reasons for doing so
- Reduce anxiety by:
  - avoiding situations that cause conflict with delusions
  - avoiding situations of condemnation and ridicule of delusions
  - giving concrete, frank explanations about changes in treatment and in the environment to enable MHCUs to interpret change realistically
  - always acting consistently
  - not making promises or 'bargaining' to get the MHCU to participate (Sadock et al, 2015)
  - introducing only one anxiety-producing situation at a time to enable MHCUs to remain in control
  - involving MHCUs in single activities at first
  - encouraging the use of healthy coping mechanisms for anxiety
- Prevent the exacerbation of delusions by:
  - correcting wrong interpretations
  - supporting doubts that the MHCU may express
  - talking about actual events and subjects
  - investigating possible reasons for false, fixed beliefs
  - encouraging the MHCU to identify behaviour that relates to delusions
  - setting fixed times for the discussion of a delusion
  - establishing whether or not the MHCU is speaking the truth
  - encouraging the MHCU to identify and express emotions
- Promote a positive self-image by:
  - assuring MHCUs that they are accepted
  - always respecting MHCUs as people
  - involving MHCUs in activities
  - giving positive feedback about activities or interpersonal responses
  - encouraging the setting of realistic goals
- In the event of a delusion or suspicion that the food is contaminated, maintain the MHCU's physical health by:
  - using disposable crockery and cutlery
  - allowing food to be sent from home
  - allowing MHCUs themselves to open containers like milk cartons
  - serving food with skin or peels that MHCUs can remove themselves
  - serving the other MHCUs first and allowing them to start eating

- allowing MHCUs to serve themselves
- suggesting that MHCUs will enjoy the meal
- Promote understanding and management of delusions by family members by
  - providing information, for example: 'The negative response of other people is of little importance, however realistic it may be. A negative response does not help to improve the situation. Always express acceptance of the MHCU and show that you care'
  - giving emotional support
  - setting realistic expectations for the MHCU
  - setting definite limits relating to conduct by making quite clear what behaviour is acceptable and what is unacceptable
  - explaining possible causes of the problem
  - giving family members emotional support by affording them the opportunity to express their experiences in relation to the MHCU.

Dealing with thought disorders

The thoughts of the MHCU with schizophrenia are often disorganised and distorted. This makes communication very difficult and may lead to nurses avoiding conversation or giving superficial answers. It is important to remember that the MHCU may be desperately trying to make sense of their thoughts, or they may be clear as to what they are thinking, but find it impossible to communicate clearly. Since social isolation is such a problem for these MHCUs, the nurse should make every effort to facilitate communication. Here are a few indications of thought disorders and how they should be handled in conversation:

- *Vagueness.* It may be difficult to follow the MHCU's conversation because the MHCU uses global pronouns, such as 'they', 'we' or 'you', without making it clear to whom they are referring. The nurse needs to clarify by questioning exactly who the MHCU is referring to. This can also be useful with generalisations ('everything is going wrong') and global adjectives ('I am a mess').
- *Circumstantiality.* The MHCU may over articulate details and take a long time to get to the point. In order to make sure that you have understood them correctly, you can restate the actual message briefly and validate with the MHCU whether this is what they meant. This will also assist the MHCU to focus and clarify their thinking.
- *Loose associations, incoherence, tangentiality.* Sometimes the thoughts of the MHCU are so muddled that they become very difficult to understand, or you may understand them up to a point, but then lose the thread. In such cases it is important to stop the MHCU politely and admit that you are finding it difficult to understand. Restate what you have understood and ask for clarification about the rest. Sometimes it might be wise to redirect the MHCU to something concrete, rather than follow them into an increasingly frustrating conversation.

- *Delusions, autistic thinking, magical thinking.* In this case it is not a problem understanding the MHCU, but the content of the thoughts does not follow the usual logic or is based on false beliefs. It is important to seek to understand the real message of the communication, which may be camouflaged in a delusion or magical thinking. 'I am Caesar' may mean 'I am important', or 'I was betrayed by a friend' or a range of other things. Try to reflect the meaning of the communication, rather than argue about the form in which it is expressed.

Assisting with self-care needs

Diminished drive, flat affect and disturbances of thought are reasons why MHCUs have difficulty in accepting responsibility for self-care.

They should be supported in their efforts to improve their personal appearance and nurses should help them with their personal grooming and ensure that they dress neatly and appropriately. They should gradually be encouraged to accept responsibility for personal grooming. Nurses should spend time with these MHCUs but should allow them to do what they can for themselves. Behaviour therapy techniques such as a token economy system, activity scheduling and shaping may be used to good effect.

Mobility should be encouraged by means of, for example, a regular exercise programme or a daily four-kilometre walk. Such a programme should provide for an average of eight hours' sleep a night to ensure that MHCUs spend their days effectively.

Support of the family and other caregivers

In addition to this section, also see 'Guidelines for families living with a family member who is mentally ill' in Chapter 5.

Hospitalisation time has been dramatically reduced during the last two decades, so that even the MHCU with schizophrenia spends more time in the community than in the hospital. The most important milieu for the treatment and rehabilitation of these MHCUs is therefore the family. Family members provide care, support, check medication and assist with multiple aspects in the life of a person with schizophrenia (Caquoe-Urízar et al, 2017).

If a close family member is diagnosed with schizophrenia and this involves having to care for that person in the long term, it places an enormous objective and subjective burden on the family. An objective burden involves problems such as financial hardship and the disruption of family functioning, while a subjective burden refers to the psychological distress engendered by the disease, such as the stigma attached to mental illness. Families often experience mental health professionals as blaming, critical and unsympathetic instead of supportive.

Studies have shown that the inclusion of the family in the treatment process, mainly through psycho-education, has the potential to reduce hospital readmission time and relapse especially if done on a more long-term basis (Motlova et al, 2006).

One of the most important functions of the nurse is therefore to enlist the family in a positive clinical alliance. In addition, families should be supported and trained and should receive counselling to deal with the caregiver burden as negative experiences could impact on their quality of life, influencing their ability to care for their family member. In turn, the caregiver's quality of life may impact on an MHCU's quality of life and psychotic symptoms (Caqeo-Urízar et al, 2017).

Family mental health education

Information eases the anxiety of both MHCUs and their families or caregivers. It gives them hope and, in general, more control of the situation, improves family cohesion and positively affects family burden, and the depressive symptoms experienced by family members (Palli et al, 2015).

Information that must be given includes the symptoms; possible causes; the course of the disorder; the prognosis; treatment that may be given, for example group therapy, behavioural therapy, medication (the type of medication, the aim/dosage, side effects, contraindications and follow-up); guidelines for the effective management of MHCUs; community resources in the family's area, such as day centres, support groups, social clubs for handicapped people; and the latest research findings about the illness and treatment. The information must be conveyed in understandable terms in order for the family to apply it meaningfully.

Giving emotional support

Family members must be given a structured opportunity to air their feelings, such as in the form of a support group. Feelings they may experience include being trapped; powerlessness; a sense of failure; a feeling of physical, emotional and social abuse, and frustration due to failure to make contact with the MHCU. These feelings may be caused by the MHCU's unpredictability and socially unacceptable behaviour and the family's inability to make and maintain contact with the MHCU. All this contributes to tension and the family must learn to cope with it effectively.

The family must be continually supported. The longer MHCUs are psychotic or ill, the greater the impact of their hospitalisation on the people with whom they live, and the older the caregivers, the greater the impact on their quality of life. There are parent support groups in various centres in the country. Some of these are You Are Not Alone (YANA) in Pretoria and Cape Support for Mental Health in Rondebosch, Cape Town. Three support groups in Johannesburg have formed a liaison committee, Friends and Family of Schizophrenics (FAFOFS).

Both the MHCU's children and other children in the family should be informed in understandable terms about the reasons for the MHCU's behaviour. Discussion groups should be held with the children to explore their feelings and practise coping mechanisms. Teachers should be informed of the situation to enable them to support the children. Teasing at school about the 'mad' family needs to be identified as early as possible, as this may lead to the development of behavioural problems. Teachers can play a supportive role in such instances. Children should know to whom they can go if the MHCU's conduct frightens them and they should be encouraged to discuss their fear with someone.

Facilitating teaching and learning of problem-solving techniques

Problem-solving techniques can be used in all family situations, not only in those involving the MHCU. Every family member shares responsibility for the success of the planned solution. If the solution does not succeed, everyone – not only one person – bears the responsibility. The family can apply this method without the aid of a therapist.

Facilitating the teaching and learning of behaviour modification principles

The effective use of behaviour modification principles by the family and the MHCU to strengthen appropriate behaviour and unlearn inappropriate behaviour gives them concrete guidelines for action. The MHCU and family will be calmer as a result of the concrete structure.

These principles promote communication. In the first place, messages are more clearly formulated. Secondly, implementation encourages positive behaviour, for example giving MHCUs positive feedback if they are well groomed. Thirdly, the principles help to set limits. MHCUs should know what is expected of them and what they can expect of others. The family must be prepared for conflict and tension if MHCUs refuse to act within the set limits. Care should be taken to ensure that the family members, including the MHCUs, cope effectively with the tension. In the fourth place, the principles are applied to negotiate a contract which binds all the family members to reaching the objectives. Lastly, the time-out technique is very useful for managing tense situations. Both the MHCU and the family may apply the technique, but care must be taken that it is not used to avoid tense situations or as a form of punishment.

Participation in group and community life

Communities are uninformed about schizophrenia. This hampers the rehabilitation of MHCUs and consequently their integration into the community. Table 14.3 points to some information that should be shared with communities to dispel common myths about people with schizophrenia.

Organisations that the MHCUs and their families may join are church groups and social clubs with specific interests. An MHCU with schizophrenia should be allowed the normal use of community services, such as libraries, sports facilities, other recreational facilities and health services, by means of a systematic integration programme.

In some cases, however, additional specific support services are required for these MHCUs and their families. Community services that may be used by MHCUs and their families are out-MHCU services, home visits by the community health nurse, and family therapy units; crisis volunteers who maintain contact with an MHCU by means of out-MHCU services can give the MHCU limited social support and will at least be able to inform the nurse if they identify a problem.

Table 14.3 Dispelling common myths about schizophrenia

Myth about schizophrenia	Reality of schizophrenia
1. Once a schizophrenic, always a schizophrenic.	There are various outcomes across time, with some well-functioning individuals who do not need medical intervention.
2. People with schizophrenia tend to live in institutions.	Institutional care may be required, usually for brief periods. It is possible to live independently in supported housing or with family members.
3. Rehabilitation can be provided only after stabilisation.	Rehabilitation should begin on day one.
4. Psychotherapy is wasted on people with schizophrenia.	Cognitive behavioural therapy and supportive psychotherapy/counselling are crucial for rehabilitation.
5. The MHCUs must be on medication all their lives.	A proportion of MHCUs do function without the use of long-term medication.
6. People with schizophrenia cannot work.	People with schizophrenia can work to varying degrees (full time or part time). Employment is an important part of rehabilitation.
7. Families or bad parenting causes schizophrenia.	Multiple factors could cause schizophrenia, many physical in nature. Families are crucial in care and rehabilitation.
8. People with schizophrenia are violent.	Incidence of violence in a person with schizophrenia is not much higher than in the general population.

Source: Adapted from Abdel-Baki et al (2011); Harding and Zahniser (1994)

Assisting with environmental needs: accommodation

Accommodation is often a problem because MHCUs cannot always be placed with their families. If accommodation means only somewhere to stay, MHCUs are inclined to wander socially and geographically.

The accommodation should be of such a nature that the occupants have opportunities to be kept busy, to become interested in finding stimulating jobs (for profit, if possible), to keep in social contact with people in their community and to develop new interests. Placements that contribute to the adjustment of MHCUs include halfway houses, day and weekend hospitals to avoid full-time hospitalisation, and hostels with single accommodation. Placements not recommended are cheap hostels, boarding houses and non-accredited and unregulated non-governmental organisations (NGOs), since these might provide circumstances that are unfavourable for optimum functioning and could be potentially harming. MHCUs should be placed in living environments that are safe and appropriately accredited. Nurses must actively advocate for the rights of MHCUs in this regard.

Assisting with occupational needs: Work patterns

Investigations have shown that MHCU's with schizophrenia who work are hospitalised less frequently than those who do not work. A job can therefore contribute to more effective functioning.

Work functioning of MHCUs with schizophrenia is largely influenced by social/communication skills (Dickinson et al, 2007) and lack of job experience. The establishment of job rehabilitation programmes that include the teaching of communication skills and general work behaviour is often necessary.

In some cases, it may also be necessary to create special job opportunities in the form of sheltered workshops. The problem is that this type of work offers little stimulation because there is so little variety – it is usually simple and repetitive. Contracts are hard to come by and the remuneration is generally too poor to meet the needs of the MHCUs. Furthermore, these facilities are not within reach of everyone, as there are only a few in the country, each of which can accommodate only a limited number of people.

The function of the nurse regarding the work rehabilitation of an MHCU is to see to it that the following aspects are built into the rehabilitation programme: self-care, communication skills, opportunities for socialising, punctuality, self-discipline, accurate performance of activities, planning of own activities and the completion of tasks. This may be done individually or in groups. The nurse should also assist in finding gainful employment for MHCU by means of appropriate referrals to services. Further, the nurse should advocate for and refer MHCUs and their families to the appropriate social services.

Utilising free time

An MHCU must be assisted in planning their activities and time economically for a day or a week, as they often require assistance in this regard. The positive use of free time is an important activity in the gradual development of a healthy lifestyle. An MHCU should be assisted to develop a positive pattern for spending their free time because lack of drive and interest in their surroundings is often a challenge.

Watching television is a common free-time activity of MHCUs with schizophrenia. This is a passive activity that can contribute to withdrawal and potentially further deterioration. It should therefore be supplemented with more social and active behaviour. This means that activities on the in-MHCU day programme need to provide for the learning of alternative skills that MHCUs must be able to use after discharge. Examples of such activities include leather work and pewter work, cane work and organised sports activities. Regular exercise has shown to be beneficial for both the physical and mental health of persons living with schizophrenia (Gorczynski & Faulkner, 2010).

Bus tours, visits to places of interest, visits to the cinema and other places of entertainment can be arranged for in-MHCUs. Funds are a limiting factor in the rehabilitation of MHCUs and the use of disability grants should be optimally managed.

Medication management

Antipsychotics (also referred to as neuroleptics) are used to treat the symptoms of schizophrenia and to prevent relapse. There are more than 60 types of antipsychotic medications that are grouped into first-generation agents (FGAs) and second-generation agents (SGAs). The FGAs were introduced in the 1950s and the SGAs in the 1990s. Antipsychotics are also referred to as typical FGAs and atypical SGAs (McCuiston et al, 2018; Roos & Burns, 2016).

Most antipsychotics are able to block the D2 receptors in the brain (also referred to as dopaminergic antagonists) and reduce psychotic symptoms. However, when dopamine is blocked, the MHCU experiences adverse reactions referred to as extrapyramidal side effects (EPS) (Baumann, 2015; McCuistion et al, 2018).

The FGAs have a high affinity for the D2 receptors and are relatively effective in managing positive symptoms and less so in managing negative and cognitive symptoms. The SGAs have progressively replaced FGAs and may improve cognitive impairments and negative symptoms. There is a general belief that SGAs are more effective than FGAs. However, it has been established that with the exception of clozapine in treatment-resistant schizophrenia, the differences in the efficacy of antipsychotics (FGAs and SGAs) are small and should not be generalised. What does differ, however, is the side effect profile of these medications. SGAs are less likely to cause EPS than FGAs are, but SGAs are more likely to cause metabolic syndrome. There are however differences within each class of drugs. Almost all antipsychotics are associated with electrocardiogram (ECG) changes (qt prolongation) which may predispose to the development of arrhythmias.

The general principles of antipsychotic treatment involve the following:
- Individualised treatment regimens must be implemented with careful monitoring of the MHCU's response and side effects, as responses are unique (McCuiston et al, 2018; Roos & Burns, 2016).
- Antipsychotic treatment should be maintained at the lowest possible dose to achieve an antipsychotic effect (Bauman, 2015; Healy, 2016).
- Treatment should start with low doses and be gradually increased (Sadock et al, 2015).
- The use of two or more medications or two or more of the same class of medications for the same condition (polypharmacy) should be avoided unless evidence-based clinical justification exists. There are more disadvantages, however, than there are advantages (Kukreja et al, 2013).

- Implement the SAIL principle: Keep the medication regimen *Simple*; know the medication's *Adverse effects*; prescribed medication should have a clear *Indication*; keep the *List* of medication names and dosages in MHCU records (Kukreja et al, 2013).
- Implement the TIDE principle: Give *Time* to address medication issues, understand *Individual variability*; avoid potentially dangerous *Drug-drug interactions*; *Educate* the MHCU about treatment (Kukreja et al, 2013).
- Abrupt discontinuation should be avoided (Taylor et al, 2015). An MHCU should be weaned slowly from medication and if stopped, it should be done slowly over a few weeks to months.
- Smaller doses should be used in older people (≥ 45 years) due to their increased sensitivity to side effects (Department of Health, 2015). Doses should be 25–50 per cent lower than they are in young and middle-aged adults (McCuistion et al, 2018).
- Children must be referred to a psychiatrist for management.

Medication management can be divided into treatment of acute psychosis and treatment during stabilisation and maintenance phases (Sadock et al, 2015). The Standard Treatment Guidelines and Essential Medicines List for primary health care and hospital level (Department of Health, 2015; Department of Health, 2018) will provide more context-specific guidelines in this regard.

Management during the acute psychotic stage

If the MHCU presents at the clinic or hospital in a very disturbed and agitated state, it might be necessary to control or prevent violence by giving an immediate intramuscular injection of an antipsychotic medication (haloperidol or zuclopenthixol acetate) or a benzodiazepine such as lorazepam, clonazepam, and midazolam (Department of Health, 2015).

The medication, dosage and route of administration depends on the severity of the condition, the size and age of the MHCU and whether other comorbid conditions are present. At all times during the administration of rapid sedation, the nurse must have access to emergency equipment as rapid sedation could lead to cardiovascular collapse, respiratory depression, neuroleptic malignant syndrome and acute dystonic reactions. This risk is increased in older MHCUs, children, persons with intellectual disability, persons with comorbid medical conditions and persons who use substances (Department of Health, 2018). An MHCU must be monitored for the development of acute dystonia and vital signs must be monitored (see 'Extrapyramidal side effects' and 'Neuroleptic malignant syndrome'). An MHCU on benzodiazepines should be monitored carefully for respiratory depression and worsening or masking of their mental state (Department of Health, 2018).

It may take up to six weeks to see the full therapeutic effect of antipsychotics (Sadock et al, 2015).

Management during the maintenance stage

Stabilisation takes place for three to six months after an initial psychotic episode. To prevent relapse, long-term maintenance treatment is needed (Taylor et al, 2015). The general period of maintenance treatment after a first episode is one to two years; after a second episode it is up to five years, and after a third episode, continuation of treatment for the rest of a person's life may be required (Sadock et al, 2015). In cases where episodes are severe and with aggression or suicidal attempts, lifelong treatment may be preferable (Taylor et al, 2015).

Maintenance treatment should be specialist initiated with review of MHCUs every six months by a psychiatrist (Department of Health, 2015). Maintenance treatment includes oral medications or longer-acting depot medications. The choice of medication depends on the MHCU's clinical presentation, response to the treatment and side effect profile. Oral antipsychotic medications commonly used and included in the essential drug list are haloperidol, risperidone and chlorpromazine (Department of Health, 2015).

Long-term treatment should be prescribed by health care providers with advanced psychiatric training and should follow the initial treatment on oral antipsychotics. Four (4) weekly (once per month) intramuscular antipsychotics could be prescribed if adherence is a problem (Sadock et al, 2015; Department of Health, 2015). Examples of these intramuscular medications are:

- flupenthixol decanoate (Fluanxol®)
- zuclopenthixol decanoate (Clopixol®) (Department of Health, 2015).

If FGAs fail to reduce psychotic symptoms or if the MHCU experiences severe unmanageable side effects, SG's such as clozapine or risperidone could be prescribed. Clozapine must be psychiatrist initiated and MHCUs should be referred to tertiary hospitals. Special care in the monitoring of the MHCU's white cell count is required (Department of Health, 2015), as can be seen in Table 14.5. Table 14.4 is a rough guide to side effects from antipsychotics.

Table 14.4 Guide to antipsychotic side effects

Medicine	Trade names	Side effects						
		Sedation	EPS	Weight gain	Diabetes	Hypotension	Anticholinergic	Prolactin elevation[1]
Chlorpromazine	Largactil ®	***	**	**	**	***	**	***
Clozapine	Leponex ®	***	-	***	***	***	***	-
Flupentixol	Fluanxol ®	*	**	**	*	*	**	***
Haloperidol	Serenace ®	*	***	*	*/–	*	*	***
Olanzapine	Zyprexa ®	**	*/–	***	***	*	*	*

Medicine	Trade names	Side effects						
		Sedation	EPS	Weight gain	Diabetes	Hypotension	Anticholinergic	Prolactin elevation[1]
Quetiapine	Seroquel XL ®	**	–	**	**	**	*	–
Risperidone	Risperdal ®	*	*	**	*	**	*	***
Zuclopenthixol	Clopixol ®	**	**	**	*	*	**	***

*/– Very low; *Low incidence/severity; **Moderate incidence/severity; ***High incidence/severity
[1] Associated with sexual side effects

Source: Taylor et al (2015)

Nursing responsibilities in relation to antipsychotics

The general management of antipsychotics will be discussed. The nurse should, however, be knowledgeable about the indications, contraindications, side effects, and monitoring of specific antipsychotics prescribed and administered to MHCUs.

Monitoring and education of MHCUs

Regular appointments are essential to monitor the continued need for medication, efficacy, side effects, and the general mental and physical health of MHCUs.

The MHCU should be educated specifically about the management of the medication that they use. However, some general principles are:
- Alcohol and other substances should not be used with antipsychotics due to the combined sedative effect.
- Health care practitioners should be informed about the antipsychotics that are used.
- The medications may not be changed without approval of a doctor or nurse, with regard to stopping or increasing the dosage.
- Regular health screens should be performed due to the risk of developing metabolic syndrome (Healy, 2016).

Managing side effects

The side effects caused by antipsychotics affect the autonomous nervous system, central nervous system, extrapyramidal system, blood, skin, eyes, cardiac system, endocrine system and sexual and reproductive health system. Careful monitoring and education of the MHCU is required (Sadock et al, 2015; Kneisl & Trigoboff, 2013). Table 14.5 summarises the commonly encountered side effects of antipsychotic medications and their management.

Table 14.5 General side effects and management of antipsychotic agents

Side effect	Management
Dry mouth	Sugar free gum, sweets and regular sips of water
Constipation	Encourage dietary fibre, exercise and taking adequate fluids Constipation in MHCUs on clozapine should be managed with a laxative as mega-colon is one of the fatal side effects of clozapine
Orthostatic hypotension	Rise from supine position gradually Monitor blood pressure lying and standing Educate to minimise falls Evaluate cardiac functioning with certain antipsychotics
Metabolic syndrome (weight gain, increased lipids and blood glucose)	Give dietary advice, dietician referral Monitor and manage: weight, body mass index (BMI), waist circumference, serum lipids and blood glucose Encourage physical activity
Sedation	Advise against activities such as driving or working with heavy machinery Consult with medical doctor about less-sedating medication Do not use alcohol and potentially harmful substances that could increase the sedation effect
Cardiac effects: QT prolongation	Use with caution in clients with cardiac disease Cardiac monitoring: baseline and during treatment
Agranulocytosis (All antipsychotics but especially with clozapine)	Routine monitoring is done for MHCUs on clozapine. Baseline and follow-up blood monitoring of white cell count (WCC) and absolute neutrophil count is required. In the case of clozapine blood monitoring of WCC: ■ weekly for first 18 weeks ■ every second week for the next six months ■ monthly thereafter ■ continue until four weeks after discontinuation ■ immediate discontinuation if agranulocytosis is detected and referral to a haematologist
Skin eruptions, photo sensitivity and discolouration of the skin and eyes	Minimal exposure to the sun Protective clothing Sunscreen
Decreased libido, anorgasmia and erectile disturbances	Assessment to exclude physical pathology Prescriber may consider dose reduction, discontinuation or switching of the medication in consultation with the MHCU
Extrapyramidal side effects	Refer to discussion below
Neuroleptic malignant syndrome	Refer to discussion below

Source: Kneisl and Trigoboff (2013); McCuistion et al (2018); Taylor et al (2015); Department of Health (2015).

Neuroleptic malignant syndrome and EPS (akathisia, acute dystonia, tardive dyskinesia and parkinsonism) present as follows (McCuison et al, 2018; Department of Health, 2015; 2018):

1. **Extrapyramidal side effects (EPS)**
    - Parkinsonism-type syndrome:
        - bradikinesia (slow, robot-like movements)
        - rigidity
        - stooped posture
        - shuffling gait
        - tremors at rest
        - pill-rolling motion of the hand
        - management involves:
            - use of anti-parkinsonism agents, for example, biperiden or orphenadrine
    - Akathisia:
        - a subjective feeling of restlessness and the need to move to relieve the feeling
        - restless movements of hands or feet, or rocking movements
        - pacing
        - inability to stand still
        - management involves:
            - consider changing to an alternative antipsychotic
            - dose adjustment
            - administration of oral propranolol (monitoring of pulse and blood pressure required) (Department of Health, 2015) *Note:* Propranolol may exacerbate the symptoms of asthma.
            - assessment of MHCUs for potential suicide risk which increases with the development of akathisia (Healy, 2016)
    - Acute dystonic reaction:
        - laryngeal spasms (may be an acute medical emergency when laryngeal spasms are present)
        - facial grimacing
        - involuntary upward eye movement
        - spasms of the large muscles at the tongue, face neck, back and eyes may occur within the first 24–48 hours of commencement of treatment but could occur thereafter
        - management involves:
            - always monitoring the MHCU for acute dystonic reaction when antipsychotics are administered.
            - administration of anti-parkinsonism such as biperiden
            - reduction of dose or change of anti-psychotic may be required
    - Tardive dyskinesia: late onset
        - facial dyskinesia
        - protrusion and rolling of the tongue

- abnormal involuntary, irregular movements of body parts
- sucking and smacking movements of the lips
- reduce or discontinue medication
- protrusion and rolling of the tongue
- chewing motion
- facial dyskinesia
- involuntary movements of the body and extremities
- management involves:
    - treatment should be planned in consultation with the MHCU and may vary based on history and clinical presentation
    - stop all anti-cholenergics
    - the specific antipsychotic dose should be reduced
    - change to an antipsychotic with less propensity for causing tardive dyskinesia
    - only 50 per cent of the cases can be reversed (Department of Health, 2018)
    - early identification and management of TD may prevent worsening

2. **Neuroleptic malignant syndrome**
   - life-threatening complication
   - hyperpyrexia, perspiration, increased pulse rate and varying blood pressure, muscle rigidity, dystonia, mutism, confusion and fluctuating level of consciousness
   - management involves:
     - immediate discontinuation of medication
     - treating symptomatically: reducing temperature and rehydration (McCuistion et al, 2018; Department of Health, 2018)
     - monitor vitals
     - benzodiazapine
     - rehydration
     - bromocriptine and dantrolene
     - ventilation and ICU admission may be required
     - refer to psychiatrist for cautious reinitiation of antipsychotic where indicated (Taylor et al, 2015).

Relapse prevention and management

Relapse prevention requires a multimodal approach, with participation of the MHCU central to the improvement of adherence. Just as in the case of diabetes, the management of this long-term illness is mainly in the hands of the MHCU. A significant amount of mental health education therefore has to be done when the diagnosis has been made and the MHCU has recovered to the level where they can understand the teaching and show improved insight (Baumann, 2015).

Adherence to antipsychotic medication is central to relapse prevention. It is estimated that that 40–50 per cent of MHCUs become non-compliant within a year or two (Sadock et al, 2015). Adherence can be enhanced by addressing the challenges facing the MHCU regarding environment, the health care system and health care providers. The relationship and trust between the health care providers and MHCUs are significant determinants of medication adherence (Healy, 2016). Some of these challenges MHCUs experience are long waiting times at health services, medication being out of stock and lack of continuation of care (frequent staff changes), polypharmacy (multiple drugs to treat the same condition leading to side effects and adverse conditions), difficult dose regimes, cost of medication, lack of information or misinformation, poor MHCU–health care provider relationships, side effects, substance abuse and stigma (Baumann, 2015). Also refer to Chapter 11 about symptom management and relapse prevention.

Psychosocial interventions such a mental health education, family support and education, cognitive behavioural therapy, motivational interviews and social skills training are important interventions to enhance medication adherence and improve the general functioning of persons with schizophrenia (Schooler, 2006; Ertem & Duman, 2107; Liu et al, 2019). All MHCUs should be taught to monitor their own symptoms to detect a threatening relapse, and to know what they should do in such a case. In addition, the family must be taught to identify these symptoms and should have a plan in place to act swiftly and seek health care, treatment and rehabilitation. The most common non-psychotic signs of impending relapse are nervousness/tenseness, trouble sleeping (either too much or too little), greater than usual fatigue and a lack of energy, depression, difficulty in thinking or concentrating, less activity than usual, an inability to get going and irritability. These early signs may differ from one MHCU to the next, and every MHCU should be encouraged to identify their own early signs.

CONCLUSION

Nurses deliver scientific nursing care as members of the multidisciplinary team on an in-MHCU and out-MHCU basis to MHCUs and their families.

Sound knowledge of the causes of the disorders that hamper the functioning of MHCUs, their consequences for MHCUs, the influence of the behaviour of MHCUs on other people, nursing interventions, treatment possibilities by other team members and available facilities form the basis on which treatment in general should be planned and implemented.

The aim of treatment is to manage symptoms optimally and to enhance optimal functioning as independently as possible within the MHCUs' personal capabilities as members of families and of the community. Even though the use of antipsychotic medications is often the backbone of treatment, nurses should be equally knowledgeable about managing disruptive behaviour and facilitating optimal functioning through non-pharmacological means (Healy, 2016).

WEB RESOURCES

http://www.psychguides.com
This website provides expert treatment guidelines for psychiatric conditions. Most of these have

been published in reputable professional journals as well. The treatment guideline for schizophrenia is available, and there is also a guide for MHCUs and families.

http://www.nsfoundation.org

This is the website of the Schizophrenia Foundation of the USA. It has very useful resources, especially the list of available videos. The site also leads you to the website of the Schizophrenia Anonymous at sanonymous.org – this organisation invites consumers to join self-help groups based on the six-step programme.

REFERENCES

Abdel-Baki, A, Lesage, A, Nicole, L, Cossette, M, Salvat, E and Lalonde, P. 2011. Schizophrenia, An Illness with Bad Outcome: Myth or Reality? *Canadian Journal of Psychiatry,* 56 (2): 92–101.

American Psychiatric Association (APA). 2013. *Diagnostic and Statistical Manual of Mental Disorders DSM-5.* 5th edition. Washington, DC: American Psychiatric Association.

Asher, L, Patel, V and de Silva, M J. 2017. Community-based psychosocial interventions for people with schizophrenia in low and middle-income countries: systematic review and meta-analysis. *BMC Psychiatry,* 12: 1–15.

Baumann, S E. 2015. 'Odd ideas, voices, disorganised behaviours and the loss of insight: the schizophrenia spectrum disorders'. In: Baumann, S E (ed). *Primary Care Psychiatry A practical guide for southern Africa.,* 2nd edition. Cape Town: Juta & Company.

Caquoe-Urízar, A, Alessandrinoi, M, Urzua, A, Zendjidjian, X Boyer, L and Williams, D R. 2017. 'Caregiver's quality of life and its positive impact on symptomatology and quality of life of MHCUs with schizophrenia'. *Health and Quality of Life Outcomes,* 15, 1: 76. doi: 10.1186/s12955-017-0652-6.

Chidarikire, S, Cross, M, Skinner, I and Cleary, M. 2018. 'Treatments for people living with schizophrenia in sub-Saharan Africa: an adapted realist review'. *International Nursing Review,* 65: 78–92.

Crismon, L, Argo, T R and Buckley, P F. 'Schizophrenia'. 2014. In: DiPiro, J T, Talbert, R L, Yee, G C et al (ed). *Pharmacotherapy: A Pathophysiologic Approach.* 9th edition. New York, New York: McGraw-Hill: 1019–1046.

Department of Health. 2015. *Standard Treatment Guidelines and Essential Medicines List for South Africa, hospital level adults.* Republic of South Africa: National Department of Health.

Department of Health. 2018. *Essential Drugs Programme. Primary Healthcare Standard Treatment Guideline and Essential Medicines List.* 6th edition. Republic of South Africa: National Department of Health.

Dickinson, D, Bellack, A S and Gold, J. 2007. 'Social/Communication Skills, Cognition, and Vocational Functioning in Schizophrenia'. *Schizophrenia Bulletin,* 33 (5): 1213–1220.

Dixon, L B, Dickerson, F, Bellack, A S, Bennett, M, Dickinson, D, Goldberg, R W, Lehman, A Tenhula, W N, Calmes, C, Pasillas R M, et al. 2010. 'The 2009 schizophrenia PORT psychosocial treatment recommendations and summary statements'. *Schizophrenia Bulletin,* 36 (1): 48–70.

Drake, R E, and Mueser, K T. 2002. 'Co-Occurring Alcohol Use Disorder and Schizophrenia'. *Alcohol research and Health,* 26 (2): 99–104.

Ertem, M Y and Duman, Z Ç. 2017. 'The effect of motivational interviews on treatment adherence and insight levels of patients with schizophrenia: A randomized controlled study'. *Perspectives in Psychiatric Care,* 55: 75–86. doi: 10.1111/ppc.12301.

Gorczynski, P and Faulkner, G. 2010. 'Exercise therapy for schizophrenia'. *The Cochrane Database Systematic Reviews* (5): CD004412. doi: 10.1002/14651858.CD004412.pub2.

Harding, C M and Zahniser, J H. 1994. 'Empirical correction of seven myths about schizophrenia with implications for treatment'. *Acta Psychatirca Scandinavica,* 90 (Supplementary): 140–146

Healy, D. 2016. *Psychiatric drugs explained.* 6th edition. Oxford: Elsevier.

Jacobs, N and Coetzee, D. 2018. 'Mental illness in the Western Cape Province, South Africa: A review of the burden of disease and healthcare interventions'. *South African Medical Journal,* 108 (3): 176–180.

Janse van Rensburg, A B R and Olorunju, S. 2010. 'Diagnosis and treatment of schizophrenia in a general hospital-based acute psychiatric ward'. *African Journal of Psychiatry,* 13: 204–210.

Kneisl, C R and Trigoboff, E. 2013. *Contemporary Psychiatric-Mental Health Nursing.* 3rd edition. New York: Pearson.

Kukreja, S, Kalra, G, Shah, N and Shrivastava, A. 2013. 'Polypharmacy in psychiatry: a review'. *Mens sana monographs,* 11 (1): 82–99. doi: 10.4103/0973-1229.104497.

Kumar, S, Soren, S and Chaudhury, S. 2009. 'Hallucinations: Etiology and clinical implications'. *Industrial Psychiatry Journal,* 18 (2): 119–126.

Liu, Y, Yang, X, Gillespie, A, Guo, Z, Ma, Y, Chen, R and Li, Z. 2019. 'Targeting relapse prevention and positive symptoms in first-episode schizophrenia using brief cognitive behavioural therapy: A pilot randomized controlled study'. *Psychiatry research,* 272: 275–283.

McCuistion, L E, Vuljoin-Dimaggio, K, Winton, M B and Yeager, J J. 2018 *Pharmacology. A MHCU-Centered Nursing Process Approach.* 9th edition. St. Louis Missouri: Elsevier.

McGrath, J., Saha, S, Chant, D and Welham, J. 2008. 'Schizophrenia: A Concise Overview of Incidence, Prevalence, and Mortality'. *Epidemiological reviews,* 30: 67–76.

Motlova, L, Dragomirecka, E, Spaniel, F, Goppoldova, E, Zalesky, R, Selepova, P, Figlova, Z and Höschl, C. 2006. 'Relapse prevention in schizophrenia: does group family psychoeducation matter? One-year prospective follow-up field study'. *International Journal of Psychiatry in Clinical Practice,* 10 (1): 38–44.

Palli, A, Kontoangelos, K, Richardson, C and Economou, M P. 2015. 'Effects of Group Psychoeducational Intervention for Family Members of People with Schizophrenia Spectrum Disorders: Results on Family Cohesion, Caregiver Burden, and Caregiver Depressive Symptoms'. *International Journal of Mental Health,* 44 (4): 277–289.

Patel, K R, Cherian, J, Gohil, K and Atkinson, D. 2014. 'Schizophrenia: Overview and Treatment Options'. *Pharmacy and Therapeutics,* 39 (9): 638–645.

Prince, M, Patel, V, Saxena, S, Maj, M, Maselko, J, Phillips, M R and Rahman, A. 2007. 'No health without mental health'. *Lancet,* 370: 859–77.

Roos, L and Burns, J. 2016. 'Schizophrenia spectrum and other psychotic disorders'. In: Burns, J and Roos, L (eds). *Textbook of Psychiatry.* 2nd edition. Cape Town: Oxford.

Sadock, B J, Sadock, V A and Ruiz, P R. 2015. *Kaplan & Sadock's synopsis of psychiatry.* 11th edition. Philadelphia: Wolters Kluwer.

Schooler, N. 2006. 'Relapse Prevention and Recovery in the Treatment of Schizophrenia'. *Journal of Clinical Psychiatry,* 76 (Supplementary 5): 19–23.

Taylor, D, Paton, C and Kapur, S. 2015. *The Maudsley Prescribing Guidelines in Psychiatry,* 12th edition. Chichester: Wiley-Blackwell.

Townsend, M C. 2011. *Nursing Diagnoses in Psychiatric Nursing.* 8th edition. Philadelphia: F A Davis.

Ward, P B. 2017. 'Addressing the scandal of early death among people with schizophrenia'. *Canadian Medical Association Journal,* 189 (37): E1175–E1176.

CHAPTER 15

Nursing the Patient with a Substance-related Disorder

L R Uys and P D Martin

Learning Outcomes

After studying this chapter, you should be able to:
- explain the core concepts to describe patterns of substance use
- assess responses associated with the more common dependence-producing substances
- participate in the implementation of primary and secondary prevention of alcoholism
- conduct an assessment using appropriate assessment tools of a patient with alcohol withdrawal
- develop a nursing care plan of a patient with alcohol withdrawal
- function as a member of the health team in the treatment and care of substance-dependent people
- give appropriate comprehensive education, instruction and counselling to substance-dependent people and their families.

INTRODUCTION

Tobacco, alcohol and illicit drug use pose a significant threat to the health, social and economic fabric of families and all communities. People use a host of substances for various purposes: to celebrate achievements, to entertain guests, to restore health, to reduce pain, to reduce anxiety, to increase energy, to create a feeling of euphoria, to induce sleep, and to enhance alertness. Alcohol consumption is a feature of every community of today, including communities where alcohol use was formerly tabooed (WHO, 2010). Global trends in the estimated prevalence for illicit drug consumption in 2006–2014 is in the range of 4.9–5.2 per cent of the total population (UNODC, 2016).

A recent study (Dada et al, 2015) on treatment admissions of young persons under the age of 20 years (n=10197), who were seen at 64 centres in the second half of 2014 in the nine provinces of South Africa, found that alcohol remained the dominant substance of abuse (73 per cent) in the Eastern Cape, Northern Cape and North West provinces. Cannabis was reported as the primary substance of abuse in all provinces except Northern Cape and North West, with KwaZulu-Natal reporting the highest number of admissions (74 per cent). Methamphetamine (also known as 'tic' or 'tik') remained the most common primary drug of abuse (35 per cent) in the Western Cape. Methcathinone ('Cat') was also noted in most sites especially in Gauteng (16 per cent), and in the

Northern Cape and North West (14 per cent in both provinces). Polysubstance abuse was found to be high in Mpumalanga and Limpopo (16 per cent in both provinces) and in the Western Cape (44 per cent). The consequences of these patterns of substance abuse include an increased risk of mental disorders.

According to the DSM-5 (APA, 2013) classification, substance-related disorders comprise two groups: the substance-use disorders (dependence and abuse) and substance-induced disorders (intoxication, withdrawal, delirium, dementia, amnesia, psychosis, mood disorder, anxiety disorder, sexual dysfunction and sleep disorders). This chapter deals with four of the conditions which are specific to use or abuse of substances: dependence, abuse, intoxication and withdrawal (other conditions are dealt with elsewhere in this book). Comorbidity between substance use and mental disorders has necessitated the need to provide care, treatment and rehabilitation within a coordinated mental health service in South Africa. Initial contact for substance users presenting with mental disorders is at primary health care services which sets in motion the contact with mental health care services (Department of Health, 2013).

COMMONLY USED SUBSTANCES

A wide variety of substances are available legally and illegally. The substances can be administered by any means or by any route into the body, bringing about impairment of mood, altered level of perception and impairment of brain function. Those in common use and associated street names are summarised in Table 15.1.

Table 15.1 Classification of the more common substances in use

Substance	Legal status	Street name
Alcohol	Freely available Available to individuals over 18 years	Juice, dop, booze, spirits
Caffeine	Freely available	Coffee, brew, joe
Cannabis	Prohibited (legal when used in private homes)	Joint, grass, zol, 'boom', weed, pipe, dope, ganja, intsangu, pot, hemp
Hallucinogenic		
Lysergic acid diethylamide (LSD)	Prohibited	Acid, black panther, candy, yellow sunshine, microdots, Kool Aid, white lightning, purple haze
PCP (phencyclidine)	Scheduled for veterinary use only	Angel dust, PCP, peace pill, magic dust, horse weed, cyclones, purple rain
Ketamine	Prescription	Blind squid, Cat, Jet, Super Acid, Vitamin K

Substance	Legal status	Street name
Mescaline		Big Chief, Blue Caps, Buttons, Moon, mexc
Inhalants		
Benzine Petrol Glue Turpentine	Found in freely available commercial products	
Nitrous Oxide	Used in anaesthetics	Laughing gas
Opioids		
(a) *Non-synthetic*		
Opium	Prohibited	O's, oupa
Heroin	Prohibited substance	Herries, horse, unga
Morphine	Prescription, schedule 7	Morph, Miss Emma
Codeine	Over the counter	Captain Cody, Little C
(b) *Synthetic*		
Pethidine	Prescription, schedule 7	Petts
Wellconal	Prescription, schedule 7	Pinks, welkies
Physeptone (Methadone)	Prescription, schedule 7	Red Rock, fizzies
Nyaope (heroin mixed with cannabis, can be laced with bicarbonate of soda, rat poison, ARVs)	Prohibited	Whoonga, wunga
Sedatives, hypnotics and anxiolytics		
Sedatives		
Diazepam	Prescription, schedule 5	Tronks, vallies, moggies
Oxazepam	Prescription, schedule 5	
Lorazepam	Prescription, schedule 5	Candy, downers, tranks
Hypnotics		
(a) *Barbiturates*		
Seconal	Prescription, schedule 5	Red devils, sleepers, candy
Vesperax	Prescription, schedule 5	Vees
(b) *Non-barbiturates*		
Methaqualone	Prohibited in South Africa	Mandies, buttons, originals, whites
Anxiolytics		
Alprazolam (Xanax)	Prescription, schedule 5	Zannies, Zan, Xanies
Chlordiazepoxide (Librium)	Prescription, schedule 5	
Clonazepam (Klonopin)	Prescription, schedule 5	
Flurazepam (Dalmane)	Prescription, schedule 5	
Stimulants		
Amphetamines		
Dexedrine	Prohibited	Dexies

→

Substance	Legal status	Street name
Benzedrine	Prohibited	Bennies
Drynamil	Prohibited	Purple hearts
Methamphetamine	Prohibited	Meth, tik, tuk, speed, crystal meth
Methylene dioxymeth-amphetamine (MDMA)	Prohibited	Ecstasy, vitamin X, XTC, E
Methcathinone	Prohibited	Kat, Cat, Khat, Cadillac Express, Wonder Star
Ephedrine	Prescription, schedule 6	–
Methylphenidate	Prescription, schedule 6	Diet coke, kiddie cocaine, skittles, smarties, vitamin R
Cocaine	Coca leaves and cocaine powder	Coke, snow, crack, rocks
Nicotine	Prescription, schedule 4. Available to persons over the age of 18 years.	Ciggies, snuff, loose
Anabolic-androgenic steroids		
Oxymetholone (Anadrol) Oxandrolone (Oxandrin) Methandienone (Dianabol) Stanozolol (Winstrol) Durabolin	Prescription needed Prohibited under the World Anti-doping Code	Arnolds, gym candy, Var Dbol Winny NPP
Painkillers (non-narcotics)		
AP Codis Paracetamol Beserol Syndol Grandpa powders	Prescription, over the counter	Downers

New substances continue to saturate the drug market. Between 2012–2014, new substances known as New Psychoactive Substances (NPS), belonging to a group of synthetic cannabinoids, were reported for the first time. However, in 2015, the trend changed with almost as many synthetic cathinones being reported. A wide range of substances not belonging to any of the major groups were also reported. These include synthetic opioids (for example, fentanyl derivatives) which are used as analgesics and anaesthetics, namely, phenethylamines, piperazines, ketamines, tryptamines, salvia divinorum and krokodil (UNODC, 2016). Dada et al (2015) found that nyaope (low-grade heroin and other ingredients smoked with dagga) continued to pose a problem with 8 per cent and 7 per cent of patients in Gauteng and in the northern region (Mpumalanga and Limpopo) respectively presenting at treatment centres. In South Africa, the Drugs and Drug Trafficking Act of 1992 was amended in April 2014 to classify nyaope or 'woonga' as illegal (United Nations, 2015).

CORE CONCEPTS ASSOCIATED WITH PATTERNS OF SUBSTANCE USE

Concepts associated with substance abuse, and explanations of these, are listed below:
- *Craving* is a term that is often used to describe some of the behaviours of individuals who abuse or are dependent on drugs. Craving relates to the feeling of wanting or needing the drug.
- *Drug use* refers to the taking of a drug and may even refer to legal use of prescribed drugs.
- *Misuse* implies that a substance is used in excess or in a way that differs from its prescribed or intended use.
- *Hazardous use* is the pattern of substance misuse that increases someone's risk of harmful consequences to themselves.
- *Harmful use* is the pattern of substance misuse that damages the person's physical or mental health.
- *Tolerance* is the need to consume more of the substance to achieve the effects of the previous consumption. It could also refer to the reduced effect when the person consumes the same amount of the substance.
- *Substance-use disorder* is defined in the DSM-5 (APA, 2013: 483) as a disorder with a cluster of 'cognitive, behavioural and physiological symptoms indicating that the individual continues using the substance despite significant substance-related problems'. In severe cases, this leads to permanent changes in the brain circuits leading to repeated relapses and intense cravings.

Other terms associated with substance use are:
- *Codependence.* Terms such as co-addiction, co-alcoholism, codependency or codependent are used to describe the dysfunctional behavioural patterns of family members who have been significantly affected by a family member's substance use or dependence. No criteria exist in the codependency.
- *Enabling.* A characteristic of codependence or co-addiction. Family members assist the substance-dependent person in maintaining addictive behaviours. For example, if a husband is unable to go to work due to a hangover, the wife calls his office to report that he is ill. The wife is an enabler as she has facilitated the abuser's addictive behaviour. She has enabled him to be irresponsible.
- *Denial.* This implies that family members and the person abusing substances themselves behave as if the substance use that is causing obvious problems is not really a problem. They are engaging in denial.

Substance dependence

This occurs when a substance becomes an integral part of an individual's life and it is becoming increasingly difficult for the individual to do without it. Dependence on a substance may be physical or psychological or both. Physical dependence is evidenced by the phenomenon of tolerance and individual's need to continue the use of the substance in order to prevent unpleasant physical effects characteristic of the withdrawal syndrome associated with that particular substance. Psychological dependence, on the other hand, occurs when the use of a substance is perceived by the user to be necessary to maintain an optimal state of personal well-being, interpersonal relations, or skill performance.

Substance-use disorders

For each of the substances, one of the following diagnoses can be made, with the diagnosis referring to the specific substance:
- substance-use disorder (for example, cannabis-use disorder)
- substance intoxication when the person has ingested the substance recently and shows clinically significant problematic behaviour (for example, inhalant intoxication)
- substance withdrawal when the person ceases or drastically reduces ingestions after heavy and prolonged use, characterised by clinically significant symptoms (for example, opioid withdrawal).

The diagnosis of a substance-use disorder is based on a set of pathological behaviours related to the use of that substance. These behaviours fall into the following four main categories:
1. impaired control
2. social impairment
3. risky use
4. pharmacological indicators which include tolerance and withdrawal.

The following factors may be present in a substance-dependent person:
- Emotional stress associated with a feeling of wretchedness and helplessness experienced as anxiety, tension, depression, loneliness, boredom
- Inability to express intense feelings of rage in a socially acceptable manner – substances offer a measure of control and lessen the patient's anger
- Inability to resolve conflict – substances provide short-term relief from the associated discomfort
- Feelings of happiness and satisfaction, resulting in improved social interaction
- Distortion of perception and sensation (especially with regard to space and time). The degree of distortion depends on the strength of the substance dosage.

Larger doses of substances may give rise to the following aberrations:
- Impaired judgement or memory
- Distortion of emotional responses
- Irritation and confusion

The following phenomena are associated with chronic use:
- Lowering of sensory thresholds, especially to optic and acoustic stimuli, resulting in more intense appreciation of art and music

- Hallucinations, illusions and delusions, usually of the paranoid type, presenting with aggression, antisocial behaviour, anxiety and sleep pattern disturbances
- Fragmentation of thoughts
- Euphoria
- Enhanced self-confidence
- Anxiety bordering on panic.

There is a relationship between substance dependence and a number of sociodemographic and psychological variables. Sociodemographic variables include, among others, unsatisfactory academic careers, smoking habits, economic status, gender (male) and genetic makeup. Psychological variables allude to unhealthy family relationships, and substance abuse among close relatives and friends and agents. Substances are taken to escape from personal and psychological problems, and conformation to social values and norms is resisted. This leads to reduced involvement in conventional activities.

It would seem that substance-dependent individuals try, because of their distrust in expectations of the future, to prevent potentially stressful situations in community, love and job circumstances.

These people avoid problem situations and acceptance of responsibility, with the result that they experience intense social maladjustment. This in turn impedes social initiative and involvement even more.

Substance abuse

In this case the person shows a maladaptive pattern of substance use resulting in a clinically significant impairment or distress within a period of 12 months, as manifested by one or more of the following:
- Failure to fulfil major role obligations at work, school or home
- Recurrent substance-related legal problems, for example arrests for substance-related disorders, or possession of illegal substances
- Substance use in situations which are physically hazardous, for example drinking and driving
- Recurrent social or interpersonal problems, for example arguments and physical fights as consequences of intoxication.

However, the condition does not include the development of tolerance to the substance, withdrawal or compulsive use. Table 15.2 indicates the conditions associated with substances in the DSM-5 (APA, 2013).

Substance intoxication

This is a reversible and substance-specific syndrome which follows recent ingestion of (or exposure to) the substance. It affects one or more of the following mental functions: memory, orientation, mood, judgement and behavioural, social or occupational functioning.

Table 15.2 Diagnoses associated with class of substances (•indicates that the category is recognised in the DSM-5)

	Psychotic disorders	Bipolar disorders	Depressive disorders	Anxiety disorders	Obsessive-compulsive and related disorders	Sleep disorders	Sexual dysfunctions	Delirium	Neurocognitive disorders	Substance use disorders	Substance intoxication	Substance withdrawal
Alcohol	I/W	I/W	I/W	I/W		I/W	I/W	I/W	I/W/P	X	X	X
Caffeine				I		I/W					X	X
Cannabis	I			I		I/W		I		X	X	X
Hallucinogens												
Phencyclidine	I		I	I				I		X	X	
Other hallucinogens	I*		I	I				I		X	X	
Inhalants	I		I	I				I	I/P	X	X	
Opioids			I/W	W		I/W	I/W	I/W		X	X	X
Sedatives, hypnotics, or anxiolytics	I/W	I/W	I/W	W		I/W	I/W	I/W	I/W/P	X	X	X
Stimulants**	I	I/W	I/W	I/W	I/W	I/W	I	I	X	X	X	
Tobacco						W				X		X
Other (or unknown)	I/W	I/W	I/W	I/W	I/W	I/W	I/W	I/W	I/W/P	X	X	X

Note. X = The category is recognized in DSM-5.
I = The specifier "with onset during intoxication" may be noted for the category.
W = The specifier "with onset during withdrawal" may be noted for the category.
I/W = Either "with onset during intoxication" or "with onset during withdrawal" may be noted for the category.
P = The disorder is persisting.
0 *Also hallucinogen persisting perception disorder (flashbacks).
**Includes amphetamine-type substances, cocaine, and other or unspecified stimulants.

Source: APA (2013)

Substance withdrawal

This is also a substance-specific syndrome following the cessation or reduction of ingestion after heavy and prolonged use. It is characterised by physiological signs and symptoms in addition to psychological changes such as disturbances in thinking, feeling and behaviour. It may cause significant distress or impairment. Please note that different substances may produce similar or identical syndromes.

Comorbidity

Comorbidity refers to the occurrence of two or more psychiatric disorders in a single patient at the same time. A high prevalence of psychiatric disorders is found in persons seeking treatment for alcohol, cocaine or opioid dependence. Common comorbid conditions include mood disorders, anxiety disorders, psychotic disorders, delusional disorders and personality disorders (Weich, 2015). Persons suffering from comorbid medical or psychiatric disorders are often referred to as having a 'dual diagnosis'. Substance abuse and a comorbid mental disorder in the same patient has a poor outcome compared to patients who present with a single diagnosis (National Institute on Drug Abuse, 2010).

Possible nursing diagnoses

The following constitutes guidelines for possible nursing diagnoses related to substance use:

Table 15.3 Guidelines for possible nursing diagnoses related to substance use

- Potential for injury RELATED TO intoxication or withdrawal EVIDENCED BY disorientation, poor judgement, unstable vital signs, seizures, etc.
- Potential for self-directed or other-directed violence RELATED TO intoxication, withdrawal, depression EVIDENCED BY history of suicide attempts or violence, anger, disturbed behaviour.
- Alternation in nutrition: less than body requirements RELATED TO drinking instead of eating, poor appetite, no money for food, malabsorption of food EVIDENCED BY loss of weight, pale mucous membranes.
- Ineffective individual coping RELATED TO inadequate support systems, unrealistic perceptions, poor social learning EVIDENCED BY low self-esteem, inability to meet role expectations, inability to meet basic needs.
- Knowledge deficit (re effects of substance abuse) RELATED TO lack of exposure to learning, lack of interest in learning EVIDENCED BY statements of misconceptions, requests for information, verbalisation of this problem.

Source: Townsend (2011)

ALCOHOL-RELATED DISORDERS

The global status report on alcohol (WHO, 2014) indicates that while alcohol consumption is declining in most of the developed countries, it is found to be rising in many of the developing countries and the countries of Central and Eastern Europe. Production of various forms of alcohol for domestic consumption is widespread and decentralised in many countries, increasing the incidence of alcoholism (or alcohol dependence, chronic alcoholism or problem drinking) in many developing countries. This trend has serious consequences for alcohol-dependent persons, their families and the community. There is sufficient evidence to indicate that alcohol poses a significant threat to the health of the millions of users across the globe. Worldwide, harmful use of alcohol is attributed to 3.3 million deaths (5.9 per cent of all global deaths) and 5.1 per cent of the global burden of disease and injury (WHO, 2014). Gender differences in these deaths have been noted. For example, in 2012, 7.6 per cent of deaths were among males and 4.0 per cent among females. Among alcoholics the death rate is two to four times higher than among the general public. Alcohol consumption, especially heavy drinking, has also been causally linked to intentional injuries such as suicide and violence.

South Africa has the highest incidence of alcohol abuse in the world, after Ukraine (Department of Health, 2013). Alcohol is also the third leading cause of death and disease in South Africa, with an estimated 30 per cent of South Africans using alcohol at risk levels. The combined tangible and intangible costs of harmful use of alcohol has cost the South African economy nearly 300 billion rand or 10–12 per cent of the 2009 gross domestic product (Matzopoulos et al, 2014).

Alcohol-related problems are very common in South Africa, especially among the youth given that almost half of South Africa's population consists of young people. In a recent study on alcohol use among learners in a rural high school in Gauteng Province, Chauke et al (2015) found that 21 per cent (n=383) of the participants reported they had engaged in binge drinking. Binge drinking is hazardous drinking where patterns of drinking increase the chances of alcohol-related risks. However, parental behaviours affected the alcohol abuse patterns of children. More than 26.9 per cent of adults drank alcohol regularly at home with 9 per cent of both parents drinking uncontrollably every day. These findings suggest that parental drinking behaviours have an influence on their children's propensity to drink alcohol. Most of the alcohol consumed was beer, followed by wine and spirits.

The impact of high-risk drinking behaviour on South African society is immense. Seggie (2012) avows that reckless driving accounting for road accidents affecting both passengers and pedestrians is on the increase. Unsafe sex and promiscuity increase the transmission of sexually transmitted diseases and human immunodeficiency virus (HIV)/acquired immunodeficiency syndrome (AIDS). Non-financial welfare costs, related to the emotional burden that premature mortality and morbidity place on people affected by the actions of misusers of alcohol, are not possible to estimate. However, Matzopoulos et al (2014) assert that this cost is likely to be substantial.

The high prevalence of alcohol problems in South Africa is related to a large number of societal factors. The colonial and apartheid history with its manipulation of social interaction, social structures and access to alcohol played a role. So did the 'dop' system of compensation with alcohol for farm workers in the Western Cape, and rapid urbanisation and industrialisation (London, 1999).

Similar conditions exist for other substances.

Alcohol dependence

The WHO uses the term 'alcohol dependence syndrome' rather than alcoholism. However, there are many definitions of dependence as there are writers on the subject. Depending on the context, dependence may be physiological, physical or psychological. Physiological or physical dependence refers to tolerance and withdrawal symptoms. Psychological dependence has to do with the experience of impaired control over drinking. The Expert Committee on Mental Health of the WHO defines alcoholics as excessive drinkers whose dependence on alcohol has reached such proportions that it is evident in psychological aberrations or interferes with their physical and mental health, interpersonal relationships, and smooth social and economic functioning. 'Heavy episodic drinking' is defined as the consumption of 60 or more grams of pure alcohol (six or more standard drinks – in South Africa a standard drink is 340ml) on at least one single occasion, at least monthly (WHO, 2014).

The International Classification of Diseases (ICD) 10 identifies features of alcohol dependence as:
- Drinking compulsively and therefore without restraint
- Drinking for a long time (chronically)
- Drinking until intoxicated, thus having difficulties in controlling behaviour related to alcohol use
- A drinking pattern which has, without exception, a negative influence on interpersonal functioning but persisting despite the consequences
- Going into a state of physiological withdrawal when alcohol use has been ceased
- Tolerance such that an increased amount of alcohol must be ingested to obtain the same effects as previously (WHO, 2014).

Stages of alcoholism

According to Jellinek (1952) and the American Addiction Centers (2018), the stages of alcoholism are as follows:
- *Pre-alcoholic phase.* Episodic and later constant drinking in response to stress. Alcohol tolerance increases.
- *Prodromal (early alcoholic) phase.* Blackouts, secret drinking and a preoccupation with alcohol. Drinks are swallowed rapidly; the person has guilt feelings about drinking and refuses to discuss the problem.
- *Crucial phase.* Loss of control over drinking ('one drink is too many and a bottle is not enough'). The behaviour is rationalised; paranoid and aggressive behaviour is evinced and the person is always remorseful. Repeated attempts are made to control drinking and more and more problems are experienced with the family and employer. Self-pity becomes evident and interest in other things, including food, begins to diminish. The person becomes unreasonably vengeful, jealously protective of liquor, suffers from tremors and begins to take a 'pick-me-up' in the morning.

- *Chronic phase.* The individual is in a protracted state of poisoning and deteriorates physically and morally. Thought is impaired, and the person suffers from indefinable anxiety and is obsessed with alcohol.

Intoxication and alcohol withdrawal syndrome

Two disorders that are part of the course of alcoholism are acute alcohol poisoning (intoxication) and the alcohol withdrawal syndrome (known as delirium tremens or DTs in its acute form). Nurses must be able not only to identify alcoholics but also to notice signs of poisoning or the withdrawal syndrome.

Alcohol intoxication

The DSM-5 criteria for alcohol intoxication are as follows (APA, 2013):

A. Recent ingestion of alcohol.
B. Clinically significant problematic beliavioral or psychological changes (e.g., inappropriate sexual or aggressive behavior, mood lability, impaired judgment) that developed during, or shortly after, alcohol ingestion.
C. One (or more) of the following signs or symptoms developing during, or shortly after, alcohol use:
   1. Slurred speech.
   2. Incoordination.
   3. Unsteady gait.
   4. Nystagmus.
   5. Impairment in attention or memory.
   6. Stupor or coma.
D. The signs or symptoms are not attributable to another medical condition and are not better explained by another mental disorder, including intoxication with another substance.

Alcohol withdrawal

Alcohol withdrawal even without delirium can be serious. Seizures and autonomic hyperactivity can be present. Symptoms usually start six to eight hours after cessation. The risk of seizures is highest in the first 48 hours but persists for more than two weeks. Delirium tremens develops after 72 hours. Sometimes the progression of the syndrome of withdrawal is skipped and the person goes directly into DTs (Trevisan et al, 1998).

Prevention of alcoholism

Prevention can occur at the primary, secondary and tertiary levels.

Primary prevention

The focus of primary prevention is to prevent the initiation of alcohol use or delaying the age at which alcohol begins. However, education and information about what should be known about alcohol abuse, and what should be understood about harmful use and the associated risks, have been shown to have very little effect. The education and information provided should focus on promoting the availability of effective interventions and support for effective policies on alcohol (WHO, 2010).

There are a number of approaches to primary prevention, which are dealt with in the following sections.

Normative manipulation

The percentage of alcoholics is low in societies that denounce moderate drinking, condemn excessive drinking and in which there is broad agreement on these norms; the norms may therefore be encouraged in a particular society to prevent alcoholism. There should be definite criteria for what is considered to be 'excessive' drinking with the suggestion that four episodes of intoxication per year should be considered a criterion of excessive drinking (Steers et al, 2016).

Integrated drinking

Integrated drinking means that the consumption of alcohol in the community is subordinated to other activities, especially family, religious and recreation activities, rather than being an organising principle of social activity. In countries and groups with few alcohol problems, the consumption of liquor may be commonplace, but it is merely one aspect of a more important activity. In Italy, for example, liquor is a necessary part of meals and Jewish people drink liquor as part of their religious observance. The French, on the other hand, structure social events around the intake of alcohol, which results in a higher incidence of alcoholism. As part of primary prevention, the consumption of alcohol should be encouraged in situations of restraint, that is, where it is restricted by coincidental activities.

Level of mental health and social conditions

Apart from the specific approaches that have been mentioned, there are also indirect measures, that is, anything aimed at enhancing the general level of mental health and improving social conditions. These include measures such as enhancing the quality of family life, helping people to cope more effectively with crises and alleviating poverty and deprivation.

Price control and distribution

The WHO (2014) recommends a number of measures aimed at reducing alcohol consumption. These include a specific domestic taxation system which takes into account the alcohol content of the beverage; a regular review of the price of alcohol in relation to inflation; the establishment of minimum prices for alcohol where applicable; and banning or restricting the use of direct and indirect price promotions. Increasing the price of alcoholic beverages is one of the most effective interventions for reducing harmful use of alcohol (WHO, 2010).

Various authors (Razvodovsky, 2016; Wagenaar et al, 2010) have proved indisputably that the lower the price of liquor, the higher the average intake per person and the greater the proportionate increase in the number of deaths from cirrhosis of the liver. This gave rise to the idea that increasing the price of liquor would prevent alcoholism. However, many authors believe that this would mean only that moderate or social drinkers would drink less, while alcoholics would drink as much as before. Others believe that price increases would lead only to the large-scale production of illicit liquor, since prices would have to be almost trebled to make a significant difference to the consumption of alcohol. It would seem therefore that price control on its own would create new problems, as was the case during prohibition in the United States in the 1920s, which caused problems like the illegal production and sale of liquor (known as bootlegging) and organised crime.

Health education
Health education takes the form of educating the total population; milestone education and educating groups at risk.
- *Total population education.* Universal prevention targets the general public. Policies and law enforcement are included as part of the prevention tactics. These include legislation related to driving. Once there is consistent and effective enforcement of laws related to driving, the prevalence of drunk driving decreases significantly. Another measure involves underage drinking. Since alcohol is abused most by the youth, raising the drinking age has also been effective (Berk, 2013). Some governments have also tried to encourage the drinking of other alcoholic substances but without success. A further suggestion has been that liquor advertisements should be prohibited. However, the WHO points out that, although advertisements make liquor more socially acceptable, people drink even when there are no advertisements (WHO, 2014).
- *Milestone education.* In this context the milestone approach means preparing children for their first drink. According to Bremmer et al (2011), although parents strongly influence the alcohol-related behaviour of their children, peer groups and the school as a socialising institution can be used for education in this regard. High-school children were first used as a target group, but it gradually became clear that teaching should begin earlier. It has also been found that children have already mastered the concept of alcohol and know the smell and behavioural manifestations of inebriation by the age of eight years. It is generally accepted that small-group discussions constitute the best teaching.
- *Educating groups at risk.* The only significant group at risk in the primary prevention context is the children of alcoholic parents. In this case, the teaching method also constitutes small-group discussions and ages vary from primary to high school.

Secondary prevention

Secondary prevention is aimed at focusing on the early stages of alcohol use (early detection) to prevent alcohol becoming a problem and causing harm to the person. Treatment is discussed separately.

The early detection and treatment of alcoholics is very difficult because they use denial as a defence mechanism, and the fact that they are alcoholics cannot be 'proved' to them. The identification of alcoholics at an early stage is therefore a strategic but difficult goal. Alcoholism develops slowly and alcoholics themselves cope with it by means of denial. The people close to them, for example a spouse, friends, colleagues and supervisors, go through various stages of recognising the problem.

First stage

Supervisors are vaguely aware of impaired performance but do not regard it as serious enough to be regarded as abnormal. Employees make sure that their abnormal behaviour is integrated in their work behaviour. The spouse and friends are vaguely concerned.

Signs include the following:
- light hand tremors
- more nervous and tense
- hangovers at work
- avoidance of supervisor and co-workers
- drinking in the mornings before going to work
- leaving their post every now and again
- unusual excuses for absence from work
- displaying deteriorating quality of work
- mood changes after lunch
- bloodshot eyes.

Second stage

This is the stage of 'blocked consciousness'. The supervisor becomes increasingly aware that the problem behaviour is associated with alcohol, but they are prevented by various factors from designating it as abnormal, for example the status of the employee or the consequences that confrontation might hold for the supervisor.

The spouse is aware of the problem, but hides it for the sake of appearances, the children or holding down a job.

The signs include the following:
- displaying increasing absenteeism and poor quality of work
- can no longer conceal hangovers
- sporadic work performance with 'good days' having to compensate for 'bad days'
- aggressiveness during bouts of intoxication.

Third stage

This is the 'see-saw' stage during which supervisors are increasingly forced to describe the deviant behaviour as abnormal, while the blocking factors ('when they work, they do a fantastic job') time and again affect the decision to act. The spouse threatens to leave but the alcoholics are 'always so penitent when sober'.

The signs include the following:
- drinking at lunch
- marked personality change after lunch
- speaking loudly
- hands tremble obviously
- more supervision required due to unpredictable work behaviour
- negative influence on work group
- children indicate that there are problems
- spouse is despondent and often depressed.

Fourth stage

The supervisor decides to acknowledge the problem. The pressure of the deviant behaviour causes alienation from co-workers and they lose their empathy. The family often breaks up.

The signs include the following:
- drinking while on duty
- more frequent absences due to physical disorders
- flushed face and bloodshot eyes.

Tertiary prevention

Tertiary prevention is aimed at ending dependence and problems that may arise. The individual is encouraged to achieve and to increase functioning to optimal levels.

Nursing Interventions with alcoholism

Many alcoholics come into contact with the general health service without anything being done about their basic problem – alcohol dependency. However, in most cases they present with other problems such as headaches which highlights the critical role that a health care professional has in identifying the substance abuse and ensuring that treatment is accessible (Muhrer, 2010).

The following recommendations could be incorporated into nursing interventions:

Talking to patients about their drinking problem

Benton (2009) identified the following response as being characteristic of such patients with an alcohol dependency problem:

'I have been in recovery from alcoholism for almost five years. I too struggled to see that I could be accomplished academically and then professionally while drinking alcohol. My image of the alcoholic was always an individual who could not hold his or her life together, and I certainly did not fit that description. The denial that I experienced was so deeply rooted and was reinforced not only from my loved ones but from society as a whole.'

Heinemann and Estes (1976) suggest that nurses should tell patients that they are glad that their physical condition is improving, but that they think they should talk about their drinking problem:

- If patients are not willing to talk about it, their decision should be respected, but an opportunity should be sought later to raise the subject again.
- If patients are willing to talk about it, they should be asked to describe it from their point of view. Do they think it is a problem or is it a solution to their problem? It should be ascertained whether there is any aspect of the problem that worries them and this should be used as a therapeutic starting point.
- During conversations the danger signs of alcoholism should be mentioned. These include: more than four episodes of intoxication per year, drinking alone, the need for a 'pick-me-up', drinking more than one's friends, the need for liquor to cope with stress, and drinking more than one wants to drink. Hearing about these signs can sow doubt and undermine denial.
- The physical aspects of alcoholism should be stressed by comparing them, for example, with those of diabetes. This emphasises both the reality of the disease and the necessity for treatment. It should be explained that the compulsion usually develops slowly, with the result that one does not become aware of it until the condition is far advanced. The difficulty of accepting the possibility that one is an alcoholic should be spoken about frankly.
- Such constructive confrontation should take place after a solid relationship has been built up with the patient. Denial should be counteracted, but preferably without using the words 'alcoholic' and 'addiction', as these may be unacceptable. Respect for the patient should always be conveyed, but at the same time it should be clearly indicated that alcoholism is regarded as a serious disease that will not go away by being ignored.

Helping patients to plan a constructive programme for obtaining assistance

Alcoholics should be helped to plan a constructive programme for obtaining assistance and they also require assistance with the implementation of the first steps to set it in motion. No two patients are alike. Alcoholics Anonymous may be the appropriate (and acceptable) recourse for one, a rehabilitation centre for a second, while the best choice for a third may be a psychologist or a psychiatrist. Nurses should be able to give their patients hope, as alcoholics often have a long history of failure. They should not, however, oversimplify the rehabilitation process, as this could foster the idea that they really do not understand. They should give realistic information about the various treatment programmes and should help patients with their first steps in that direction.

Detoxification

When a diagnosis of alcohol dependence is made and the patient wishes to be detoxified, this can be done on an outpatient basis if there is adequate family support. This may, however, not be feasible in cases of severe dependence over a very long time, or where return to the clinic or hospital in case of complications is not possible or too difficult. Also, if there is a history of DTs or convulsions, the patient should be admitted for detoxification.

If outpatient detoxification is undertaken, the family should be told to make the patient take lots of fluid (three litres per day or more), and to bring the patient back if they have convulsions or become delirious.

The patient usually presents in a state of sympathetic nervous system hyperarousal, with a rapid pulse, tremors, nausea, sweating and a raised blood pressure.

The role of nurses in treatment of alcoholism

This section looks at the way nurses should approach patients with alcoholism and at assessment tools.

Approach to patients

Nurses who work with alcoholics should realise that feelings of superiority and domination have no place in the care of these patients. Alcoholics already have very poor self-esteem and the attitude of their nurses can make a major contribution to their regaining their self-respect. In a study of registered nurses' perceptions and actions regarding the care of alcoholics in primary care services in Brazil, Vargas et al (2010) reported that nurses treated the alcoholic with disrespect as they were perceived to be usually aggressive. Care should nevertheless be taken not to be overly sympathetic or accepting, thereby bolstering the pathology.

Assessment of people with alcohol problems

A nursing history can be taken in one or more sessions, depending on the patient's condition. If the problem is understood and accepted to be an alcohol-related one, the drinking history can be taken as a starting point, but if it is not acknowledged, the history must begin with related problems. Heinemann and Estes (1976: 787–788) constructed and tested the nursing history form set out on the following pages. The questions with asterisks refer to emergencies and threatened withdrawal syndrome.

Table 15.4 Nursing history form

Nursing history form for patients with alcohol problems
Demographic data
Date:
Place of interview:
Patient's name:

→

- Age:
- Sex:
- Place of birth:
- Occupation:
- Education level:
1. Why did you come to this institution/organisation?
2. In what way would you most like to be helped right now?

Drinking history
3. How old were you when you began drinking alcohol regularly?
4. How long have you had problems with alcohol?
5. How often do you drink alcoholic beverages?
6. What types of liquor do you drink?
7. How much of each alcoholic beverage do you drink?
8. When did you have your last drink?*
9. When did your last drinking bout begin?*
10. What did you drink during your last drinking bout?*
11. How much alcohol did you consume each day during your last drinking bout?*
12. Has your drinking caused problems in any of the following areas?
    - With your spouse
    - At work
    - With your children
    - With your friends
13. Have you ever been injured as a result of drinking?
    - Yes
    - No
    - Fighting
    - Road accident
    - Accidental falls
    - Other reasons
14. Have you ever been arrested as a result of drinking
    - Yes
    - No
    - On what charge?
       - Driving under the influence
       - Fighting
       - Other (specify)
15. Have you ever been in prison as a result of drinking?
    - Yes
    - No
16. What previous treatment have you had for alcohol problems?
    - Date:
    - Place:

Symptoms relating to the gastrointestinal system
17. What did you eat during your last drinking bout?*

→

18. What is your normal eating pattern:
    - When drinking?
    - When not drinking?
19. Have there been recent changes in your appetite?
20. Has your weight changed recently?
21. Are you on a special diet?
22. What fluids, other than alcohol, do you drink?
    - Coffee
    - Tea
    - Water
    - Milk
    - Fruit juice
23. Do you often have mouth or throat irritations?
24. Do you have stomach-ache?
25. Are you bothered by heartburn or flatulence?*
26. Are you nauseous?*
27. Do you vomit or gag without bringing up anything?*
28. Have you ever vomited blood? If so, when?*
29. Have you ever had gastric ulcers or other stomach problems?
30. How often and for what reason do you take aspirin?
31. What medication do you take for stomach-ache?
32. Do you suffer from pain in your abdomen?
33. Do you suffer from diarrhoea or constipation?
34. Do you have piles?
35. Have you ever had blood in your stools?
36. Have you noticed a change of colour in your stools?
    - Clay-coloured
    - Black
    - Bright red
37. What problems have you experienced in the past with your bowels?
38. What medication do you take for abdominal pain?
39. Have you ever had pancreatic problems?*
40. Has your skin or the whites of your eyes ever turned yellow?*
41. Have you ever had problems with your liver?*
42. Do you have diabetes? If so, what medication do you take?

Symptoms relating to the neurological system

43. Have you noticed how much more alcohol it takes to obtain the effect you desire? If so, describe the change.
44. What reactions do you have when you stop drinking?
    - Tremors
    - Hear or see things
    - Other convulsions
    - DTs
45. Have you ever taken medication for the convulsions?

46. Have you ever had periods of loss of memory after a drinking bout?
47. Have you ever experienced tingling, pain or numbness in your hands or feet?
48. Do you ever have muscle pains in your arms or legs?
49. Do you have any trouble keeping your balance?
50. Do you have any problems with your vision?*
51. Do you have problems with sleeping?
52. How many hours a night do you usually sleep?
    – When you drink
    – When you don't drink
53. Do you feel rested after a night's sleep?
54. What do you do if you are unable to sleep?
55. Have you noticed any change recently in your sex life? If so, describe the change.

Symptoms relating to the cardiovascular and pulmonary systems

56. Do you have heart trouble? If so, describe the trouble.
57. Do your hands and feet swell?
58. Are you often short of breath?
59. Do you have chest pains?
60. Do you take any medicine for heart disease?
61. Have you ever had pneumonia?
62. Have you ever had tuberculosis (consumption)?
63. Do you often get infections (for instance, colds, boils or sores that do not heal easily)?
64. Do you have a persistent (chronic) cough? If so, describe the cough.
65. Have you ever coughed up blood or phlegm?
66. Describe any other lung problems that you might have.
67. Do you smoke? If so, how many a day?

Psychosocial status

68. What is your marital status?
69. With whom do you live?
70. Does this person use alcohol regularly?
    – Yes
    – No
71. To whom do you feel closest?
72. Do your neighbours, family and/or friends use alcohol regularly?
    – Yes
    – No
73. How many children do you have?
74. How often do you see your children?
75. Describe your home:
    – Type (for example, house, flat or room)
    – Cooking facilities
    – Number of stairs
    – Availability and type of transport
76. Have you ever had mental or emotional problems?
    – Depression

- Suicide attempts
- Loneliness
- Nervousness (anxiety)
- Other

77. Are you currently involved in a counselling programme?
78. Are you currently taking medication for a psychiatric problem? If so, describe the medication.
79. Are you affiliated to a religious group?
80. What is your present employment status?
81. Do you have any specific occupational skills?
82. If you have a job, how does this period of treatment affect it?
83. If you are unemployed, what is your present source of income?
84. What are your hobbies or special interests?
85. How do you spend a typical day at home?

Drug-taking

86. What medication do you take that you have not yet mentioned?
    - Prescribed drugs
    - Over-the-counter drugs
    - Drugs obtained on the street
87. What is your usual manner of taking medication?
    - As prescribed
    - More than prescribed
    - Less than prescribed
88. Are you allergic to any medication?*

Final questions

89. How do you plan to control your drinking when you are discharged?
90. Would you like to make any further remarks?
91. Would you like to ask any questions?

(* Refers to emergencies and threatened withdrawal syndrome)

This interview schedule includes the most important problem areas of alcoholics, that is, drinking habits, symptoms of damage-prone systems and psychosocial status. Alcoholics often give less than accurate histories, especially about their drinking, so it is useful to confirm this aspect by interviewing family or friends. Patients may also be examined for signs of physical damage.

Table 15.5 The CAGE questionnaire

> **The CAGE questionnaire**
> This questionnaire is a very simple tool that can be used to identify persons at potential risk for alcohol dependency. The actual diagnosis must be made by a medical doctor or a nurse. It consists of four questions from which the acronym CAGE is extracted. The questions focus on Cutting down, Annoyance by criticism, Guilty feeling, and Eye-openers:
> 1. Have you ever felt you ought to **C**ut down on your drinking?
> 2. Have people **A**nnoyed you by criticising your drinking?
> 3. Have you ever felt **G**uilty about your drinking?
> 4. Have you ever had a drink first thing in the morning to steady your nerves or get rid of a hangover (**E**ye-opener)?
>
> Scoring: Two 'yes' answers indicate probable alcoholism

Source: Ewing (1984: 1905); O'Brien (2008).

A fairly accurate history of drinking is important, as it enables the nurse to anticipate the nature and degree of withdrawal symptoms and to evaluate the chronicity of the alcoholism. All the other questions relate to specific complications of alcoholism. It has been found, for instance, that alcohol prevents the type of sleep that is necessary for rest that is rapid eye movement (REM) sleep. Rapid eye movement sleep deprivation results in poor concentration and memory, and causes anxiety, fatigue and irritability. Information about these aspects is consequently necessary, not only for planning nursing interventions but also for planning patient education. Enquiry into the use of medication is also important, as some substances are incompatible with alcohol, for example some oral hypoglycaemic substances. The action of some substances, such as the anticoagulant Warfarin, is impaired by alcohol, while others, such as aspirin, can cause serious damage if taken with alcohol. Another reason why nurses should know what medication patients are taking is that withdrawal symptoms may occur if certain drugs are suddenly discontinued. The action of some substances, such as psychotropic drugs, is enhanced by alcohol.

Nursing care during acute intoxication and withdrawal

This section provides guidelines for nursing care during acute intoxication and withdrawal.

Acute intoxication

Breath that smells of liquor together with a drunken appearance do not necessarily imply intoxication. A thorough examination is always required to eliminate other causes for the signs and symptoms. This is particularly important in patients who are subsiding into a coma.

Patients who are in a coma due to too much alcohol are always in danger of dying of circulatory collapse or depressed respiration. Medical assistance should be sought in such cases and aspiration should be prevented by nursing the patients on their side with the head slightly higher than the body. An airway may be required. Vital signs should be monitored and respiratory secretions suctioned if necessary.

Alcohol metabolism takes place at a constant rate and no medication or substance can speed it up. The rate is, however, higher in alcoholics. Remedies such as cold showers, strong black coffee, forced activity or vomiting evidently contribute nothing to sobriety.

Withdrawal

According to the American Addiction Centers (2018) alcohol withdrawal may follow three stages and present with the following signs and symptoms:
1. *Stage 1 (mild).* Anxiety, insomnia, fatigue, gastrointestinal signs and symptoms such as nausea, abdominal pain and/or vomiting, loss of appetite, psychomotor restlessness, altered mood and heart palpitations
2. *Stage 2 (moderate).* Increased blood pressure, body temperature and respiration, irregular heart rate, confusion, sweating, irritability, and increased mood disturbances
3. *Stage 3 (severe/delirium tremens).* Hallucinations, delusions, disorientation and delirium, fever, seizures, severe confusion, and agitation.

The nursing care of such patients includes the following:
- *Keeping the patient as calm as possible.* Re-orienting the patient to time, date, and place reduces anxiety. In addition, evaluating and treating the patient in a well-lit room while providing reassurance is advised (Schuckit, 2014), Procedures should be planned in such a way that these patients are disturbed as little as possible while asleep to avoid startling them and making them uncontrollable all over again. An intravenous infusion is often set up to avoid having to wake the patient to take fluids. An in-dwelling catheter may also be passed to obviate the necessity of disturbing the patient for urine specimens. Insomnia may be a problem after the acute phase, but narcotics must be administered with great circumspection as addiction is a distinct possibility. The patient's fearfulness should not be disregarded, and even the simplest procedure must be properly explained.
- *Keeping the patient well hydrated.* Most people who have been drinking for a long time are dehydrated. In addition, patients suffering from the withdrawal syndrome perspire profusely and are very agitated; both conditions cause further dehydration. The oral fluid intake of patients with mild to moderate withdrawal is increased: at least 180 ml milk is given every half hour until 1 440 ml has been taken, followed by fluids ad lib. If patients with threatened or true DTs can keep to this regimen, they are kept on it, but nausea often precludes oral fluid intake. In such cases fluids are given intravenously, with milk, fruit juice and other fluids administered orally ad lib.

An accurate record of fluid intake and output must be kept. Output must be checked at least four-hourly or hourly if it is low.
- *Checking vital signs and symptoms to prevent complications.* Hypertension is a common, but not inevitable, sign of imminent DTs. Both systolic and diastolic pressure rises, and this is particularly dangerous in patients who are already hypertensive. Hypotension occurs if sufficiently high doses of sedatives are given in the treatment of DTs. Hypotension and a raised pulse rate can also be indications of internal haemorrhage, for example from oesophageal varices. Patients with DTs often have a subnormal temperature unless an infection somewhere in the body complicates the condition. Hyperthermia is a very serious prognostic sign and demands immediate intervention to lower the temperature. Vital signs are consequently taken every hour for 12 hours, two-hourly thereafter for another 12 hours and as often as dictated by the patient's condition after that.

  Another important observation is to test the urine for albumin every four hours, since this may give an indication of renal function. Nurses should also be mindful of signs and symptoms of pending hepatic coma or bleeding oesophageal varices. These two disorders are complications of liver cirrhosis, which is common in alcoholics (refer to texts on medical and surgical nursing for nursing care).
- *Keeping the patient well nourished.* Most alcoholics suffer from malnutrition and they are put onto a normal, balanced diet as soon as the acute phase is over. A low-fat diet, rich in proteins and carbohydrates, is sometimes prescribed, especially for people who cannot tolerate fatty foods. Patients with gastritis sometimes require a soft, bland diet.
- *Observing side effects and toxic effects.* These patients are on many forms of medication and should be observed for side effects and toxic effects.
- *Treating convulsions.* Convulsions, which sometimes occur, are managed in the same way as epileptic convulsions and the same preventive measures are taken for the patient's safety.

Patient education regarding alcoholism

Most alcoholics are surprisingly uninformed about the influence of their drinking on their health and about factors that influence their drinking habits. Structured patient teaching consequently often forms part of treatment programmes, especially for inpatients, and this function is frequently delegated to nurses. The broad outlines of such a teaching programme are as follows.

What is alcoholism?

A number of authors emphasise that the concept that alcoholism is a disease that is most acceptable to patients, since it allows them to retain a modicum of self-respect and self-confidence. However, the therapeutic philosophy of the institution will dictate the approach of the nurses, since the illness concept does not, for example, fit in with the transactional-analysis approach. This approach focuses on analysing the content of social interactions between people.

Physical consequences of alcohol abuse

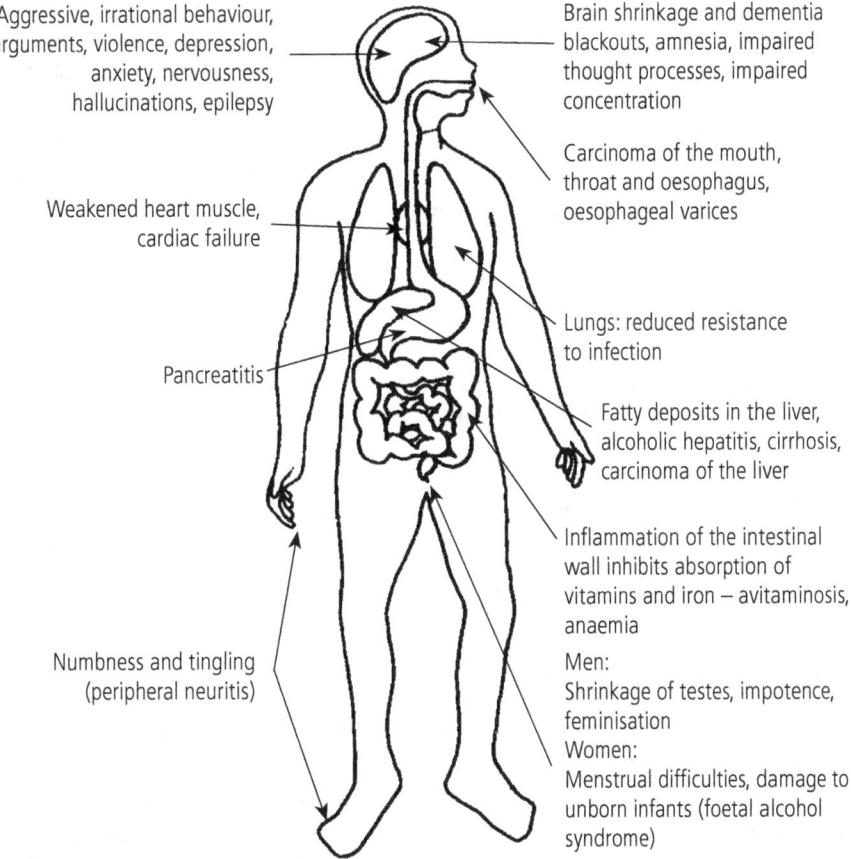

Figure 15.1 Physical effects of alcoholism

Source: Adapted from Cole (1990); Barclay et al (2008)

The effect of alcohol on general health must be pointed out, particularly on the following:
- gastrointestinal system
- cardiovascular system
- liver and pancreas
- nervous system (see Figure 15.1).

Information should be made more comprehensible by the use of diagrams and photographs; and should be supported by statistical data.

Dietary habits

Alcoholics usually follow very poor diets, which may even exacerbate their drinking problem. A breakfast and lunch consisting of mainly carbohydrates may lead to fatigue by mid-morning or mid-afternoon, and this increases the chances of drinking. Alcoholics often eat a lot of sweets to cope with their anxiety and this leads to a sharp rise in blood sugar. When the blood sugar declines sharply again, they generally feel weak and tremulous, which once again increases their chances of drinking. Coffee often has a detrimental effect on alcoholics – it increases tremors and impedes sleep. This and other information should be given to patients without demands being made that they change their eating habits. It should be remembered that these patients have already given up alcohol, and they may become rebellious if too many demands are made. The desired habits (a balanced diet and eating habits) must be emphasised, rather than the undesirable ones.

Sleeping habits

Sleep disturbances should be discussed in detail. Information should be given about the effect of alcohol on sleep, and about measures to improve sleep.

Promotion and maintenance of general health

The importance of an annual general medical examination, including chest X-rays, needs to be stressed. The effects of alcohol on the body must be given special emphasis.

Assisting the family of the alcoholic

The four stages through which alcoholics and their families pass are summarised as follows (Antai-Otong, 2008):

1. At first all the members of the family cope with the drinking problem by pretending that it is not a problem (denial). Tension increases and emotional security diminishes, but they try to give the impression that they are a 'normal' family and that there is nothing wrong.
2. As the frequency and level of the drinking bouts increase, the pretence becomes impossible and the family members concentrate their efforts on hiding the problem.
   All the family members reduce their social activities. This leads to isolation and introversion and their lives become alcoholic-centred. Home remedies to resolve the problem are used repeatedly. The alcoholic tries very hard to hide the supply of liquor, while the family colludes in efforts to find and destroy it. The efforts of the family to persuade the alcoholic to stop drinking vary from sentimental requests to quarrels.
3. The intrapsychic conflicts of each member of the family become apparent during this stage. The alcoholic feels guilty because they repeatedly disappoint the family.

The spouse feels guilty because of accusations that they are causing the alcoholic's drinking problem. The children feel guilty for various reasons, for example because they feel disloyal or because they think that their behaviour causes the drinking. Hostility, frustration, quarrelling and fear are common in this stage.
4. In the fourth stage the family members stop their fight against alcoholism in an effort to retain a measure of individual inner stability. Although they do not experience the problem themselves, they tolerate it without trying to hide it any longer. The spouse now has the confidence to seek help. The family no longer functions as a unit. If a combined effort is needed, however, role interchange takes place. The alcoholic's role in the family is assumed by the spouse and the alcoholic is no longer involved in planning and decision making.

Counselling for the spouse

The spouse needs to be counselled in order to prevent complete disintegration of the family. It also helps to teach the family not to encourage the drinking habits of the alcoholic. Estes (1974) divides this type of counselling into stages.

Early phase

During this stage, the aim and procedure of the counselling are defined and the spouse is given the opportunity to unburden themselves while information about alcoholism is given all the time.

- The goal is clearly defined as an opportunity for the spouse to learn to know themselves better. No other results are promised. The spouse often hopes that the counselling will by some miraculous means make the alcoholic stop drinking. In fact, however, the alcoholic has to practise self-control to remain sober. This fact must be frankly and clearly stated, even if it takes some time before the spouse truly accepts it.
- The spouse is encouraged to air feelings of guilt, rage and frustration. At the same time the spouse is helped to describe important incidents in daily life in minute detail. At first these descriptions are used merely to formulate thoughts, feelings and behaviour, but they are used later to seek alternatives.
- The counsellor counteracts any tendency to a negative self-image from the beginning. This is done by asking questions that extract positive and realistic self-appraisals. The relationship between the nurse and the spouse can, in itself, lead to greater self-confidence and a feeling of worth.
- After the initial unburdening, a didactic process is commenced in order to establish the idea of alcoholism as a disease. Misconceptions about alcoholism (associated with denial) are thoroughly and systematically eliminated. The spouse must learn what alcoholism is and must be able to recognise physical manifestations in the alcoholic. The spouse must also learn to recognise the alcoholic's usual defence mechanisms, for example denial and rationalisation, as disease symptoms and not as shameless lies, meanness or laziness. This insight enables the spouse to be less judgemental.

Middle phase

The middle phase commences when the spouse is able to examine problem areas in their own life frankly and consistently. The spouse acts purposefully and is emotionally willing to work at themselves in their situation. The aim of this phase is to identify, examine and, where necessary, change the way in which the spouse copes with their problems. According to Senthil (2016), the family responsibilities shift to the spouse who may display behaviours which are inconsistent, demanding and neglecting of the children. The spouse is often unaware of their conduct and should be helped to gain insight into their own behaviour.

After the type of conduct has been identified, its effect on the marriage relationship, on the development of the children, on the drinking behaviour and on the spouse's own personality is examined. This is a lengthy process and eventually certain behaviour patterns are modified and others completely eliminated.

Krimmel (Bourne & Fox, 1973: 306) emphasises that the spouse should be encouraged to follow a creative approach. By this he means that the non-alcoholic family members should stop playing roles complementary to the role of the alcoholic. The non-alcoholics should release the alcoholic emotionally and should completely stop trying to control their drinking or protecting them from its consequences.

Final phase

The final stage commences when it becomes clear that the spouse has more self-respect and has a better understanding of alcoholism. The spouse is able to make good decisions after considering the alternatives and sticks to them even if they are resisted or questioned. The spouse looks better and is calmer and more relaxed. The spouse is also more meticulous about grooming. The aim of this phase is to help the spouse to plan the future realistically, after which counselling is terminated.

The spouse may decide to confront the alcoholic regarding the need for treatment in this stage. The spouse should be well prepared for this confrontation, so that they do not make idle threats. If the alcoholic agrees to accept help, the spouse could put them in immediate touch with appropriate sources. The spouse should, however, leave as much initiative as possible to the alcoholic themselves.

The spouse should also know what to do if the alcoholic does not agree to accept assistance, as such a decision would require reconsideration of the situation. The spouse also considers alternatives such as divorce or separation during this stage. The spouse often requires spiritual help for this decision and may be advised to discuss it with a minister, pastor or priest.

At the end of the counselling, the spouse may be referred to an Al-Anon group for further support.

Al-Anon family groups

Al-Anon groups are similar to Alcoholics Anonymous (AA) but members are the spouses of alcoholics. They originated in the United States in 1945 and by 1974 there were 6 500 registered groups throughout the world. Groups began meeting in South Africa in 1953 and by 2004 AA South Africa had general service offices in eight areas and 314 groups. Alateen groups, specially intended for the children of alcoholics, were first established in South Africa in 1970.

Al-Anon groups meet regularly (usually weekly), generally in the form of discussion groups. Members share their experiences openly with peers who have been through the same trauma. The 'Twelve Steps' of AA are used in a modified form to enable non-alcoholics to understand that they cannot make alcoholics stop drinking but that they can improve their own and their children's lives with the help of a higher power.

Members have very high opinions of the groups and professionals recommend them in cases where long-term counselling is impossible. They may also be of great value in conjunction with or after counselling. Al-Anon groups may be contacted through local AA branches.

Employee assistance programmes (EAPs)

The highest incidence of alcoholism occurs in people between the ages of 35 and 45 years when most adults are active in their occupations.

Employment organisations offer both an opportunity for the early identification of problem drinkers and good reasons for constructive intervention. The following factors make this situation eminently suitable for early intervention.

Alcohol dependence impairs occupational functioning from an early stage of a worker's drinking history. Matzopoulos et al (2014) undertook a study to determine the cost of harmful alcohol use in South Africa. These authors found that although the SA alcohol industry contributes substantially to the economy in terms of jobs, output and export earnings, the social and emotional cost of harmful alcohol use was enormous. These costs relate to alcohol-related illness, violence, death through drunk driving and the related disabilities. The costs could not be calculated given that the data is incomplete in several cost categories.

However, the relationship between employer and employee offers valid grounds for interference by the employer with regard to a poor performance record. The employer has the 'right' to try to do something about the drinking behaviour, whereas very few other people in an alcoholic's life have this right.

Programmes like EAPs address alcoholism and other forms of dependence, as well as emotional and social problems. For further information on EAPs and workplace alcohol prevention, see https://pubs.niaaa.nih.gov/publications/arh26-1/49-57.htm.

OTHER COMMON DEPENDENCE-PRODUCING SUBSTANCES

Up to the early 1990s so-called 'hard drugs' (heroin and cocaine) were a very small problem in South Africa. This changed rapidly during the 1990s and into the new century. A combination of methaqualone (mandrax) and marijuana ('white pipe') remains very common. There has also been a dramatic change in the patterns of abuse with the introduction of crystal methamphetamine (tik) in the Western Cape within the last two or three years. The use of heroin (in addition to nyaope), cocaine and crack cocaine, and 'recreational drugs' such as ecstacy (3.4–methylenedioxymethamphetamine) has also increased in South Africa (Weich, 2015).

The use of dagga (cannabis or marijuana)

Dagga is the substance most used by young people in South Africa. It is obtained from the dried flowers and leaves of the *Cannabis sativa* plant. The active intoxicating ingredient in dagga is 9-delta-tetrahydrocannabinol (THC) and it acts in conjunction with other chemical compounds called cannabinoids. Dagga can be taken in the form of cakes, hash oil and tea, but it is generally smoked in cigarettes or pipes. THC is a lipid soluble drug, therefore stored in body fat and the time it takes to clear the system is dependent on how much of the drug was used and the period of time of abuse: single use: 2–4 days; moderate use: 4 days; chronic use: 3–6 weeks. In September 2018, dagga was decriminalised for private possession, consumption and cultivation in South Africa after a protracted legal battle between civil society and government. The Constitutional Court found that the dagga ban infringed section 14 of the South African Constitution which alludes to the right to privacy.

Medicinal uses of dagga include relief of anxiety and tension, reduction in inflammation and relief from spasms, control of nausea and vomiting during chemotherapy, killing cancer cells and slowing tumour growth. Dagga may also stimulate appetite and improve weight gain in people with cancer and HIV/AIDS (Scott, Dalgleish & Liu, 2014).

The signs and symptoms related to the use of this substance are set out in Table 15.6.

Effects of long-term use of dagga

Although many people believe that dagga is not a harmful substance, long-term use has the following adverse effects:
- Dagga damages the respiratory system, which may lead to bronchitis, lung damage and a higher risk of lung cancer.
- It has a negative effect on the body's immune system.
- Dagga harms the foetus of a pregnant woman who uses it.
- It affects the sex hormones by:
  - suppressing ovulation in young women, resulting in infertility
  - delaying sexual development in young men (Crean et al, 2011).

Effects and symptoms of dagga intoxication

The effects of dagga intoxication and consequently the associated symptoms are the following:
- People experience extreme happiness or euphoria, with giggling and laughing.

- Others become quiet and introspective, thinking about and discussing what they think are wonderful topics; however, they may not be making sense to the listener.
- There might be a loss of short-term memory.
- There is hunger, especially a craving for sweet foods, and thirst.
- People have reddened eyes.
- They have slower reaction time and perception.

Hallucinating while taking dagga is a sign of overdosage, while 'bad trips' in the form of acute anxiety or psychosis also occur. With long-term use, people develop an 'amotivational syndrome', in which they lose interest in most activities, drop out of social, occupational and other circles, and do very little.

Twelve questions
The Marijuana Anonymous group suggests a dagga smoker ask the 'Twelve Questions' listed below to decide whether they have an abuse problem.
1. Has smoking pot stopped being fun?
2. Do you ever get high alone?
3. Is it hard for you to imagine a life without marijuana?
4. Do you find that your friends are determined by your marijuana use?
5. Do you smoke marijuana to avoid dealing with your problems?
6. Do you smoke pot to cope with your feelings?
7. Does your marijuana use let you live in a privately defined world?
8. Have you ever failed to keep promises you made about cutting down or controlling your dope smoking?
9. Has your use of marijuana caused problems with memory, concentration, or motivation?
10. When your stash is nearly empty, do you feel anxious or worried about how to get more?
11. Do you plan your life around your marijuana use?
12. Have friends or relatives ever complained that your pot smoking is damaging your relationship with them?

(Marijuana Anonymous)

Detoxification guidelines

No medication is generally required.

The use of mandrax

The active ingredient in mandrax is the synthetic chemical, methaqualone. Mandrax causes physical addiction, which soon leads to tolerance. This substance is forbidden in South Africa. It is usually taken by mouth in tablet form, but in southern Africa it is generally smoked with dagga, a method practically unique to this part of the world.

The drug appears in the urine for up to 14 days but can be present for up to 21 days for chronic users.

Mandrax is used mainly for the relief of insomnia and anxiety. It causes a strong physiological dependence, and the physical effects include impaired functioning of the respiratory and circulatory systems. Many users of the substance die of an overdose or in accidents, the latter due to the fact that mandrax reduces vigilance and causes mental apathy.

The use of inhalants (industrial and household substances)

This heterogeneous group of substances can cause general suppression of the central nervous system. It includes glue, benzene, petrol, nail polish remover, naphtha, fluorocarbons, turpentine and paint thinners. These substances belong to the groups of chemicals known as volatile hydrocarbons and volatile fluorocarbons. Inhalants are used for the euphoric sensation that they induce within 15 to 45 minutes. They are freely available, cheap and legal, and easily hidden. They are used to alter the state of consciousness and cause sensations of light-headedness and disorientation. They are inhaled from plastic bags or directly from cloths, tissues or handkerchiefs (Weich, 2015). This form of addiction occurs mainly among young children who cannot afford more expensive substances.

Inhalants can engender strong psychological and physiological dependence and can cause serious physical damage. They damage the central and peripheral nervous systems, kidneys, liver and mucous membrane of the airways. They can also result in death from asphyxiation as they cause spasm of the larynx. Cardiac failure may also occur.

Table 15.6 Symptoms associated with common dependence-producing substances

Physiological signs	Psychological signs and symptoms	Withdrawal symptoms
Dagga (cannabis or marijuana)		
<ul><li>Fine tremors</li><li>Slight reduction in temperature</li><li>Decreased muscle strength and balance</li><li>Decreased motor coordination</li><li>Dry mouth</li><li>Bloodshot eyes</li><li>Nausea and headache</li><li>Nystagmus</li><li>Slight hypotension</li><li>Elevated respiratory rate</li><li>Tachycardia</li></ul>	<ul><li>Euphoria</li><li>Feelings of relaxation and drowsiness</li><li>Increased libido</li><li>Distorted perception of time, distance and control</li><li>Uncontrollable laughter</li><li>Loss of contact with reality</li><li>Disintegration of body image</li><li>Somatosensory disturbance</li><li>Depersonalisation</li><li>Disorientation</li></ul>	<ul><li>Restlessness</li><li>Aggression</li><li>Insomnia</li><li>Lack of self-control</li><li>Moodiness</li><li>Irritability</li><li>Listlessness</li><li>Nausea</li><li>Loss of appetite</li><li>Headache</li></ul>

Physiological signs	Psychological signs and symptoms	Withdrawal symptoms
	▪ Anxiety that may lead to panic ▪ Paranoid delusions sometimes occur ▪ At behavioural level, conduct may vary between drowsiness and hyperactivity ▪ Chronic use may cause fluctuations of conduct and mood ▪ Feeling of irritation and aggressive outbursts ▪ General inadequacy ▪ Impaired occupational functioning and capacity for work ▪ Possible internalisation of an apathetic and unmotivated way of life	
Mandrax		
▪ Drowsiness ▪ Retarded thought processes ▪ Dull, thick-headed feeling ▪ Noticeable loss of weight ▪ Emaciation	▪ Feelings of relaxation and unreality ▪ Improved social interaction ▪ Absence of sexual inhibitions ▪ Lack of concentration ▪ Retarded thought ▪ Poor judgement ▪ General emotional instability	▪ Insomnia ▪ Nervousness ▪ Anxiety ▪ Nausea and vomiting ▪ Abdominal cramps ▪ Hallucinations ▪ Convulsions
Inhalants		

▪ Sensory
  – Light sensitivity
  – Eye irritation
  – Diplopia
  – Buzzing of the ears
▪ Respiratory
  – Sneezing
  – Sinus discharge
  – Cough
	▪ Forgetfulness
	▪ Inability to think logically and clearly
	▪ Disorientation
	▪ Ataxia
	▪ Visual and tactile hallucinations
	▪ Aggressive outbursts
	▪ Decreased inhibitions
	▪ Floating sensation
		▪ Hallucination
		▪ Depression
		▪ Anxiety
		▪ Impaired intellectual functioning
		▪ Delirium
		▪ Headache
		▪ Muscle spasms
		▪ Gastric distress
		▪ Aggressive outbursts
		▪ Sensation of cold

Physiological signs	Psychological signs and symptoms	Withdrawal symptoms

• Gastrointestinal
  – Nausea
  – Vomiting
  – Diarrhoea
  – Poor appetite
• Ataxia
• Chest pain
• Abnormal heart rhythm
• Muscle and joint pains
• Pallor
• Lethargy
• Tremors
• Thirst
• Drowsiness
• Rash round the nose and mouth
	• Incorrect perceptions or illusions
	• Amnesia
	• Behavioural disturbances	

Amphetamines including methamphetamine (tik) and cocaine		
• Hyperactivity • Increased vigour • Stereotypical behaviour • Hallucinations	• Euphoria • Gregariousness • Interpersonal sensitivity • Tension • Talkativeness • Grandiosity • Impaired judgement	• Withdrawal starts within 24 hours, and peaks within 2–4 days • Fatigue • Depression • Nightmares • Insomnia • Headaches • Sweating • Muscle cramps • Craving
Hallucinogens		
Sympathomimetic, so intoxication leads to: • Tachycardia • Hypertension • Sweating • Dilated pupils • Hyper-reflexia • Pyrexia	• Anxiety or depression • Ideas of reference • Impaired judgement • Perceptual abnormalities	• Craving • Hangover after ecstacy use • Insomnia • Fatigue • Drowsiness • Loss of balance • Headaches

→

Physiological signs	Psychological signs and symptoms	Withdrawal symptoms
Opioids		
- Flushing, orgasmic sensation - Drowsiness, lethargy - Constricted pupils - Respiratory depression - Hypotension - Bradicardia - Hypothermia - Impaired concentration and memory - Slurred speech - Long-term use leads to lowered sex drive and appetite, constipation and weight loss	- Euphoria and contentment - Long-term use leads to personality changes, mood swings	- Withdrawal starts within 10–48 hours, mild to severe - Lacrimation - Sweating - Yawning - Piloerection - Hypertension - Tachycardia - Hot and cold sweats - Muscle and joint pain - Nausea and vomiting

Source: UNODC, 2016

Cocaine and amphetamines

These drugs are used recreationally and lead to feelings of euphoria. They include the popular 'tik' (or 'tic'), currently the scourge of many individuals, families and communities in South Africa. People intoxicated with cocaine can have a variable heart rate and/or blood pressure, dilated pupils, perspiration or chills, nausea or vomiting, weight loss, psychomotor agitation or retardation, muscular weakness, respiratory depression, chest pain, confusion, seizures, dyskinesias, dystonias or coma. In terms of psychological indicators, one can also see aggression, and wildly irrational behaviour, which is called 'cocaine-agitated delirium'. The behaviour should be controlled as described in Chapter 11, 'Dealing with anger and aggression.'

The use of methamphetamine

This is a powerfully addictive stimulant that affects many areas of the central nervous system. It is a white, odourless, bitter-tasting crystalline powder that readily dissolves in water or alcohol. The drug can be easily made in clandestine laboratories from relatively inexpensive, over-the-counter ingredients such as ephedrine or pseudo-ephedrine and can be purchased at a relatively low cost. It can be smoked, snorted, orally ingested or injected intravenously. In South Africa it is typically smoked by placing the powder/crystal in a light bulb from which the metal thread has been removed. A lighter is used to heat the bulb and the fumes are inhaled. The drug appears in the urine after two to seven hours and is present for two to five days or longer, depending on pH (alkaline urine for up to nine days).

Methamphetamine triggers the release of epinephrine, norepinephrine and dopamine in the sympathetic nervous system.

Acute intoxication and/or overdose

Common effects of intoxication include euphoria, increased energy and self-confidence, insomnia, restlessness, irritability, heightened sense of sexuality and tremors. Overdose is characterised by dehydration, hyperthermia, convulsions, renal failure, stroke and myocardial infarction.

Long-term/chronic use

Prolonged use can result in severe weight loss/anorexia, severe dermatological problems, higher risk of seizures and uncontrollable rage/violent behaviour. Chronic mental health effects include confusion, impaired concentration and memory, hallucinations, insomnia, depressive reactions, psychotic reactions, paranoid reactions and panic disorders. Long-term use also increases the risk of contracting HIV/AIDS due to risky sexual behaviour.

Detoxification guidelines (cocaine, amphetamines, including tik)

No medical detoxification is required. Patients need a range of interventions such as motivational counselling, support and occasionally pharmacotherapy to manage symptoms.

Hallucinogens

Most of the hallucinogens are synthetically made and used for their effect on moods. Ecstasy or MDMA (3,4methylenedioxy-methamphetamine) is the most common drug of this kind in South Africa; it is used especially by young people at 'raves'. Heavy users may spend hours each day using or recovering from an episode of use. During acute intoxication or withdrawal, one needs do little more than keep the person safe, and make sure they do not become dehydrated or overheated. Diazepam can be used to calm the person if they are very restless.

Opioids

Dipipanone HCL (Wellconal), Pethidine HCL and heroin are the main opioids used in South Africa. While these drugs are very good for pain control, abusers usually use them for the euphoric feelings they induce. Due to their easy access to such drugs, health care professionals are among the most common abusers of these substances (Annagür, 2012). These drugs are extremely addictive, and although few people are involved in their abuse, the costs to such people, their families and communities are very high. The substances can be taken orally, smoked or administered by injection. The drugs lead to tolerance, so that the person needs higher and higher doses to satisfy the craving.

Detoxification guidelines

Detoxification must be coupled with rehabilitation. The person should move directly from a detoxification to a rehabilitation programme. The duration of withdrawal symptoms depends on the half-life of the drug: pethidine, onset within four to six hours; heroin, onset within six to eight hours; morphine, onset within eight to twelve hours; codeine after 24 hours; methadone after 36 hours.

Uncomplicated and mild symptoms can be managed with an antispasmodic, for example hyoscine for abdominal cramps, ibuprofen for muscle pains and diazepam for the irritability and anxiety associated with withdrawal. Moderate to severe withdrawal requires methadone detoxification and hospitalisation. (Weich, 2015)

TREATMENT OF SUBSTANCE-DEPENDENT PEOPLE

The treatment of substance-dependent individuals is a complex problem, since psychological, social and medical aspects must be taken into account. The following aspects emphasise the importance of active treatment:
- the social costs of treatment programmes
- the harm that dependent individuals do to themselves.

People who are substance dependent are frequently members of subcultures that are poorly integrated with the broader community and often reject social norms. This makes it difficult to involve them in treatment.

The aim of treatment is not so much an immediate cure as gradual improvement of the behaviour. To this end, realistic but simple and limited objectives which patients will accept as being within reach, should be set.

Treatment depends on factors such as the abilities of the individual, the duration of the dependence, the type of substance used, the available treatment facilities, the objectives of the dependent person and the presence of physical and psychological complications.

Motivational interviewing has been found to be effective in the management of addiction in randomised trials across a range of conditions and settings (Smedslund et al, 2011). Key strategies in motivational interviewing (Resnicow & McMaster, 2012) which are effective in the management of patients with an addiction, include:
- *Reflective listening.* These begin with the phrase, 'It sounds like...'. However, others use words like, 'You are having trouble with...'. Through reflection, the nurse demonstrates that the patient has been heard, thereby affirming the patient's thoughts and feelings without judgement. It is important to suppress the instinct to respond with questions or advice. Reflection tests whether the nurse has understood the content of the patient statement.

- *Rolling with resistance.* Rather than confronting patients about their alcohol abuse which may result in an argument, the nurse should 'roll with resistance'. An example could be: 'You really enjoy drinking alcohol. You look forward to relaxing with a few drinks when you are stressed and giving up seems very difficult.' Statements such as this capture the patient's reasons for not changing their behaviour and allows them to express their resistance without feeling pressured to change or worrying about being judged.
- *Change talk.* Patients are more likely to accept and act on opinions that they voice. The more the patient argues for a position, the greater their commitment to it often becomes. Patients are encouraged to express their own reasons and plans for stopping alcohol use. This process is referred to as eliciting change talk.

The short-term objectives of treatment are the initiation and support of uncomplicated withdrawal or detoxification of the substance, as well as treatment of any physical complications that may be present. Detoxification may be facilitated by blocking the dependence-producing appetite by means of chemical agents such as methadone or a narcotic antagonist. Criminal activity, such as theft to obtain money for the substances, should be stopped from the outset.

As soon as withdrawal is completed, patients are involved in a therapeutic programme that covers the physical, psychological and social aspects of functioning. The will to avoid the substance and not to try to obtain it is reinforced in every possible way. New, healthy behaviour patterns are established and reinforced at the same time.

During treatment, attempts are made to break the pathological structure of substance dependence. This means that patients should be removed from their substance-centred culture and, if appropriate, also from their pathological family structure. This helps to reduce their negative effects. Guidelines for a less substance-centred way of life should be given in this phase.

One of the most important factors in the management of substance-dependent patients is the reduction of anxiety and confusion about their own value systems. Problem areas in the management of these patients consequently centre on their reliance on a lifestyle of substance dependence, which affords them a constant source of excitement, challenge and adventure, while authority, responsibility and emotional pain are suppressed. This is why the attainment of independence and confidence is stressed. Patients also have to be freed of their overwhelming anxiety in order to establish a more adaptable lifestyle.

Tertiary prevention emphasises the functions and contributions of social support systems. The most important contributions of a social network are emotional support, task-oriented aid and communication that focus on evaluation and expectations, particularly the establishment of a sense of belonging. Support groups, whether they be the family, friends or members of the community, therefore have the task of rendering assistance in order that patients may learn to cope more effectively with their environment. Their assistance enables patients to assess problem areas, plan and implement problem-solving methods, and evaluate the results with the aid of feedback information.

CONCLUSION

Alcohol and substance dependence constitute a tremendous problem in South African society. Because of the interweaving of these problems with other socioeconomic and political problems, prevention and treatment are more problematic. This needs to be addressed on a broad front by society itself.

The key position of nurses in the health services and their wide distribution in the community demand that they play a cardinal role in the fight against this debilitating disorder.

WEB RESOURCES

http://www.sahealthinfo.org/admodule/sacendu.htm
> This is the website of the South African Community Epidemiology Network on Drug Use (SACENDU) which is funded by the Medical Research Council and the National Department of Health. This website gives you data on alcohol and other drug (AOD) use and associated consequences on a six-monthly basis from specialist AOD treatment programmes.

http://www.addictions.org
> This website not only directs you to specific sites for different addictions, it also offers resources to assist a person in recovering from a range of addictions, including drugs and alcohol.

http://www.niaaa.nih.gov
> This is the website of the National Institutes of Alcohol Abuse and Alcoholism, which is the major research organisation of the USA government. It is a very useful site, with answers to frequently asked questions, databases on the topic, and publications. It also has a graphics gallery, where you can access all kinds of illustrations for talks and lectures. One such a diagram is the ecological model of drinking behaviour, which is very useful for teaching.

http://www.who.int/substance_abuse/facts/alcohol/en/
> This is the WHO's 2017 information on the topic of alcohol.

The following sites represent some of the consumer websites in this area:
www.alcoholic-anonymous.org: Alcoholic Anonymous
www.na.org: Narcotics Anonymous
www.ca.org: Cocaine Anonymous
www. Sancanational.info: South African Council on Alcoholism and Drug Dependence.

REFERENCES

American Addiction Centers. 2018. 'Alcohol withdrawal treatment, symptoms and timelines: Learn if detox is needed'. www. americanaddictioncentres.org (Accessed September 2018).

American Psychiatric Association (APA). 2013. *Diagnostic and Statistical Manual of Mental Disorders – 5TM*. Washington, DC: American Psychiatric Association.

Annagür, B B. 2012. 'A Nurse with Pethidine Addiction'. *European Journal of General Medicine*, 9 (1): 59–61.

Antai-Otong, D. 2008. *Psychiatric Nursing: Biological and behavioural concepts*. 2nd edition. New York: Delmar.

Barclay, G A, Barbour, J, Stewart, S, Day C P and Gilvarry, E. 2008. 'Adverse physical effects of alcohol misuse'. *Advances in Psychiatric Treatment*, 14: 139–151. doi: 10.1192/apt.bp.105.001263.

Benton, S. 2009. *Understanding the High-Functioning Alcoholic: Professional Views and Personal Insights (Praeger Series on Contemporary Health & Living)*. Connecticut: Greenwood Publishers. https://www.soberrecovery.com/forums/ (Accessed December 2018).

Berk, B. 2013. 'Effective Substance Abuse Prevention: why it matters, what works, and what the experts see for the future'. Community Prevention Initiative. http://www.ca-cpi.org/docs/Publications/Other/EffectiveSubstanceAbusePrevention_March2013.pdf (Accessed December 2018).

Bourne, P G and Fox, R. 1973. *Alcoholism: Progress in research and treatment*. New York: Academic Press.

Bremmer, P, Burnett, J, Nunney, F, Ravat, M and Mistral, W. 2011. 'Young people, alcohol and influences: A study of young people and their relationship with alcohol'. Joseph Rowntree Foundation. www.jrf.org.uk (Accessed June 2017).

Chauke, TM, Van der Heever, H and Hoque, ME. 2015. 'Alcohol use amongst learners in rural high school in South Africa'. *Africa Journal of Primary Health Care Family Medicine*, 7 (1). doi: 10.4102/phcfm.v7i.755.

Cole, D. 1990. 'Identifying the alcohol misuser'. *Nursing Times*, 86 (16): 58–59.

Crean, R D, Crane, N A and Mason, B J. 2011. 'An Evidence-based Review of Acute and Long-Term Effects of Cannabis Use on Executive Cognitive Functions'. *Journal of Addictive Medicine*. 5 (1): 1–8.

Dada, S, Harker Burnhams, N, Erasmus, J, Parry, C, Bhana A, Timol, F and Fourie, D. 2015. 'Monitoring alcohol, tobacco and other drug abuse trends in South Africa (July–December 2014)'. *South African Community Epidemiology Network on Drug Use (SACENDU)*. www.mrc.ac.za/intramural-research-units/ATOD-sacendu (Accessed June 2017).

Department of Health. 2013. *National Mental Health Policy Framework and Strategic Plan 2013-2020*. Department of Health: Pretoria.

Estes, N J. 1974. 'Counselling the wife of an alcoholic spouse'. *American Journal of Nursing*, 74 (7): 1251–1255.

Ewing, J A. 1984. 'Detecting alcoholism: The CAGE questionnaire'. *JAMA: The Journal of the American Medical Association*, 252 (14): 1905–1907.

Heinemann, E and Estes, N. 1976. 'Assessing alcoholic patients'. *American Journal of Nursing*, 76 (5): 785–789.

Jellinek, E M. 1952. 'Phases of alcohol addiction'. *Journal of Studies in Alcohol*, 13 (4): 673–684.

London, L. 1999. 'The "dop" system, alcohol abuse and social control amongst farm workers in South Africa: a public health challenge'. *Social Science & Medicine* 48, 10: 1407.

Marijuana Anonymous. 'The Twelve Questions of Marijuana Anonymous'. https://www.marijuana-anonymous.org/the-twelve-questions-of-marijuana-anonymous/ (Accessed December 2018).

Matzopoulos R G, Truen S, Bowman B and Corrigall J. 2014. 'The cost of harmful alcohol use in South Africa'. *South African Medical Journal*. 104: 127–32.

Muhrer, J C. 2010. 'Detecting and dealing with substance abuse disorders in primary care'. *Journal of Nurse Practitioner*, 6: 597–605.

National Institute on Drug Abuse. 2010. *Research Report Series, Comorbidity: Addiction and Other Mental Illnesses*. US Department of Health and Human Services. United States of America.

O'Brien, C P. 2008. 'The CAGE Questionnaire for Detection of Alcoholism'. *JAMA*, 300 (17): 2054–2056. doi: 10.1001/jama.2008.570.

Razvodovsky. Y E. 2016. 'Affordability of Vodka and Liver Cirrhosis Mortality Rates in Russia'. *ARC Journal of Addiction*, 1 (1): 16–20.

Resnicow, N and McMaster, F. 2012. 'Motivational Interviewing: moving from why to how with autonomy support'. *International Journal of Behavioral Nutrition and Physical Activity,* **9** (9).

Scott, K A, Dalgleish A G and Liu W M. 2014. 'The combination of cannabidiol and Δ9-tetrahydrocannabinol enhances the anticancer effects of radiation in an orthotopic murine glioma model'. *Mol Cancer Therapy.* 13 (12): 2955–2967. doi: 10.1158/1535-7163.MCT-14-0402.

Schuckit, M A. 2014. 'Recognition and management of withdrawal delirium (delirium tremens)'. *N Engl Journal of Medicine,* 371: 2109–2113. doi: 10.1056/NEJMra1407298.

Seggie, J. 2012. 'Alcohol and South Africa's Youth'. *South African Medical Journal,* 102 (7): 587.

Senthil, M. 2016. 'Family interaction pattern and co-dependency in spouses of alcohol dependence in comparison with normal control'. *International Journal of Research,* 4 (2): 121–128.

Smedslund, G, Berg, R C, Hammerstrøm K T, Steiro, A, Leiknes, K A, Dahl, H M and Karlsen, K. 2011. 'Motivational Interviewing for Substance Abuse'. *Campbell Systematic Reviews* 6. http://www.campbellcollaboration.org/lib/project/100/.

Steers, M L N, Coffman, A D Wickham, R E, Bryan, J L and Caraway L. 2016. 'Evaluation of alcohol-related personalized normative feedback with and without an injunctive message'. *Journal of studies on alcohol and drugs,* 77 (2): 337–342.

Townsend, M C. 2011. *Nursing Diagnoses in Psychiatric Nursing.* 8th edition. Philadelphia: F A Davis.

Trevisan, L A, Boutros, N, Ismene, L, Petrakis, M D and Krystal, J H. 1998. 'Complications of alcohol withdrawal; pathophysiological insights'. *Alcohol Health & Research World,* 22 (1).

United Nations (UN). 2015. *Report of the International Narcotics Control Board for 2014.* Vienna.

United Nations Office on Drugs and Crime (UNODC). 2016. *World Drug Report 2016.* United Nations publication, Sales No. E.16.XI.7.

Vargas, D, de Oliveira, M A F and Luís, M A V. 2010. 'Care of alcoholic persons in primary care services: perceptions and actions of registered nurses'. *Acta Paulista de Enfermagen,* 23 (1).

Wagenaar, A C, Todler, A L and Komro, K A. 2010. 'Effects of alcohol tax and price policies on morbidity and mortality: a systematic review'. *American Journal of Public Health,* 100 (11): 2270–2277.

Weich, L. 2015. 'Alcohol and other substance-use disorders'. Chapter 25. In: Bauman, S E (ed), *Primary Care Psychiatry: A Practical Guide for Southern Africa.* 2nd edition. Cape Town: Juta.

World Health Organisation (WHO). 2010. *Global Strategy to reduce the harmful use of alcohol.* Geneva: WHO.

World Health Organisation (WHO). 2014. *Global Status Report on Alcohol and health.* Geneva: WHO.

CHAPTER 16

Nursing the Patient with a Neurocognitive Disorder

L R Uys, L Middleton and V van Zyl

Learning Outcomes

After studying this chapter, you should be able to:
- explain the different concepts and aetiology relating to neurocognitive disorders (NCDs)
- distinguish between delirium and major NCD; mild and major NCD; and major NCD and major depressive disorder
- outline the cognitive domains and levels of functioning
- perform a mini-mental state examination (MMSE) and interpret results
- apply appropriate nursing interventions for individuals living with neurocognitive disorders
- liaise with family members and caregivers
- describe the guidelines when using medicine in the elderly
- assist the person with epilepsy to adjust and cope with the condition.

INTRODUCTION

An individual's cognitive function is directly related to quality of life. The number of people developing an NCD is increasing as the population ages. The prevalence of dementia is anticipated to rise exponentially, with an estimated 35.6 million people living with dementia worldwide in 2010, and numbers expected to almost double every 20 years, to 65.7 million in 2030 and 115.4 million in 2050 (Tay et al, 2015). Previously termed cognitive disorder, the term was changed in the DSM-5 to NCD. The DSM-5 classifies the NCDs and presents diagnostic criteria in order to identify and distinguish between the three clusters: delirium; mild NCD, and major NCD. Figure 16.1 illustrates how the NCDs comprise these three syndromes.

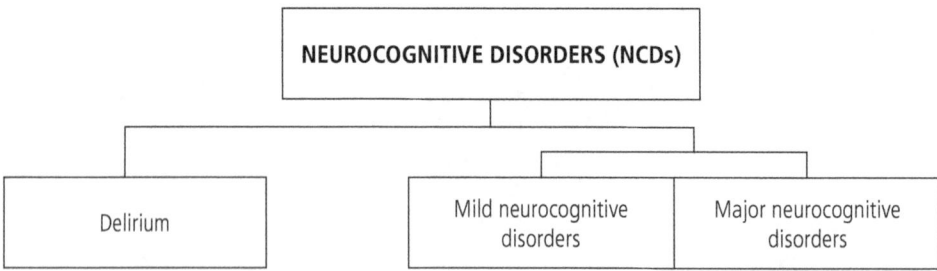

Figure 16.1 The three clusters of NCDs

The high incidence, irreversibility and co-existence with other psychiatric illnesses, together with misconceptions, myths and stereotypes, increase the stigma associated with NCDs. Although dementia is still retained in the DSM-5, the preferred usage is major NCD. This is to decrease the stigma which can impact negatively on the care, treatment and rehabilitation of people and families affected by NCDs.

This chapter focuses on explaining the different subtypes and outlines their diagnostic criteria, identifying causes, nursing care problems, and implementation of appropriate and effective nursing interventions for individuals living with NCDs. The last part of the chapter will focus on people living with epilepsy. Nurses and psychiatric nurses practising in hospitals, clinics and community settings are well placed to identify vulnerable individuals early, understand the trajectory of their NCD, and intervene with effective individual and family-centred psychosocial treatment and support programmes. Early recognition, therapeutic intervention and environmental manipulation can save lives, improve the quality of life of a person living with an NCD, and minimise the burden of care (Simpson, 2014).

INCIDENCE AND PREVALENCE OF DELIRIUM AND MILD AND MAJOR NCDs

Delirium is common in elderly patients and there is a profound increase in cases where cognitive impairment, because of NCDs, already exists (APA, 2013). The DSM-5 (APA, 2013) reports that delirium is prevalent in up to 60 per cent of individuals in nursing homes or post-acute care settings and can be present in up to 83 per cent of all individuals at the end of life. Substance intoxication or withdrawal, human immunodeficiency virus (HIV)/acquired immunodeficiency syndrome (AIDS), Parkinson's disease, hypertension, hospitalisation, post-operative and intensive care admissions increase the prevalence of delirium and pose a medico-legal risk. This risk stems from possible injuries, because of perceptual disturbances (hallucinations, illusions) and unpredicted and rapid shifts in emotions and behaviour.

Delirium may progress to stupor, coma, seizures, or death, particularly if the underlying cause remains untreated. Mortality among hospitalised individuals with delirium is high, and as many as 40 per cent of individuals with delirium, particularly those with malignancies and other significant underlying medical illness, die over the ensuing year (APA, 2013; Uys & Middleton, 2014). Delirium in the elderly may be associated with longer hospital stays, more intensive caregiving, and higher mortality up to a year after hospitalisation. Correct identification, and proper management of delirium is therefore important.

The incidence of major NCD (dementia), on the other hand, increases steeply with age, with a prevalence as high as 30 per cent by the age of 85 years. It is significant that several of the NCDs frequently coexist with another NCD (APA, 2013). In South Africa the high incidence and comorbidity of substance abuse, chronic diseases, HIV/AIDS, and other stressors, which include challenging socioeconomic conditions and high levels of violence, increase the risk of NCDs and contribute significantly to the global burden of disease (Western Cape Department of Health, 2013). The elderly are particularly vulnerable to both delirium and NCDs. Cognitive changes in the elderly, especially in those with mild NCDs, are considered by many health workers and family members to be part of the normal process of ageing and are often overlooked. Health workers, specifically nursing staff and care workers, should be observant when caring for the elderly.

UNDERSTANDING NCDs

The prevalence of NCDs is worldwide. According to Larner (2017), populations worldwide are ageing due to many factors such as industrialisation, living a healthier lifestyle and the prevention and treatment of illnesses. The disorders are acquired rather than developmental, meaning that they would not have been present since birth or early life. The key clinical concern of these syndromes is a decline in cognitive functioning from a previously attained level of functioning, in one or more of the six neurocognitive domains.

Cognition consists of three components: perception, thought and memory. Perception refers to the way in which the brain receives information through the five senses, thought involves the way in which the brain interprets this information, and memory (and learning) consists of stored knowledge and the ability to recall information (Baumann, 2015). The domain of social cognition has only recently been included in the DSM-5. The person with an NCD can also present with psychological and behavioural problems at some point during the course of the illness (Regier & Gitlin, 2017). Socially inappropriate behaviour is a prominent feature of NCDs and was previously referred to as personality change (Sachdev et al, 2014). In a person with an NCD, the interaction between input-and-output processing is affected and changes in the individual's perceptual-motor functions, language skills, executive skills, learning and memory, attention and social cognition (the neurocognitive domains) influence their ability to interact meaningfully with the environment. Figure 16.2 represents the six neurocognitive domains which form the basis on which a diagnosis for NCDs is made.

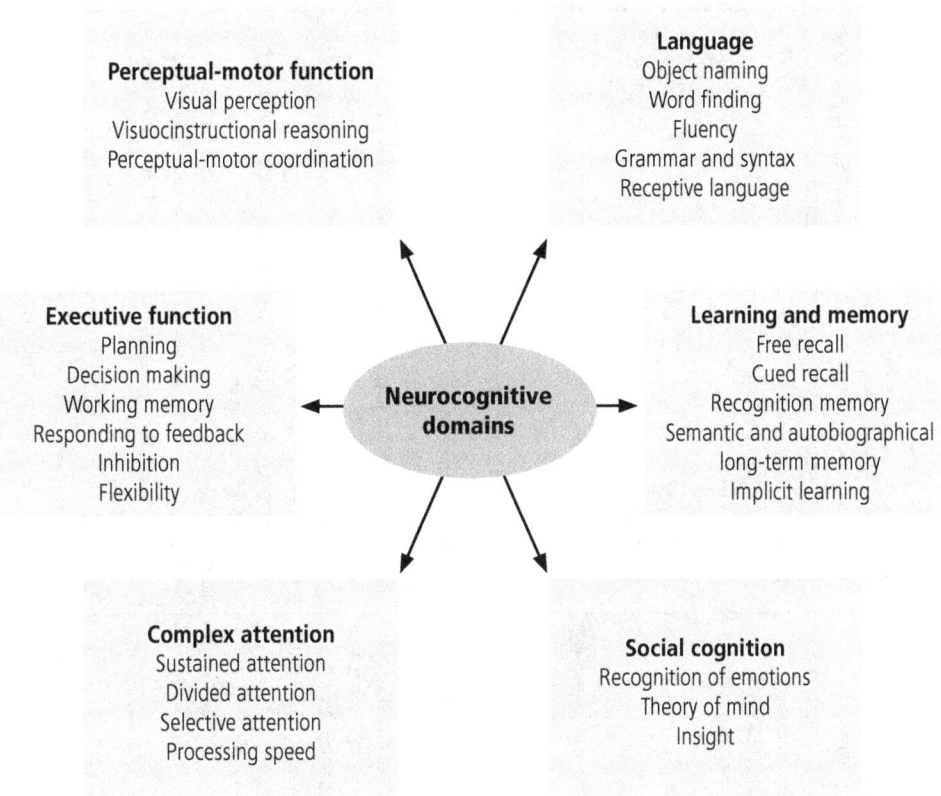

Figure 16.2 Neurocognitive domains

Source: Sachdev et al (2014)

An assessment that shows there has been a decline in the cognitive functioning of the different domains and related deficits in everyday activities would indicate an NCD (Sachdev et al, 2014). Table 16.1 illustrates the six neurocognitive domains and assessment examples.

Table 16.1 The neurocognitive domains

Cognitive domain	Examples of symptoms or observations	Examples of assessments
Complex attention (sustained attention, divided attention, selective attention, processing speed)	*Major:* Has increased difficulty in environments with multiple stimuli (TV, radio, conversation); is easily distracted by competing events in the environment. Is unable to attend unless input is restricted and simplified. Has difficulty holding new information in mind, such as recalling phone numbers or addresses just given, or reporting what was just said. Is unable to perform mental calculations. All thinking takes longer than usual, and components to be processed must be simplified to one or a few. *Mild:* Normal tasks take longer than previously. Begins to find errors in routine tasks; finds work needs more double-checking than previously. Thinking is easier when not competing with other things (radio, TV, other conversations, cell phone, driving).	*Sustained attention:* Maintenance of attention over time (e.g., pressing a button every time a tone is heard, and over a period of time). *Selective attention:* Maintenance of attention despite competing stimuli and/or distractors: hearing numbers and letters read and asked to count only letters. *Divided attention:* Attending to two tasks within the same time period: rapidly tapping while learning a story being read. Processing speed can be quantified on any task by timing it (e.g., time to put together a design of blocks; time to match symbols with numbers; speed in responding, such as counting speed or serial 3 speed).
Executive function (planning, decision making, working memory, responding to feedback/ error correction, overriding habits/ inhibition, mental flexibility)	*Major:* Abandons complex projects. Needs to focus on one task at a time. Needs to rely on others to plan instrumental activities of daily living or make decisions. *Mild:* Increased effort required to complete multistage projects. Has increased difficulty multitasking or difficulty resuming a task interrupted by a visitor or phone call. May complain of increased fatigue from the extra effort required to organize, plan, and make decisions. May report that large social gatherings are more taxing or less enjoyable because of increased effort required to follow shifting conversations.	*Planning:* Ability to find the exit to a maze; interpret a sequential picture or object arrangement. *Decision making:* Performance of tasks that assess process of deciding in the face of competing alternatives (e.g., simulated gambling). *Working memory:* Ability to hold information for a brief period and to manipulate it (e.g., adding up a list of numbers or repeating a series of numbers or words backward). *Feedback/error utilisation:* Ability to benefit from feedback to infer the rules for solving a problem. *Overriding habits/inhibition:* Ability to choose a more complex and effortful solution to be correct (e.g., looking away from the direction indicated by an arrow, naming the color of a word's font rather than naming the word). *Mental/cognitive flexibility:* Ability to shift between two concepts, tasks, or response rules (e.g., from number to letter, from verbal to key-press response, from adding numbers to ordering numbers, from ordering objects by size to ordering by color).

Cognitive domain	Examples of symptoms or observations	Examples of assessments
Learning and memory (immediate memory, recent memory [including free recall, cued recall, and recognition memory], very-long-term memory [semantic; autobiographical], implicit learning)	*Major*: Has significant difficulties with expressive or receptive language. Often uses general-use phrases such as "that thing" and "you know what I mean," and prefers general pronouns rather than names. With severe impairment, may not even recall names of closer friends and family. Idiosyncratic word usage, grammatical errors, and spontaneity of output and economy of utterances occur. Stereotypy of speech occurs; echolalia and automatic speech typically precede mutism. *Mild*: Has noticeable word-finding difficulty. May substitute general for specific terms. May avoid use of specific names of acquaintances. Grammatical errors involve subtle omission or incorrect use of articles, prepositions, auxiliary verbs, etc.	*Immediate memory span*: Ability to repeat a list of words or digits. *Note*: Immediate memory sometimes subsumed under "working memory" (see "Executive Function"). *Recent memory*: Assesses the process of encoding new information (e.g., word lists, a short story, or diagrams). The aspects of recent memory that can be tested include 1) free recall (the person is asked to recall as many words, diagrams, or elements of a story as possible); 2) cued recall (examiner aids recall by providing semantic cues such as "List all the food items on the list" or "Name all of the children from the story"); and 3) recognition memory (examiner asks about specific items—e.g., "Was 'apple' on the list?" or "Did you see this diagram or figure?"). Other aspects of memory that can be assessed include semantic memory (memory for facts), autobiographical memory (memory for personal events or people), and implicit (procedural) learning (unconscious learning of skills).
Language (expressive language [including naming, word finding, fluency, and grammar, and syntax] and receptive language)	*Major*: Has significant difficulties with expressive or receptive language. Often uses general-use phrases such as "that thing" and "you know what I mean," and prefers general pronouns rather than names. With severe impairment, may not even recall names of closer friends and family. Idiosyncratic word usage, grammatical errors, and spontaneity of output and economy of utterances occur. Stereotypy of speech occurs; echolalia and automatic speech typically precede mutism. *Mild*: Has noticeable word-finding difficulty. May substitute general for specific terms. May avoid use of specific names of acquaintances. Grammatical errors involve subtle omission or incorrect use of articles, prepositions, auxiliary verbs, etc.	*Expressive language*: Confrontational naming (identification of objects or pictures); fluency (e.g., name as many items as possible in a semantic [e.g., animals] or phonemic [e.g., words starting with "f"] category in 1 minute). *Grammar and syntax* (e.g., omission or incorrect use of articles, prepositions, auxiliary verbs): Errors observed during naming and fluency tests are compared with norms to assess frequency of errors and compare with normal slips of the tongue. *Receptive language*: Comprehension (word definition and object-pointing tasks involving animate and inanimate stimuli): performance of actions/activities according to verbal command.

Cognitive domain	Examples of symptoms or observations	Examples of assessments
Perceptual-motor (includes abilities subsumed under the terms visual perception, visuoconstructional, perceptual-motor, praxis, and gnosis)	*Major:* Has significant difficulties with previously familiar activities (using tools, driving motor vehicle), navigating in familiar environments; is often more confused at dusk, when shadows and lowering levels of light change perceptions. *Mild:* May need to rely more on maps or others for directions. Uses notes and follows others to get to a new place. May find self lost or turned around when not concentrating on task. Is less precise in parking. Needs to expend greater effort for spatial tasks such as carpentry, assembly, sewing, or knitting.	*Visual perception:* Line bisection tasks can be used to detect basic visual defect or attentional neglect. Motor-free perceptual tasks (including facial recognition) require the identification and/or matching of figures-best when tasks cannot be verbally mediated (e.g., figures are not objects); some require the decision of whether a figure can be "real" or not based on dimensionality. *Visuoconstructional:* Assembly of items requiring hand-eye coordination, such as drawing, copying, and block assembly. *Perceptual-motor:* Integrating perception with purposeful movement (e.g., inserting blocks into a form board without visual cues; rapidly inserting pegs into a slotted board).
Social cognition (recognition of emotions, theory of mind)	*Major:* Behavior clearly out of acceptable social range; shows insensitivity to social standards of modesty in dress or of political, religious, or sexual topics of conversation. Focuses excessively on a topic despite group's disinterest or direct feedback. Behavioral intention without regard to family or friends. Makes decisions without regard to safety (e.g., inappropriate clothing for weather or social setting). Typically, has little insight into these changes. *Mild:* Has subtle changes in behavior or attitude, often described as a change in personality, such as less ability to recognize social cues or read facial expressions, decreased empathy, increased extraversion or introversion, decreased inhibition, or subtle or episodic apathy or restlessness.	*Recognition of emotions:* Identification of emotion in images of faces representing a variety of both positive and negative emotions. *Theory of mind:* Ability to consider another person's mental state (thoughts, desires, intentions) or experience-story cards with questions to elicit information about the mental state of the individuals portrayed, such as "Where will the girl look for the lost bag?" or "Why is the boy sad?"

Source: APA (2013: 593–595)

THE AETIOLOGY OR CAUSES OF NCDs

A diagnosis of an NCD is determined by its cause, as well as cognitive, functional and behavioural symptoms. The DSM-5 describes the causative factors (see Table 16.2); the specific features or diagnostic criteria (see Tables 16.4 and 16.5); and the cognitive and functioning decline according to the neurocognitive domains (see Table 16.6).

Table 16.2 The aetiology or causes of delirium and major and mild NCDs according to the DSM-5

DELIRIUM	NCD Mild and major NCD
▪ Substance intoxication: Alcohol, cannabis, phencyclidine, other hallucinogen, inhalant, opioid, sedative, hypnotic, or anxiolytic, amphetamine (or other stimulant), cocaine, or other (unknown) substance ▪ Substance withdrawal delirium ▪ Medication-induced delirium ▪ Delirium due to another medical condition ▪ Delirium due to multiple etiologies ▪ The course: acute or persistent and psychomotor activity: hyperactive, hypoactive or normal	▪ Alzheimer's disease ▪ Frontotemporal lobar degeneration ▪ Lewy body disease ▪ Vascular disease ▪ Traumatic brain injury ▪ Substance/medication use ▪ HIV/AIDS infection ▪ Prion disease ▪ Parkinson's disease ▪ Huntington's disease ▪ Another medical condition ▪ Multiple etiologies ▪ Unspecified

Source: APA (2013)

Causative and risk factors for delirium

In delirium (see Table 16.2) there is disturbance in awareness which can be caused by substance intoxication or withdrawal, an underlying medical condition, exposure to toxins or a combination of factors (Sachdev et al, 2014). Delirium is seldom caused by a single factor and attention should be given to predisposing or general risk factors such as: age (younger than 10 years and older than 65 years); cognitive impairment (dementia, previous head injury); visual or hearing impairments; dehydration and malnutrition; an underlying medical condition; substance intoxication or withdrawal or a combination of these factors (Baumann, 2015). Some of the causes of delirium are also outlined in Table 16.3, represented by the mnemonic, MENDAMIND. While the DSM-5 mainly focuses on substance withdrawal and intoxication, the focus in this table is more on the physiological/medical conditions.

Table 16.3 Causes of delirium as represented by MENDAMIND

	Cause	Examples
M	**M**etabolic and endocrine disorders	Electrolyte disturbances (dehydration) Acid/base disturbances Organ failure (hepatic, respiratory, cardiac, renal); pituitary problems (thyroid, adrenal, pancreas, hypoglycaemia)
E	**E**pilepsy	Generalised, ictal, post-ictal
N	**N**eoplasma and tumours	Primary; secondary; non-metastatic
D	**D**eficiency disorders	Thiamine; Niacin; B12; Folate
A	**A**ge **A**rterial diseases	Younger than 10 years; older than 65 years Large or multiple infarcts, emboli, arteriosclerosis
M	**M**echanical	Head injuries (trauma, subdural and extradural haemorrhages); dementia
I	**I**nfections	Cerebral (encephalitis/meningoencephalitis, abscesses, neurosyphilis, HIV/AIDS) Extracerebral (urinary tract infections, pneumonias, tuberculosis)
N	**N**utritional deficiencies	Malnutrition (lack of protein)
D	**D**rugs and toxins (either intoxication or withdrawal)	Most common to least common: alcohol, and other proactive agents, such as hypnotic, anxiolytic, anticonvulsants and analgesics; anticholinergic drugs, antituberculosis drugs, cytotoxins and anti-Parkinson's drugs; industrial poisons and heavy metals

Source: Adapted from Baumann (2015); Uys and Middleton (2014)

Causes and symptoms of mild and major NCDs

In mild and major NCDs, the decline in performance, consistent memory and executive functioning is a concern for the individual, a knowledgeable informant or the clinician. In some major and mild NCDs, the cause or aetiology supports the diagnosis, as portrayed in Table 16.2. The general causes for mild and major NCDs are Parkinson's or Huntington's disease, or traumatic brain injury, stroke or neurodegenerative disease (APA, 2013). An NCD due to an infection from HIV/AIDS is usually more prevalent in individuals with prior episodes of severe immunosuppression.

Individuals with advanced NCDs may experience prominent neuro-motor features such as severe incoordination, ataxia, and motor slowing. There may be loss of emotional control, including aggressive or inappropriate affect or apathy. The influence of many factors like comorbid secondary infections, medical illness, substances and the fact that HIV/AIDS can affect a variety of brain regions, makes a confirmed diagnosis more challenging (APA, 2013).

These NCDs can be caused by Alzheimer's disease which is a neurodegenerative disorder with an insidious onset and gradual progression. The cognitive deficit includes amnesia and feature as a decline in learning and memory (Sachdev et al, 2014). The prominence of memory loss can cause significant difficulties relatively early in the course. Social cognition (and thus social functioning) and procedural memory (for example dancing, playing musical instruments) may be relatively preserved for extended periods. Some individuals can live with the disease for as long as 20 years (APA, 2013).

A vascular-related NCD is caused by cerebrovascular disease and includes both ischaemic and haemorrhagic lesions (Sachdev et al, 2014). The lesions may be focal, multifocal, or diffuse and occur in various combinations (APA, 2013). Neuroimaging (MRI or CT scans) support the diagnosis. Risk factors for vascular NCDs are hypertension, diabetes, obesity and metabolic syndrome, and they also increase the risk for AD (APA, 2013).

An NCD with Lewy body disease (NCDLB) is a gradually progressive disorder with insidious onset. There are early changes in complex attention (Sachdev et al, 2014). Individuals with NCDLB are more functionally impaired than a person living with AD. The motor and autonomic impairments cause problems with toileting, mobility, eating and sleeping, which markedly decrease a person's quality of life (APA, 2013).

Frontotemporal NCD is characterised by the progressive deterioration in behaviour, personality and/or language (aphasia). Individuals present with varying degrees of apathy or disinhibition and may lose interest in socialisation, self-care, and personal responsibilities, or display socially inappropriate behaviours. Insight is usually impaired (APA, 2013).

DSM-5 CLASSIFICATION OF DELIRIUM AND MAJOR NCDs

The DSM-5 diagnostic criteria for delirium and dementia are reflected Tables 16.4 and 16.5.

Table 16.4 DSM-5 diagnostic criteria for delirium

DSM-5 diagnostic criteria for delirium
A. A disturbance in attention, ie reduced ability to direct focus, sustain, and shift attention and awareness (reduced orientation to the environment).
B. The disturbance develops over a short period of time (usually hours to a few days), represents a change from baseline attention and awareness, and tends to fluctuate in severity during the course of the day.
C. An additional disturbance in cognition (for example memory deficit, disorientation, language, visuospatial ability or perception).
D. The disturbances in Criteria A and C are not better explained by another pre-existing, established, or evolving NCD and do not occur in the context of a severely reduced level of arousal, such as coma.
E. There is evidence from the history, physical examination, or laboratory findings, that the disturbance is a direct physiological consequence of another medical condition, a substance intoxication or withdrawal (ie due to a drug of abuse or to a medication), or exposure to a toxin, or is due to multiple aetiologies.

Specify whether:
- Substance intoxication delirium or substance withdrawal delirium (specify substance)
- Medication-induced delirium/delirium due to another medical condition (specify)
- Delirium due to multiple aetiologies

Specify if:
Acute: Lasting a few hours or days.
Persistent: Lasting weeks or months.

Specify if:
Hyperactive: The individual has a hyperactive level of psychomotor activity that may be accompanied by mood lability, agitation, and/or refusal to cooperate with medical care.
Hypoactive: The individual has a hypoactive level of psychomotor activity that may be accompanied by sluggishness and lethargy that approaches stupor.
Mixed level of activity: The individual has a normal level of psychomotor activity even though attention and awareness are disturbed. This also includes individuals whose activity level rapidly fluctuates.

Source: APA (2013: 596–598)

Table 16.5 DSM-5 diagnostic criteria for major NCDs

DSM-5 diagnostic criteria for major NCD

A. Evidence of significant cognitive decline from a previous level of performance in one or more cognitive domains (complex attention, executive function, learning and memory, language, perceptual-motor or social cognition) based on:
   1. Concern of the individual, a knowledgeable informant, or the clinician that there has been a significant decline in cognitive function and
   2. A substantial impairment in cognitive performance, preferably documented by standardised neuropsychological testing or, in its absence, another qualified clinical assessment.
B. The cognitive deficits interfere with independence in everyday activities (ie at a minimum, requiring assistance with complex instrumental activities of daily living such as paying bills or managing medications).
C. The deficits do not occur exclusively in the context of a delirium.
D. The cognitive deficits are not better explained by another mental disorder (ie major depressive disorder, schizophrenia).

Specify whether due to:
- Alzheimer's disease
- Frontotemporal lobar degeneration
- Lewy body disease
- Vascular disease
- Traumatic brain injury
- Substance/medication use
- HIV infection
- Prion disease
- Parkinson's disease
- Huntington's disease
- Another medical condition

- Multiple aetiologies
- Unspecified

Specify:
- With or without behavioural disturbance

Specify current severity:
- Mild, moderate or severe

Source: APA (2013: 602–605)

DISTINGUISHING NCDs

The differences between delirium and major NCDs; and between mild and major NCDS will be explored.

Difference between delirium and major NCDs

Cognitive disturbances occur in both delirium and major NCD (dementia). In delirium, the essential feature is a disturbance in attention or awareness and in major NCD the cognitive decline is evident in one or more cognitive domains. Table 16.6 differentiates delirium from the major NCDs based on categories of onset, cause, duration, course, level of consciousness and effect on the major cognitive domains.

Table 16.6 Differences between delirium and major NCD

Category	Delirium	Major NCD
Onset	Abrupt, rapid (over a short period of time)	Insidious (months to years)
Cause	Medical condition, substance intoxication or withdrawal, use of a medication, or exposure to a toxin, or a combination of these factors	Trauma, degenerative illnesses (Alzheimer's disease, substances, Parkinson's, etc, causing damage to the brain tissue)
Duration	Usually less than one month	Months to years
Course and reversibility	Fluctuating and reversible	Fluctuating and progressive, not reversible
Level of consciousness	Reduced, clouded, fluctuating	Clear, alert
Orientation Perception Memory	Impaired; disorientation Sensory misperceptions, including illusions or hallucinations (especially visual) Memory impairment (recent memory)	Initially intact; first loses orientation to time, then place and person. Hallucinations less common (except in 'sundowning') Short-term memory loss; precedes long-term memory loss

→

Category	Delirium	Major NCD
Thinking	Disorganised, incoherent, rambling, disordered	Impoverished, decreased in amount
Attention/concentration	Prominently impaired (hard to direct or sustain)	Initially intact, later impaired
Executive functioning	Markedly impaired	Relatively preserved
Sleep–wake cycle	Usually disrupted which can include daytime sleepiness, difficulty falling asleep	Normal for age; cycle disrupted as the disease progresses

Source: Adapted from Uys and Middleton (2014); Baumann (2015)

Difference between mild and major NCDS

Normal ageing is a degenerative process. In some individuals, only a subtle impact on cognitive functioning and everyday activities are visible. Nowadays the term mild NCD is used more often, because individuals are more aware and knowledgeable and seek treatment earlier (Sachdev et al, 2014). Diagnosing mild and major cognitive disorders is a specialised field. The criteria for mild NCD and major NCD run parallel to each other. The margin or threshold of cognitive and functioning decline is depicted on a continuum, which makes it difficult to measure (Simpson, 2014). The level of cognitive and functioning decline determines whether the diagnosis is major NCD, or mild NCD (Sachdev et al, 2014).

Major NCD includes the degenerative dementias, usually affecting older adults. While the incidence of major NCD increases with age, major NCD is not a normal consequence of ageing. Younger individuals can also be diagnosed with an NCD after, for example, a traumatic brain injury or HIV/AIDS infection (Sachdev et al, 2014). In Table 16.7 the deficits in everyday activities in persons with mild and major NCD within the six cognitive domains are compared.

Table 16.7 Differences in the functioning abilities and deficits in mild and major NCD within the neurocognitive domains

Neurocognitive domain	Mild NCD	Major NCD
Perceptual-motor function (includes visual perception, visuo-constructional, perceptual-motor, praxis and gnosis)	May rely more on maps or others for directions. Uses notes and follows others to get to a new place. Is less precise in parking. Needs to expend greater effort for spatial tasks such as carpentry, sewing or knitting.	Has significant difficulties with previously familiar activities (using tools), navigating in familiar environments.
Complex attention (sustained attention, divided attention, selective attention, processing speed)	Normal tasks take longer than previously; errors arise in routine tasks; needs more double-checking. Thinking is easier when not competing with other things (radio, driving, cell phone).	Has increased difficulty in environments with multiple stimuli; easily distracted by competing events in the environment. Has difficulty in recalling information (telephone numbers or what was just said). Unable to perform mental calculations. All thinking takes longer than usual.
Learning and memory (immediate memory, recent memory, very long-term memory)	Has difficulty recalling recent events and relies increasingly on making lists. Needs occasional reminders or re-reading to keep track of characters in a novel or movie. Occasionally repeats the same story. Loses track of whether bills have been paid.	Often repeats self within the same conversation. Cannot keep track of short list of items when shopping or of plans of the day. Requires frequent reminders to orient to task at hand.
Executive function (planning, decision making, working memory, responding to feedback/error correction, overriding habits/inhibition, mental flexibility)	Increased effort required to complete multistage projects; increased difficulty multitasking or resuming a task when interrupted (phone call, visitor). May complain of fatigue from the extra effort required to organise, plan or make decisions. May report that large social gatherings are less enjoyable because of increased effort to follow shifting conversations.	Abandons complex projects. Needs to focus on one task at a time. Relies on others to plan activities of daily living or to make decisions.

→

Neurocognitive domain	Mild NCD	Major NCD
Language (expressive language and receptive language)	Noticeable word-finding difficulty. May avoid use of specific names of acquaintances. Grammatical errors involve subtle omissions or incorrect use of articles, prepositions, auxiliary verbs, etc.	Significant difficulties with expressive or receptive language. Often uses general-use phrases such as 'that thing' and 'you know what I mean', and prefers general pronouns rather than names. With severe impairment the following occur: inability to recall names of close friends and family; idiosyncratic word use; grammatical errors; stereotypy of speech; echolalia; automatic speech ending in mutism.
Social cognition	Subtle changes in behavioural attitude – described as change in personality. Less able to recognise social cues or read facial expressions, decreased empathy, increased extraversion or introversion, decreased inhibition or subtle or episodic apathy or restlessness.	Behaviour clearly out of social range; shows insensitivity to social standards of modesty in dress or political, religious, or sexual topics of conversation. Focuses excessively on a topic despite group's disinterest or direct feedback. Behavioural intention without regard to family or friends. Makes decisions without regard to safety. Has little insight into these changes

Source: APA (2013: 626–628)

ASSESSING NCDs

Comprehensive screening and evaluation are necessary when dealing with a person presenting with an NCD. Such an assessment entails the following: a thorough and complete history involving medical and physical examinations and investigations; a psychiatric assessment involving a mental state examination (MSE) and screening tests in the form of a mini-mental state examination (MMSE); diagnostic tests (neuroimaging) and blood tests; a functional assessment and a social assessment. In order to assess the various features of the functional and social aspects, collateral information from a reliable source (family member, friend or carer) is of great significance (Baumann, 2015; Sachdev et al, 2014). Careful questioning about specific symptoms is necessary as the problem is usually raised as a concern and not as a complaint which would be voiced spontaneously. The history and physical examination go hand-in-hand. A full history of medical problems, course of the illness, risks, substance use or abuse, and the reason for seeking professional help is necessary to assess the individual holistically.

An evaluation of the patterns of functioning completes the nursing assessment. The extent of the decline (see Table 16.5) and examples of assessments that can be given to determine the functioning abilities within the six neurocognitive domains have been documented in Table 16.1. This also reveals the nursing problems which require individualised nursing interventions and the specific amount of care needed.

The nursing assessment focuses on:
- identifying risks
- use of screening tools like the MMSE
- recognising depression and other mental disorders
- recognising social and lifestyle functioning problems.

These different aspects will be covered in the following sections.

Identifying risks

Part of the nursing assessment is to identify predisposing and risk factors for delirium and for mild and major NCDs (see the respective sections under 'The aetiology or causes of NCDS'); and also to detect elder abuse or the risk of abuse (see 'Ethical issues' under 'Family and carer liaison'). Medications with anticholinergic effects are particularly problematic for the elderly and can cause cognitive impairment that is reversible by discontinuing the medication (Uys & Middleton, 2014). A sudden deterioration in functioning in an elderly person can indicate a minor medical illness. A minor medical illness (for example, a urinary tract infection or upper respiratory tract infection) in a person with underlying dementia can precipitate delirium (Baumann, 2015). Nursing staff should keep this in mind and check that the medical problem is being treated before referring a client for specialised psychiatric evaluation.

Patients posing a risk should be identified and monitored and abnormal behaviour reported and recorded in order for prompt and effective interventions to be made. Correct identification, proper referral and appropriate interventions of NCDs can reduce medico-legal risks, prevent death, reduce the hospitalisation period and increase independent functioning which would alleviate the burden of care.

The elderly are soft targets in the community and vulnerable to abuse and neglect from family members, care givers and other members in the community and in institutions. The Older Persons Act 13 of 2006 deals with the plight of older persons and aims to empower, protect and maintain their status, well-being, rights, safety and security (South Africa, 2006). In South Africa, elder abuse is a crime which should be reported. Any suspicion of elder abuse should be reported to the Department of Social Development and to the nearest police officer or SAPD. Alternatively, the abuse can be reported anonymously to Halt Elder Abuse line (HEAL) at 0800 003 081.

Use of screening tools like the MMSE

Cognitive screening instruments remain an integral part of the assessment of any patient with cognitive complaints. The MMSE is a screening instrument that is most commonly used in the assessment of a variety of cognitive disorders (Larner, 2017). It is a relatively simple and practical tool to screen for cognitive impairment. Patients should be literate and the test should not be repeated within a three-month interval (Baumann, 2015).

The tool comprises a short battery of 20 individual tests covering 11 domains and totalling a score of 30 points. The MMSE can reveal cognitive functioning deficits in orientation, registration, attention, calculation (serial sevens or spelling), recall, naming, repetition, comprehension (verbal and written), writing, and construction (Larner, 2017). Normal time for completion is eight minutes, but a person with dementia can take up to 15 minutes (Larner, 2017). Table 16.8 explains three examples of the types of questions in the MMSE.

Table 16.8 Samples of questions in the MMSE

Question	Score	Cognitive functions involved
"What day is today? or What is the… date?"	1	Orientation to Time
"What is this?" [*Point to an object.*]	1	Naming
"Now I am going to ask you to repeat what I say. Ready? It is a lovely, sunny day but too warm. Now you say that. [*Wait for examinee response and record response verbatim. Repeat up to one time.*]	1	Repetition

Adapted and Reproduced by special permission of the Publisher, Psychological Assessment Resources, Inc., 16204 North Florida Avenue, Lutz, Florida 33549, from the Mini-Mental State Examination, by Marshal F. Folstein, MD and Susan E. Folstein, MD, Copyright 1975, 1998, 2001 and the Mini-Mental State Examination-2, Copyright 2010 by Mini Mental LLC, Inc. Published 2001, 2010 by Psychological Assessment Resources, Inc. Further reproduction is prohibited without permission of PAR, Inc. The MMSE-2 can be purchased from PAR, Inc. by calling (813) 968-3003.

In the MMSE a range of questions are asked and each correct question scores one mark. Orientation to time and place receives much focus as it scores the highest marks (5 and 5), with attention/concentration/calculations (5 marks) and lower emphasis is placed on registration, memory (3 marks), and reading, writing and copying (1 mark each) (Larner, 2017). An extensive neuropsychological and clinical evaluation is indicated when scoring is below the acceptable range.

The MMSE is particularly useful in distinguishing dementia from pseudo-dementia or depression as depressed patients usually attain a normal score (Baumann, 2015). Delirious patients rarely complete the test, largely because of attention difficulties. There is no time limit for completing the test. Table 16.9 reflects an interpretation of MMSE scores.

Table 16.9 Interpreting MMSE scores

▪ A score of 24 or less indicates global cognitive impairment
▪ Impairment can be either from delirium or dementia

▪ The level of education and age determine the MMSE scores:
  − Average score for adults:
    ○ up to the age of 50 = 29
    ○ over the age of 80 = 25
    ○ with high school education and higher = 29
    ○ with one to five years of schooling = 22
  − In SA, people with grade 7 = 28

▪ The test is less sensitive to frontal lobe problems and subcortical dementia than cortical impairments
▪ Testing anxious, thought-disordered, intoxicated or delirious patients − results not meaningful or valid

Source Baumann (2015)

There are a few other screening tests available. The Montreal Cognitive Assessment (MoCA) is more sensitive in detecting early cognitive decline. The test is relatively easy and takes about 10 minutes to complete. It is a paper and pencil test that assesses the cognitive domains including memory, language, executive functions, visuospatial skills, calculation, abstraction, attention, concentration, and orientation (Larner, 2017). MoCA is used as a cognitive screening instrument which is grounded in a thorough clinical evaluation and the sound interpretation of MoCA test results. MoCA can also predict Alzheimer Disease (AD) conversion in patients with mild cognitive impairment (MCI) (Larner, 2017). According to Larner (2017), MoCA would be better suited in the assessment of patients who present with cognitive complaints and who have no functional impairment in their activities of daily living (ADL).

According to Larner (2017), other screening tests, such as the Clock Drawing Test (CDT), can also be used in the assessment of cognitive functions. The CDT is easy to use and screens a wide range of cognitive abilities which makes it a popular tool. The CDT screen many cognitive functions, including selective and sustained attention, auditory comprehension, verbal working memory, numerical knowledge, visual memory and reconstruction, visuospatial abilities, on-demand motor execution (praxis), and executive function (Larner, 2017).

Recognising depression and other mental disorders

Patients living with NCDs may present with mood disturbances, including depression, anxiety and elation (APA, 2013). Individuals in the mild to moderate stages of NCDs are particularly vulnerable to depression and anxiety. Older adults and younger persons are similarly affected by major depressive disorder (MDD), but there are some important differences in the way MDD affects the elderly. In the past, the term pseudo-dementia was used for patients who mimicked dementia, but who actually suffered from depression (Baumann, 2015). The MMSE is a useful tool for distinguishing between a depressed mood and dementia. A patient with a depressed mood will not have a lower MMSE score. Dementia and depression can coexist. Depression is fairly common early in the course of an NCDs (including a mild NCD), and especially in NCDs caused by Alzheimer's and Parkinson's disease (APA, 2013), as the person may realise they are losing abilities. The presence of depression may exacerbate an underlying cognitive impairment.

It is important that nurses are able to identify depression and other mood symptoms in the elderly because misdiagnosis can lead to mismanagement. The DSM-5 makes it very clear that the clinician must rule out depression before making the diagnosis of an NCD. Individuals with a history of depressive episodes earlier in life are prone to present with episodes of depression and or an NCD later in life. Table 16.10 indicates the difference between an NCD and depression.

Table 16.10 Differences between an NCD and depression

	NCD	**Depression**
Onset	Cognitive deficits predate depressive symptoms	Depressive symptoms antedate cognitive deficits
Presentation of memory symptoms	Patient minimises or denies; often will guess or evade the question if does not know the answer	May answer simple questions such as name or date, with 'I don't know'
Appearance and behaviour	Social skills are preserved until the later stages	Often neglected or slovenly
Intellectual skills	Consistently impaired	Inconsistent and often associated with poor effort
Affect	Usually normal	Flat
History	Possible depressive episodes earlier in life, which might not even have required treatment	Previous periods of major depressive disorder

Source: Adapted from Uys and Middleton (2014)

Individuals with NCDs can present with psychiatric symptoms such as psychosis with symptoms of delusions (usually with a persecutory theme) and hallucinations (visual hallucinations are more common) as well as mood changes (emotional lability) (DSM-5, 2013).

Recognising social and lifestyle functioning problems

Neurocognitive symptoms are noticed in individuals who engage in complex occupational, domestic, or recreational activities. As already mentioned in this chapter, the decline in functioning abilities in individuals living with NCDs is assessed according to the six neurocognitive domains: complex attention; executive function; learning and memory; language; perceptual-motor and social cognition (see Figure 16.2). Table 16.1 depicts the normal functioning abilities and Table 16.7 indicates the decline in the functioning abilities.

As the NCD progresses, it consequently impacts on the execution of everyday activities and on the independence of the individual. It is important to recognise and to be aware of the problems relating to social and lifestyle functioning of the person with an NCD.

The person can present with different behavioural and emotional problems, including aggression, inappropriate affect or apathy, which impact on their interaction with themselves, the environment and others. Patterns of communication become impaired to the extent that the person is no longer able to interact meaningfully with others or to communicate needs. Use of language, which one takes for granted, is gradually undermined. The consequences could be dysphasia (impairment in language communication), aphasia (an inability to express oneself), and impairment in the comprehension of messages.

Individuals with advanced NCDs may experience prominent neuro-motor features such as severe incoordination, ataxia (problems with balance and coordination), motor slowing and apraxia. Apraxia is the inability to carry out learned purposeful movement in the absence of weakness, incoordination, sensory loss or impaired comprehension ea. brush teeth or a series of sequential actions (Baumann, 2015).

Agitation is observed in a wide variety of people suffering from NCDs and can feature as inappropriate verbal, vocal or motor activity. It is often present when there is confusion or frustration (APA, 2013). Agitation can also manifest as wandering behaviour, inability to sit still, short attention span, picking at clothing, dressing and undressing and constant hand movements.

Other problems are sleep disturbances such as insomnia or hypersomnia. The individual loses a sense of cued time and the normal sleep–wake cycle may be disrupted. Restlessness and confusion may be noted as twilight approaches. This is also referred to as 'sundown syndrome'. According to Cipriani et al (2015) 'sundowning' presents at a specific time of the day and may affect people with dementia. The syndrome shares similarities with symptoms of delirium, such as attention deficits and activity disturbances.

Apathy is common in mild and mild major NCDs. It is observed particularly in persons who have an NCD due to Alzheimer's disease and may be a prominent feature of NCD due to frontotemporal lobar degeneration. Apathy is typically characterised by diminished motivation and reduced goal-directed behaviour, accompanied by decreased emotional responsiveness or aboulia (APA, 2013). Symptoms of apathy may manifest early in the course of NCDs when a loss of motivation to pursue daily activities or hobbies may be observed (APA, 2013).

One of the important functions of cognition is reality testing. As disorientation increases, the ability to assimilate, retain and use cues in the environment is lost. Agnosia is the inability to identify and recognise an object (Baumann, 2015). Disorientation with regard to place and person may become so extensive that the identity of the person concerned is eventually obliterated. Impairment of the ability to retain and recall information is a prominent symptom of NCDs. The person may be absent-minded and forgetful, but may spend a great deal of time reminiscing about events and experiences of the past.

Personality changes, now referred to as a decline in social cognition (see the section under 'Understanding NCDs') and challenging behavioural symptoms, which include inappropriate social behaviours such as lack of inhibition, shoplifting, promiscuity, exhibitionism and hoarding of seemingly meaningless articles, can be a stressful experience for family members and friends and can lead to a strain in relationships. Initially the person might resort to defence mechanisms to hide or compensate for the impairment. These include denial, regression, rationalisation, somatisation, hypochondriasis and aggression, and as the disease progresses, the person might engage in more primitive defences, as seen in rigid, negativistic behaviours. Other changes can involve emotional lability, impaired impulse control, suspiciousness, being overly dependent and helpless, distorted judgement or indiscretion and unreliability. In some cases premorbid personality traits are accentuated. In others, changes may be dramatic, for example a previously outgoing and sociable person might become withdrawn, rude or paranoid.

Other noticeable features are physical changes, psychomotor slowing and executive dysfunction. Cognitive deterioration gradually erodes the person's ability to perform the basic activities of daily living and as the cognitive impairment progresses, the person's ability to fulfil biological needs or self-care are reduced and supervision in respect of eating, drinking and elimination is necessary. Patients usually resist caregiving duties around personal hygiene, such as bathing, and dress may be inappropriate or slovenly. Abnormal appetite or excessive ingestion of food (hyperphagia) may occur. The person's ability to handle money, organise their time constructively and engage meaningfully in social and work-related activities is diminished.

Disorientation, memory loss, impaired judgement, impaired communication patterns and alterations in affect, self-image and personality all combine to reduce the person's ability to interact meaningfully with self and the environment.

Nursing staff can assess the problems or features associated with NCDs by mapping the abnormal behaviour in order to find out what triggers or worsens the behaviour of the person living with an NCD. From this, specific interventions can be planned.

INTERVENING IN NCDs

Psychosocial and environmental interventions have positive outcomes for individuals living with mild and major NCDs (Regier & Gitlin, 2017). The aim of intervention is to delay the course of the illness, maintain quality of life, improve cognitive functioning and behaviour and preserve independent functioning for as long as possible. The nursing or caring interventions are guided by the impact of the problem on the individual and the ability of the person to function independently. Interventions when a patient has delirium, and interventions focusing on mild and major NCDs will be examined in the next sections.

Intervening when a patient has delirium

The identification of delirium is the crucial first step in its treatment. Nursing staff should therefore be knowledgeable and be alert to the risk factors for delirium. Once recognised, the underlying cause must be diagnosed and addressed. Emergency medical treatment together with supportive nursing care are essential in the management of delirium. Guidelines to reduce the risk of delirium during hospitalisation are outlined in Table 16.11.

Table 16.11 Guidelines to reduce the risk of delirium during hospitalisation

- Ensure early identification of predisposing factors.
- Identify co-existing medical conditions and treat accordingly.
- Recognise prodromal symptoms like restlessness, anxiety, irritability or sleep disturbance before delirium appears.
- Implement early mobilisation after surgery and during rehabilitation.
- Ensure adequate pain management.
- Minimise use of new or multiple medication/drugs.
- Maintain hydration and electrolyte balance – encourage and assist with fluid intake and eating.
- Minimise bladder catheter use.
- Avoid physical restraints.
- Nurse the patient in a safe (prevent self-harm), calm, quiet environment, with adequate light and as little disturbance as possible.
- Provide sensory devices such as glasses, hearing aids.
- Alleviate distress and limit factors that aggravate condition.
- Allow uninterrupted period of sleep.

Source: Adapted from Baumann (2015)

Nursing interventions focusing on mild and major NCDs

Interventions are geared towards minimising the psychiatric and physical complications that can accompany these disorders, relieving treatable symptoms of the disorder and creating an environment in which the individual can live a productive and comfortable a life for as long as is possible. Psychosocial nursing interventions might not reverse the process of NCDs, but they can do much to minimise the maladaptive responses associated with neurocognitive disorders. Health care workers should focus on maintaining normality and convey a positive attitude during the establishing of a sound nurse–patient relationship with the individual living with an NCD.

Different nursing interventions include those focusing on language, creating a therapeutic environment, reality orientation, validity theory, other non-pharmacological interventions, intervening in wandering behaviour, behaviour modification and reward, and maintaining the physical well-being of a patient. These various interventions are dealt with in the following sections.

Language

As indicated in Tables 16.1 and 16.7, one of the neurocognitive domains affected in NCDs is language. Sound communication skills form the basis of the nurse–patient relationship. Nursing staff therefore need to practise sound communication skills to improve interaction and understanding, and to establish a therapeutic relationship with the individual living with an NCD. Table 16.12 shows the principles of verbal and non-verbal communication.

Table 16.12 Principles of verbal and non-verbal communication

Principles of verbal communication
▪ Get the person's attention before speaking.
▪ Address the person by name and identify yourself by name each time that you interact with the patient.
▪ Messages should be clear, concise and unhurried.
▪ Pronouns are often misunderstood. Short sentences that convey one idea at a time should be used ('Ms X, it is time for lunch' is clearer than 'Ms X, I want you to walk to lunch with me').
▪ Questions that require yes/no answers are more appropriate than open-ended questions. If you are concerned that a person may resist you, do not ask a question, but supply direction ('Would you like to have breakfast?' can be answered, 'no'. It is better to say, 'Come with me, Mr X, it is time for breakfast').
▪ When making requests of the person, present the steps of the task one at time.
▪ Allow the patient ample time to respond to statements and requests.
▪ If the question or statement needs to be restated, exact repetition should be used, so that the person has only one statement to decode.
▪ If the patient does not understand the request or statement after it has been repeated a few times, rephrase the content or change the subject to decrease frustration.
▪ Do not increase voice tone because it can be interpreted by the person as an aggressive overture.
Non-verbal communication
▪ Non-verbal and verbal communication should be congruent so that the person's confusion is minimised.
▪ Allow the person ample time to respond to statements and requests.
▪ Non-verbal gestures should be clear and unhurried; they can be used to enhance verbal communication and to cue appropriate responses from the patient, for example pointing at the cup while asking the patient to pick it up.
Physical stroking, hugging, patting and holding are valuable means of conveying caring and establishing contact.

Source: Uys and Middleton (2014)

Creating a therapeutic environment

Interventions relating to mild and major NCDs are also aimed at creating a therapeutic environment where optimal care can be provided, cognitive deficits and specific problems addressed, and the overall well-being and quality of life of the person improved. Studies have shown that non-pharmacological interventions have improved the quality of life of people living with dementia (Cabrera et al, 2014).

The environment can be manipulated to bring about positive changes in the functioning of individuals living with NCDs, prevent injuries and improve the quality of life. The term 'sheltered freedom' is used to describe an environment that is supportive of the person's emotional, social, physical and cognitive abilities and deficits (Uys & Middleton, 2014). Environmental manipulation is based on the principle of normalisation and encompasses the following concepts (Uys & Middleton 2014):

- Patients are consistently encouraged to engage with reality.
- The environment compensates for gaps in patient functioning.
- Meaningful therapeutic activities and stimulation encourage optimal functioning.
- Activities take place in small groups.
- Patients are encouraged to exercise some degree of personal control within the context of their particular disability.
- Patient interaction and mutual help are encouraged.
- Appropriate behaviour is consistently reinforced.
- Ward staff are actively involved with patients and demonstrate attitudes of respect and acceptance in their verbal and non-verbal communications with patients.

The environment should be flexible enough to accommodate fluctuating levels of cognitive and functioning decline, and stable enough to provide the person with a sense of consistency and continuity. The principles which apply in a therapeutic environment for individuals living with an NCD are indicated in Table 16.13.

Table 16.13 Principles of a therapeutic environment for individuals living with an NCD

- **Pleasant and safe physical facilities**
  The environment should ensure:
  - safety (prevention of harm, injuries and abscondment)
  - an attractive, cosy and homely atmosphere which allows comfort
  - adequate privacy and social well-being
  - acceptable living standards (feeding, sleeping, hygiene)
  - an increase and/or sustaining of social interaction and social skills.
- **Democracy and humanity**
  To implement the principles of democracy and humanity, caregivers should:
  - Respect and accept individuality. Encourage the individual to make choices, although limited at times, and allow the keeping of some personal possessions.
  - Give adequate information and education. Allow individuals to voice their opinion and involve them in decision making. Allow the taking of initiative and sharing the responsibilities.
  - Display attitudes of empathy and respect in order to maintain dignity – do not treat the individual like a child.
  - Involve family and ensure that they are adequately informed.

→

> - **Positive staff attitude**
>   - Staff attitudes are an important aspect of the psychosocial environment because they can influence positively and/or negatively the quality of care the patients receive. Essential and worthy qualities are flexibility, casualness, active and passive friendliness, vigilance and friendly firmness.
>   - Staff placement changes should be reduced to a minimum to ensure consistency, for example a six-monthly rotation could be implemented, as opposed to a monthly rotation.
> - **Family involvement and contact with friends**
>   - Encourage contact with family and friends. Place photos and mementoes of family in their room. Allow phone calls, visits (flexible visiting hours), leave, outings.
> - **Encouraging participation in activities**
>   - Make available a wide variety of activities for physical and cognitive stimulation.
>   - Allow for choice in these activities.
>   - Use/spend time meaningfully.
>   - Establish an unhurried and consistent daily schedule. Mealtimes, medication administration, therapeutic activities, rest times, bath times, etc, should take place at the same time each day.
>   - Allow patients sufficient time to complete the various activities. It is vitally important that the ward programme matches the patient's needs and abilities. Staff should refrain from completing the activities as this would not have the intended therapeutic value.

Source: Adapted from Uys and Middleton (2014: 257–260.)

Intervening in the social and interpersonal atmosphere of the unit, ward or facility can support, maintain and enhance appropriate lifestyle functioning in individuals living with an NCD. Staff attitudes are an important aspect of the psychosocial environment as they can influence the quality of care the patients receive. Meaningful interaction and showing empathy, respect and understanding also forms part of reality orientation (see Table 16.14) – to be discussed in the next section – which increases positive emotions. This positivity will create feelings of well-being which will improve cooperation and performance in daily activities (Cabrera, 2014).

Caregivers should refrain from contributing to negative behaviour of individuals living with an NCD through the following actions:

- Treating the patient as 'senile', which encourages disorganised thinking and behaviour.
- Assuming that progressive cognitive deterioration implies an inevitable worsening of the condition and believing that a stimulating environment is of no real value.
- Treating the patients as incapable of making choices which fosters dependency and a loss of self-esteem. Examples of this would be talking about a patient as if they were not there because 'they won't understand', leaving the toilet door open because 'they don't know what is going on anyway', giving patients nicknames they have not chosen themselves or calling all patients 'darling/dearie/love'. This might reinforce the loss of dignity and self-esteem the patient might already be mourning (Uys & Middleton, 2014).

The quality of the physical environment will influence, to some degree, the quality of the psychosocial environment. As the NCD progresses the person can become more disorientated and can experience difficulty with interpreting the meaning of abstract concepts. Environmental manipulation increases the success of reality orientation and social interaction and decreases wandering behaviour.

Reality orientation (RO)

The interventions of RO, remotivation therapy and validation therapy are integrated, complement one another and reflect normalisation. Creating a bridge to reality forms part of RO, remotivation and validation therapy. Reality orientation is based on a technique to help individuals engage and connect with their surroundings (Heersema, 2017a). The technique uses a basic communication approach where the current environment (location or surroundings), people, and time or dates are frequently included in conversations with the person. The aim is to increase awareness of time, place and person and maintain a link with reality. It is a 'continual process whereby staff present current information to the person in every interaction, reminding the patient of time, place and person and providing a commentary on events' (Uys & Middleton, 2014). Every interaction with the patient is an opportunity for RO. Routine activities such as waking the patients, serving meals and helping them to the bathroom are invaluable opportunities for RO. During the process of RO nursing staff and carers can use the opportunity to monitor and evaluate individuals living with an NCD.

Some studies show that RO not only delays cognitive decline, but also improves cognitive functioning and challenging behaviour in people living with NCDs (Heersema, 2017a). Appropriate behaviour and personal appearance (dress, grooming) help to maintain dignity and increase self-esteem. Maintaining a link with reality also encourages optimal and meaningful participation in everyday activities and ensures remotivation. Recognising and identifying the people with whom they interact can lead to a sense of belonging. The focus of remotivation is to establish a climate of acceptance and success which increases self-esteem and hope. Individuals living with NCDs might resist interaction and attempts to get them to join in certain activities might be met with aggression and hostility. The individual should be constantly motivated to continue with independent lifestyle functioning and be allowed to make decisions, handle money, organise their time and engage in meaningful activities. Structured RO sessions (group therapy) are very effective in remotivation.

It is important that information be presented in an interactional style and that the patient is given an opportunity to respond. The manipulation of the physical environment and the provision of environmental supports are important components of RO. Some strategies for RO and environmental support are depicted in Table 16.14.

Table 16.14 Strategies for RO and environmental support

▪ Talk about orientation, including the time of day, the date, and the season. ▪ Use the person's name frequently. ▪ Comment on current events and encourage response. ▪ Use clear visual, tactile, sensory prompts. ▪ Ask concrete, simple questions. ▪ Refer frequently to clocks, calendars, season, ward programme and staff on duty. ▪ Ask questions about personal possessions such as photos and other decorations. ▪ Increase spatial orientation by using signs, arrows and colour coded routes. Place signs, pictures and labels on doors and cupboards to indicate their function. ▪ Apply prosthetic devices to compensate for sensory and motor deficits (visual or hearing aids, walking aids). ▪ Involve all staff in routine activities (waking, serving meals, personal hygiene activities, hobbies). ▪ Always ensure the person's dignity is retained. ▪ Respond appropriately to confused or rambling talk and correct misconceptions tactfully. ▪ Protect the person by not over-accentuating inability or decline. Do not tease when the person show distress or agitation, but rather ignore and change the topic. ▪ Create a bridge to reality by linking to experiences that have meaning for the person and/or re-orientate to the present by referring to the past. ▪ Recognise the person's need to feel productive and useful (acknowledge and appreciate previous occupation, hobby). ▪ Encourage humour. The individual living with an NCD should be motivated to continue with cognitive functioning and activities of daily living for as long as possible

Source: Adapted from Heersema (2017a)

Structured group activities serve multiple purposes which include RO and remotivation therapy. Participation in community life and interacting in group activities form part of maintaining normality. Group sessions or structured RO sessions should be scheduled at times when the participants are least likely to be fatigued (for example, in the early morning or after naps). The aim is to increase awareness of the surroundings, to maintain a link with reality and to protect the individual from undue exposure and growing deficits. Through active socialisation in the group sessions, asocial behaviour, withdrawal and deterioration of thinking are discouraged (Uys & Middleton, 2014). Table 16.15 describes the guidelines for structured group activities to increase RO and remotivation.

Table 16.15 Guidelines for structured group activities to increase RO and remotivation

- The setting should be as informal and as pleasant as possible.
  A small corner of a room can be screened off and decorated with plants, colourful pictures and so on, to simulate a comfortable, homely environment.
- Group size depends on the patients' level of functioning. As a general rule, the numbers should be restricted to two or three patients, but the size of the group could be increased for people who are less disorientated.
- All members of the group should be involved and their input acknowledged. Questions should be direct questions to the group.
- Members should make physical and personal contact in the group session, through introduction and by shaking hands, calling members by name and visible name tags. Create a climate of acceptance, enthusiasm and optimism. Apply verbal and non-verbal communication skills to attract and sustain attention. Media aids or equipment should be large, clear, colourful and uncluttered. Use a large, portable weatherboard with a collection of smaller slot-in pieces on which names of the days and months, and comments and pictures about the weather, are written. For patients who can still write, personal diaries can be handed out for the purposes of copying down the information.
- Prompts to stimulate recall and the various senses can also be used to reinforce verbal information. This may include fresh fruit, flowers, food (sweet, sour, cold, hot or savoury), maps of places, picture cards illustrating occupations, pets, places, cars, birds or real-life models and songs appropriate to the situation.

Source: Uys and Middleton (2014)

Validation therapy

In contrast to RO, the focus of validation therapy is on the underlying feelings behind the statements or behaviours. Studies have revealed contradicting results on the effectiveness of validation therapy as depicted in the Cochrane Library (Heersema, 2017b). Some benefits are that the individual gets the opportunity to reflect on their memories, rephrase feelings and express emotions.

Focusing on feelings and experiences can uncover the issues with which the individual may be grappling. Talking with individuals on their terms and discussing the subjects they raise can help them to resolve past conflicts and to integrate these indirectly into their self-concepts. On the other hand, this approach could have a potentially destructive influence, especially if feelings of despair are aroused and the realities in the individual's life are avoided.

Other non-pharmacological interventions

Non-pharmacological interventions should be seen in context. According to Cabrera (2014), non-pharmacological interventions are best-practice strategies, or a first-line approach to manage behavioural and psychological symptoms in NCDs (Regier et al, 2017).

Activities are more beneficial if they are tailored around the individual's preferences, interests and abilities. According to Regier et al (2017), the individuals were more cooperative and revealed less negative behaviour when their needs, abilities and interests were accommodated. Other non-pharmacological interventions which proved to be effective are:

- *Sensory stimulation.* Studies by Regier et al (2017) indicated that sleep improved with the use of bright light therapy, while Cabrera et al (2014) found that bright light therapy assisted in the management of agitation. Behavioural and psychological symptoms were more effectively controlled by group music therapy than by music on its own.
- *Physical activity.* Physical activity improved functioning ability and decreased apathy, agitation and passivity. Regier et al (2017) revealed that meaningful activities increased positive emotions and feelings of well-being and improved performance in daily activities.
- *Cognitive interventions.* Studies showed that cognitive interventions improved cognitive performance and neuropsychiatric symptoms of depression and delusions (Regier et al, 2017).
- *Animal-assisted therapy.* Positive results were reported from previous studies on animal-assisted therapy which could not be substantiated by Regier et al (2017). However, a study by Menna et al (2015) reported positive outcomes regarding multimodal stimulation (verbal, visual and tactile) and on mood and cognition.
- *Staff-focused interventions.* Cabrera et al (2014) reported that training programs for staff members had a positive effect on nursing outcomes. The individuals' overall behaviour improved to such an extent that a significant decrease in the number of restraints used in the institutions was reported and the attitudes of the staff members were more positive.

Intervening in wandering behaviour

Wandering behaviour is a common outcome of disorientation and memory loss in individuals living with mild and major NCDs. According to Gu (2015), up to 60 per cent of persons with an NCD display wandering behaviour, which is one of the most challenging behaviours to manage as it is problematic and dangerous.

Wandering is defined as aimless movement, walking and or fidgeting which can be associated with stress and coping patterns, previous work roles and the seeking of familiar places, people and security (Gu, 2015). Sensory deprivation, in the form of a monotonous environment or an absence of therapeutic activities, can increase confusion and wandering behaviour in individuals living with NCDs. Wandering behaviour tends to increase as the cognitive decline progresses. Sleep disturbance, unfamiliar environments, loneliness, separation, boredom, frustration, extrapyramidal side effects or paradoxical agitation caused by psychotropic medications are associated aspects of wandering behaviour.

Wandering behaviour is not always random and is to some degree under external, environmental control. One study mapped the patterns of wandering as experienced by three institutionalised wanderers. The results showed that these people developed consistent patterns of travel and would rest at points of interest, stimulation or potential reinforcement, such as at an untended food tray, around other people, near windows with views outside and in areas of high activity like the nurses' station and/or tearoom (Uys & Middleton, 2014).

Caring staff can therefore map the wandering behaviour in order to identify the triggers, route and time of day. Identification of at-risk individuals may prevent the adverse consequences of wandering and ensure effective interventions (Ali et al, 2015). Good physical health is a positive outcome of wandering, as the effects of physical exercise and increased appetite ensure that the individual maintains mobility and physical independence However, the adverse consequences of wandering may outweigh the benefits (Ali et al, 2015). The person with dementia may not be able to identify dangerous situations and may sustain falls, fractures, bruises, injuries and can get lost and/or even die. Attempts and actions to prevent them from eloping can result in institutionalisation (Ali et al, 2015).

The physical environment can be modified to promote social interaction, increase reality engagement and decrease wandering behaviour. Caregivers should manipulate the environment to be safe and in ways to increase stimulation, socialisation and meaningful activities. Table 16.16 gives specific guidelines for intervening in wandering behaviour which should coordinate with the therapeutic milieu.

Table 16.16 Specific guidelines for intervening in wandering behaviour

- Set up a structured ward programme where each person is involved.
- Arrange lounge chairs in small groups of six or seven to increase social interaction.
- Set specific meal times and encourage interaction by arranging the room to cater for small groups.
- Ensure adequate lighting to decrease sharp contrasts and shadows and prevent illusions, disorientation or confusion (night-lights can reduce nocturnal confusion).
- Decrease noise levels. Excessive noise and hearing problems can increase feelings of tension and thus contribute to agitation, wandering and confusion.
- Offer distraction and self-stimulation activities. Place an activity barrel or container filled with plastic objects and toys to engage the attention of wanderers.
- Place chairs in areas of high activity, for example outside the duty room and next to the front door, which can distract wanderers.
- Prevent wide-open spaces and lengthy corridors as they are not 'user friendly' and may inhibit exploratory behaviour and mobility.
- Screen or camouflage unsafe areas. Wanderers are easily distracted by anything that is perceived as a barrier:
  - Access routes leading to exits, unsafe or undesirable areas can be camouflaged with room dividers, screens. Use stop signs or a black tape or carpet on the floor. Gu (2015) found that a mirror placed in front of the exit door was most effective.
  - Door knobs or locks on doors can be camouflaged with a panel to prevent eloping.
- Provide an enclosed outdoor area in which patients are able to wander safely. The hazards associated with being outdoors should be taken into account; for example, suntan lotions, hats and umbrellas to prevent sunburn, and the provision of enough fluids and some shelter are necessary.

Source: Adapted from Uys and Middleton (2014)

Behaviour modification and reward

There is evidence to suggest that people with cognitive disorders are capable of learning, given the right environmental conditions. These studies show that the use of positive reinforcement is effective in increasing the frequency of desirable behaviours such as independent eating skills, mobility, social and verbal interaction, participation in activities and continence (Uys & Middleton, 2014).

Some principles applicable in behaviour modification are depicted in Table 16.17.

Table 16.17 Principles of behaviour modification and reward

- Unacceptable behaviour should be identified.
- Behaviours to be modified must be carefully defined.
- The person's assets, abilities, interests, and likes and dislikes must be identified, because these are potential sources of positive reinforcers.
- Inconsistencies in the person's behaviour should be noted.
- The behaviour modification plan consists of a set of goals or target behaviours, together with a set of procedures to achieve the target behaviours.
- The individual should be involved and acknowledged in the decisions and setting of goals.
- The target behaviours should be specific enough to measure and should relate to the problem.
- Behaviour modification techniques need to be adapted to maximise the possibility that learning will take place.
- Reward should follow immediately after the desired behaviour has occurred. This is especially important when dealing with confused people, because they tend to forget quickly and the impact of the reinforcement is then lost.
- The patient should not be allowed to become frustrated and rewards should never be withheld. Each time a reward is given, the reason for it should be explained to the person.
- Positive reinforcers include consumable reinforcers (food or drink); activity reinforcers (things the person likes to do, for example, hobbies, crafts, pouring the tea, watching TV, listening to the radio, walking or wandering); possessional reinforcers (things the person likes to possess, for example, perfume or a hairbrush); social reinforcers (verbal and physical stimulation, for example verbal praise, hugging or touching).
- Reward and modelling are the basic methods that can be used to bring about change.
- The environment and psychosocial interventions should constantly be monitored to ensure that they aid learning and contribute to the well-being of the individuals.

Source: Adapted from Uys and Middleton (2014)

Maintaining the physical well-being of the patient

This aspect will be mentioned briefly because it is assumed that the person caring for the individual living with NCD should be competent to intervene appropriately where there is a decline in fulfilling biological needs. The degree of disruption determines the amount of supervision necessary. Patterns of nutrition, elimination, mobility, sleep, rest and hygiene can be maintained in the following ways (Uys & Middleton, 2014):

- *Ensure adequate hydration and nutrition in the form of nourishing drinks and light, well-balanced diets.* Patients are often given liquidated food because it is assumed that, even though they may have their own teeth or dentures, they are incapable of chewing and digesting firm foods. In addition 'sloppy' food is often given because patients take less time to swallow than to chew their food. The implications of this for the emotional and physical well-being of patients need to be seriously considered.

- *Prevent constipation by increasing the amount of fibre in the diet, regular toileting, exercise and, if necessary, the use of mild laxatives.*
- *Employ stimulating daytime activities* (patients are often allowed to doze all day in chairs and then spend at least ten hours a night in bed) thus reducing daytime doziness and the need for night sedation, which in itself might contribute to nocturnal confusion and disorientation. Regular 'nap periods' built into the daily programme might help to restore energy for activities.
- *Reinforce the importance of personal cleanliness, grooming and dressing in the overall well-being of the person.* Patients who appear dishevelled or who are dressed in an odd assortment of clothes are less likely to be treated with dignity and respect than those who are appropriately dressed. Dean (Adams, 1987: 42, in Uys & Middeton, 2014) investigated the clothing of elderly patients in hospital. He reported that '… to be fully dressed is good for morale, helps to maintain dignity, independence and status, delays institutionalisation and in mental illness helps to mitigate disturbance and to provide resistance to deterioration'. Self-help in daily bathing and grooming should be encouraged and patients should be allowed to select their own clothing.
- *Monitor the physical health of the person carefully.* Because urinary tract infection is one of the most common causes of delirium in the elderly, the nurse should be alert to symptoms of urinary tract infection (dysuria, lower abdominal pain, foul-smelling urine, haematuria, sudden onset of incontinence, change in behaviour).
- Ensure safety through other devices, such as nonslip mats for plates, thick-handled utensils for eating and Velcro fasteners to replace buttons. These are useful when motor deficits interfere with eating and dressing skills. Use cot sides to prevent the individual from falling out of bed.

Self-care activities should not be seen as insignificant chores to get out of the way quickly. They represent opportunities for remotivation, reality orientation, validation and retraining and are an integral part of the psychosocial environment.

Assessing pain in people with cognitive impairment can be difficult, as individuals living with NCDs are not reliable in relaying pain experienced over a period of time. Several pain scales have been developed to help in assessing pain through the observation of behaviours.

FAMILY AND CARER LIAISON

Intervening with families can be done with individual families or by arranging for a number of families to meet together as a group. The latter approach is especially useful because families can share their problems as well as any successes and obtain support from other families in the same position.

The aim of family liaison is to assist the family in continuing their caregiving role for as long as possible. According to Regier et al (2017), the use of non-pharmacological approaches, which encompass environment simplification and communication techniques, can decrease the burden on the caregiver and limit the occurrences of behavioural symptoms. Conveying an attitude of normality might help to maintain sound relationships, and physical and psychological health, which would enable individuals with 'dementia' to remain in their community for longer (refer to therapeutic milieu and re-orientation therapy). The family and carers might not understand the varying functioning abilities as the individual can have better and 'brighter' days in between others, even though their cognitive functioning would be progressively declining. Mild and major NCDs are irreversible which can contribute to frustration and despondency in the family and carer. This leads to challenges regarding the individual's capacity to make decisions, live alone, drive and manage their own affairs. Working with a person who lives with an NCD can be extremely challenging and stressful for nurses, family members and carers and it is extremely important that carers could be relieved and receive support to help them to cope with the burden of caring (Roach et al, 2016).

Challenges encountered by families/carers looking after individuals living with NCDs

Increasing cognitive decline interferes drastically with the pattern of building and maintaining relationships and independent functioning. Person–family interactions become strained as the family battles to adjust to the loss of a significant relationship and to the increasing need to provide supervision for the person. Exhaustion, demoralisation and the degree of strain experienced by family caregivers have been cited as common reasons for referral to hospital services (Steffen & Grant, 2015). Caregivers are prone to have a higher rate of illness, disability, stress and symptoms than non-caregivers. The stress associated with increased physical work, sleepless nights, constant vigilance, social isolation, frustration and intra-family conflict can lead to family strain.

Caregivers may be aware that there are no 'cures' and that the individual's functioning will deteriorate over time which leaves them with feelings of hopelessness and impotence despite every caring effort. Behaviours such as emotional and physical withdrawal, distancing or avoidance and benign neglect are some of the ways to deal with their own feelings of helplessness, impotence and frustration. These behaviours, although understandable, further serve to alienate the family and caregiver. This can lead to insufficient care and even abuse. The individuals are deprived from much-needed interpersonal contact and support, which can increase disorientation and confusion lead to a loss of self-esteem. Being equipped with the relevant knowledge, skills, logic and reason might help family members, carers and nurses to manage their frustration, anger, depression and prevent stigmatisation.

Problem-solving methods

The most useful framework for family intervention is the problem-solving method. This method has the added advantage that, if used correctly, it can help the family gain a sense of mastery and control in the face of an otherwise unpredictable condition. A positive nurse–family relationship is central to the well-being of the family caring for a demented person at home. Hertzberg and Ekman (in Uys & Middleton, 2014) suggest that nurses talk about 'we' and not 'us and them' to facilitate this process. Much can be accomplished by the following:

- Acknowledging family distress and exploring feelings associated with the condition. These feelings might include sadness related to the loss of a significant relationship, feelings of anger and resentment towards the person, guilt about having these feelings, denial of the condition, feelings of helplessness in the face of the person's declining abilities
- Asking family members to narrate, in their own words, aspects of the person's life-history they wish the staff to know about
- Making uninterrupted time to sit with family members and to talk about issues of concern, changes in treatment and so on
- Identifying and exploring problem areas and establishing how the family copes with the person and their behaviours
- Reinforcing positive coping strategies
- Exploring the extent of the family's knowledge about the condition and providing necessary and desired information
- Involving the family in the care process and in decisions relating to care
- Helping the family to find alternate ways of coping with the patient and any problem behaviour, as well as with the family's own level of distress
- Making use of respite care to relieve the carer
- Other helpful interventions are:
  - Teaching the family stress-management skills
  - Devising time away from caregiving
  - Reallocating physical and emotional caregiving tasks among family members for periods of time
  - Providing simple activities for the person that create immediate pleasure, re-establish connections with family members, provide meaningful tasks and enable friendships. Examples include reviewing family photographs, playing simple, homemade rhythm instruments and doing puzzles made out of old family photographs
  - Developing environmental manipulation skills
  - Facilitating psychosocial support meetings
  - Eliciting outside help where necessary, for example from community nurses.

Coping abilities

Most individuals with NCDs are cared for in their homes. Caregivers' responses depend to a large extent on their understanding of the disease process and on their coping abilities. Assessing the impact of the cognitive disorder on the family and identifying the attitude and coping mechanisms can assist in the giving of sound advice and support for the family members and carers. Table 16.18 shows an assessment of the family's coping abilities.

Table 16.18 Assessing the coping abilities of the family

- Is the family involved in the care of the individual or is there hostility and rejection?
- What was the nature of the relationship between the caregiver and the individual before the onset of the disease?
- Have all family members accepted the diagnosis?
- Are some denying the diagnosis and, if so, how is this affecting interaction with the individual?
- Is only one member responsible for the care or is the responsibility shared?
- Does the caregiving person feel burdened and unable to obtain relief?
- Does the individual require constant supervision?
- How is the individual's condition affecting the family financially and/or socially?
- Are those members not directly involved in the care supportive of those who are?
- Are family members able to talk about their feelings, fears and fantasies?
- Does the behaviour of family members aggravate or minimise the patient's coping?
- What coping behaviours – namely, problem-focused and/or emotion-focused – do the family use and to what degree are these behaviours effective?
- How do family members feel about the eventual institutionalisation of the individual?
- Have they discussed this and who is to make the decision?
- Is the caregiver able to have time free from supervising the individual?
- Is there potential or actual abuse related to individual-care exhaustion?

Source: Adapted from Uys and Middleton (2014)

Ethical issues

Family members can encounter different ethical issues which have to be resolved by them, but at the same time they might trigger many emotions and can leave them in a predicament. At some point in the caring process, family members, carers or friends have to decide whether the individual is still capable of managing their own finances, affairs and or driving a vehicle.

The extent of the functioning decline requires interventions which might not carry the approval of all involved. The individual should be referred for assessment to a panel of expert health professionals specialising in NCDs, who can decide on the capacity of the person. Initially the individual can appoint a proxy, such as a family member or lawyer, to act on their behalf by appointing a 'power of attorney' (Kaliski, 2006). Power of attorney lapses when the individual is not mentally capable or competent or if they lose capacity, which necessitates a durable or enduring power of attorney, which should be legally appointed. This process can be costly and time-consuming to implement, and is called curatorship. Kaliski (2006), differentiates between three types of curatorship:

1. *Curator personae.* Usually a family member, who is appointed by the court, to assist a person who lacks capacity to conduct their personal and daily affairs.
2. *Curator ad litem.* A person appointed by the court to act as legal guardian for a person who lacks capacity.
3. *Curator bonus.* A person, usually a lawyer, appointed by the court to administer the property of a person who lacks capacity to administer their own affairs.

Another ethical dilemma is whether the individual is capable of driving their own vehicle. The individual usually does not give up driving without protest as this is part of their independence. The individual would continue to drive their vehicle despite the advice or warning of family members, carers or even a medical practitioner. The person's lack of insight and judgement makes them unable to understand the consequences of their impairment. The individual could be referred for a specialised assimilated driving test, which should be conclusive about their driving capabilities. Other ethical issues involve issues that have to do with abuse (see 'Identifying risks' and 'Physical restraint').

Striving to maintain the person's quality of life might help to reduce some of their problematic responses and the family and carer's sense of helplessness.

SOCIAL CONTROL

According to Gray and Smith (2009), social control has to do with the managing of aggressive patients, also referred to as restraint. Physical control forms part of social control. Constant supervision is the most effective form of physical control and should be the first choice in caring for the individual living with an NCD. Other forms of social control are physical restraint and psychotropic medication. Psychotropic medication is helpful in curbing wandering behaviour, treating psychotic symptoms, depression and aggressive behaviour.

Physical restraint

The use of physical restraint is a controversial issue. Restraint should be avoided because it can aggravate the delirious elderly and cause untold physical problems like abrasions and pressure sores.

If restraint is used, the person's dignity and self-esteem should remain intact. The following principles should be adhered to:
- Patients should be restrained in an upright position.
- Restrained patients should be placed in a position where staff are able to observe them and in an environment that is therapeutic.
- Patients should be ambulated and toileted two-hourly and on demand.
- Restraints should be made of soft, non-abrasive material.

- Restrained patients should be included in therapeutic activities where possible, or staff should ensure that they spend frequent, short periods sitting and talking quietly with the patient.
- Restraints should be removed immediately when the behaviour decreases and should never be used as a preventive measure.
- Patients should be positively reinforced for desirable behaviour.
- Restraints should not be used to punish patients for undesirable behaviour.

Psychopharmacology

In general, pharmacological treatment is prescribed to treat symptomatic, psychotic and aggressive symptoms and should be prescribed by a medical doctor or specialist. In South Africa, the only medications now available to slow the degenerative process of cognitive decline are acetylcholinesterase inhibitors (like Donepezil for people with dementia due to Alzheimer's disease); cholinesterase inhibitors (like Galantamine); and N-methyl-D-aspartate (NMDA) receptor antagonists (like Memantine). These can only be prescribed after a comprehensive assessment has been completed by a multidisciplinary team.

The elderly are particularly responsive to pharmacological agents. Over-sedation (snowing) is not uncommon and contributes to increasing confusion, agitation and disorientation.

Medication should therefore be prescribed judiciously and nurses should monitor the effects of medication and report these carefully. Refer to the *Maudsley Prescribing Guidelines 12th edition*, 2015.

Table 16.19 encompasses some guidelines and principles when using psychotropic medication in the elderly (Baumann, 2007; 2015).

Table 16.19 Guidelines and principles when using psychotropic medication in the elderly

- Avoid drugs that block alpha adrenergic receptors if possible (anticholinergic, very sedative, long half life)
- Use with particular caution, because the elderly can suffer from concurrent illnesses and have a higher risk of adverse side effects.
- Adherence can be problematic due to cognitive and communication problems, and hearing and visual impairment.
- Pharmacodynamics changes should be considered as reactions to medication can be more severe and can include falls, fractures, pulmonary embolus, constipation, distress, agitation, anticholinergic sensitivity and even death.
- Pharmacokinetic changes include reduced absorption, slower onset of action, increased volume of distribution and longer duration of action of certain drugs which can lead to drug accumulation and toxicity.
- Drug interaction can lead to altered metabolism with either a loss of efficacy or increased effect.
- Basic principles are:
  - Use medication sparingly and only when strictly necessary.

→

- A 'start low, go slow' method is advised – meaning that you start with low doses and titrate cautiously upward, as well as gradually withdrawing medication – but be careful not to under-treat.
- Avoid treating side effects of one drug with another drug.
- Use a simple regime and aim for a once-a-day administration.
- Avoid treating symptoms before a diagnosis has been made.
- The need for ongoing treatment should be regularly reviewed.
- Be aware of medical problems and cognitive decline.
- Ensure that the client, family member and carer receive clear instructions and that they are knowledgeable about the indications and side effects of the medication. Avoid statements like 'necessary or required'.
- Avoid using drugs that cause sedation or have anticholinergic or alpha-adrenergic side effects.
- Be aware of covert use of over-the-counter medication or other drugs or substances.

Source: Adapted from Baumann (2007; 2015)

COPING WITH EPILEPSY: PRINCIPLES FOR PSYCHOSOCIAL NURSING INTERVENTION

According to Baumann (2015), epilepsy is the most common chronic neurological condition in the general population, with 30–50 per cent of individuals who live with epilepsy developing psychiatric problems. This section focuses on assisting the individual living with epilepsy as well as the family in order to manage the psychosocial implications of the condition. The different types of epilepsy and the medical and nursing treatments will not be covered. Table 16.20 encompass a case study of Ruth, a person living with epilepsy.

Table 16.20 Case study

Ruth, a busy mother and community worker, knew her life had changed when she suffered an epileptic seizure for the first time last year. She writes:
> I was a coward for not writing this a year ago and seeing the full horror in print. I did not want to leave writing about it till the time when I could say 'the first few months were dreadful' or 'I've got used to it now, it doesn't bother me'. I realise that my emotions are as strong as ever. They well up at a chance remark, a minor difficulty, a frustrated whim.

She was at work when she had the seizure and ever since the incident some of her co-workers seemed to distance themselves from her and it feels as though they do not take her comments seriously or listen to her input during meetings. She wanted to apply for a senior post, but her supervisor advised her to attend first to her medical problems. She does not want to follow up on the job opportunity as she fears she might 'faint' during the stressful situation.

There were periods when Ruth forgot to take her medication as prescribed, skipped her appointments or blamed the doctor for the weight that she picked up since being on treatment. She initially ignored the advice that she should not drive her car and when she was confronted, said that her family members must not expect anything from her. She makes excuses not to play with her children, or go to the shop, because the exercise might trigger a 'fit'. She isolated herself in her room.

Source: Uys and Middleton (2014)

Ruth's statement illustrates two of the most important and yet least understood characteristics of epilepsy. The first is that epilepsy as a chronic illness involves adjustment, not a cure. The second is that adjustment involves successfully negotiating a change in self-image to accommodate this new aspect of self. This process of adjustment is often a difficult and painful one. Coping underlies the process of adjustment. Coping has been variously defined, but within the context of nursing, coping refers to the behaviours people apply to control, master or resolve problems and their negative emotional consequences (Uys & Middleton, 2014).

The psychosocial nursing management of the person with epilepsy is reflected within the context of a coping model. This model is shown in Figure 16.3.

Cognitive appraisal

The ways in which people perceive their condition and their coping options are the most significant factors in adjustment. People with epilepsy tend to view themselves and their condition as unacceptable and are thus less likely to seek support. This negative appraisal is influenced by a number of factors. First, people are more likely to evaluate their condition as threatening if they have tonic-clonic seizures, if their seizures are poorly controlled, if they experience unpleasant side effects from medication and if they have previously experienced rejection as a result of their condition (Uys & Middleton, 2014).

Secondly, the attitudes of others significantly influence the appraisal process. Although negative attitudes towards people with epilepsy have decreased, stigmatisation still exists and individuals are perceived as abnormal and capable of violent crime who should not go out without an escort.

People living with epilepsy have difficulties finding and maintaining employment or are underemployed. Employers were less likely to hire people who experienced seizures than those with cancer in remission, depression, history of heart problems, AIDS, mild mental retardation, and spinal cord injury (Uys & Middleton, 2014: 525).

Family reactions vary and range from overprotection to scapegoating and rejection. A comparison study of epileptic and diabetic families showed that epileptic families perceived themselves to be less close with less family involvement, family interaction and activities (Uys and Middleton, 2014: 525). Considering the wide range of personal and social implications epilepsy has for people living with epilepsy, it is thus hardly surprising that they evaluate themselves, their condition and life events in a negative way.

Coping behaviours

The second step in the coping process focuses on the actual behaviour people use to manage the stressful appraisal. Depending on their function, they can be classified as emotion-focused or problem-focused strategies.

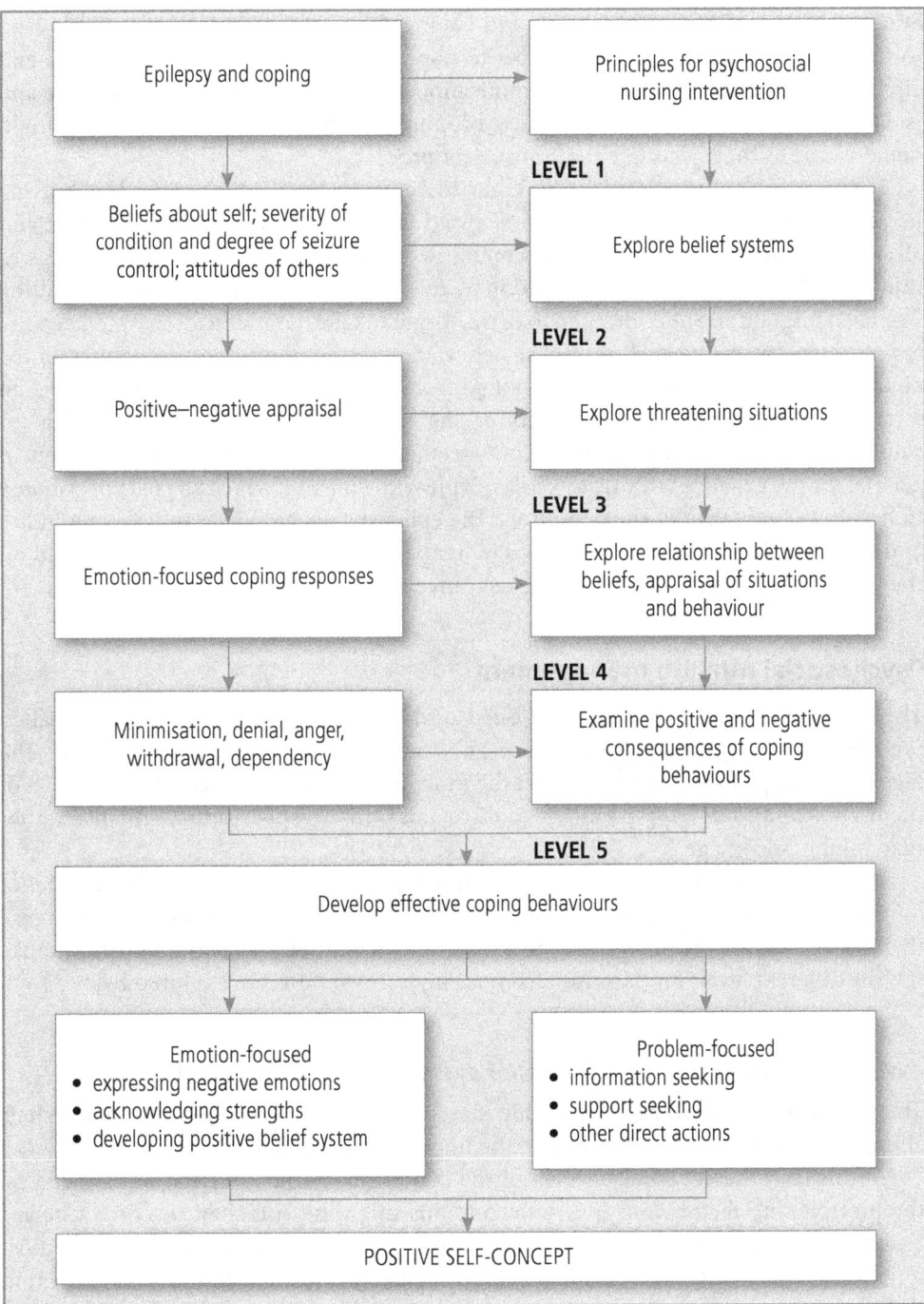

Figure 16.3 Epilepsy and coping: strategies for psychosocial nursing intervention
Source: Uys and Middleton (2014: 524)

Studies in the area of chronic illness and coping show that chronically ill people tend to use more emotion-focused defences to cope and adjust with their condition and circumstances. Denial, avoidance, minimisation, dissociation, resentment, blaming and isolation are some of the emotion-focused coping responses people with epilepsy might demonstrate as they negotiate the adjustment process.

In the case study referred to in Table 16.20, Ruth was initially afraid of hurting herself, afraid of dying during a seizure, afraid of what others would think of her, and afraid of losing her job. Her way of coping with the emotional consequences was to minimise the true nature of the condition by referring to her seizures as faints, resulting from bad migraines. She continued to drive, forgot to take her medication or to keep her appointments at the local clinic. These behaviours can be interpreted as a denial of the condition. It was only after she was banned from driving that she began developing an awareness of the reality of the situation. She became resentful of the condition for causing her pain, embarrassment and inconvenience. She also began blaming society in general for the negative attitude towards people with epilepsy, which she felt contributed to her slow acceptance of the condition. The epilepsy triggered fear and anxiety in her and she began isolating herself. This led to her becoming more and more dependent on the family for comfort, support and reassurance.

Psychosocial nursing management

The behaviours and responses mentioned under 'Coping behaviours' may be called maladaptive if they interrupt, retard or halt the adjustment and coping process. The biggest challenge for nurses is to assist the individual to accept the condition as part of themselves and to develop coping responses and utilise resources that enhance rather than inhibit self-image.

If the coping model is reviewed from a nursing management perspective, a number of intervention strategies emerge, all of which are interrelated and based on the premise that the way someone thinks about an event, influences their behaviour and emotions.

The different levels for psychosocial nursing interventions are explored below.

Level 1: Exploring the person's belief system

The supportive counselling relationship starts with the person exploring their beliefs about the condition, their abilities and the implications for their lifestyle.

At this level, health education about the condition, medication and its side effects, the precipitating factors and injury precautions might be sufficient to correct beliefs based on lack of knowledge. Adherence to epilepsy controlling medication is the most important aspect with the individual being adequately informed and involving them in the decision-making process. Active participation and a collaborative relationship have proved to be most effective. Ruth (from the case study) described how she was not fully informed about her condition and the role of medication in controlling her seizures. Inadequate health education led to Ruth believing that less medication and taking the medication at irregular intervals or only when she remembered, would still effectively control the seizures. This resulted in a lowering of her seizure threshold after being non-compliant and taking her medication at irregular intervals.

Another false perspective is that mental and physical strain precipitates seizures. For many people this can lead to unnecessary passivity and a restricted way of life. On the contrary, it has been shown that moderate amounts of physical and mental activities have the tendency to reduce epileptiform activity and seizure frequency.

Assessing the individual's beliefs about themselves and the condition is a useful strategy, because the person is forced to clarify and make abstract ideas concrete. At this stage, the idea of being a 'public relations official' for people with epilepsy rather than a victim of prejudicial attitudes might be introduced.

This level leads to the second level of intervention, where the person is assisted in identifying events and situations they find threatening, as well as situations in which they feel competent.

Level 2: Identifying threatening situations

People with a negative self-image tend to view all situations as threatening. This perception does not always have its roots in reality and the person needs to learn to differentiate between situations which pose a real threat and those that do not. It would be helpful for the person to make a list of situations in which they feel competent and those in which they feel threatened.

Ruth was anxious about going back to work because she believed her colleagues would avoid her and be unsupportive. In reality, her colleagues had been visiting her regularly and had clearly stated that they missed having her at work. As Ruth came to realise that her beliefs about her work environment were products of her own thinking, her anxiety began to diminish and she was able to consider returning to work.

Level 3: Exploring the relationship between beliefs, appraisal of situations and behaviour

The third level of intervention is to assist the person in understanding that beliefs influence the appraisal of situations and, consequently, behaviour. A useful strategy would be to ask the person concerned to match the beliefs with the identified situations and then, next to each pair, to list the ways in which they behave and the feelings they have in each situation. Ruth compiled the list shown below. She was able to recognise that the beliefs she held about herself in various situations influenced her behaviour. See Table 16.21.

Table 16.21 Ruth's beliefs

Beliefs	Situations	Feelings, behaviours
Worthless	Work	Inferior, avoiding applying for job
Exercise causes fits	Playing with children	Anxious, finding excuses not to play with them, feeling guilty
Social outcast	Social events	Inferior, resentful, angry, blaming others, avoiding social situations, for example going to the shop

Again, to reinforce the idea of epilepsy as only one aspect of self, it would be important for the person to focus on the positive as well as on the negative. Ruth believed she was a social outcast. This led to her interpreting all situations involving other people as threatening, and consequently she isolated herself at home. At the same time, Ruth saw herself as a caring mother and wife. Highlighting this aspect of herself helped to increase her sense of self-worth.

Level 4: Examining the positive and negative consequences of coping

As the person begins to develop an understanding of how they respond emotionally and behaviourally to events, the fourth level of intervention is introduced. At this point, the nurse should explore with the person the positive and negative consequences of the coping responses.

Just as people with negative self-concepts tend to interpret all situations as threatening, they also tend to evaluate their coping behaviours as ineffective. Again, this evaluation needs to be carefully challenged. Not all coping behaviours are ineffective. Coping is a shifting process and, to some extent, is determined by the situation. Minimisation might be a useful response in a situation involving strangers. On the other hand, if the person constantly uses minimisation, some of the negative consequences could be medication non-compliance, leading to increased seizure frequency, which could in turn lead to further isolation.

Sometimes people with epilepsy express a great deal of resentment and anger at having to take medication regularly, eat sensibly, monitor their seizures and be aware of factors that precipitate seizures because it means having to make lifestyle adjustments.

In this case, the nurse could point out the positive consequences of these coping behaviours, such as seizure control and increased mastery of the condition.

Level 5: Developing effective coping behaviours

The goal of this level of intervention is for the person to develop and strengthen effective emotion-focused and problem-focused coping responses. Developing the ability to engage actively in the problem-solving process is particularly important since the aim is to facilitate a sense of mastery and control. Depending on the area of need, this would involve health education around a variety of alternate emotion and problem-focused coping behaviours.

Emotion-focused strategies

These may include learning to express negative emotions appropriately, to acknowledge the positive aspects of self and to develop a positive belief system. Ruth learned the positive self-statements each time she felt anxious in situations involving other people. She would say to herself, over and over, 'My seizures are only one part of me. There are other parts to me; I am a good mother, a competent worker and I like talking to people.'

With continued practice, these positive beliefs became a part of her self-image and she was able to put her epilepsy into perspective.

Problem-focused strategies

These may include information-seeking strategies such as learning more about the condition, precipitating factors, medication and its side effects, legal restrictions on driving, and alternative transport services, such as bus routes, and possible safety precautions. Other strategies may include seeking support from social agencies, family and friends; learning how to tell relevant people about what to do and what not to do in the event of a seizure; and learning how to monitor seizures in terms of frequency and precipitating events and how to report this information in the course of clinic visits. Epilepsy South Africa have branches throughout South Africa which can be contacted for useful information and support. Learning strategies such as relaxation training to deal with feelings of anxiety, assertiveness skills, and ways of developing a realistic exercise plan can also prove useful.

Ruth started to keep a seizure calendar. She would record the seizure type and frequency and any side effects she felt from her medication. When she attended the clinic, she was able to report her findings concisely. Being able to participate in her treatment in this way gave her a sense of control over the condition.

Epilepsy and coping: conclusion

Too much emphasis has been placed on an individual's seizures and deficiencies rather than on strengths, abilities and overall capacity. This approach needs to be remedied if the person is to negotiate a successful change in self-image to accommodate epilepsy as only one aspect of themselves. Placing the psychosocial management of the person concerned within the context of a coping model is one way of correcting this approach, since coping by definition implies mastery and control.

CONCLUSION

In this chapter the different concepts, causes, diagnostic criteria and the assessment of NCDs were explained. Different nursing interventions and family liaison and medication guidelines were discussed. The principles of coping with epilepsy were also covered. Working with individuals living with NCDs offers a unique challenge to the nurse. Although NCDs are degenerative with cognitive decline and progressive functional impairment, the environment and quality of care is important. Considering that quality of life is the basic ethos of nursing, the opportunity to practise this philosophy should inspire nurses in creating a therapeutic environment where tailored and individualised care can be rendered for the individual living with an NCD.

WEB RESOURCES

https://www.alzheimers.org.za
> This is the official site of the Alzheimer's Association of South Africa. The site offers education, news, and information about support groups.

http://www.dementiasa.org/
> This is the site of Dementia South Africa. It offers education, training, research and information about support groups.

https://epilepsy.org.za
> This website offers information and support.

https://www.tafta.org.za/about.html)
> This is the website for Tafta (The Association for the Aged) which is a useful website advocating the well-being of older persons.

Another organisation, Action on Elder Abuse South Africa (AEASA) is a national non-governmental organisation focused on elder abuse prevention.

REFERENCES

Ali, N, Luther, S L, Volicer, L, Algase, D, Beattie, E, Brown, L M, Molinari, V, Moore, H and Joseph, I. 2015. 'Risk assessment of wandering behaviour in mild dementia'. *International Journal of Geriatric Psychiatry, 2015*, 31: 371-378.

American Psychiatric Association (APA). 2013. *Diagnostic and Statistical Manual of Mental Disorders – DSM-5*. Washington, DC: American Psychiatric Association.

Baumann, S E. 2007. *Primary Care Psychiatry A practical guide for southern Africa*. Cape Town: Juta.

Baumann, S E. 2015. *Primary Care Psychiatry A practical guide for southern Africa*. 2nd edition. Cape Town: Juta.

Cabrera, E, Sutcliffe, C, Verbeek, H, Saks, K, Soto-Martin, M, Meyer, G, Leino-Kilpi H, Karlsson, S and Zabalegui, A. 2014. 'Non-pharmacological interventions as a best practice strategy in people with dementia living in nursing homes. A systematic review'. On behalf of the RightTimePlaceCare Consortium School of Health Sciences TecnoCampus, University Pompeu Fabra, Avda. Ernest Lluch 32, 08332 Mataro´, Barcelona, Spain. *European Geriatric Medicine*, 6: 134–150.

Cipriani, G, Lucetti, C, Carlesi, C, Danti, S and Nuti, A. 2015. 'Sundown syndrome and dementia'. *Elsevier Masson SAS and European Union Geriatric Medicine Society*, 6(2015): 375–380.

Folstein, M F, Folstein, S E and McHugh, P R. 1975. 'Mini-mental state examination'. https://www.parinc.com/products/pkey/237 (Accessed June 2019).

Gray, B and Smith, P. 2009. 'Emotional labour and the clinical settings for nursing care: the perspectives of nurses in East London'. *Nurse Education in Practice, 9:* 253–261.

Gu, L. 2015. 'Nursing Interventions in Managing Wandering Behavior in Patients with Dementia: A Literature Review'. *Archives of Psychiatric Nursing, 29:* 454–457.

Heersema, E. 2017a. 'Using Reality Orientation in Alzheimer's and Dementia. Strategies and Cautions in its Use'. https://www.verywellhealth.com/treating-alzheimers-disease-with-reality-orientation-98682 (Accessed June 1019).

Heersema, E. 2017b. 'Using Validation Therapy for People with Dementia. Definition, History and Techniques'. https://www.verywellhealth.com/using-validation-therapy-for-people-with-dementia-98683 (Accessed June, 2019).

Kaliski, S. 2006. *Psycholegal Assessment in SOUTH AFRICA.* Cape Town: Oxford.

Larner, A J. 2017. *Cognitive Screening Instruments A Practical Approach.* 2nd edition. Switzerland: Springer International Publishing.

Menna, L F, Santaniello, A, Gerardi, F, Di Maggio, A and Milan, G. 2015. 'Evaluation of the efficacy of animal-assisted therapy based on the reality orientation therapy protocol in Alzheimer's disease patients: a pilot study'. *Japanese Psychogeriatric Society. Psychogeriatrics,* 16: 240–246.

Regier, N G and Gitlin, L N. 2017. 'Psychosocial and Environmental Treatment approaches for Behavioral and Psychological Symptoms in Neurocognitive Disorders: An Update and Future Directions'. *Geriatric Disorders. Current Treatment Options in Psychiatry,* 4: 80–101. Springer International.

Roach, P, Drummond, N and Keady, J. 2016. 'Nobody would say that it is Alzheimer's or dementia at this age': Family adjustment following a diagnosis of early-onset dementia. *Journal of Aging Studies,* 36: 26–32. doi: 10.1016/j.jaging.2015.12.001.

Sachdev, P S, Blacker, D, Blazer, D G, Ganguli, M, Jeste, D V, Paulsen, J S and Petersen, R. 2014. 'Classifying neurocognitive disorders: the DSM5 approach'. *Nature Reviews/Neurol.* advance online publication 30 September 2014. doi: 10.1038/nrneurol.2014.181. Macmillan Publishers Limited.

Simpson, J R. 2014. 'DSM-5 and Neurocognitive Disorders'. *The Journal of the American Academy of Psychiatry and the Law,* 42 (2): 159–64.

South Africa. 2006. *Older Persons Act. No, 13 of 2006.* Pretoria: Government Printer.

Steffen, A and Gant, J R. 2015. *International Journal of Geriatric Psychiatry,* 31: 195–203.

Tay, L, Lim W S, Chan, M, Ali N, Mahanum, S, Chew, P, Lim, J, Chong, M S. 2015. 'The new DSM-5 Neurocognitive Disorders criteria and its impact on diagnostic classifications of mild cognitive impairment and dementia in a Memory Clinic setting'. *The American Journal of Geriatric Psychiatry* (2015). doi: 10.1016/j.jagp.2015.01.004.

The Maudsley Prescribing Guidelines in Psychiatry, 12th Edition, David M. Taylor, Carol Paton, Shitij Kapur, 2015, Wiley Blackwell.

Uys, L and Middleton, L. 2014. *Mental Health Nursing. A South African Perspective.* 6th edition. Cape Town: Juta.

Western Cape Department of Health. 2013. *Healthcare 2030.* Cape Town: Western Cape Government. www.capegateway.gov.za/health (Accessed 27 July 2017).

CHAPTER 17

Nursing Care of Persons with Intellectual Disabilities

L R Uys, L Middleton and R Ramalisa

Learning Outcomes

After studying this chapter, you should be able to:
- analyse the concept of intellectual disability and approaches to caring for the person with an intellectual disability
- differentiate the most common disorders associated with intellectual disability
- assess levels of functioning of the person with an intellectual disability through utilising an appropriate and relevant assessment tool
- compile and implement stimulation and skill-teaching programmes in the cognitive, social, occupational and motor areas of development
- provide relevant information to parents and family with regard to caring for a person with an intellectual disability
- promote the prevention of learning disabilities at primary, secondary and tertiary levels by compiling mental health education and rehabilitation programmes for target population groups
- assess the impact of intellectual disability on the family and provide therapeutic interventions to assist the family.

INTRODUCTION

The DSM-5 (APA, 2013: 31) classifies intellectual disability under neurodevelopmental disorders. These disorders manifest in early development, often before the child starts school.

Nurses have been involved in the care of people with intellectual disabilities for many years. The attitude of the community to these people has varied over the years, ranging from disregard, and even rejection, to positive involvement.

The last 50 years have seen tremendous progress in the care of people with intellectual disabilities. The greatest breakthrough was probably the general acceptance of a developmental perspective in this regard. A task group of the National Institute for Child Health and Human Development (1986: 2) put it this way:

The major empirical finding has been that in the majority of domains of infant behaviour little relationship has been found between assessments or diagnosis in the first year of life and assessments later in childhood. The major theoretical achievement has been the explanation for the lack of these relationships. A developmental approach has emerged that recognises that child progress is a product of both the capacities of the child and the experiences of the child.

This approach is based on the assumption that no diagnostic label can forecast what a child will or will not be able to do. The emphasis is therefore on the development of capabilities and not on the making of forecasts.

There are some problems with the terminology used in this area of psychiatry. Persons who have the disability feel that the term 'mental retardation' is stigmatising and derogatory. However, the DSM-5 has replaced the term mental retardation with intellectual disability, which is acceptably used by medical and other professions, as well as by the lay public and advocacy groups. Some people and organisations, including the World Health Organisation, used terms with stipulated definitions like impairment, disability and handicap, which gave them a defined meaning (WHO, 1980). However, the revised version of this text used the term 'disability' as an umbrella term for all three perspectives – for impairments, activity limitations or participation restrictions (WHO, 2001). In the United Kingdom (UK), the term 'learning disability' is now generally used but this causes confusion in terms of 'learning disabilities' as defined by the DSM-5. In South Africa's Mental Health Care Act 17 of 2002, the term used is 'intellectual disability', hence the decision to use it in this chapter, except when referring specifically to the diagnostic system. Intellectual disability is a term that best describes the problem and is correct in terms of the WHO classification.

Similarly, in terms of anti-stigma language usage, one should not equate the person with the condition. Therefore, one should not talk of 'mentally retarded people', but of 'people with intellectual disabilities'. This approach is followed in this chapter. The views of consumers are expressed below (Hewitt & O'Nell, 1998: 1).

Who we are is as much about how others see us as it is about our physical beings. We can eat right, exercise, and believe in ourselves all we want, but if no one ever notices it won't last for long. So what does it mean to be 'a person with mental retardation'? Does it say something about a person that is meaningful and relevant? Does it tell people something about that person that is valuable, helpful, or essential?

When asked, most self-advocates with intellectual disabilities will make it clear that the label 'mentally retarded' is stigmatising and limiting. If the label comes before the person then a large part of who that person is has already been defined.

Despite clear indications from self-advocacy groups that the words mental retardation should be 'retired', support professionals and agencies that oversee support systems struggle with how to provide the necessary assistance to people who need it, without defining who is eligible (ie, creating a label). By its very nature service provision hangs onto labels in order to know where to best put resources. The dilemma of dropping all labels and still accurately describing who can receive supports through state agencies is not solved. But there is a clear mandate from the people who receive these services and supports that people – not labels – always come first.

Recent developments in South Africa have seen major transformation in terms of the protection and rights for people with disabilities. The Mental Health Care Act 17 of 2002 makes reference to this and is inclusive on the care, treatment and rehabilitation of persons with intellectual disabilities. Furthermore, the White Paper on the Rights of Persons with Disabilities was approved in 2015, which updates the Integrated National Disability Strategy and encompass the rights of people with physical, intellectual or neurological disabilities (South Africa, 2015).

PREVENTION

Issues related to primary, secondary and tertiary prevention, and the role that mental health nurses can play, are examined in this section.

Primary prevention

Kromberg et al (2008) screened a total of 6 692 children in rural South Africa, between two and nine years of age, and reported that the cause of intellectual disability in 20.6 per cent of the children was congenital; in 6.3 per cent, the cause was acquired, while the cause in 73.1 per cent of the children was undetermined. According to Adnams (2010: 437), the prevalence rate for conditions that are associated with intellectual disability in the prenatal and developmental period indicates a higher total prevalence of intellectual disability in South Africa compared to that in other developed countries. The most obvious way in which nurses can be involved in the primary prevention of intellectual disability is by ensuring good antenatal and maternity services. And despite conducive policies and high coverage of antenatal care in South Africa, prenatal mortality rates are largely caused by the inadequate implementation of guidelines and programmes (UNICEF). This means that birth injuries may be expected to remain an important cause of intellectual disability in this country. Other causes of intellectual disability include nutritional deficiencies, infectious diseases such as mother-to-child transmitted human immunodeficiency virus (HIV)/acquired immunodeficiency syndrome (AIDS), tuberculosis and meningitis, foetal alcohol spectrum disorder, violence and injury (Adnams, 2010: 437). Most of these conditions are preventable and manageable.

Other important preventive measures include genetic counselling, educating the public on abstinence from alcohol during pregnancy and a continuous effort by primary health care nurses to follow and adhere to national guidelines. Genetic counselling prevents genetic abnormalities, more so in families with a history of genetic disorder. The most common genetic abnormalities causing intellectual disability, in South Africa, are Down syndrome and 'Fragile X'. Prevention is, however, not easy. Early genetic counselling aimed at the prevention of high-risk pregnancies would probably not achieve much greater acceptability. Only long-term strategies, such as the improvement of the socioeconomic status of families and improved literacy, would make genetic counselling a more successful strategy for the overwhelming majority of the population.

Secondary prevention

Secondary prevention involves rehabilitating children and focuses on avoiding any secondary complications, teaching children to manage their disabilities, and enhancing their psychological adjustment (Sobralske, 2013: 36).The early detection of intellectual disability, in order to commence stimulation and learning programmes as soon as possible after birth, could play an important role in optimising the capabilities of all children. This type of programme originated in the United States of America (USA) in the 1970s and spread rapidly. Early detection means the early identification of groups at risk because of developmental delays. The diagnosis only indicates a risk and focuses attention on the need for stimulation and learning and should not be seen as a forecast of future capabilities. The programme usually includes comprehensive teaching and counselling of the parents. There is evidence that such programmes do not limit the educational, motor, sensory, language and social ability of these children (State of Washington, 2012). This is more especially so when sensitive and responsible care is provided before the age of nine months. This can remedy skills deficits and ultimately results in these children being indistinguishable from their typically developing classmates by the time they begin school (Weis, 2015: 97).

The establishment of programmes for early detection, stimulation and learning in South Africa is hampered by the following factors:

- There are few psychiatric nurses in primary health services who could launch this type of programme. Alternative staff, such as primary school teachers and clinical psychologists, are just as scarce, if not more so.
- A large proportion of the population is very poor and some are illiterate, and home environments in such circumstances do not facilitate the early recognition of developmental delays.
- Specialised services for children with developmental disabilities – and even for other children – are not generally available in large parts of the country.

Despite the inaccessibility of specialised services for persons with intellectual disabilities, certain medical conditions in these persons, such as hyperthyroidism, can be effectively treated early to prevent complications.

Tertiary prevention

This means that adequate, goal-directed programmes and services should be available for the optimum development of all identified people with an intellectual disability, throughout their lives. This is an ideal that has not yet been remotely realised.

Considering the fact that the South African population is made up of about 55 million people, according to the census of 2011, about 1 per cent of the population (South Africa, 2015: 24) can be expected to have mild or moderate developmental disabilities, which involves limitations in self-care. Thus the need for service is evident. The policy of 'mainstreaming' or inclusion in typical classrooms might go a long way to addressing the need.

Within the broader educational system, the process of inclusion by which all learners, with or without disabilities, are educated together, with sufficient support, in age-appropriate, regular education programmes in their neighbourhood schools, can be incorporated. Support is often provided on a 'push-in' (in-class aid or assistant to teacher), or 'pull-out' (visits of the child to a resource room) basis. This approach became the rule rather than the exception in the USA in the late 1970s, when the Education for All Handicapped Children Act (USA, 1975), amended to the Every Student Succeeds Act (USA, 2015), made educational provision a right for all children in the 'least restrictive environment' (Rynders & Low, 2003).

In a national study commissioned by the USA National Down Syndrome Society (NDSS), the majority of participating teachers reported that entire classes benefit from working with a learner with Down syndrome (NDSS, 2003). Almost all teachers who responded found inclusion enjoyable, with some calling it the single most interesting and rewarding experience of their careers. Overall, both parents and teachers found current inclusive practices successful, but there is room for improvement. The study found that more appropriate teacher preparation and more time for conferences between teachers, therapists, parents and support personnel would be beneficial to all involved (NDSS, 2003).

In this study, factors directly affecting the success of an inclusive experience, as measured by both parents and teachers, included a match of teacher personality and style to the skills of a learner. Teachers who were flexible, willing to modify classroom materials, and who utilised hands-on learning tools, were the best catalysts for achievement. Those parents whose children with Down syndrome had friends in class rated the inclusion experience the most successful and reported great benefits in the areas of communication, self-esteem and independence. Teacher preparation was important for success, but surprisingly, formal training from the school district did not appear to be relevant (NDSS, 2003).

This approach to rehabilitation and social integration of persons with intellectual disabilities is the direction in which the future lies. This inclusive education is, furthermore, promoted by the National Development Plan and will enable everyone to participate effectively in a free society (South Africa, 2015).

INTELLECTUAL DISABILITY

Over the past decade, as stated earlier, the term intellectual disability has been preferred instead of mental retardation, covering the same population of individuals who were diagnosed previously with mental retardation (Schalock et al, 2007). Intellectual disability refers to conditions that have to do with cognitive functioning, adaptive behaviour, and learning that is age-appropriate (Salvador-Carulla et al, 2011: 177). The DSM-5 criteria for intellectual disability are as follows (APA, 2013: 33):
A. Deficits in intellectual functions, such as reasoning, problem solving, planning, abstract thinking, judgement, academic learning and learning from experience,

confirmed by both clinical assessment and individualised, standardised intelligence testing.
B. Deficits in adaptive functioning that result in failure to meet developmental and sociocultural standards for personal independence and social responsibility. Without ongoing support, the adaptive deficits limit functioning in one or more activities of daily life, such as communication, social participation, and independent living, across multiple environments, such as home, school, work, and community.
C. Onset of intellectual and adaptive deficits during the developmental period.

The DSM-5 defines severity levels for intellectual disability according to the following four subtypes reflecting the degree of intellectual impairment:
1. mild
2. moderate
3. severe
4. profound (APA, 2013: 33)

Most persons with intellectual disability have mild intellectual disability; approximately 20 per cent of persons with intellectual disability have moderate disability and 5 per cent have severe or profound disability. A figure of 4 per 1 000 of the population is used for the planning of services for learning disabled persons. This condition is often associated with others, such as epilepsy, cerebral palsy, sensory impairment and behavioural problems. A survey in 2001 found that the prevalence of intellectual disability in South Africa was 0.5 per cent and in a 2007 survey, the prevalence of severe intellectual or learning disability was 0.27 per cent (Adnams, 2010).

People with intellectual disabilities have the same wide variety of characteristics as people with a normal IQ, and persons with intellectual limitations have their own preferences just as others do. It is therefore important to treat every person with an intellectual limitation as an individual and without prejudice. People with such a limitation sometimes have a limited range of emotions, and lack personality traits such as self-control and perseverance due to their intellectual disability. They find it difficult to grasp abstract concepts and they have a limited understanding of the choices that may be put before them. They usually have less drive, energy and motivation than people with a normal IQ, although such traits vary enormously even in the 'normal' population.

A limited intellect impairs normal development. This in turn makes this group more vulnerable to personal and emotional problems such as poor self-esteem, acting-out behaviour and excessive attachment. Because of their cognitive and affective limitations, they are unable to give adequate meaning to the realities surrounding them and it is almost impossible for them to interpret abstract reality. They have a fragmented perception of their world and often miss the meaning of complete experiences.

Table 17.1 Development features of subtypes of persons with intellectual disabilities

Degree of intellectual disability	Preschool age: 0–5 years	School age: 6–5 years	Adult: 21 years and over
Mild: IQ 50–55 to about 70	Can develop social and communication skills; minimal impairment in sensory motor areas; often not distinguishable from normal children	Can master academic skills; often taught in special classes in normal schools; can be guided into social adjustment	Can usually master vocational skills well enough to be self-supporting, but require guidance and support when under unusual social or economic stress; open job market; are in unskilled or semiskilled employment
Moderate: IQ 35–40 to 50–55	Can talk and learn to communicate; poor self-awareness; fair motor development but reach milestones later; profit from training in self-help procedures by means of early detection and stimulation and learning programmes; placement in day centres from the age of three years	Profit from training in social and occupational therapeutic skills; can learn to travel alone in familiar places; trained in training centres	May be self-supporting and able to do sheltered employment in special workshops; require supervision and guidance when under moderate social or economic stress
Severe: IQ 20–25 to 35–40	Poor motor development; speech minimal; profit little from training in self-help procedures; few or no communication skills; early detection, stimulation and learning programmes	Can talk or learn to communicate; can be trained in elementary hygiene skills; profit from systematic habit training in stimulation centres	May contribute partially to self-care under full-time supervision; can develop self-protection skills to a minimally useful level in a controlled environment; spend their lives in stimulation centres
Profound: IQ below 20 or 25	Minimal capacity for sensor-motor functioning; require total physical care	Limited motor development; may respond to minimal or limited training in self-care; admission to care facilities often necessary	Limited motor and speech development; may develop very limited self-help skills; require total care for life

Source: Adapted from Kaplan and Sadock (1985)

ASSESSMENT

In keeping with the developmental approach, assessment focuses on function and development and not on the DSM-5 diagnosis. A complete assessment of a person with an intellectual disability includes more than the assessment of the individual. It also includes an assessment of the parents or caregivers and the environment.

The Washington State Early Learning and Development Guidelines provide essential information to support and enhance children's development and learning (State of Washington, 2012: 2). The developmental stages and chronological ages are compared, offering guidelines for the support of parents. This instrument is included as an example (see Table 17.2).

Table 17.2 Washington guide for the evaluation of the development of young children

Motor skills	Eating skills	Play
1–3 months • Head erect briefly when prone • Head erect and bobbing when supported in sitting position • Follows object through all planes • Palmar grasp • Moro reflex	• Sucking reflex • Rooting reflex • Swallows strained food • Coordinates sucking, swallowing and breathing	• Quietens when picked up • Regards face of others
4–8 months • Sits with minimal support and stable head and back • Sits alone steadily • Plays with hands which are usually open • Grasps rattle or bottle with both hands • Picks up small objects, for example a cube • Transfers toys from one hand to other • Neck-righting reflex	• Uses tongue in moving food in mouth • Hand to mouth motions • Recognises bottle on sight • Gums or mouths solid foods • Feeds crackers to self	• Plays with own body • Distinguishes strangers from family • Seeks out objects • Grasps, holds and manipulates objects • Repeats enjoyable activities • Bands toys or objects together
9–12 months • Rises to sitting position • Creeps or crawls, maybe backwards at first • Pulls self to standing position • Stands alone • Cruises, holding on to furniture	• Holds own bottle • Drinks from cup or glass with assistance • Finger-feeds • Begins to hold spoon	• Puts objects in containers and takes out • Explores objects in hand • Plays interactive games (peek-a-boo) • Holds toys out to others without letting go

Motor skills	Eating skills	Play
<ul><li>Uses index finger to poke</li><li>Parachute reflex</li><li>Landau reflex</li><li>Grasps objects with index finger and thumb</li><li>Can catch self from falling sideways, backwards, or forwards while sitting</li></ul>		<ul><li>Makes an effort to get hold of toys which are out of reach</li></ul>
13–18 months<ul><li>Walks several steps without support</li><li>Balanced when walking</li><li>Walks upstairs with help and crawls downstairs</li><li>Turns pages of book</li></ul>	<ul><li>Holds cup and handle with digital grasp</li><li>Lifts cup and drinks well</li><li>Begins to use spoon, may turn bowl down before reaching mouth</li><li>Difficulty in inserting spoon into mouth</li><li>May refuse food</li></ul>	<ul><li>Plays alone, may play near others</li><li>Has preferred toys</li><li>Enjoys walking activities, pulling toys</li><li>Throws and picks up objects, throws again</li><li>Imitates, for example reading newspaper, sweeping</li></ul>
19–30 months<ul><li>Runs</li><li>Walks up and down stairs one at a time (not alternating feet)</li><li>Imitates vertical strokes</li><li>Imitates building tower of four or more blocks</li><li>Throws ball overhand</li><li>Jumps in place</li><li>Rides tricycle</li></ul>	<ul><li>Drinks without spilling</li><li>Holds small glass in one hand</li><li>Inserts spoon in mouth correctly</li><li>Distinguishes between food and inedible material</li><li>Plays with food</li></ul>	<ul><li>Parallel play, not interactive but plays alongside another child</li><li>Uses both large and small toys</li><li>Rough-and-tumble play</li><li>Play periods longer than before, interested in manipulative and constructive toys</li><li>Enjoys rhymes and singing (TV programmes)</li></ul>
31–48 months<ul><li>Walks downstairs, alternating feet</li><li>Hops on one foot</li><li>Swings and climbs</li><li>Balances on one foot for 10 seconds</li><li>Copies circle</li><li>Copies cross</li><li>Draws person with three parts</li></ul>	<ul><li>Pours well from jug</li><li>Serves self at table with little spilling</li><li>Rarely needs assistance</li><li>Interested in setting table</li></ul>	<ul><li>In playing with others, begins to interact, shares toys and takes turns</li><li>Dramatises and expresses imagination in play</li><li>Combines playthings, more use of constructive materials</li><li>Prefers two or more children to play with, may have a special friend</li></ul>

Motor skills	Eating skills	Play
49–52 months • Balances well • Skips and jumps • Can heel-toe walk • Copies square • Catches bounced ball	• Feeds self well • Sociable and talkative during meal	• Dramatic play and interested in going on excursions • Fond of cutting and pasting, creative materials • Completes most activities
Language	**Toilet training**	**Dressing and undressing**
1–3 months • Smiles when socially stimulated • Has facial, vocal and generalised bodily responses to faces • Makes pre-language vocalisations that consist of cooing, throaty sounds, for example 'goo' • Makes 'pleasure' sounds • Crying can be differentiated from discomfort, pain and hunger sounds		
4–8 months • Eyes locate source of sounds • Responds to 'hi there' by looking up at face across and in front • Turns head to locate sound at 90-degreee angle from head • Laughs aloud when stimulated • Produces vowel sounds and chained syllables, for example baa, goo-goo and didi • Makes 'talking sounds' in response to others talking • Vocalises to toys • Babbles to produce consonant sounds		

→

Language	Toilet training	Dressing and undressing
9–12 months • Ceases activity when name is pronounced or 'no no' is said • Gives toys on request when accompanied by facial and bodily gestures • Attends to simple commands • Imitates definite speech sounds such as tongue-clicking, lip-smacking or coughing • Uses two words that are specific for parents, for example 'mama' and 'dada'	• Begins to show regular patterns in bladder and bowel elimination • Has one to two stools daily • Interval of dryness does not exceed one to two hours	
13–18 months • Attends to person speaking • Finds 'the baby' in picture when requested • Indicates wants by gestures • Looks towards family members or pets when named • Uses three words other than mama and dada to denote specific objects	• Will have bowel movement if put on toilet at approximate time • Indicates wet pants	• Cooperates in dressing by extending arm or leg • Removes socks, hat and shoes • Can unzip zips • Tries to put shoes on
19–30 months • Points to one named body part • Follows two or three verbal directions not accompanied by gestures • Combines two different words, for example 'play ball', 'want cookies' • Names objects in picture • Refers to self by pronoun rather than by name	• Anticipates need to eliminate • Same word for both functions • Daytime control (occasional accident) • Requires assistance (reminding, dressing and wiping)	• Can undress • Can remove shoes if laces are untied • Helps dress • Tries to unbutton • Pulls on simple clothes
31–36 months • Attends longer to stories and TV programmes • Demonstrates understanding of two prepositions by carrying out two commands, one at a time, for example	• Takes responsibility for toilet if clothes are simple • Continues to verbalise need to go, ability to hold urge to go for longer periods • May have occasional accident	• Interested in dressing and is more skilled • Tries to fasten shoes, usually incorrectly • Does not know back from front

Language	Toilet training	Dressing and undressing
'Put the block under the chair' - Follows commands asking for two objects or two actions - Demonstrates understanding of concepts of big and little - Gives first name and surname - Names what has been drawn after scribbling - Tells you what gender on request - Repeats few rhymes or songs - Tells what action is going on in picture	- Needs help with wiping	- Washes and dries hands, brushes teeth - Buttons
38–48 months - Expresses appropriate responses when asked if tired, cold or hungry - Tells story - Common expression: 'I don't know' - Repeats sentences composed of 12 or 13 syllables - Masters phonetic sounds of p, k, g, v, tf, d, z, lr, hw, j, kw, l, e, w, qe and o		
49–52 months - Points to 1 cent, 5 cents or 10 cents on request - Carries out command containing three parts - Counts three objects, pointing to each in turn - Defines simple words, for example hat and ball - Asks questions - Can identify or name four colours	- General independence	- Dresses and undresses with care except for tying shoes and buckling belts - May learn to tie shoes - Combs hair with assistance

Using these guides, nurses are able to screen young children through early identification of developmental delays which should prompt access to essential services with timeous, efficient and appropriate assistance. According to the Department of Basic Education and UNICEF (2015), the Ten Question Disability Screen (TQS) is the most appropriate disability screening tool for children. Other screening tools and developmental assessments include developmental milestone charts, the Road to Health Booklet (RtHB) and the Strive Towards Achieving Results Together (START) programme.

SUPPORT FOR PARENTS OF CHILDREN WITH INTELLECTUAL DISABILITIES

This section examines the effect on the family if a family member has an intellectual disability; methods of supporting the parents of such a child and support regarding specific aspects like discipline, sexuality and schooling.

Effect of a member of the family having an intellectual disability

The gravity of the problems experienced with a family member who has an intellectual disability depends on the degree of disability, the concomitant emotional and physical impairment and the values, interests and circumstances of the rest of the family.

Parenthood is a challenge and is viewed as an enriching and uplifting experience. Consequently, the birth of a child with a disability is extremely disillusioning. The hopes and expectations that the parents have for the child are shattered and they have to make tremendous adjustments. The most common responses of families with a member who is intellectually disabled are the following:
- denial, apathy, shock and tension
- anger, bitterness and rejection
- bargaining and going from service to service
- depression, sadness, grieving, despair and guilt
- acceptance and planning.

Even after initial acceptance, such families find that raising a child with an intellectual disability is far more complicated than raising a normal child. Among the factors that cause additional pressure in the life of the family are the following:
- the specific disability of the child
- slow development
- the necessity of making special arrangements for the child's physical care, training and comradeship
- the family's expectations of the future.

These problems easily cause disequilibrium in the family. Financial problems are also common.

Methods of supporting the parents of a child with an intellectual disability

Professionals who work with the parents of children with intellectual disabilities should be knowledgeable about the medical, social, educational and behavioural aspects of the disability. They should also be well informed about available agencies and services, and about written information and aids that are useful in the home. Essential attributes demanded of these professionals include sensitivity to the needs of the families, and a great deal of patience and skill in solving short-term family problems.

Olsson (2016: 65) discussed the support needs for parents of children with an intellectual disability:

- Most of the parents reported the need for information, particularly information about available services for their child
- About 63 per cent of parents reported needs concerning information about their child's impairment
- A further 63 per cent requested information on how to handle their child's behaviour and how to teach their child various skills
- It was also 63 per cent of the parents who expressed needing more time for themselves – opportunities for respite from caring for their child
- There was a need to meet and share experiences with other parents of children with impairments and to read about the experiences of parents with children with the same impairment
- Another need was for regular meetings with a psychologist, psychiatrist or counsellor for advice and support
- Some 24 per cent expressed their need for financial support.

Douglas et al (2016: 2743) outlined three key themes regarding the support needed by parents caring for children with intellectual disabilities in the first year of diagnosis. These include the following:

- *Adjusting.* This refers to the emotional journey that underlay the other experiences of the first year as parents grappled with what it meant to be the parent of a child with a disability. Parents by necessity took charge of their child's care whether or not their emotional needs were met. Providing emotional, psychosocial and practical support enables a smoother adjustment.
- *Quest for knowledge.* This is significant in parents regarding their need for information. Parents sought a range of information related to their child's condition and the support and services they could access to meet their child's needs. Parents needed information to enable them to take charge of their child's care.
- *Connecting in.* Parents benefitted from connecting with other parents of children with intellectual disabilities who provided practical advice and psychosocial support. This was particularly helpful for parents as it built both their confidence and their knowledge base.

Among the most effective sources of support are parent groups, such as the Down Syndrome South Africa (DSSA) and the Sunshine Association, which offer support, information and services to members. Parents with similar problems readily accept one another because they understand one another's problems and can talk about them. Parents find a sympathetic ear for their anxiety and stress in these groups, as well as support to work through and cope rationally with their problems.

Support for parents of children with intellectual disabilities is a long-term undertaking, as these children may always be dependent on some level of support. Support is required to enable them to fulfil their role as a permanent unit in a functioning family and to prevent family dysfunction and disintegration. Furthermore, Mohsin, Khan, Doger and Awan (2011), stated that parents can play a vital role in the training and development of children with intellectual disabilities. The following are methods that parents can use when involving themselves in educating their children.

- Parents should break down each activity into small steps. Reward helps to increase the possibility of desired behaviour.
- The child learns by repetition and drill methods.
- The parent has to demonstrate the task to the child first.
- Different activities can be demonstrated by parents during their daily interaction with children.
- Learning through games is recommended and parents can play different games with their children.
- Parents should seek professional guidance and support.

Support regarding specific aspects

The different aspects looked at in this section include discipline, sexuality and schooling.

Discipline

The parents of a child with an intellectual disability often have difficulty in disciplining the child because of their response to the child's condition.

- *The child's condition.* These children do not learn as easily as normal children do because of their limited intellectual capacity. They require stronger, more organised and more repeated stimuli than their brothers and sisters. When they realise that normal discipline is unsuccessful, parents may begin to believe that these children are incapable of learning the desired behaviours, instead of understanding that they merely need more help.
- *Response of the parents.* Overprotection is often one of the responses of parents to a child's disability. They do not want to be strict, as they are afraid that this will be construed as rejection or cruelty and they feel sorry for the child. This, together with the belief that the child has too little understanding to profit from discipline in any case, results in a lack of discipline.

Intervention is essential. Persons with intellectual disabilities are not readily accepted in the community at the best of times and to be further debilitated by inappropriate behaviour is an almost certain recipe for rejection. The future of such children therefore depends on successful discipline.

The following interventions are necessary:
- *Help the parents to discuss their own feelings about the problem.* Work through feelings of guilt or pity, and correct misconceptions about the child's capabilities.
- *Identify problem behaviour and help the parents to plan and implement a consistent response.* It is often necessary to acquaint parents with techniques such as time out, as these are seldom used with normal children. Time out means that the child is removed from a situation for up to five minutes so that undesirable conduct is not reinforced by attention. It may be necessary to equip a special room in the house for this purpose. It may also be necessary for parents to use a particular technique, for example ignoring a temper tantrum, by means of role play.
- *Ensure adequate support for discipline.* The parents must support each other, and others in the immediate circle must understand and support the discipline. Older brothers and sisters, grandparents, domestic helpers and play-group leaders should all be involved to ensure consistent discipline.

Sexuality

Matters to do with sexuality have historically either been ignored or actively suppressed for persons with intellectual disabilities (Bleazard, 2010: 1). Over the years, the emphasis that persons with intellectual disabilities should understand their sexuality has become a matter of contention, more especially in a South African context where the society is affected by HIV/AIDS. The sexuality of persons with intellectual disabilities therefore presents special challenges. Sexuality is not limited to sexual intercourse, homosexuality or masturbation. It is defined as the quality of being sexual and is one way in which individuals express their personality. This can be seen in the person's choice of clothing, use of cosmetics and hairstyles, interaction in social settings and use of leisure time.

Health workers can be encouraging and in the first instance promote healthy sexuality by assisting the person with an intellectual disability to look as attractive as possible. This can be achieved by attending to personal hygiene and grooming, by encouraging the choice of appropriate clothing and by teaching acceptable social skills. Opportunities for males and females to interact socially in an age-appropriate manner should be encouraged.

A few guidelines should be kept in mind in this respect:
- Sexuality is part of every person's being. It is not possible to encourage the development of a strong and healthy self-image in persons with intellectual disabilities if their sexuality is denied. They must be helped to know and accept themselves as men and women.
- The sexual drives and needs of persons with intellectual disabilities seldom differ from those of normal people. They enjoy sex and view marriage in a very positive light, and some would like to have children. They are seldom hypersexual or asexual.
- Acceptable sexual conduct and morality needs to be learned by persons with intellectual disabilities from an early age. The denial or avoidance of this aspect of life leaves these people very vulnerable in the adult world.

There are many myths, fears and beliefs in the wider community and among those involved in the care of persons with intellectual disabilities. These impede healthy learning and development in this respect. Some of these problems are the following:

- The community denies the dignity of persons with intellectual disabilities and therefore has an aversion to associating highly regarded human behaviour, such as sexual intimacy and motherhood, with them. Remarks such as 'It's not right' or 'They don't understand' are typical of this view.
- Parents and caregivers are afraid that girls with intellectual disabilities will be vulnerable to sexual exploitation and unwanted pregnancies. They fear that boys and girls will express their sexual curiosity and drives in an unacceptable manner and that this could lead to rejection and even prosecution. This fear often results in the denial of sexual maturity, for instance by addressing adults with intellectual disabilities like children, or by teaching them that all sexual behaviour is wrong.
- Professionals are often unwilling to make provision for normal sexual activities within the services for which they are responsible, as they are afraid of rousing the ire of families or the community. An extramarital sexual relationship or even a pregnancy could result in serious accusations against the service. Most institutions still do not provide married quarters, and this exacerbates the problem for the staff.
- Some people question the ability of persons with intellectual disabilities to accept the responsibility of parenthood and there is a belief that sterilisation should be enforced. It is important to examine this argument thoroughly and from an ethical viewpoint. Furthermore, Coren et al (2010: 11) suggest that parents with intellectual disabilities can be trained to learn a range of parenting skills which they might not otherwise master. There are few research findings containing accurate figures and estimates of the number of parents with intellectual disabilities vary widely (Coren et al, 2010: 9).

It is not easy to find answers to this aspect of persons with intellectual disabilities. However, it is important to broach the subject with the parents early in the lives of such children, and to help them to sort out their own feelings in this regard. In this way it will be possible to help the children to experience this enriching aspect of human life in a positive way.

Schooling

By the age of six years, children with intellectual disabilities also have to enter the school system. At this stage parents have to decide whether to place the child in a special school or not; many opt for integration into a mainstream school. It is very useful to have a thorough assessment conducted by an agency experienced in this field. To identify such agencies, contact a parent support group in the area and social service department, since they usually have the most experience. If parents decide on integration, the most appropriate school needs to be identified. Not all schools and/or teachers are equally 'disability friendly', and some who might be very willing have class sizes that make it more difficult to cope. All these factors need to be taken into account when making a choice.

Once a decision has been made, the child and parent need careful preparation for entry into the school. This might mean, for example, that the parents initially accompany the child, and then gradually reduce time with the child at school.

If the child is in a mainstream school, Henderson (2001) makes the point that it might be necessary during adolescence for parents to organise social events where the child can interact with others who have the same disability. The after-school programmes strive to build community and foster interdependence among young people who can become a peer group for one another. The activities emphasise communication skills, group affinity, decision making, personal empowerment, self-help, financial responsibility, opportunities for service and recreation, lifetime fitness, outdoor adventure, creative movement, and the arts. Each group has 6–12 participants and meets roughly once a week for an hour and a half for a duration of nine months, following the academic calendar. In addition, the groups plan and take field trips or go on outdoor adventures together several times each year.

STIMULATION OF DEVELOPMENT

Home stimulation programmes are based on the assumption that children with an intellectual disability develop better in stable, loving families than in institutions. The reasons for this are that sustained attention, a familiar environment, and a consistent model exhibiting the same opinions, gestures and attitudes day after day are an advantage.

Parents should be encouraged to act as teachers to their child with an intellectual disability for the following reasons:
- parents are powerful agents of reinforcement
- parents know their children better than anyone else and usually devote more time to them
- the effectiveness of interventions can be enhanced if parents use the skills they have learned
- teaching children at home reduces expense
- parents experience satisfaction by contributing to the development of their children.

A home stimulation programme can be described as one in which parents are taught how to stimulate and teach a child who is living with an intellectual disability. A home stimulation programme consists of the steps outlined in Figure 17.1 and is based on the following components:
- early stimulation of all senses
- teaching self-care.

Early stimulation of senses

Infants and toddlers with intellectual disabilities require more repeated and stronger stimulation for development. Their environment should therefore be more stimulating than that of normal children – and this is seldom the case in institutions. Ideas for stimulating infants up to the age of three years are given in Table 17.3.

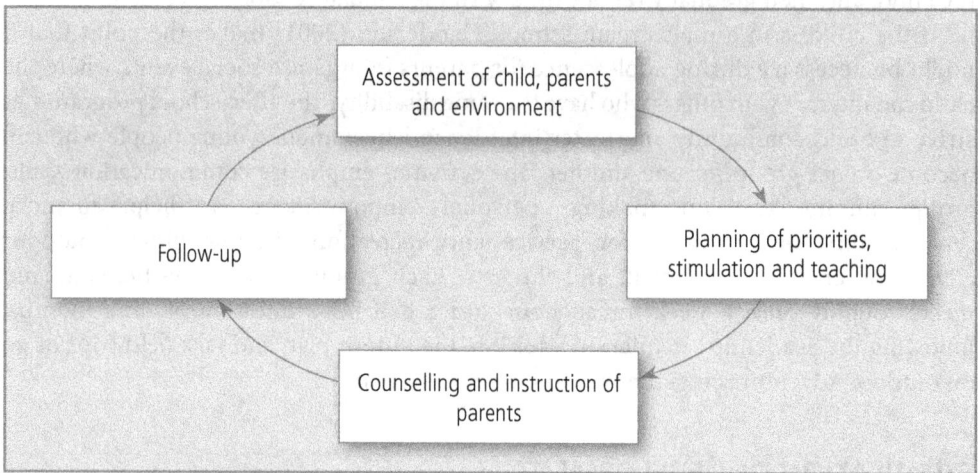

Figure 17.1 Home stimulation cycle: assessment of child, parents and environment

Table 17.3 Development stimulation chart

Age in months	Communication and sound	Smell and touch	Vision	Gross motor skills	Fine motor skills	Feeding	Toilet training
0	Call child by name. Use full sentences and words; do not use baby talk. Tell child what you are doing; name objects you use. Parents must cooperate in every way. Leave child with baby-sitter once in a while. Sing to child. Play radio softly near crib for short periods. Introduce child to sound of running water, musical toys, household utensils, whistling, rattles.	Hug, hold, kiss, stroke. Rub with different textures, for example cotton, silk, feathers, sandpaper, wood, thread. Introduce to odour of fruit, vegetables, cereals, perfume, spices. Rub down vigorously with towel after bath. Feed and change from both sides.	Move crib around in room. Move child round to windows. Hang a single-object mobile 22 cm from eyes. Use bright sheets, pillowcases, clothes.	Exercise arms and legs in bath (passively if necessary). Place prone on hard surface for one to two minutes (tummy time).	Povide objects with different textures.	Make meals relaxed and pleasant. Give bottle and teach to suck and swallow.	

Age in months	Communication and sound	Smell and touch	Vision	Gross motor skills	Fine motor skills	Feeding	Toilet training
1	Stitch bells to bracelets and shoes with dental floss. Encourage smiles and laughter.		Change mobile weekly. Use mittens in bright colours. Move objects in air in circle and arc for eyes to follow.	Help to sit up on mat on floor. Stimulate to raise head. Use infant seat. Place in sitting position for short periods.	Brings hands together round bottle. Show bright colours and objects for eyes to follow.	Feed cereals and strained food.	
2				Take outside weather permitting. Roll over and over. Tilt in all directions. Swing in blanket. Bounce on bed.		Supply good variety of tastes. Feed fruit.	
3						Feed vegetables	
4	Speak loudly, softly, in high pitch, in a low pitch, whisper. Reinforce sound with facial expression and posture.	Introduce hot, cold, hard, soft. Bring into kitchen when cooking.	Hang multiple object mobile 30–37 cm from eyes. Still change weekly.	Allow to stretch for objects out of reach.	Give objects to hold in hands (to grasp and let go). Allow to reach for small objects.	For supper, feed egg yolk, meat (food containing iron). Feed more coarse foods. Offer cup.	

Age in months	Communication and sound	Smell and touch	Vision	Gross motor skills	Fine motor skills	Feeding	Toilet training
5	Clap child's hands. Play peek-a-boo. Repeat child's own sounds. Play finger and toe games. Start scrapbook with one object. Parent to name pictures in book.	Teach how to finger foods.		Rock prone back and forth on beach ball. Support in sitting position. Allow to sit alone. Allow to sit on low stool in front of table. Parent to play rough-and-tumble games. Let swim if possible.			
6	Reward all language attempts. Give toys that make noise to hold.		Play mirror games. Fasten balloons to wrist and feet.	Allow to play with belly board.		Allow finger foods, for example crackers, cereal, toast. Encourage dipping fingers in food and bringing to mouth.	

Age in months	Communication and sound	Smell and touch	Vision	Gross motor skills	Fine motor skills	Feeding	Toilet training
7	Play hide-and-seek. Allow to stay with family during meals.		Alternate toy collection. Divide toys in two–three groups. Change groups every two–three weeks.	Allow to ride on parent's shoulders. Allow to play with blocks, aeroplanes.	Allow to bang on blocks, saucepans, lids. Use kitchen utensils as toys.		
8	Play hide-and-seek (with parents and toys). Stay with parents during meals. Introduce to animal sounds.	Smell and touch trees, shrubs, flowers, grass, etc.	Show outdoor objects in motion, for example cars, lawn mowers, aeroplanes. Change toy collection. Divide toys into two–three groups.	Hang mirror above cot. Use Jolly Jumper; support feet. Allow to crawl on various surfaces, for example floor and mat.			
9				Teach to kneel. Play dropping and throwing games.	Allow to play with rag dolls, pack things in and out of boxes (aids visual coordination). Play water games.	Feed tactile foods. Try to get child to eat with spoon. Use bowl instead of plate. Offer cup frequently.	Check regularity of bowel actions. Put on potty when elimination is expected. Praise for success, ignore failure. Use correct terms for body functions. Use same words every time child goes to potty.

Chapter 17: Nursing Care of Persons with Intellectual Disabilities

Age in months	Communication and sound	Smell and touch	Vision	Gross motor skills	Fine motor skills	Feeding	Toilet training
10		Allow exploration within boundaries of safety.	Hang notice board in child's room instead of pictures. Change pictures on board often. Use large, single pictures with objects.		Wants to know what everything does. Allow to slash, stir, pour; feed self, drink from cup. Wean off bottles one at a time.		
12	Name toys with single words. Name and point to body parts. Let child point to pictures.	Encourage to return affection.		Allow to play in sandpit with spades, buckets, cars. Teach to transport objects.		Help to brush teeth.	
14	Allow to play with toy telephone, listen to real telephone. Read simple stories. Help to follow simple commands.		Encourage to touch textured pictures.	Allow to push and pull toys. Give opportunity to help in house. Provide swing in garden. Help to climb up stairs. Allow to undress. Ask to fetch and carry.	Encourage to open, close, explore functions. Allow to play with crayons, build towers with blocks.		

Age in months	Communication and sound	Smell and touch	Vision	Gross motor skills	Fine motor skills	Feeding	Toilet training
				Encourage walking, holding onto shirttail, walking on various surfaces, for example grass, mattress, walking backwards, doing somersaults.			
16				Teach to balance on one foot. Play jumping games. Imitate pets. Allow to play with tricycle, in paddling pool with supervision.	Teach to trace, finger-paint, put on shoes (without fastening), wash and dry hands.		Check on regularity of voiding urine: 1. Fairly regular times. 2. Holds urine for hours. 3. Bothered by wet nappy. Keep written record of voiding for two–three weeks. Sit on potty when voiding is expected. Praise for success, ignore failure.

Age in months	Communication and sound	Smell and touch	Vision	Gross motor skills	Fine motor skills	Feeding	Toilet training
20	Teach to say please and thank you. Play blowing games. Teach to use plural, combine two words, play with others, name desired object, name object in picture.			Walk on stepping stones.		Gradually teach neatness and table manners. Do not try to teach rapidly. Teach to drink through a straw.	
24	Simple how and why of daily activities. Allow to play with puppets. Imitate other people, animals, objects.			Teach to dress with help, without help.	Teach long, short, big, small, to trace circle, to build bridge with blocks.	Teach to brush teeth without help.	
30	Teach basic colours, opposites, to share, to fill in words in stories, name and address.		Teach concept of shapes. Let play with form box. Teach names of colours. Teach concepts like under, in, on top.	Play walking games on well-marked route. Play follow-my-leader. Allow to play with large cardboard box.	Allow to play with busy board, clay.	Make dental appointment.	
36					Teach to set table.		

Snoezelen multisensory stimulation

Snoezelen was first introduced in the 1970s by staff working at two Dutch centres as an intervention for persons with intellectual disabilities (Chung & Lai, 2009). It allows an individual to receive sensory input in the type and amount desired by visual, auditory, olfactory, tactile, vestibular and proprioceptive sensory input using different objects (Kaplan et al, 2006: 443).

Snoezelen has been found to increase time spent on task during a session. Furthermore, a study conducted by Kaplan et al (2006) supports the hypothesis that there is a carryover effect of Snoezelen-based sessions upon subsequent on-task behaviour. This means that there is significant improvement in the attention spent on vocational activity or on training in activities involving daily living skills. The findings also suggest its effectiveness on alleviating maladaptive behaviours during sessions in persons with intellectual disabilities. These include aggression, self-harm and destructive behaviours (Shapiro et al, 1997).

Elements of a Snoezelen room involves identifying a therapeutic space that will allow the individual to choose whichever stimuli they enjoy. Materials and the environment should be stimulating and bring peace and quietness. Another aspect is playing calm music with dimmed lights to create a special atmosphere (Verheul, 2014).

TEACHING SELF-CARE AND OTHER SKILLS

Observation and assessment form the first link in the chain of skills development. Teaching a skill merely because it is the next skill on a checklist – regardless of its relevance to the individual's life – is frustrating and useless to the person with an intellectual disability. For example, a child may be taught to tie shoelaces and is then given slip-on shoes to wear. This section discusses approaches to and the content of teaching self-care.

Approaches to teaching self-care

Much of the care and treatment of persons with intellectual disabilities has to do with teaching, and sometimes also with helping them to unlearn negative behaviour. Learning is very dependent on intellectual capacity, and special skills and techniques are therefore necessary when teaching persons with intellectual disabilities.

The following are effective teaching behaviours when working with persons with intellectual disabilities:
- Remove distractions from the teaching environment, for instance other people or noises.
- Ensure basic needs, such as toileting, are attended to first, before commencing teaching.
- Ensure eye-contact by positioning yourself at the level of the patient and within his/her direct view. This improves focusing on what you present.

- Develop a trusting relationship, so that the person is comfortable with the teacher. The learning process should be fun.
- Use short declarative sentences, supported by your body language and actions. For instance: 'Shake my hand firmly' accompanied by an outstretched hand.
- Use open-ended questions to avoid acquiescence. Persons with intellectual disabilities are very prone to agreeing and trying to please the questioner. Ask: 'How should you greet me?' rather than 'Should you greet me by hand?'
- Provide corrective feedback in a friendly, non-judgemental manner. 'Just shake my hand and let it go. Don't hold on to it.'
- Teach a skill that is one step above competence or at a level of competence.
- Ensure continuity of the teaching programme in a specific direction, so that gains are not lost.
- All teaching should be a building-on process, moving from simple to complex tasks.
- Establish a baseline (measurement of what the person can do before any intervention to change).
- Routine, reward and repetition are important in teaching the persons with intellectual disabilities.
- Break tasks into simple steps (task analysis).

Specific teaching techniques

Contingency management and chaining are two specific teaching techniques that are relevant.

Contingency management means that you make sure that positive or desired behaviour is followed by a reward and that negative or undesirable behaviour is not followed by a reward. It has been found that people are inclined to repeat behaviour that is rewarded, for instance when a child smiles at a nurse, the nurse can reward the child by smiling back. A smile is an example of a social reward, but a reward may also be physical, such as giving a person a cookie when they have correctly completed a task. The reward, which is contingent on desired behaviour, reinforces that behaviour.

It is important to remember that attention is a powerful reward to most people, and they will even be willing to engage in behaviour that leads to negative attention (a scolding or a fight) rather than doing without attention. When a child (or adult) has a temper tantrum in a public place, giving attention rewards the behaviour, and this may lead to the behaviour being repeated. The first important technique in modifying negative behaviour is therefore to make sure it is not rewarded in any way.

In contrast, one should make sure that positive behaviour, which you want the person to learn, is rewarded immediately. Persons with intellectual disabilities, especially severe or profound disabilities, cannot make the connection between the reward and the behaviour unless the reward follows very quickly upon the behaviour. This link between behaviour and reward also needs to be repeated very many times before the behaviour is learned.

Chaining is a technique used to teach a number of behaviours that, when linked together, form a complete skill, for example 'feeding/eating with a spoon'. The task is broken into small steps that can be taught to the individual. The procedure of teaching a skill from the beginning to the end is termed 'forward chaining' or 'progressive chaining'. This technique is not often used with people with intellectual disabilities as it can make learning difficult. Backward chaining refers to first teaching the person to complete the last step of the chain, and then working backwards. This is more successful, since the reward can be given immediately upon completion of the task.

Content of self-care teaching

The following are the most important aspects of self-care:
- motor skills, which eventually enable the child to walk and without which independence is impossible
- feeding skills
- dressing and undressing
- toilet training.

These self-care skills are outlined in the following sections.

Motor skills

Children's early motor skills develop in the following sequence. Children are able to:
1. Lift their heads when lying prone
2. a. Lift their heads with their weight on their elbows
   b. Keep their heads in line when pulled into a sitting position
3. Lift their heads with their weight on their hands (and arms straight)
4. a. Lean forward when sitting
   b. Roll over from prone to supine
5. a. Creep on the floor in the prone position
   b. Crawl on arms and legs
   c. Crawl contralaterally
6. Stand with support
7. Pull themselves into a standing position
8. Stand without support
9. a. Walk with support
   b. Walk without support
10. Do the following regarding balance and maintenance of posture:
    – static balancing stunts
    – balancing beam activities
    – umbling and gymnastics
    – playing games requiring balance
    – going through an obstacle course

11. Undertake locomotion in the following ways:
    - executing basic motor skills such as walking, running, hopping, skipping, jumping and landing
    - playing games of touch
    - playing relay games
    - doing stunts
    - repeating rhythms
    - participating in play that entails movement
    - going through an obstacle course.

Teaching step 1: Control of the head – lifting the head when prone

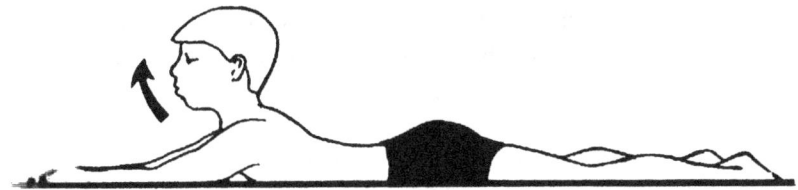

1. Place the child prone on a firm surface such as a carpet.
2. Stimulate the child lift to his/her head by calling the child's name or shaking a rattle in such a position that the child has to lift his/her head to identify the origin of the sound. Give plenty of reinforcement (smile, kiss and become excited) for every attempt to lift the head.
3. Kneel on the floor behind the child. Hold the child's head in your hands and lift it so that the child can focus on an object 30 cm in front of his/her eyes. The object must be directly in front of the child. Hold the child's head in this position for 15 to 30 seconds before lowering it. Allow the child some rest before repeating. Repeat the exercise three times a day (lift the head five times during each exercise session) to strengthen the child's neck muscles.
4. As soon as the child can lift his/her head and hold it upright for one minute, he/she is ready for the next step.

Teaching step 2: Lifting the head with the weight on the elbows

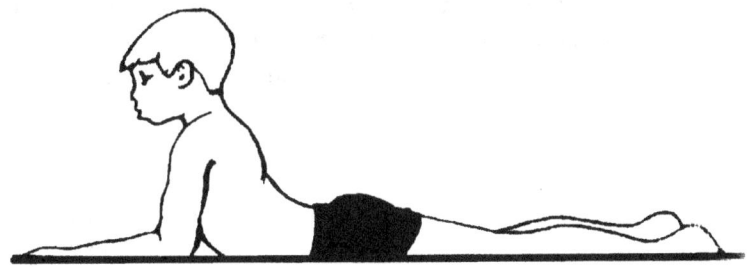

A.
1. Place the child prone on the floor.
2. Place a blanket or rolled towel under the child's chest in such a way that the child's elbows and forearms rest on the floor. The roll strengthens the neck muscles and also those of the trunk and shoulders.
3. With much of the child's weight now on the elbows, place a toy nearby in such a position that the child can see, grasp and move it. The child may also enjoy looking in a mirror.
4. Engage in play, call the child's name, hang an object in front of and above the child's head, ring bells, anything to make the child lift his/her head.
5. Reinforce this behaviour by singing, clapping your hands and kissing the child. Gradually demand more from the child before showing that you are satisfied.
6. Place the child on the floor without the rolled blanket under his/her chest. Exert slight pressure on the sacrum; this stimulates the spine to straighten and lift the head.

B.
When the child has mastered the steps above, attention must be given to opening fists, as this is a prerequisite for placing weight on the hands. The following steps lead towards the child's opening his/her fists.
1. Hold the child on your lap or place the child prone on the floor and carefully massage a closed fist. Massage away from the knuckles until the hand begins to relax. Open the hand and let it rest on a smooth surface for a few moments.
2. While bathing the child, follow the same procedure in the water. Warm water is relaxing and the child's hand will open more readily.
3. Every day place a face cloth or small toy in each hand for 20 to 30 minutes. Roll up a face cloth (or other absorbent material) and place it in the child's hand in such a way that the thumb is pushed out straight. If necessary, use masking tape or sticking plaster to ensure that the hand stays in this position.
4. Every time you pick up the child, place your middle and index fingers in the child's fist to encourage a more open-hand position. Carefully pull the child up into a sitting position to take him/her into your arms. Put your arms out and encourage the child to imitate you. Initially accept any attempt at an open-hand technique, but gradually demand more before you show your satisfaction.
5. Place your thumbs in the child's hands and bring both arms to the midline position or bring the child's hands (with your thumbs inside them) to the child's eyes and play peek-a-boo. Always show your pleasure at all attempts to do what you wish, in this case opening the hands.

C.
When the child's hands are open most of the time, the arm and upper trunk muscles must be strengthened before the child is able to place his/her weight on the arms. The following procedures strengthen these muscles and help the neck to remain stable while the child is pulled to a sitting position:

1. Take hold of the child's upper arms and elbows and slowly pull the child to a sitting position. Now bring your hands to the child's chin and use them to lift the head gently to a normal position. Initially repeat this procedure five times twice a day, but gradually increase the number as the child's strength increases. Also shift your support to the child's elbows and then to his/her hands.
2. Place the child on your lap facing you. Lift the child's arms above his/her head and slightly away from the body. The child will be inclined to lift his/her head.
3. Place the child on your lap facing away from you. Bring his/her hands together directly in front. It is more fun if you allow the child to clap his/her hands or place an interesting object between his/her hands.
4. Place the child on your lap facing you. Lift the child's outstretched arms (with the elbows straight) to shoulder height and move them slightly backwards.
5. Inflate a large inflatable plastic ball to about three-quarters of its full size and let the child lie on the ball. Sit in front of the child and hold his/her arms out to the sides like wings. Carefully rock the ball and the child forwards, backwards and sideways. Be prepared for initial signs of fear such as crying. Gently encourage the child to overcome this fear and enjoy the experience.
6. Hug the child and suddenly release your firm grip.
7. Swing the child in a blanket and play rough-and-tumble; the other parent can be of great help in this regard. Continue with these procedures until the child holds his/her head steady when pulled into a sitting position.

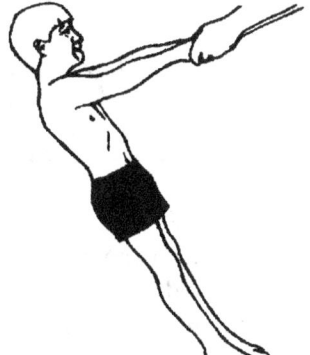

Teaching step 3: Placing weight on the hands
A.
1. Place the child prone on the floor.
2. Place a rolled blanket under the child's chest. The roll must be large enough to keep the child's elbows off the floor. (Make a large roll like this: use masking tape to attach two one-kilogram-sized coffee tins to each other lengthways and cover the roll with foam rubber.)
3. Place the child's hands flat on the floor and in front.
4. Place toys with colourful designs in front of the child and encourage him/her to place weight on his/her hands. Shake a rattle or other noisy toy above and slightly behind the child's head so that he/she has to use his/her hands as support to look at it.

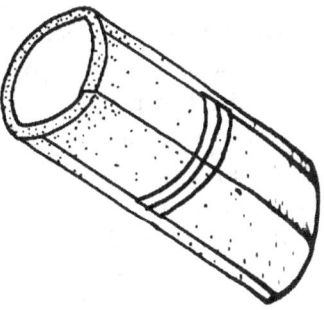

5. Place the child prone on the floor with a cloth under his/her chest. Kneel over the child and use the cloth to lift his/her trunk until the arms are straight and the hands rest on the floor (crawling position). Gradually allow the child to take more weight on his/her hands.
6. Play the 'aeroplane' game with the child to improve the parachute reflex. This reflex usually appears at 12 months and must develop before the child can walk. Hold the child in the air (face down) and make a swooping motion down to a firm surface without touching the surface. Note whether the child puts out his/her arms as though to stop (this is the parachute reflex). Initially work at getting the child to put out his/her arms – this may take a few weeks. As soon as this has been achieved, allow the hands to touch the surface when playing. Also gradually allow more weight to be placed on the hands. The ideal position aimed at in this step is shown below.

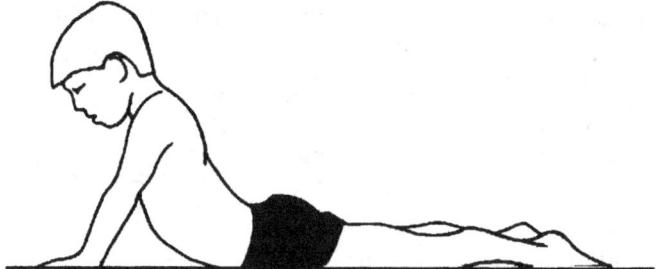

B. Preparing to sit
1. *Put the child in an infant's chair for 30 minutes a day. Adjust the chair in such a way that the child advances from a reclining to sitting position over a period of weeks. Take the child from room to room in this position, while you talk to the child and allow him/her to watch you at work.
2. *Place the child prone on the floor for at least 15 minutes a day.
3. *The child must develop a sense of balance, as this is essential for sitting. Let the child sit on the floor. Kneel in front of the child and gently rock him/her to and fro. Watch whether the child tries to stop by stretching their arms out to the sides. It may be necessary for you to do this for the child at first. (This exercise may initially require two people – one to move the child's arms and the other to rock the child.)

*These activities should be part of the daily routine of all infants from the age of two weeks

4. Place the child on his/her back and allow the child to touch and play with his/her toes. This strengthens the muscles of the lower trunk and will also help the child to become aware of his/her legs and feet.

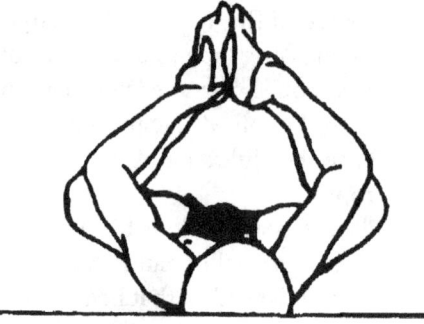

The latter is important for the development of self-image and for standing and walking.

5. Let the child sit on the floor with his/her legs wide apart, knees bent and hands on the feet. Support the child in this position for a few minutes, taking care not to let him/her fall over.
6. When the child can sit reasonably well but still requires support, place him/her in a Jolly Jumper for short periods. Ensure that the feet are firmly on the floor. If the Jolly Jumper is too high, place a cardboard box underneath it. Encourage the child to bounce up and down by pushing with his/her feet. Initially set the example by pushing the seat down. Smile 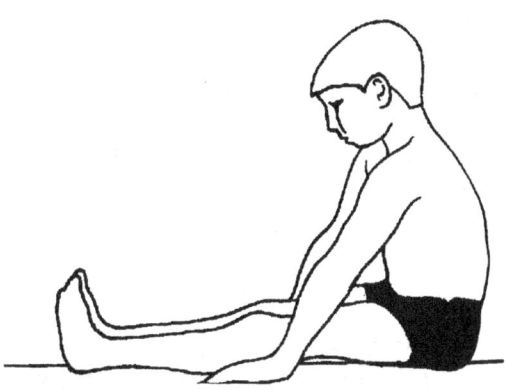 and give praise for every bounce. Gradually decrease your help but continue giving praise. Continue with these procedures until the child can sit as shown here.

Teaching step 4: Rolling over

This is an important preparatory step to mobility.

A. Supine to prone
1. Place the child on the floor on his/her right side. Move the left leg over the right and encourage the child to roll over onto his/her abdomen. It may be necessary to roll the child over at first, but your assistance should gradually be diminished. As soon as the child can turn from his/her side to their abdomen, place the child on his/her back, place your hands in the hollow of the back and encourage the child to roll over. Make sure that the head is turned in the direction they are to roll, as this will help a great deal.
2. Repeat the procedure with the child placed on their left side. In both cases a rattle can be used to give the child something to work towards.

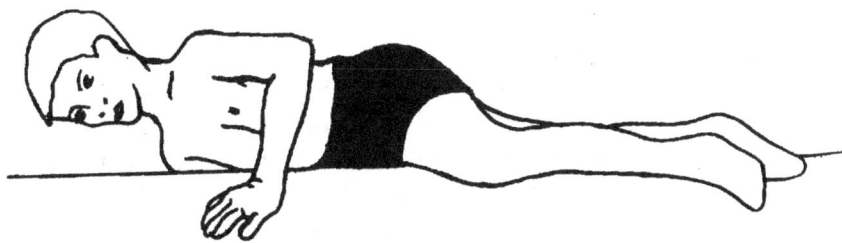

B. Prone to supine
1. Place the child prone on the floor and kneel alongside him/her. Lift one arm; bend it at the elbow and let the palm press down flat on the floor. Place the other arm underneath, making sure that the child's head is turned in the direction of the bent arm. Encourage the child to use the arm, which has its hand pressing on the floor, to help him/her turn over onto his/her back. It will probably be necessary to show the child what you want by placing one of your hands on the flat hand and your other hand under the child's back in order to roll him/her over. Say 'Push yourself over' while doing this so that the child knows what you expect. Let the child roll to both sides.
2. This exercise is best done with the child wearing only a vest and nappy. Allow the child to roll over on various surfaces, such as the carpet, the floor tiles, grass, paper and a blanket.

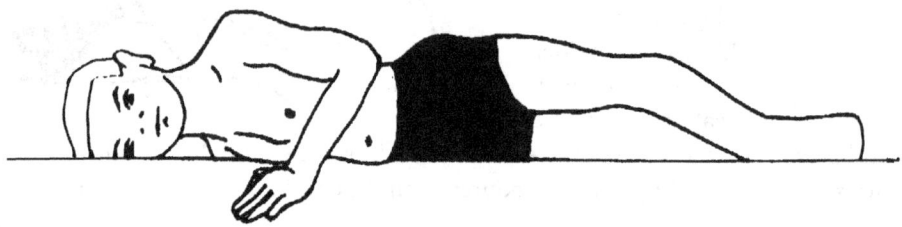

Teaching step 5: Crawling
A.
The child should crawl with the abdomen on the floor (start this simultaneously with step 3 B).
1. Place the child prone on the floor with a favourite toy in front of him/her, but just out of reach. Kneel behind the child and encourage him/her to move forward. Initially two people may be required, one to kneel behind the child and one in front. Both must move the child's arms and legs in opposing motions, that is, left arm forward, then right leg, then right arm, then left leg. Encourage the child to move forward and talk all the time so that he/she knows what you want. Praise every little success.
B.
Start the exercises for crawling on all fours when the child can do 3 B and 5 A fairly well.
1. Place the child prone on the floor. Place a cloth under the child's chest, kneel and pull up the cloth until the child is on his/her hands and knees. Retain this position for a few minutes and then rock the child back and forth. Talk all the time, saying what it is you want. Gradually decrease your help. Practise until the child can rock to and fro on his/her hands and knees without support.
2. Place the coffee tin roll of step 3 under the child's waist so that his/her knees reach the floor in a normal crawling position.
Note: The tin rolls well if it is covered with plastic material.

C.
As soon as the child can carry his/her own weight in the crawling position or can remain in this position with the support of the tin roll, contralateral crawling can commence.
1. Do this activity with the child in the crawling position and with two people helping (one behind and one in front). Move the child's arms and legs in a contralateral pattern, that is, right arm and then left leg, then left arm, then right leg. When moving the child's leg forward, first press gently against the foot. This pressure will later be sufficient to induce the child to move the leg forward. Always explain what you want and break the activity down into small sections.
2. As soon as the child is fairly skilled at moving his/her arms forward, the person in front may leave. Place a favourite toy in front of the child, but out of reach, and encourage him/her to move towards it. At this stage it will generally still be necessary to move the legs.
3. If the child has no particular interest in toys, a favourite food may be used instead. Initially this food can serve as reward for each small success, but use it together with a social reward (praise, a kiss or a hug). The child will soon discover the advantages of crawling, and then the artificial reward (food) can be withdrawn.

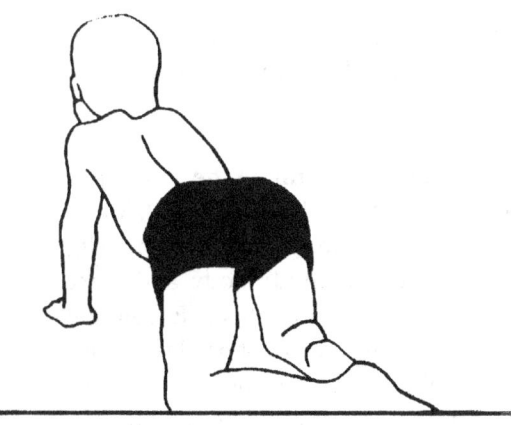

Teaching step 6: Standing with support
1. Place the child on a plastic ball that has been three-quarters inflated. Carefully rock the ball back and forth so that the child is forced to balance with his/her arms and legs. Take hold of the child's hands and lift them above his/her head so that the feet reach the ground and the body is partially supported by the ball. Bring the hands down to the ball so that the child gets the feeling of support. A second person holds the child by the knees and ensures that the feet are resting firmly on the floor. Initially hold the child in this position for a few seconds and later for a few minutes.

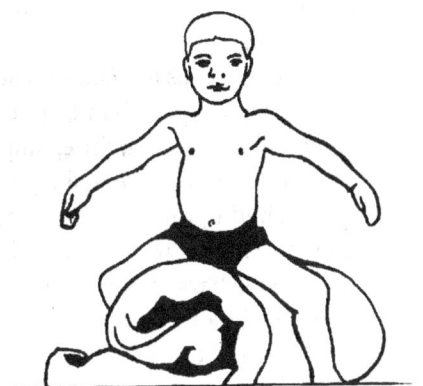

2. Place the child on the floor in a crawling position. Kneel behind the child – close enough for your knees to support the child's lower legs. Place a cloth around the child's waist and pull on it carefully to bring the child to a kneeling position.
3. Place a large blanket roll on the floor and let the child sit on it. Support the child to prevent his/her falling.
4. Place the child in a Jolly Jumper so that his/her feet rest flat on the floor. Encourage the child to jump.
5. Sit on a chair. Let the child sit in front of you with his/her back against your lower legs. Place a cloth around his/her chest and pull him/her upright.

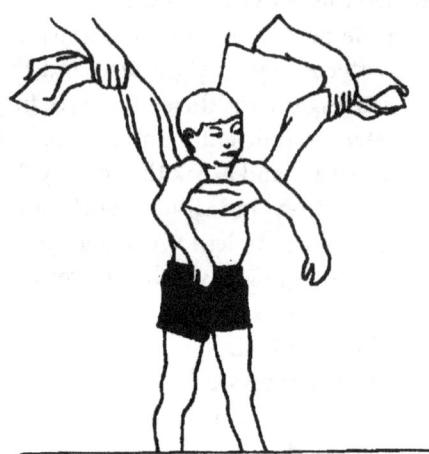

Note: Do not hold the child by the arms or hands, as he/she must use these to balance him/herself.

Teaching step 7: Pulling the child up into a standing position
1. Kneel next to the sitting child. Move one arm (with the elbow straight) slightly behind the child's body and place an open palm on the floor. Encourage the child to rest the wrist partly on that arm.
2. While in this position, encourage the child to reach out with the other hand. This may be done by offering a toy or something to eat. Praise attempts at reaching out.
3. When the child has learned to reach out with the unoccupied hand, guide this hand to a firm support, for example the armrest of a chair, and encourage the child to pull him/herself up. Say 'Pull up' and help the child upright at first. Decrease your help but continue to praise.

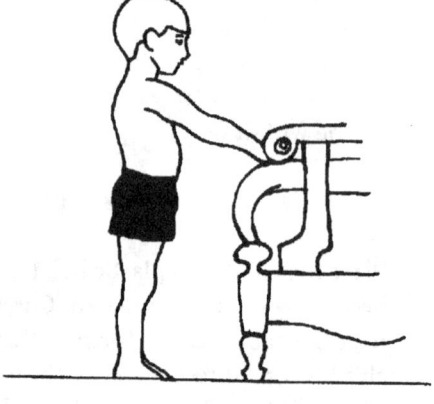

4. When the child is in his/her cot, show him/her how to reach up with a free hand and grasp the bars of the cot. Tie a favourite toy or 'busy board' to the bars, initially at knee height and later at standing height.
5. When the child begins to pull him/herself up, fix a small mirror (20 cm × 25 cm) to the backrest of a chair just above the seat. Allow the child to stand upright to look in the mirror. Place the child in front of the chair in a sitting position and encourage and help him/her to pull him/herself up so as to stand and look in the mirror.

Teaching step 8: Standing without support
1. Stand with the child in a standing position in front of you, with the child's back resting against your legs.
2. With the child in this position, place a cloth around his/her chest. Hold cloth close to the child's body and move away slightly. Give praise for slightest attempt at standing alone. As the child becomes steadier on his/her feet, continue using the cloth but hold it further away from the child's body, as illustrated in (b) below. Gradually reduce your support over the next few sessions and later remove the cloth. By this time the child should be able to stand alone for a few seconds.
3. Let the child stand facing you while you sit. Place your hands at the child's sides. Let go for short periods but give support when necessary. Allow the child to lean forward against your legs for support if necessary. A toy in your lap may help the child relax and make him/her more willing to stand.
4. Let the child stand facing away from you and repeat step 3. Give the child a toy to hold to help him/her relax and make him/her more willing to stand.

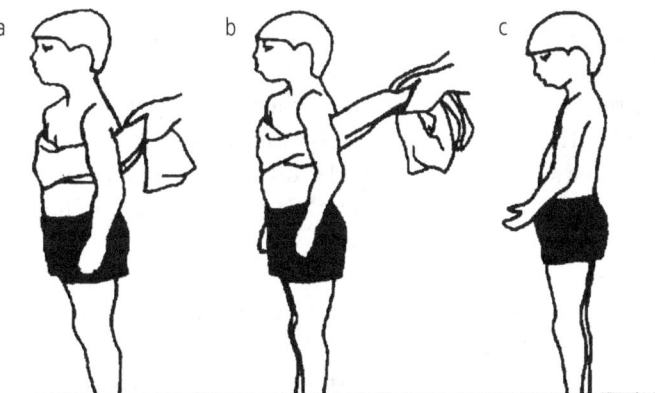

Note: Never support the child with his/her arms outstretched and his/her hands in yours. The child needs support near the waist and arms should be free to balance.

Teaching step 9: Walking with help and then without
A.
1. When the child has learned to stand using furniture as support, kneel and move the child's leg to the side at the knee (side-step). Place a toy just out of reach and encourage the child to step sideways to reach it. Say 'Step' when you move the child's leg sideways.
2. Place the child in a standing position. Stand in front of the child and gently pull him/her forward by his/her hands. If the child does not take a step, a second person may be required to kneel behind the child and move his/her legs forward in an (a), (b), (c) walking movement. Even if you started the movement, show enthusiasm for the child's attempts, no matter how small. The assistance of the person behind the child should be gradually decreased.

3. Stand behind the child and give support with your legs when he/she leans back. Take the child's hands and gently push-kick forward.

B.
1. When the child takes steps with support, two people are required for the following exercise: support the child from behind with a cloth tied around his/her chest. The second person stands in front and offers an object in such a way that the child must take two steps in order to reach the object. Show your approval if this is done. Gradually hold the toy (or something to eat) further away and grasp the cloth further and further from the child's body. Verbally encourage the child to walk. Practise until the child can walk unaided.

Feeding skills

Feeding skills develop in the following sequence:
1. Sucking and swallowing are coordinated and the child sucks fluid from a bottle.
2. The child puts his/her hands around a bottle and holds it.
3. The child learns to eat with a spoon; is fed.
4. The child is ready to start finger-feeding when he/she puts his/her hands or toys into his/her mouth. This may involve two separate activities:
   - The child dips a finger into strained food and licks the finger.
   - The child takes solid food, for example a piece of bread, in his/her hand and puts it in his/her mouth.
5. The child drinks from a glass.
6. The child feeds him/herself with a spoon. This develops in the following sequence:
   - The child bangs the spoon when he/she gets hold of it.
   - The child holds the caregiver's wrist when he/she feeds him/her.
   - The child holds the spoon while the caregiver guides his/her hand to his/her mouth.
   - The child holds the spoon, with the caregiver's hand on his/her arm for guidance.
   - The child holds the spoon while the caregiver observes and encourages.
   - The child feeds him/herself with very little supervision.
7. The child drinks through a straw.

Teaching steps 1 and 2: Strong and coordinated sucking and holding a bottle

A.
The child is first taught to suck if he/she is still unable to suck from a bottle.
1. Dip a clean, hemmed linen cloth in milk and allow the child to suck it. Very little sucking is necessary to ensure a pleasant result for the child, and this encourages the child to try again.
2. When the child is sucking fairly strongly, pour part of the feed into a bottle with a teat with an enlarged hole. Chill the teat in ice and dip it in a sugar solution. Place

it between the child's lips and at the same time let the child smell some ammonia, vinegar or clove oil. This technique combines all the stimuli required for sucking.

B.
The child is then taught strong and coordinated sucking from a bottle.
1. Hold the child in your arms or let the child recline in an infant's seat.
2. Use a bottle with a teat with a hole just large enough to let through about 12 drops a minute when the bottle is held upside-down.
3. If the child's mouth does not open when the bottle is brought near, tap the child's lips lightly with the teat or gently press the child's cheeks together to force the lips apart. It may sometimes be necessary to pull the child's chin down firmly but gently to open the mouth.
4. When the teat is in the child's mouth, put your fingers round the lips and gently stretch them outwards. This usually causes the lips to move in the opposite direction, thus pouting around the teat.
5. Place your fingers under the child's chin and over the upper lip and move the jaw up and down to initiate sucking. It may be necessary to move the jaw up and down occasionally to remind the child to continue sucking. Continuous upward pressure on the lower jaw also encourages a stronger sucking reflex.
6. Occasionally pull lightly at the bottle while the child is sucking to encourage stronger sucking.
7. Begin holding the child's hands around the bottle at every feed, even if the child does little or nothing to help.

C.
Some children dribble a lot and cannot close their mouths properly. To encourage better lip control and to reduce dribbling, the following may be done:
1. Massage the area around the mouth with your index finger as follows:
   – Place your finger horizontally, parallel to the mouth above the upper lip, directly under the nose. Massage the area above the upper lip with downward strokes of the finger. Use firm pressure but do not massage the lip.

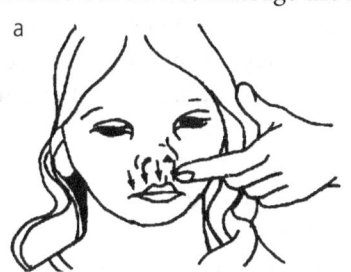

- Place your finger on the area lateral to the corner of the child's mouth and rub with rapid strokes to the corner of the mouth. Repeat on the other side.

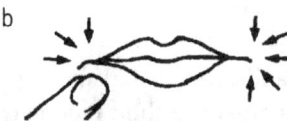

- Place your finger horizontally to the mouth on the chin beneath the lower lip and massage this area.

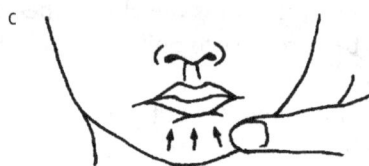

- Massaging must be done at least once a day or before every feed.
2. If the skin above the upper lip is short because of an undershot jaw, it must be stretched before the lips can close properly. In this case perform step (a) more regularly.
3. If the child dribbles, the aim is to develop subcortical, automatic control. If the child concentrates all day on whether or not dribbling occurs, this impedes functioning. If the child dribbles, push up the lower jaw and maintain the pressure until the child swallows, without comment.

Teaching step 3: Learning to eat with a spoon and to be fed
A.
Infants should start eating solids by the age of three months (for example, cereals with iron, strained vegetables and fruit).
1. Be absolutely consistent in your feeding routine in order to facilitate learning. The slightest deviation in the order in which you put on the bib, place the child in the chair, etc, is upsetting. Make sure that at least one other person in the household knows the feeding routine in order to relieve the caregiver once in a while.
2. Feed the child in a highchair. Support his/her feet. Begin by offering solid food once a day when the child is hungriest and make the food more or less the consistency of a milk pudding.
3. Sit directly in front of the child with your thumb on his/her chin, your middle finger under the chin and your index finger alongside the jaw. Use your thumb to open the child's mouth and your index finger to close it. Open and close the mouth a few times before offering food.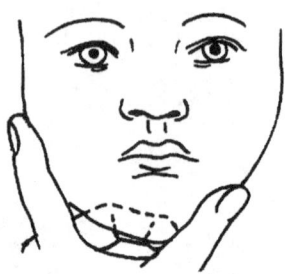
4. While the child's mouth is open, put a very small amount of food on the tip of a teaspoon and bring the

spoon near enough to touch both lips. Do not give food while the child's neck is stretched backwards. This can be stopped by gently patting the child's chest with the back of the hand.
5. Open the child's mouth (not too wide) and place the spoon on the middle of the tongue. Gently press the spoon to the tongue for a few seconds until the child's lips begin to close. Verbally encourage the child to close his/her mouth and/or use manual manipulation.
6. Pull the spoon out straight without scraping it against the upper teeth, the upper lip must learn to take food from the spoon.
7. Close the child's mouth with your middle finger as soon as the spoon has been removed and keep it closed until the child has swallowed.
8. If swallowing is slow, gently stroke the throat towards the chest and say 'Swallow'.
9. Do not continue with a feeding attempt for longer than half an hour. Stop and try again at the next feed or the following day.
10. Gradually reduce your assistance; withdraw help with the middle finger last of all.
11. Give small portions; rather offer second helpings. Do not force the child to eat to satisfy you, as this may lead to emotional problems and teaches poor habits such as overeating.
12. If the child refuses all food and you are sure that he/she is physically healthy, do not force the food. You can remove the food after a thorough attempt and offer only small amounts of water until the next meal. Missing a few meals will cause no harm.
13. If the child gags on or vomits the food, make sure that there are only small amounts of food in his/her mouth at a time and that the child swallows before the next mouthful. Try smaller feeds five or six times a day in the case of a child who vomits. Do not give fluids with meals. If the child vomits, clean up and immediately give a smaller amount more slowly.

B.
The child is taught to inhibit strong tongue thrusting.
1. The tongue step procedure is followed twice a day as follows:
    - With the tip of the child's tongue behind the lower teeth, put the bowl of a teaspoon on the tip of his/her tongue and push it down.

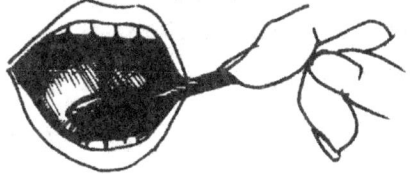

    - Place it a little further back and push down again. Continue until the child gags.
    - Open the mouth quickly by means of upward pressure under the chin to encourage swallowing.
2. Teach the child to imitate a yawn and to do so throughout the day. This pushes the tongue down.

Teaching step 4: Finger-feeding

A.
The first step is to teach the child to chew.
1. Help the child to achieve better control of his/her tongue by placing something sticky, such as peanut butter, on the tip of the tongue and lips. Place grapes, nuts, pieces of cake or raisins on and under the tongue or between cheek and gums. This teaches the tongue to move food around in the mouth.
2. Place something that makes a crackling sound under a large molar. If you are afraid that the child might choke, use a long piece of food that you hold onto (a carrot stick, finger of bread or piece of tough biltong). If choking is not a problem, try a piece of water biscuit, hard sweet, potato crisp or apple.
3. Close the child's mouth.
4. Place your hand on the child's jaw and move it up and down in a chew movement. Say 'Chew' and demonstrate.
5. If the child refuses to swallow, gently massage the throat upwards or downwards, or place upward pressure under the jaw with the back of two fingers.
6. Make sure that the child's mouth is closed when swallowing.
7. Gradually make the child's food more bulky: add small pieces of bread or toast and leave a few lumps in mashed potato and other foods.

B.
The second step is to teach the child to finger-feed.
1. When you serve the food, give the child a chance to lick some of it from his/her forefinger. Put the finger in the food and allow the child to lick it. This may sound messy but it teaches the child plate-to-mouth movement. Offer finger-feeding when the child is hungry.
2. Put the child in the highchair, put on a large feeder and spread newspaper on the floor. Place pieces of buttered bread, fruit or cheese directly on the tray of the highchair. Encourage the child to grasp and eat them. Do not worry about a little mess, as long as the child gradually learns to eat with his/her hands.

C.
The child is taught lip and jaw control. Once the child starts eating, these techniques will not be willingly accepted. Follow the following brush-and-ice procedure once a day very consistently for a few months.

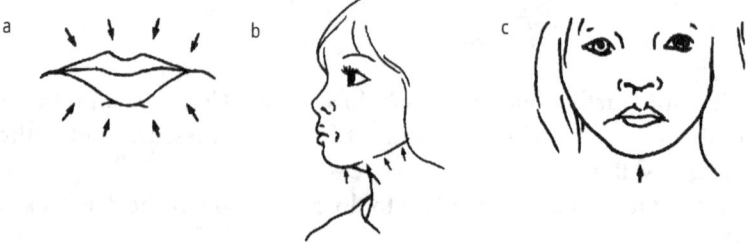

1. Brush the area around the mouth as shown in diagram a without brushing the lips. Repeat about 10 times.
2. Brush under the lower jaw with upward strokes (diagram b).
3. Brush the throat area under the chin with upward strokes (diagram c).
4. Take an ice cube in your hand (protecting your hand by covering it with a paper towel or face cloth). Rub the ice cube seven times around the outer edge of the lips. Do not rub the lips. Periodically dab the mouth area as you work to prevent dripping.
5. Rub the throat area as described in step 3 above. Dab regularly.
6. Hold the ice cube in the hollow above the breastbone for five seconds and dab as soon as you remove the ice.

Teaching step 5: Drinking from a glass/tumbler
A.
The child should learn to drink from a glass with help at about five to six months.
1. Use the normal jaw control grip or stand behind the child and hold his/her chin from the back. Keep a feeder under the chin.
2. Use a small plastic tumbler without handles. Pour a little of the child's favourite drink into it – only a teaspoonful at first. From now on the child must drink this fluid only from this glass.
3. Place the rim of the glass between the child's lips (not against the teeth, as this stimulates a child to bite) and pour in a little of the fluid. Do not remove the glass because the child must learn to take a few sips in succession. Tip the glass very slightly and apply a little pressure under the jaw to encourage swallowing.
4. If the child refuses to swallow, gently stroke up and down the throat area or show the child how you swallow and say 'Swallow'.
5. Rest after two or three sips and gradually increase the volume of fluid in the glass.

B.
Teach the child to drink independently.
1. Use the same glass and fluid.
2. Stand behind the child, place your hands over the child's hands around the glass and help the child to bring it to his/her mouth.
3. Let the child practise with an empty glass between meals.
4. Take the child off the bottle as soon as he/she can drink well from the glass. Gradually decrease bottle feeds; first omit the meal-time bottles and last of all those at bedtime.

Teaching step 6: Eating independently with a spoon
1. Make the child comfortable with his/her feet and back well supported and put on a feeder that covers the child up to the waist.
2. Place the feeding bowl in front of the child and fix it to the table with plasticine. Start with fairly thick food that will not fall off the spoon.

3. Sit comfortably next to the child so that you can see his/her arm and head movements.
4. Draw the child's attention to the spoon by using it to tap the food bowl and by saying: 'Look at the spoon' and/or turning the child's head in that direction. Give plenty of verbal approval if the child takes the spoon. If not, place your hand over the child's hand and bring it to the bowl.
5. Help the child scoop up the food and bring it to his/her mouth. Do not allow finger-feeding at this stage and do not go passively through the movements if the child does not look at the spoon or bowl. The child will learn nothing if he/she does not watch what is being done.
6. Gradually decrease your assistance; first place your hand over the child's wrist, then on his/her elbow and eventually remove your hand altogether.
7. Remember to praise the child lavishly for these attempts and not to help for too long, as this makes the child lazy. Try feeding every other mouthful, making a game of it, then every third mouthful, and so on. The child will probably require most assistance in scooping up the food.
8. Avoid all behaviour that interrupts the spoon-to-bowl, bowl-to-mouth sequence, for example by keeping other children out of the room.
9. Do not be concerned about eating neatly at first; table manners can be learned later.

Teaching step 7: Drinking through a straw
This is a very important activity because the sucking movement gives the mouth and tongue muscles essential exercise.
1. Use a plastic straw. Dip it into a favourite drink and put your finger over the opening to keep the fluid, which has been drawn up into the straw, in place. Hold the straw in the child's mouth and let the fluid run into it. Repeat a few times until the child begins to associate the drink with the straw. Do not allow the child to obtain the fluid in any other way.
2. Hold your side of the straw a little lower so that the child has to suck a little to obtain the fluid.
3. Place the straw in a plastic bottle with the top cut off just enough to admit the straw. Encourage the child to suck, and help the child by squeezing the bottle. Demonstrate the sucking movement and encourage the child to put only his/her lips, not his/her teeth, around the straw. Use your hand to help close the child's mouth around the straw.
4. Give plenty of praise for sucking and gradually withdraw your assistance.
5. Eventually offer all drinks with a straw and gradually thicken the fluids to force the child to suck more strongly. Children with cerebral palsy must continue to drink through a straw at least twice a day.

Dressing and undressing

Undressing is taught first, as it is easier than dressing. The sequence is not important and the child does not need to be able to distinguish between the inside and outside of garments. As is the case with other tasks, it is important to divide the activity into very small steps. Chaining is the usual method used to teach dressing and undressing. This means that the child starts by performing only the last part of an activity. For instance, pull down the child's pants until both legs are halfway over his/her feet and then allow the child to pull them off the rest of the way. Gradually allow the child to pull the pants down further and further. Place your hand over the child's hand if necessary, to show him/her how it is done. Praise every attempt lavishly.

Dress the child in simple, loose-fitting clothes during the training period. A front zip may initially be easier to undo than buttons. Show the child how to fasten and undo buttons by starting with large ones and gradually decreasing the size. To help put the correct shoe on the correct foot, mark the heel of one with a dab of paint.

Persons with intellectual disabilities often find dressing a very difficult skill to learn. Besides breaking up the process into small steps, the child can be further assisted by keeping to a very strict sequence, for example by always laying out the clothes on a chair and doing so in the same order. The child should always stand facing the chair and should put on the garments in the same way and in the sequence in which they have been laid out. Chaining is once again the teaching method of choice. An easy way of teaching a child how to put on shirts, jerseys and jackets follows:

1. Hang the shirt over the back of the chair.
2. Let the child sit on the chair.
3. Make the child look right and put one arm into the sleeve.
4. Make the child look left and put the other arm into the sleeve.
5. Let the child lift the shirt over the back of the chair and put it on by pulling both arms forward.

The child requires about twenty minutes at a time to learn to dress and undress. This exercise should also be included in playtime, for example dressing and undressing dolls, fastening and undoing buttons, and threading shoelaces.

Toilet training

Toilet habits cannot be taught before the child can walk. The ability to walk demonstrates that the spinal pathways are myelinated as far as the level of the bowel and bladder sphincters and that the child is physiologically capable of sphincter control.

Preparations for teaching toilet habits

1. Keep the following record for three or four days:
   Times wet or soiled: 9.30 soiled
   Child's response: tearful
   Your response: cleaned immediately
   Intake: porridge and milk hour before
   Keep the record in a convenient place, for example pasted to the bathroom door.

2. If the child urinates more than once an hour, take him/her for a medical examination to exclude the possibility of a physical problem.
3. Baseline data should not be gathered if the child is ill or if the fluid intake pattern is temporarily disturbed.
4. Toilet habits can be taught if the child:
   - can hold urine for about two hours and has one or two stools a day
   - can walk (except if the child has a physical handicap)
   - shows signs of being aware of elimination, for instance changing facial expression, becoming quiet, pulling at clothes, making other sounds, crossing legs and being irritable
   - can feed him/herself
   - is not ill.
5. Make sure that the child wears clothes that are easy to handle, such as pants with elastic.
6. The bathroom must be convenient for the child. Leave the door open and put a footstool next to the toilet so that the child can reach it. If a potty is used, it must be kept in the bathroom.
7. Flushing may frighten the child; initially avoid this while the child is in the bathroom.
8. Toilet training must commence when social interruptions are at their minimum, for example when there are no visitors.
9. Determine what reinforcers you are going to use, for example smile, touch, verbal praise or food (such as raisins).
10. Always dry the child immediately to make him/her used to being dry; being wet then becomes unpleasant.

Teaching toilet habits
1. Study the record you have kept and use it to determine the most likely time that the child will eliminate. This is usually after a meal, exercise or long nap. These are the times that the child should be taken to the toilet as a regular routine.
2. Lead the child to the bathroom, take down his/her pants and put him/her on the toilet.
3. Stay and keep the child's attention to the task at hand. If the child has done nothing after five or ten minutes, take him/her off the toilet. It is important not to punish or scold or even to change your facial expression if the child does nothing or wets his/her pants between visits to the toilet.
4. If the child does eliminate, reinforce (reward) him/her with food or praise.
5. Take the child off the toilet, pull up his/her pants and wash his/her hands.
6. Watch for signs that the child is beginning to indicate needs and take him/her to the toilet immediately.
7. Gradually allow the child to pull down his/her pants, climb on to the toilet, wipe and wash his/her hands. In the end you will only be required to stand by. Never forget to give a reward.

INSTITUTIONAL CARE

A single principle that could be of great help to nurses in judging and planning a department or institution for persons with intellectual disabilities is the normalisation principle. This principle originated in Sweden but has since become accepted throughout the world. It means that the lives of people with intellectual disabilities should be as normal as possible.

In fact the normalisation principle implies normalisation of the total environment, of activities, attitudes and the atmosphere surrounding the intellectually disabled person to such a degree that life in the open community will have become understandable to them. The application of the normalisation principle will 'not make the subnormal normal', but will make life conditions of the intellectually disabled person normal as far as possible, bearing in mind the degree of disability, competence and maturity, as well as the need for training activities and availability of services (Gunzburg, 1973: 30).

Key elements of the normalisation principle

The normalisation principle comprises the following eight elements:

1. *Normal rhythm for every day*. This means that patients get up at a normal time, dress and go to work (regardless of the type of work). They eat under normal circumstances, that is, relaxed and sociably at a family table. They do not go to bed earlier than normal people and allowance is made for their personal rhythm. *Example*: Bedtime is regulated and laid down by a 'lights out' order; or largely left to the discretion of the patients.
2. *Normal rhythm for every week*. Normal people live in one place, work somewhere else and relax in other places. Patients with an intellectual disability should be able to choose their recreation and should, as far as possible, make use of facilities outside the institution as soon as possible. Working hours should be normal. *Example*: Sundays follow the same pattern as other days; or patients may sleep in on Sundays if they wish.
3. *Normal rhythm for every year*. The recreation, food, clothes, etc, of normal people change with the seasons, but seasonal changes usually have little impact on persons with intellectual disabilities. In addition, normal people generally have an annual holiday, which includes physical and psychological rest and a change of environment. Days of personal significance are also commemorated. *Example*: No distinction is made between winter and summer underwear and clothes except for the addition of jerseys and/or coats in winter; or different underwear and clothes for summer and winter.
4. *Normal life cycle*. The environment of normal people changes as they grow older, for example toddlers have warmth and continual stimulation and encouragement, school children have educational institutions with all the necessary facilities, adults have job opportunities and social events, and the elderly have a more restful but familiar environment. All these facilities and opportunities should also be available to people with intellectual disabilities.

5. *Normal respect for the choicest wishes and wants of individuals.* Persons with intellectual disabilities should be consulted as much as possible about rules, routines and events in their own environment. They should have their own personal belongings. *Example:* Personal belongings in lockers are regularly inspected by staff to prevent the accumulation of rubbish; or considered private and clearing out is done by discussion and persuasion.
6. *Normal heterosexual world.* To normalise the lives of institutionalised persons with intellectual disabilities and to prepare them for heterosexual society, the two sexes must mix as much as possible within the constraints of normal control. Sex education must be given as part of the education programme.
7. *Normal economic standards.* Persons with intellectual disabilities must be considered for normal financial benefits such as old-age pensions and minimum wages. Even though most of the money is spent on board and lodging, a portion should be available as pocket money.
8. *Normal standards for physical facilities.* Normal standards of living, working and recreational facilities in the community should also hold good for persons with intellectual disabilities. The size of living quarters should correspond with those in the community, the underlying principle being that the longer the tenure, the smaller they should be. The standard of decoration and furniture should also be the same. *Example*: Staff use separate toilet facilities; or staff use the same toilet facilities as patients/residents.

If the normalisation principle were to be implemented in the total organisation for those with an intellectual disability, it would have far-reaching consequences for them, for health workers, for parents and for the community.

Various modalities for promoting socialisation and preventing institutional neurosis can be used in institutions where people with intellectual disabilities live permanently.

Group activity therapy

Activity groups develop self-respect as well as social and interpersonal skills. They offer individuals living with an intellectual disability an opportunity to develop a feeling of acceptance and an outlet for aggressive impulses.

Group activity therapy may comprise the following: action games, volleyball, clay modelling, story-telling, role play, finger-painting, excursions, starch work, care of pets and plants, gardening and needlework. These activities strengthen the interests and attention span of a person with an intellectual disability to ensure pleasure, fulfilment and personal development.

Play or games

Play is beneficial for a number of reasons, as outlined in the following points:
- Play is one of the most effective ways of learning, according to Marzollo (1984).

- Play is a natural way in which persons with intellectual disabilities can learn to concentrate and use their imagination. They can also use play to test new ideas and adult behaviour. Another benefit is that play develops their thinking and teaches them a measure of control over their world.
- The body is developed by means of play.
- Play promotes social adjustment and offers a safe means of giving vent to frustrations.
- Play means far more than mere amusement or a pastime.

Important aspects during play activities include the following:
- Nurses must begin with something that the patient can already do and gradually build on this; success stimulates the learning process.
- The play of people with individual learning styles is adapted to their needs.
- Nurses must create effective learning opportunities. This means that the right activity must be introduced at the right time, with a specific aim, at each individual's level of functioning.
- Games equipment must be easily manageable, simple and strong. The patients should not be frustrated by equipment that constantly breaks or is too complicated to master.

Music therapy

Music therapy is defined as the systematic use of music (rhythmic, melodic and harmonious) in a therapeutic environment to bring about behavioural change.

Music provides pleasure to most people, whether or not they are disabled. Music provides an atmosphere of unity and group identity – it communicates without words. Music should be adapted to the category of disability, for example:
- *Passive music (listening)*. The profoundly intellectually disabled person shows signs of pleasure such as smiling, clapping hands and relaxation at hearing music.
- *Active music (dancing, percussion band, singing, exercising to music)*. This promotes coordination, balance and rhythm in persons with mild and moderate intellectual disabilities.

ADULT PERSONS WITH INTELLECTUAL DISABILITIES

Adult persons with intellectual disabilities are greatly dependent on learning and development during the childhood years and whether the persons have other disabilities or problems, such as epilepsy or blindness. It should be possible for the majority of people with an IQ of 35 and above to be relatively independent as adults. In such cases, all the principles of psychosocial rehabilitation come into play.

The Technical Assistance Guidelines on the Employment of Persons with Disabilities published by the Department of Labour (South Africa, 2017: 16) states that persons with intellectual disabilities may require support and accommodation that may include access to a job coach; more frequent rest periods; consideration of the side effects of medication; possible adjustment of working hours; and consideration of the effect or tolerance of environmental factors such as noise levels and interruptions, and how these could be managed best. In the following sections, guidelines are given for how to prepare persons with intellectual disabilities for the world of work at various stages of their lives – at elementary and primary school ages; and at 14–16, 17–18 and at 19–21 years of age.

Pre-primary school age

When the person with an intellectual disability is at this age, these guidelines should be implemented:
- The concept of work should be introduced into everyday activities.
- Learners should become familiar with all types of careers.
- They should develop self-care and daily living skills and routines.
- There should be a focus on developing good human relationships and good social skills at home and school.
- They should explore the available vocational opportunities at the upper grade levels and beyond.
- The child should be made a productive part of the household, doing chores and receiving an allowance.

Primary school age

At the age of attending primary school, these guidelines can be implemented:
- Career exploration can begin through activities like watching movies, reading books, going to work with adults..
- The teacher's efforts to provide job training as part of the school programme should be supported.
- Information should be gathered about the types of education programme options, such as inclusion, vocational or combination programmes.
- At home, parents can also help their children explore careers by getting them to do chores around the house, volunteer in the community and participate in community service projects.

Age 14 to 16 years

These are the recommendations for preparing people who are 14–16 years of age for the working world:
- Parents should participate in a transition programme for themselves, which assists them in planning for their children after school.
- Vocational training should be built into the educational programme in which the child is placed.
- Recreation and leisure interests can be explored.

- Information can be obtained about funding sources (for example, skills development levies and learnerships) and financial assistance programmes (for example, disability grants) and how these may benefit the person.
- Independent living skills should be developed.

Age 17 to 18 years

During this period of the person's life, these recommendations can be put in place:
- The person could find and hold a part-time job in the school or in the community.
- There should be a discussion about how long the learner will attend high school – for the required number of years or until the age of 21.
- Information about future planning can be obtained.
- The learner could enrol in vocational education classes.
- Where relevant, the learner should establish a graduation date.
- Guardianship procedures should be investigated to determine what is in the best interest of the learner.
- A vocational evaluation can be scheduled to help determine the learner's interest and to set a vocational goal.
- The learner could be encouraged to attend a job fair.

Age 19 to 21 years

During this period of the person's life, the following steps can be implemented:
- They should be introduced to budgeting and the real cost of 'living on your own'.
- Suitable employment should be found, with desired work hours and salary.

Housing and work

Housing and work are major issues, since the person should not only be safe and happy but should also have adequate resources for life. In the USA and the UK, supported employment has become the approach of choice. This means that employment is found for the person in the open labour market, and the person is supported to enable them to learn and maintain the job. This approach works well for persons with intellectual disabilities, since they are reliable and consistent workers. Similarly, the South African Department of Labour has made guidelines available for the employment of persons with disabilities, including intellectual disabilities. According to the guidelines, persons with intellectual disabilities may learn vocational skills through observation, role play and breaking a complex job down into small steps, which can be mastered (South Africa, 2017: 2).

In the UK, 4 800 people with learning disabilities are employed through such programmes (Jenkins, 2002: 40). However, the same author cautions against over-emphasising employment for this group. He points out that the demands of employers might be too onerous for the persons with disabilities, and conditions at work might influence their health negatively. They might also be worse off financially if the social support system (disability grants, etc) is not geared to encouraging employment.

Group homes seem to be the approach of choice for adults who might otherwise find total independence – that is, financially, physically and emotionally – impossible. Such homes can accommodate a small number of individuals with different strengths and weaknesses. Pooling their resources might make them more able to cope and living together makes it easier to provide them with social support on a cost-effective basis.

Very few such homes are currently available and there is much room for growth in this sector. The organisation DSSA has been providing training in supported employment to a core group of parents and professionals, and it will be interesting to see whether they manage to implement this modality more widely in South Africa.

People with intellectual disabilities are generally less physically healthy than their non-disabled counterparts. They are also less physically active, with one study indicating that as many as 56 per cent engage in no physical activity as opposed to about 36 per cent in the general population (Stanish et al, 2006). According to the Centers for Disease Control and Prevention (cited by Stanish et al, 2006: 16) the overall conclusion of a review of studies indicates that only a third of intellectually disabled adults engage in adequate physical activity and this leads to many health problems related to inactivity. It is therefore important that health promotion receives adequate attention when working with adult people in this group. Such health promotion should include a strong focus on physical activity.

MANAGEMENT OF CHALLENGING BEHAVIOUR

(Also see 'Limit setting' and 'Dealing with anger and aggression' in Chapter 11.)

The most common challenging behaviours among institutionalised patients with intellectual disabilities are hyperactivity, destructive behaviour, aggression, absconding and self-harm. These types of behaviour occur fairly regularly among about a quarter of all patients with intellectual disabilities (Weis, 2015: 99). Weis (2015: 99) further states that challenging behaviour is problematic because it affects children and families in the following ways:

- It can be physically harmful.
- It can strain relationships with parents and cause children to be rejected by peers.
- It can limit children's access to developmentally appropriate social experiences, such as birthday parties, sleepovers, and participation in sports.
- It can interfere with learning and cognitive development.
- It can place a financial burden on families and the public.

Psychosocial treatment

When trying to manage challenging behaviour, it is important in the first instance to understand that most behaviour is motivated. One of the instruments used to investigate challenging behaviour classifies the motivation for behaviour as follows:

- *Attention behaviour.* The person seeks to get attention and personal contact. Negative attention behaviour includes disturbing others, speaking when others are speaking and repetitive vocalisations.
- *Escape behaviour.* This is used to escape from a situation or from people. Negative escape behaviour includes isolating self, being non-compliant and cursing.
- *Tangible behaviour.* This deals with a specific person or object in the environment. Negative tangible behaviours include temper outbursts, aggression and ignoring instructions.
- *Non-social behaviour.* This is behaviour for which no specific social reason can be found, such as odd mannerisms, inappropriate noises and not attending to the environment (Matson et al, 2002).

Research has indicated that the poorer people's social skills and self-care skills are, the more they use negative behaviour to achieve their social goals and express their frustration (Matson et al, 2002). One of the most important interventions to decrease problem behaviour is therefore training in self-care and social skills. This can be very challenging in severely and profoundly disabled people, but simple social skills such as making positive physical contact like holding hands, returning an item, or greeting a person, can be taught. This not only leads to increased skill in dealing with emotions, but also to more positive interactions with people. A simple self-care skill such as being able to get something to drink or to eat can greatly reduce discomfort and frustration. (Also see 'Social skills and learning' in Chapter 11).

Pharmacological treatment

Treatment approaches must be multidisciplinary and include medicine, psychology, education, rehabilitation, nursing, and social work (Katz & Lazcano-Ponce, 2008:139). Persons with intellectual disabilities are at risk for developing comorbid psychiatric conditions. Medication is often administered to persons with intellectual disabilities, more so when there are dual diagnoses of psychiatric symptoms and disorders. Pharmacological treatments for challenging behaviour and the effect they might have are listed below:

- *Antipsychotics*
    - Act by blocking certain dopamine and/or serotonin receptors
    - Used for broad range of behavioural and affective challenges in ID, including aggression, destructive behaviour, oppositional behaviour, irritability, lability and self-injury in people with intellectual disabilities
    - Options include: first generation antipsychotics (eg haloperidol or depot antipsychotics such as fluphenazine, flupenthixol or zuclopenthixol decanoate) or second-generation antipsychotics (eg risperidone; olanzapine)

- *Anticonvulsants/mood stabilisers*
  - In addition to seizure control, may also be used for aggression, mood lability, impulsivity and self-injurious behaviour in intellectual disabilities
  - Most common medication used is sodium valproate
- *Antidepressants*
  - Used to treat anxiety, depressive and obsessive symptoms or disorders in both adults and adolescents with intellectual disabilities
  - May be used as alternative/adjunctive to antipsychotics for treatment of aggression, impulsivity and self-injurious behaviour
  - Most common class used are SSRIs
- *Stimulants*
  - Methylphenidate may be used to treat attentional deficits and/or co-morbid ADHD.

CONCLUSION

The limitations in lifestyle functioning and self-care of persons with intellectual disabilities make stimulation, support, motivation and love imperative for their development into becoming more independent individuals. The effective assessment of and planning for such patients will result in the implementation of appropriate interventions to optimise their functioning.

WEB RESOURCES

http://www.thearc.org
　This website is for people with intellectual and developmental disabilities in the USA. It has a range of very useful resources for persons with intellectual disabilities and their caregivers.

www.sunshine.org.za
　This is a non-profit organisation specialising in the field of intellectual disability by providing early intervention projects and therapeutic services to parents and caregivers of children with disabilities and delays.

http://www.downsyndrome.org.za/
　This is a South African association which helps to improve the lives of people with Down syndrome and other intellectual disabilities as well as their families.

http://www.nichy.org
　This site allows access to information provided by the National Information Center for Children and Youth with Disabilities. Intellectual disability is one of the topics addressed and the information is up to date and relevant.

http://www.ndss.org
　This is the website of the National Down Syndrome Society (NDSS) and is a wonderful resource for parents and professionals. It provides basic information, emerging research and chat rooms.

REFERENCES

Adnams, C M. 2010. Perspectives of intellectual disability in South Africa: epidemiology, policy, services for children and adults. *Current Opinion in Psychiatry*, 23: 436–440.

American Psychiatric Association (APA). 2013. *Diagnostic and Statistical Manual of Mental Disorders*. 5th edition. Washington, DC: American Psychiatric Press.

Bleazard, A V. 2010. 'Sexuality and intellectual disability: perspectives of young women with intellectual disability'. PhD Thesis. Stellenbosch: Stellenbosch University.

Coren, E, Hutchfield, J, Thomae, M and Gustafsson C. 2010. 'Parent training support for intellectually disabled parents'. *Campbell Systematic Reviews*, 2010: 3.

Chung J C C, and Lai C K Y. 2009. 'Snoezelen for dementia'. *Cochrane Database of Systematic Reviews*, 2002 (4). Art No: CD003152. doi: 10.1002/14651858.CD003152.

Department of Basic Education and UNICEF. 2015. *Study on Children with Disabilities from Birth to Four Years Old*. Pretoria: UNICEF South Africa.

Douglas, T, Redley, B and Ottmann, G. 2016. 'The first year: the support needs of parents caring for a child with an intellectual disability'. *Journal of advanced nursing*, 72 (11): 2738–2749.

Gunzburg, H C, ed. 1973. *Advances in the Care of the Mentally Handicapped*. London: Bailliére Tindall.

Henderson, N. 2001. 'Being in sync with teens and young adults: a guide to relationships'. *National Down Syndrome Society (NDDS) Compendium*. http://www.ndss.org/content.cfm?fus eaction=Inf oResSchEduArticle&article=166 (Accessed July 2003).

Hewitt, A and O'Nell, S. 1998. 'Speaking up – speaking out'. *US Department of Health and Human Services*. http://www.acf.hhs.gov/programs/pcmr/ (Accessed June 2003).

Jenkins, R. 2002. Value of employment to people with learning disabilities. *British Journal of Nursing*, 11 (1): 38–45.

Kaplan, H I and Sadock, B J. 1985. *Comprehensive Textbook of Psychiatry IV, Volume two*. 4th edition. Baltimore: Williams & Wilkins.

Kaplan, H, Clopton, M, Kaplan, M, Messbauer, L and McPherson, K. 2006. 'Snoezelen multi-sensory environments: Task engagement and generalization'. *Research in Developmental Disabilities*, 27: 443–455.

Katz, G and Lazcano-Ponce, E. 2008. 'Intellectual disability: definition, etiological factors, classification, diagnosis, treatment and prognosis'. *Salud Publica de Mexico*, 50 (2): S132–S141.

Kromberg J, Zwane E, Manga P, Venter, A, Rosen, E, Christianson, A. 2008. 'Intellectual disability in the context of a South African population'. *Journal of Policy and Practice in Intellectual Disabilities*, 5 (2): 89–95.

Marzollo, J. 1984. *Learning Through Play*. Guernsey: Guernsey Press.

Matson, J L, Mayville, E A and Lott, J D. 2002. 'The relationship between behaviour motivation and social functioning in persons with intellectual impairment'. *British Journal of Clinical Psychology*, 41 (2): 175–184.

Mohsin, M N, Khan, T M, Doger, A H and Awan, A S. 2011. Role of parents in training of children with intellectual disability. *International Journal of Humanities and Social Science*, 1 (9 Special Issue): 78–88.

National Down Syndrome Society (NDSS). 2003. 'National study finds inclusive education rewarding for all involved'. http://www.ndss.org/content.cfm?fuseaction=InfoResSchEduArticle&article=166 (Accessed July 2003).

National Institute for Child Health and Human Development. 1986. *Early Diagnosis and Intervention Subcommittee Report*. Washington.

Olsson, L. 2016. *Children with mild intellectual disability and their families – needs for support, service utilisation and experiences of support.* Göteborg: Jönköping University.

Rynders, J E and Low, M L. 2003. '"Adrift" in the educational mainstream: the need to structure communicative interactions between students with Down Syndrome and their nondisabled peers'. *Down Syndrome Quarterly,* http://www.denison.edu/ (Accessed July 2003).

Sadock, B J, Sadock V A & Ruiz, P. 2015. *Kaplan and Sadock's synopsis of psychiatry. Behavioural sciences/ clinical psychiatry.* Philadelphia: Wolter Kluwer. p1472.

Salvador-Carulla, L, Reed, G M, Vaez-Azizi, L M, Cooper, S, Martinez-Lea, R, Bertell, M, Adnams, C, Cooray, S, Deb, S, Akoury-Dirani, L, Girimaji, S C, Katz G, Kwok, H, Luckasson, R, Simeonsson, R, Walsh, C, Munir, K and Saxena, S. 2011. 'Intellectual developmental disorders: towards a new name, definition and framework for "mental retardation/ intellectual disability" in ICD-11'. *World Psychiatry,* 10: 175–180.

Schalock, R L, Luckasson, R A and Shogren, KA. 2007. 'The renaming of mental retardation: understanding the change to the term intellectual disability'. *Perspective of Mental retardation to intellectual disability,* 45 (2): 116–124.

Shapiro, M, Parush, S, Green, M and Roth, D. 1997. 'The efficacy of the "Snoezelen" in the management of children with mental retardation who exhibit maladaptive behaviors'. *The British Journal of Developmental Disabilities,* 43 (85): 140–155.

Sobralske, M C. 2013. 'Common physical or sensory disabilities'. In Eddy, L L, ed. *Caring for Children with Special Healthcare Needs and Their Families: A Handbook for Healthcare Professionals.* Washington: Wiley-Blackwell.

South Africa. Department of Social Development, 2015. *White Paper on the Rights of Persons with Disabilities.* Government Printer, Pretoria.

South Africa. Department of Labour, 2017. *Technical assistance guidelines on the employment of persons with disabilities.* Pretoria.

Stanish, H I, Temple, V A and Frey, G C. 2006. 'Health-promoting physical activity of adults with mental retardation'. *Mental Retardation and Developmental Disabilities,* 12: 13–21.

State of Washington. 2012. 'Washington State Early Learning and Development Guidelines'. https://www.dcyf.wa.gov/sites/default/files/pdf/guidelines.pdf (Accessed June 2018).

Verheul, A. 2014. 'Snoezelen –"niet moet, alles mag"'. 'Snoezelen –'nothing has to be done, everything is allowed"'. *Everyday Multisensory Environments, Wellness Technology and Snoezelen.* ISNA-MSE's XII world conference.

United Nations International Children's Emergency Fund (UNICEF: nd). 2015. 'Child and maternal health. Mother and child healthcare'. *UNICEF South Africa.* https://www.unicef.org/southafrica/survival_devlop_759.html (Accessed September 2019).

United States of America (USA), 1975. *Education for All Handicapped Children Act.* Public Law 94-142–Nov 1975.

United States of America (USA), 2015. *Every Student Succeeds Act.* Public Law 114–95–Dec 2015.

Weis, R. 2015. *Introduction to abnormal child and adolescent psychology.* 2nd edition. Los Angeles: SAGE Publications.

World Health Organisation (WHO). 1980. *International classification of impairments, disabilities, and handicaps. A manual of classification relating to the consequences of disease.* Geneva: World Health Organisation.

World Health Organisation (WHO). 2001. *International Classification of Functioning, Disability and Health.* Geneva: World Health Organisation.

CHAPTER 18

Nursing the Mental Health Care User Diagnosed with a Personality Disorder

A Fourie

Learning Outcomes

After studying this chapter, you should be able to:
- develop an understanding of the common characteristics and difficulties that persons diagnosed with a personality disorder experience
- use a psychodynamic and a transactional analysis model to understand these characteristics and difficulties, and to help direct treatment
- diagnose the more commonly presenting personality disorders, using DSM-5 criteria
- reflect on the skills needed to establish and maintain long-term therapeutic relationships with persons suffering from various personality disorders
- consider various therapeutic modalities in the care of persons diagnosed with personality disorders.

INTRODUCTION

Working with people who have been diagnosed with personality disorders can be one of the most challenging areas of mental health nursing. Mental health practitioners are often confronted by persons who have difficulty in relating to others and managing their emotions. It can be difficult to understand what the person is struggling with emotionally and hard to be around such strong emotions. Such a situation can evoke very strong feelings, such as anger and frustration or hopelessness and helplessness.

The mental health nurse needs to have the inner strength and maturity to experience and manage strong emotions within the mental health care user (MHCU) and themselves. The nurse would need to keep thinking about the difficult inner world of the MHCU that sits behind a 'protective amour' or what is clinically called a defence or defensive system. These defences can be difficult to understand and penetrate.

The difficulties mentioned above can be further exacerbated if the mental health practitioner feels solely responsible for the management and treatment of the MHCU.

At the outset, two guiding therapeutic principles are proposed which can assist in the treatment of MHCUs with personality disorders.
1. Whether working in a community or in a hospital setting, the mental health nurse should make full use of a team approach. The nurse should ensure there is the necessary supervision and support, and that it is possible to work together with

other members of the team. The issues that develop around MHCUs can often feel overwhelming, and if not shared with others, can lead to burnout.
2. When caring for a person with a personality disorder it is important to be realistic about what change is possible in the person. Such persons have often had a long, traumatic and complicated history in relation to interpersonal relationships. Constant support and validation in the face of these difficult dynamics are often needed rather than cure.

There is often the tendency in those working with persons with personality disorders to label and judge such persons negatively. This can serve to separate one from these difficulties because of the parts within oneself that struggle at times to relate to others arising from one's own strong emotions. Such labelling can lead to avoiding people in the work and can reinforce the patterns of difficulties people have experienced in the past and continue to experience in current relationships. It is always helpful to think about what lies beneath an MHCU's difficulties and to take care not to be dismissive of the person with a personality disorder.

The mental health nurse's task, then, is to understand and support those diagnosed with personality disorders, rather than to judge or condemn them.

UNDERSTANDING THE PERSON WITH A PERSONALITY DISORDER

Persons diagnosed with personality disorders are not easy to understand. In contrast to persons diagnosed with other psychiatric conditions, who are for the most part aware of their problem and willing to adapt through changing themselves, the person with a personality disorder is more likely to be unaware of their difficulties and deny their problems. Such persons are also more likely to refuse psychiatric help and to 'blame' the external environment for their problems. There is often the expectation or wish that the environment, rather than themselves, should change.

The external environment here would include others, the family, the therapist, the mental health care professional team and the mental health nurse.

What, then, does a mental health nurse need to know about MHCUs diagnosed with personality disorders in order to facilitate an understanding and assessment of the difficulties and to create a sense of anticipation and readiness when working with such persons?

1. First, the mental health nurse needs knowledge about the characteristics common to persons with personality disorders.
2. Secondly, a knowledge of the broad classification of personality disorders in terms of the DSM-5 is essential.
3. Thirdly, it is important to know about the ways, albeit maladaptive, in which persons diagnosed with personality disorders cope with distress from overwhelming emotions and relationship difficulties.

4. Finally, the mental health nurse needs to be aware of the natural emotional reactions, which may arise in themselves and other staff who deal with persons suffering from personality disorders.

Common characteristics of all personality disorders

There are four common characteristics of all personality disorders, which include the following:

1. There is a longstanding, inflexible, and maladaptive response or way of coping with stress and distress that is recognisable at the time of adolescence or before, and which continues throughout adulthood.
2. Problems manifest in most areas of the person's life such as work and social functioning.
3. The person struggles with awareness and understanding of their difficulties and how others might be experiencing them.
4. The person often evokes strong emotions in other people, which exacerbates interpersonal difficulties further.

Classification of personality disorders

The DSM-5 (APA, 2013) defines the general criteria for personality disorder as:

- An enduring pattern of inner experience and behaviour that deviates markedly from the expectations of the individual's culture. This pattern is manifested in two (or more) of the following areas:
  - Cognition (ie ways of perceiving and interpreting self, other people, and events)
  - Affectivity (ie the range, intensity, lability, and appropriateness of emotional response)
  - Interpersonal functioning
  - Impulse control
- The enduring pattern is inflexible and pervasive across a broad range of personal and social situations.
- The enduring pattern leads to clinically significant distress or impairment in social, occupational, or other important areas of functioning.
- The pattern is stable and of long duration, and its onset can be traced back at least to adolescence or early adulthood.
- The enduring pattern is not better explained as a manifestation or consequence of another mental disorder.
- The enduring pattern is not attributable to the physiological effects of a substance (for example, a drug of abuse, a medication) or another medical condition (for example, head trauma).

Within these general criteria, for each personality disorder, specific impairment and traits are required for a diagnosis. Currently the DSM-5 defines 10 specific personality disorders which will be discussed in more detail later in this chapter.

(*Reprinted with permission from the* Diagnostic and Statistical Manual of Mental Disorders, Fifth Edition (Copyright ©2013). *American Psychiatric Association.* All Rights Reserved.)

The DSM-5 classification system for psychiatric conditions is not without its limitations. Although it has succeeded in giving practitioners a common language in which to discuss patients, which does not require agreement on the causes or the meanings of symptoms, this common language fails to take into account the subjective experiences of persons (Mc Williams, 2011). What is unique to the individual or what remains as their strengths, despite their difficulties, is not highlighted.

With this in mind one should look at the ways in which not only MHCUs, but all people, try to protect themselves in the world. These attempts at self-protection, both from difficulties one experiences in the outside world and one's internal worlds, are termed *defences* or *defence mechanisms* within psychological theory.

Although an MHCU diagnosed with a personality disorder will exhibit a predominant defence, most MHCUs will use several defences. Consequently, the management of defences will be dealt with globally, rather than under each specific disorder.

It is also important to have an understanding of the terminology of defences, as other mental health practitioners, such as social workers, psychologists and psychiatrists, will often speak about the difficulties of MHCUs using these terms.

Important factors to be taken into account when dealing with defence mechanisms include:

- The predominant defence used by the MHCU is observable through interactions with the MHCU, either on an individual basis or in a group setting and is exhibited by, or can be inferred from, their behaviour.
- However maladaptive the defence, it represents unconscious efforts on the part of the MHCU to protect themselves, rather than an intention to be difficult.
- The person with a personality disorder uses defences as an attempt to manage unbearable emotional states. However, when the defence is directly confronted, the difficulty is often made worse. The main reason why persons with personality disorders struggle to change their behaviour is that this will involve giving up their defences, thereby increasing the possibility of being overwhelmed by negative emotions.
- Early recognition of the predominant defences used by the MHCU enables the mental health nurse to respect the underlying fear and to anticipate the use of the defences in future interactions.
- The mental health nurse should be aware of their own feelings when interacting with MHCUs, as these feelings provide a valuable source of information regarding the defences used by the MHCU, particularly a person with personality difficulties.

Table 18.1 Some defence mechanisms used by MHCUs with personality disorders and management of possible responses evoked by these.

Defence	Possible subjective experience within MHCUs	Possible response of the mental health nurse and management recommendations
Fantasy Person seeks inner comfort by creating an imaginary life of persons and places in their mind.	Fear of intimacy or closeness to others.	The mental health nurse could feel rejected by the behaviour of the MHCU which may not feel reciprocal. The nurse should rather respect the fear and maintain a quiet, reassuring approach that acknowledges the fear of being close.
Projective identification Person unconsciously 'puts' or transfers an aspect of themselves onto another person. This person then accepts this aspect unconsciously and identifies with it as part of themselves. This is often a defence used by borderline, narcissistic, paranoid and schizoid personality disorders.	Struggling to own aspects of themselves, often related to early interpersonal trauma that is unbearable.	Mental health nurses could react in accordance with projected aspect of the MHCU and abuse the MHCU. Instead, the nurses should be aware of feelings evoked by the MHCU in themselves. Ask what is being re-enacted here? What is the MHCU trying to 'make one' into at that moment? Mental health nurses act as a repository for the projected parts of MHCUs and consciously need to separate this from themselves.
Isolation/distancing Intensified self-restraint; overformal social behaviour when stressed; commonly used by the person with obsessive-compulsive personality disorder and schizoid personality disorder.	Fear of losing control and/or fear of intimacy.	Mental health nurses could feel frustrated with the MHCU's need for self-control or feel rejected by MHCU's distancing. Rather than engaging in a power struggle, nurses should allow the MHCU to control their own care and try to work collaboratively later.
Projection Attributing one's own unacceptable motives/feelings or characteristics to others in the form of fault finding and criticism of others; often found	Fear of trusting others and their motives during interaction.	Defensiveness and arguments should be avoided by the mental health nurse. Instead the nurse should try to validate the MHCU's feelings in accordance with their perception

→

Defence	Possible subjective experience within MHCUs	Possible response of the mental health nurse and management recommendations
in the paranoid personality disorder.		of the situation. The nurse does not have to agree with the MHCU's feelings of injustice or with their perception of the situation; the nurse should empathise with the MHCU's feelings and try to perceive the situation as they do.
Splitting Viewing oneself or others as 'all good' or 'all bad', without integrating the positive and negative qualities that all people have. This leads to idealising some people while devaluing others. This is often used by the borderline personality and by narcissistic, paranoid and schizoid personalities.	Fear that the 'badness' within or without will destroy the 'good'; hence the need to keep it separate and apart.	Conflict might arise between the staff team as they unconsciously assume these polarised positions of 'good' and 'bad' in staff discussions about the MHCU. For the treating team to remain cohesive they need to be aware of the splitting and understand their positions in relation to the MHCU's internal world.
Passive aggression Involves directing one's anger inwards and takes the form of self-defeating behaviours of self-harm or directing one's anger outwards. This is done in an indirect way that is perceived by others as manipulative and obstructive.	Can be a fear of one's own and other's anger, which is experienced as destructive and unmanageable.	There might be anger and frustration in the staff who feel as though they are failing in their work or that the MHCU is manipulating them. It is important to assist the MHCU to become aware of their angry feelings and get them to talk about the anger, rather than acting it out.

Reactions of mental health care professionals

It is clear from the above table that the treatment of MHCUs with personality disorders is a complex and difficult area to work in, since these MHCUs display the following behavioural patterns:

- Tendency not to seek help or are often not able to perceive their difficulties as being in need of help
- Difficulty in taking responsibility or ownership of their problems and locate the 'problem' in others with the expectation that others need to change

- Longstanding maladaptive patterns of coping in the world which cause significant distress for themselves and those around them, such as family and mental health care professionals
- Use of the above-mentioned defences in ways that can lead to breakdowns in the personal and professional boundaries between them and mental health care professionals and affect the professionals' abilities to make sound professional judgements
- Direction of anger at mental health care professionals through what is experienced as demanding, unreasonable and manipulative behaviours.

Among mental health care professionals, negative feelings and reactions are natural and normal, and include getting angry with the MHCU, feeling defensive, wishing to control the MHCU, losing the ability to concentrate or think rationally, feeling helpless, frustrated and impotent. These types of reactions are often called countertransference within psychological theories.

However, the mental health nurse needs to develop an ability to accept that it is normal to experience such feelings and not to react to these feelings. Only by anticipating and understanding these feelings will the mental health nurse be able to retain their own sense of self and create enough distance from the patient to maintain a professional and therapeutic role. Support and supervision from the team form an essential part in aiding the development of these abilities.

USING A TRANSACTIONAL ANALYSIS MODEL WHEN TREATING PATIENTS WITH PERSONALITY DISORDERS

Because of the challenges faced when working with people with personality disorders, it is important to be grounded in a theoretical framework. This framework can be used to help further understanding of the person and the frequently overwhelming feelings one might feel in relation to the person. Such a theory or framework is transactional analysis.

Although there are numerous conflicting viewpoints regarding the nature and treatment of MHCUs with personality disorders, most theorists agree that each person is a conglomerate of mutually influencing thoughts, feelings and behaviour, some of which are maladaptive and have a reciprocal effect on the interpersonal environment.

The transactional analysis model is an approach that is logical and based on concepts that are user-friendly and easy to understand for both mental health practitioners and MHCUs. It can serve to empower patients and practitioners and can be taught and applied in the treatment of any personality disorder.

Although this model is introduced and used here to help with of the difficulties encountered with personality disorders, it is a model that can be implemented in any interactions with other people, MHCUs and colleagues. In coming to an understanding of this model it may be helpful to think about all one's relationships with others, friends, family members and co-workers to see how one is able to apply this framework to these interactions too.

The transactional analysis model

This model was initially devised by Eric Berne (1961) and has been further developed by other personality theorists in their work on what they have termed 'redecision therapy', and by Paul Ware (1983) in his theory of personality adaptations. In 2016, the *Transactional Analysis Journal* published a list of recently published books of an ever-growing library of resources to mark the 50th anniversary of the International Transactional Analysis Association. Although this model has undergone changes since its inception it is based on the premise that we can understand our personality as having three functional parts called the parent, adult and child ego states – which together make up the whole person.

Each ego state is identified by a characteristic system of feelings, thoughts and behaviour patterns. Within each person is a parent, adult and child that together makes up one's personality.

The parent ego state (see Figure 18.1) is further divided into a nurturing part and a more critical aspect. It contains moral and value judgements one takes in from outside sources, mainly from one's parents.

The nurturing parent (NP) is that part of oneself that has the potential to:
- be caring
- be loving
- be encouraging
- be guiding
- be supportive
- be attentive
- be protective
- be affectionate
- allow the above feelings within oneself and in others.

The critical parent (CP) is that part of oneself that has the potential to:
- be critical
- be a strict disciplinarian
- be questioning
- be comparing
- have high expectations
- display little affection
- be uncomfortable with feelings
- use words such as 'should', 'must', 'will', 'can't', 'won't' with the self and others in terms of all the above.

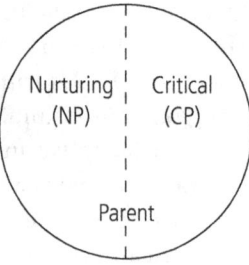

Figure 18.1 Parent ego state

The adult ego state (A) (See Figure 18.2) is that part of oneself that looks at reality more objectively and rationally, and has the potential to:
- be logical
- be rational

- be responsible
- process information about the world and people in it
- look at this information carefully
- be decisive
- be assertive
- express feelings appropriately that are felt by the child ego state
- be compromising in conflict situations.

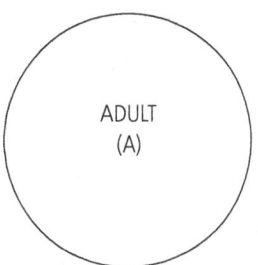

Figure 18.2 Adult ego state

The child ego state (see Figure 18.3), in contrast with the other ego states, consists of our inner impulses and feeling states. Like the parent ego state, it is also divided into two parts, namely the adapted child (AC) and the free child (FC):
1. The AC is that part of ourselves which consists of a set of feelings and behaviours developed in response to parental and societal demands and the general demands placed on us through living in the world. It is further divided into two parts:
    - *Rebellious child* (RC) is the part of our AC self which can:
        - be impulsive
        - be blaming
        - act out feelings, for example have a tantrum or sulk, or abuse substances
        - be reckless
        - be demanding and unreasonable in response to CP messages from others or from our own CP part within our personality
    - *Conforming child* (CC) is the part of our AC self which
        - is shy
        - pleasing
        - withdrawn
        - gives in to others demands and
        - bottles up feelings in response to CP messages from others/ from one's own crucial parental part.
    - *Natural/FC* is that part of ourselves which is the spontaneous expression of our personality and has the capacity to:
        - be creative
        - have fun
        - be expressive
        - be trusting of others
        - be energetic
        - be original
        - experience feelings
        - be decisive and aware of choices.

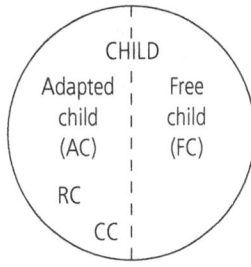

Figure 18.3 Child ego state

The development of the three ego states

To understand these ego states further it is helpful to think about how they are formed and become distinct from each other during our development. First, we are born to parents or caregivers who have all three ego states, to a greater or lesser extent, as part of their personalities. The mother, or primary caregiver, has the responsibility for taking care of their helpless new-born infant. When the baby cries, the mother must think for it, figure out what is wrong and respond to its problems. If its biological and emotional needs are met, the child grows both physically and emotionally and, in the process, learns to think for itself. However, this initial thinking is very basic and intuitive rather than careful, objective or complex. As the child continues to grow, it also learns how to take care of others and, in doing so, learns to take care of itself. Much of learning how to think, as well as how to take care of others and the self, is a natural outgrowth of the child's relationship with its parents and other important adult figures in its life.

Analysis of intrapersonal and interpersonal problems

As mentioned, the three ego states are present in all of us to a greater or a lesser degree and develop within our interpersonal relationships and in response to both parental and societal messages and the messages from the reality of the world. By way of example, a person who often feels anxious and has negative thoughts about their self-worth may have introjected or 'swallowed' very critical messages from their parents while growing up. This introjection happens outside of awareness or unconsciously.

Such a person would have an unhealthy egogram as illustrated in Figure 18.4. This diagram demonstrates that the person has introjected a large CP from their parent(s). Even in the parents' absence, this critical part continues to affect the person. This critical part activates or 'hooks' the AC and this results in the individual behaving in a maladaptive way. Such a person would need to develop a gentler, more nurturing parenting of themselves. This will enable their FC to feel the feelings which have been 'bottled up' or acted out. The adult part can then give these feelings a 'voice' in their relationships with others.

What is going on inside the person (intrapersonally) can also be described or explained as an interpersonal or transactional problem. Three basic transactional patterns are recognised within this theory and will be discussed here with examples. These are complementary, crossed and ulterior transactional patterns.

Complementary transactional patterns

Complementary transactions involve a parallel communication between two ego states of two people. One of the ways in which this pattern can be problematic is when a transactional pattern occurs between a critical position in one person and a rebellious or conforming position, identified as AC, in another.

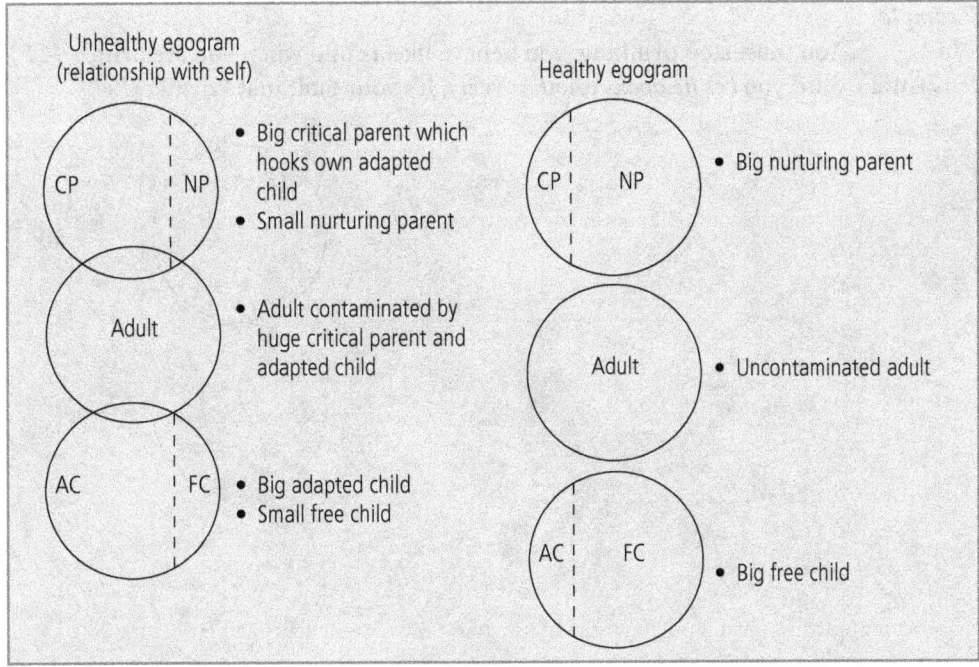

Figure 18.4 Egograms of differing ego states

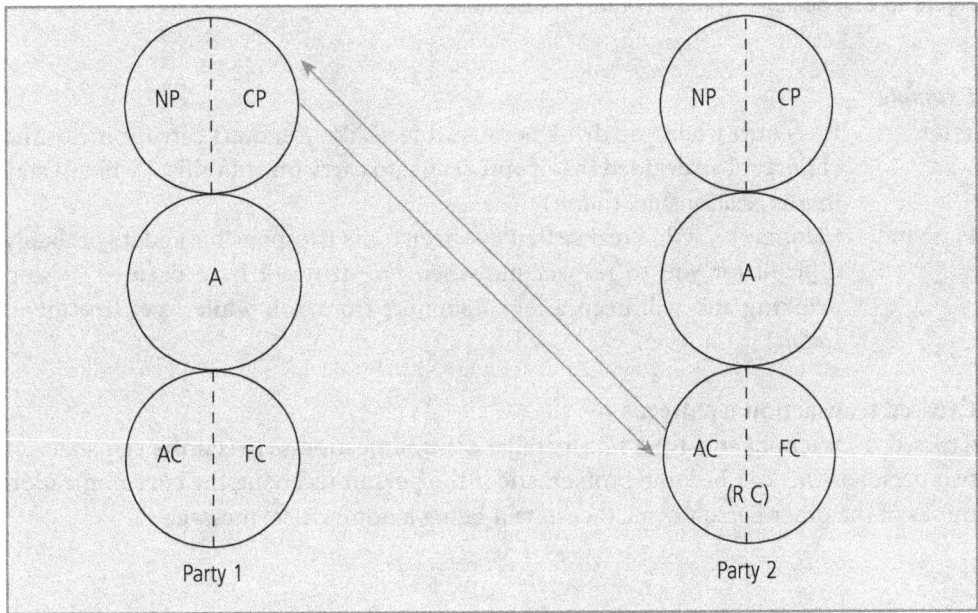

Figure 18.5 Problematic complementary transaction

Example

Wife: You must stop drinking; you behave like a child when you are drunk. *(CP)*
Husband: Stuff you (*as he opens another beer*). It's your fault that I drink. *(RC)*

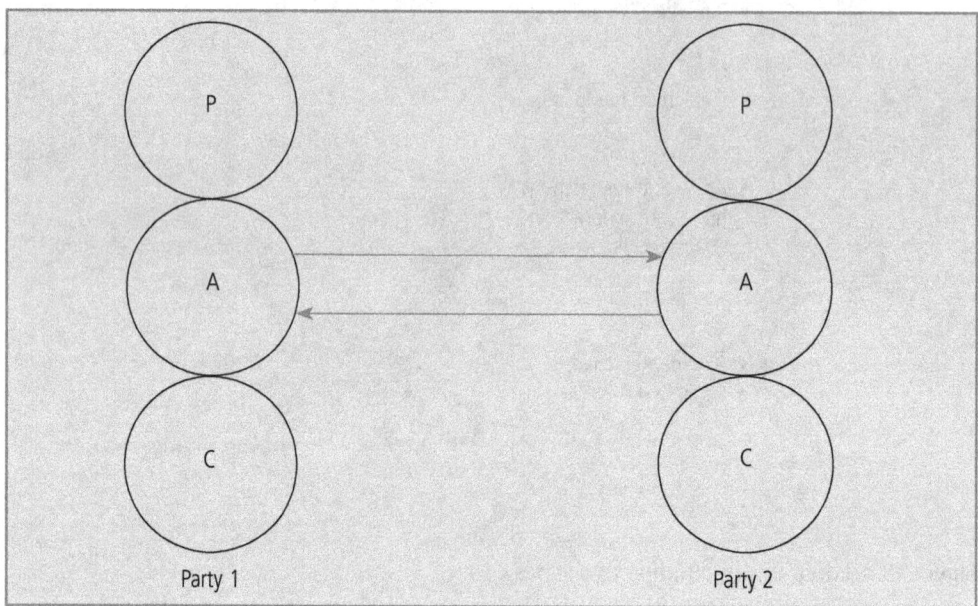

Figure 18.6 A healthier complementary transaction

Example

Wife: I feel hurt when you drink because it feels like you don't care for me or the children. I've decided that if you decide to carry on with this, I will not stay in this relationship. (*adult*)

Husband: (*hesitates*) ... Oh, I realise that I've been quite irresponsible and it's probably difficult for you to respect me when I'm drunk. I have decided to stop drinking and will need a lot of support from you while I get treatment. (*adult*)

Crossed transactional patterns

Crossed transactions involve a non-parallel communication between the ego states of two persons. This can become problematic if the person receiving the communication thinks of the other person as a CP despite it being a non-critical message.

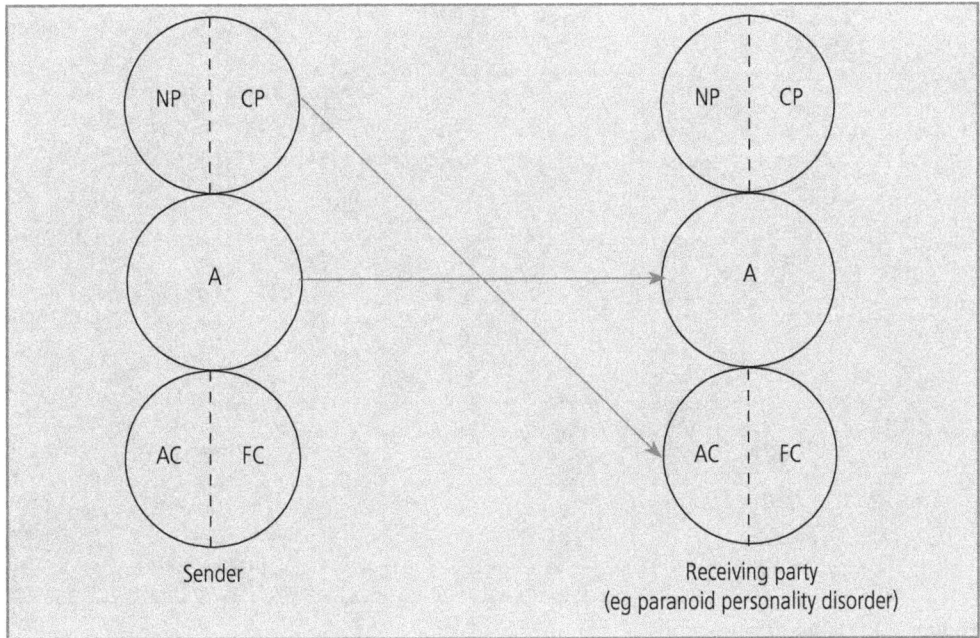

Figure 18.7 Crossed transactions

Example

Sender: I feel frustrated when you constantly question me because it feels like you don't trust me. (*adult*)

Receiver: Well, it's your fault, you always let me down and you probably arrived late because you are having an affair with Eric. (*RC blaming, suspicious; projects a critical element onto the sender of a non-critical message*)

Ulterior transactional patterns

Ulterior transactions involve communication between three or four ego states of people. Often the messages are hidden messages and could be non-verbal and incongruent with the verbal message. People can frequently be made aware of the hidden messages behind the direct message in their transactions.

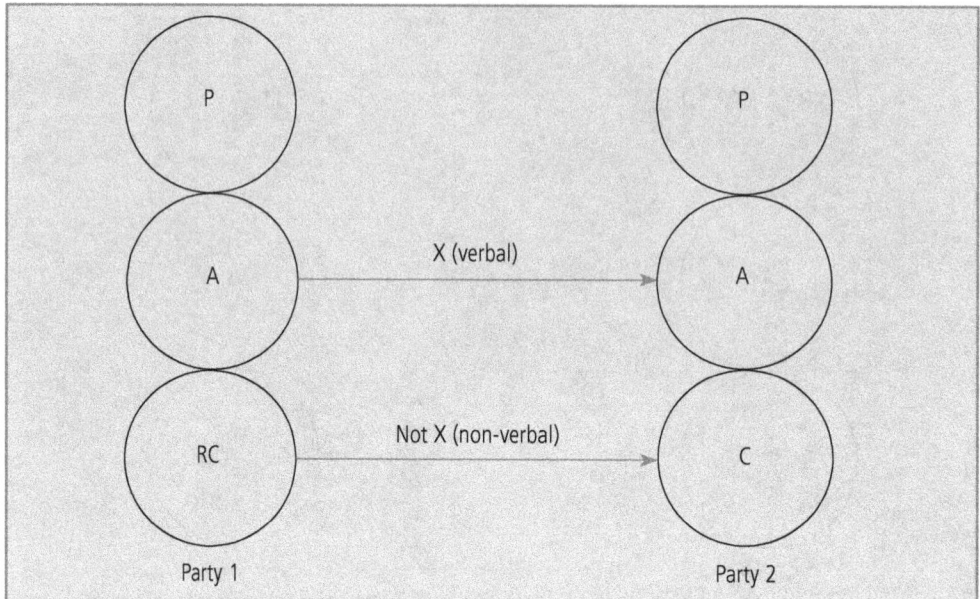

Figure 18.8 Ulterior transactions

Example
Husband: 'You are important to me (*while fiddling with the TV remote*).'

Other important concepts related to the theory of transactional analysis

There are several other concepts that are relevant to the theory of transactional analysis. These concepts and explanations of what they mean are listed below.

- *Injunctions.* Parental messages internalised by the child part of oneself and which can be positive or negative in content. Examples of negative injunctions are:
  - 'don't feel'
  - 'don't think'
  - 'don't be close'
  - 'don't be weak'.
- *Scripts.* Opinions we form about ourselves and the world as children through internalised parental messages: 'You are worthless; others are more important than you.'
- *Rackets.* Bad feelings most frequently felt by oneself, often related to negative injunctions received and decisions made by the child part of oneself.
- *Games.* Behaviour patterns which reinforce the bad feelings and used to support the racket.

- *Existential position.* Belief about oneself and others which one forms at the end of the 'game'.

Application of the concepts

The following example illustrates these concepts.

Dineo often experiences the 'bad' feelings (racket) associated with depression; this is related to the parental message (injunction) of 'don't feel'. She then plays the 'game' of holding on to her feelings in her here-and-now relationships. This leaves her feeling more depressed, which reinforces her existential position: 'I'm not important; others are more important.'

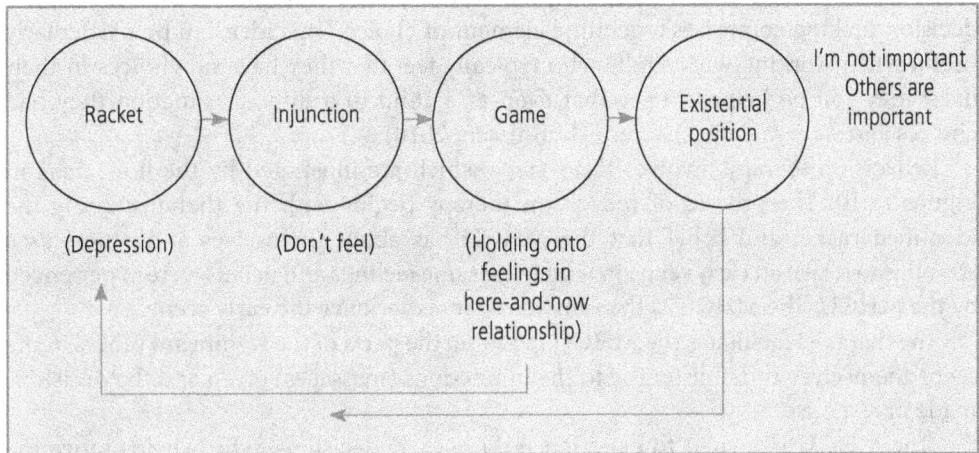

Figure 18.9 An example of the dynamics of depression

Using transactional analysis therapeutically: Redecision therapy

Goulding and Goulding (1979) have expanded on the transactional analysis model. They are best known for their view of children as imaginative decision makers who react innovatively to injunctive family messages and learn to use emotions as tools in interpersonal relationships.

> **The child is viewed as:**
> capable of making choices
> in arriving at creative decisions
> as to how he/she will be in order
> to feel secure and loved
> in his/her unique family environment.

Example

> **The child decides either to:**
> act out (RC)
> conform (CC)
> be spontaneous (FC)
> use his/her adult reasoning
> any of which may gain him/her attention from his/her
> parents (positively reinforced).

Goulding and Goulding (1979) recognise that the child's developmental level limits the range of choices at their disposal, but still emphasise that the child's capacity for decision making comprises a genuine element of choice. This idea can be particularly useful when working with adults who typically feel that they have no choices in their lives; they can be helped to see that even as a child in a difficult situation they had choices and were making choices (Thunnissen, 2010).

Redecision therapy involves three steps which are illustrated by the flow chart in Figure 18.10. The process of redecision therapy begins with the therapist using the identified racket and belief that the MHCU has about themselves and others as a stimulus to evoke an early scene in which the same feelings and beliefs were experienced by the MHCU. The MHCU is then invited to re-experience the early scene.

The therapist facilitates the MHCU in taking the parts of the significant others in the scene themselves and in listening to the injunctions (messages) given and the decisions made in response.

- The MHCU is invited to experience these early decisions, which helps move the MHCU from an AC position to an FC position.
- The MHCU stays with this early decision until a redecision emerges spontaneously.
- The redecision facilitates new behaviours, which will need practice in order to become comfortable to the MHCU.
- The therapist operates from specific ego states (their own) so as to develop specific ego states in the MHCU (see Tables 18.2 and 18.3).

In brief, then, the process of redecision involves the MHCUs doing something, so that they can enter the FC ego state. This may entail, for example, regressing to early childhood and re-experiencing the feelings, the scene, the words, the action involved in an initial, early decision and then, while still reliving the experience, changing the decision.

In essence, the overall aim of the therapist is to:
- replace parent
- educate adult
- deconfuse child, so that the person can be:
  - energetic
  - creative

- intuitive
- sensual
- intimate
- original
- now!

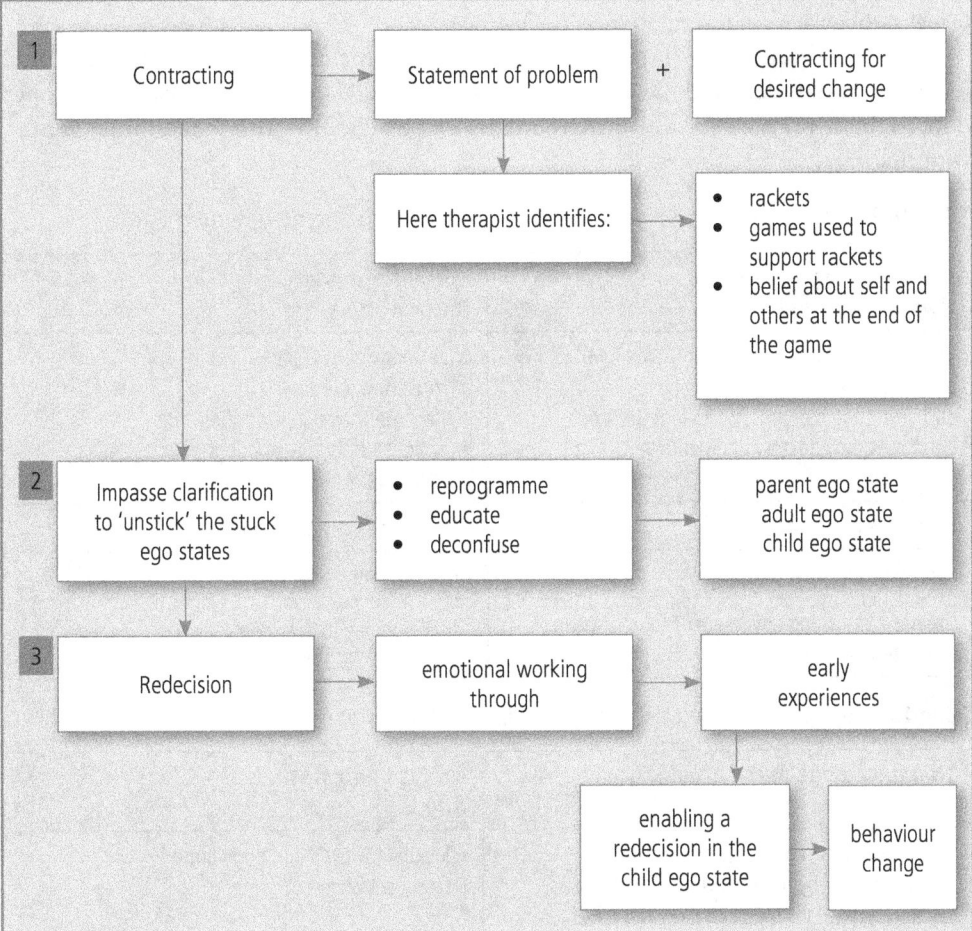

Figure 18.10 Flow chart of redecision therapy

Understanding personality disorders within the transactional analysis model

Persons diagnosed with a personality disorder often feel vulnerable in an individual setting and even more so in a group setting. As a result, they often react strongly to any show of vulnerability and to the risk taking required for a redecision to emerge. Ware's (1983) information on personality adaptations and what he calls 'doors for intervention' is useful when using redecision therapy to facilitate change in MHCUs.

The personality types and the intervention approach applicable to each type are presented in the conceptual framework of six personality adaptations and 'doors to therapy'. The six personality adaptations within this framework are referred to as hysterical, obsessive-compulsive, schizoid, antisocial, passive-aggressive and paranoid, each of which requires different approaches when making contact (the open door) with the MHCU. Those to avoid (the trap door) and the ongoing direction for change (the target door) are also described (see Table 18.4).

Since each personality type has its own pattern, mental health practitioners must recognise and understand the area in which each MHCU invests the most energy (open door) – be it primarily in feelings, thoughts or behaviour – and make initial contact with this area.

Table 18.2 Ego states in the MHCU and therapist: nurturing parent–natural child

Therapist's ego state Nurturing parent	MHCU's ego state Natural child
Protects the MHCU, emphasising their own personal power and responsibility and giving them permission to feel/think or behave as they do now and did then	Enables the MHCU to: ▪ trust and feel safe ▪ feel the therapist is on their side ▪ take risks and re-experience early scene ▪ redecide
Reinforces new behaviour	MHCU feels comfortable with new behaviour
Exhibits healthy behaviour	Models healthy behaviour
Creates a nurturing environment for change in group setting (specific norms)	Person has a stage to redecide

Table 18.3 Ego states in the MHCU and therapist: adult–adult

Therapist's ego state Adult	MHCU's ego state Adult
Separates myth from reality in terms of old decisions made by the MHCU as a child, which assisted survival for the child then, but which are now outdated	Educates MHCU's adult ego state Deconfuses child ego state.
Draws script diagrams to illustrate what child ego state experienced	Provides adult ego state reinforcement of what child state experiences

Table 18.4 Personality adaptation therapy and doors for intervention

Adaptations	Doors		
	(Open door) Contact door	Target door	Trap door
Schizoid (Cluster A)	Behaviour	Thinking	Feeling
Antisocial (Cluster B)	Behaviour	Feeling	Thinking
Paranoid (Cluster A)	Thinking	Feeling	Behaviour
Histrionic (Cluster B)	Feeling	Thinking	Behaviour
Obsessive-compulsive (Cluster C)	Thinking	Feeling	Behaviour

WORKING WITH MHCUs WITH SPECIFIC PERSONALITY DISORDERS

In this section we look more specifically at the personality disorders as laid out in the framework of the DSM-5. It is important to remember that no person fits neatly into any one category or cluster. People generally have difficulties characteristic of many of the categories discussed here. When working with a person, rather than trying to fit them into a narrow understanding and treatment model, a mental health practitioner should consider all the information here and take what may be of use to their understanding and treatment of the person.

Cluster A personality disorders

This grouping of personality disorders includes the paranoid, schizoid and schizotypal personality disorders that share oddness and aloofness as common features.

Schizoid personality disorder

The DSM-5 (APA, 2013) classifies the schizoid personality disorder according to the following criteria:
A. A pervasive pattern of detachment from social relationships and a restricted range of expression of emotions in interpersonal settings, beginning by early adulthood and present in a variety of contexts, as indicated by four (or more) of the following:
   1. Neither desires nor enjoys close relationships, including being part of a family
   2. Almost always chooses solitary activities
   3. Has little, if any, interest in having sexual experiences with another person

4. Takes pleasure in few, if any, activities
5. Lacks close friends or confidants other than first-degree relatives
6. Appears indifferent to the praise or criticism of others
7. Shows emotional coldness, detachment, or flattened affectivity.

B. Does not occur exclusively during the course of schizophrenia, a mood disorder with psychotic features, another psychotic disorder, or a pervasive developmental disorder and is not due to the direct physiological effects of a general medical condition.

Note: If criteria are met prior to the onset of schizophrenia, add 'premorbid', for example 'Schizoid personality disorder (premorbid)'.
(*Reprinted with permission from the* Diagnostic and Statistical Manual of Mental Disorders, Fifth Edition (Copyright ©2013). *American Psychiatric Association. All Rights Reserved.*)

Understanding the psychology of the person with a schizoid personality disorder

A person diagnosed with a schizoid personality disorder characteristically has an underlying fear of closeness. As an infant such persons experienced rejection from the primary care giver and withdrew into themselves. This cycle of rejection, withdrawal and the difficulties in negotiating basic needs from others can be represented diagrammatically (see Figure 18.11):

Common defences used

- Fantasy
  - to comfort self
- Distancing
  - to push others away so as to avoid feelings of needing others and others needing them
  - others feel rejected
- Splitting
  - to keep perceived 'good' and 'bad' parts of self and others apart
- Projective identification
  - world becomes rejecting towards MHCU as mother did, leaving person alone.

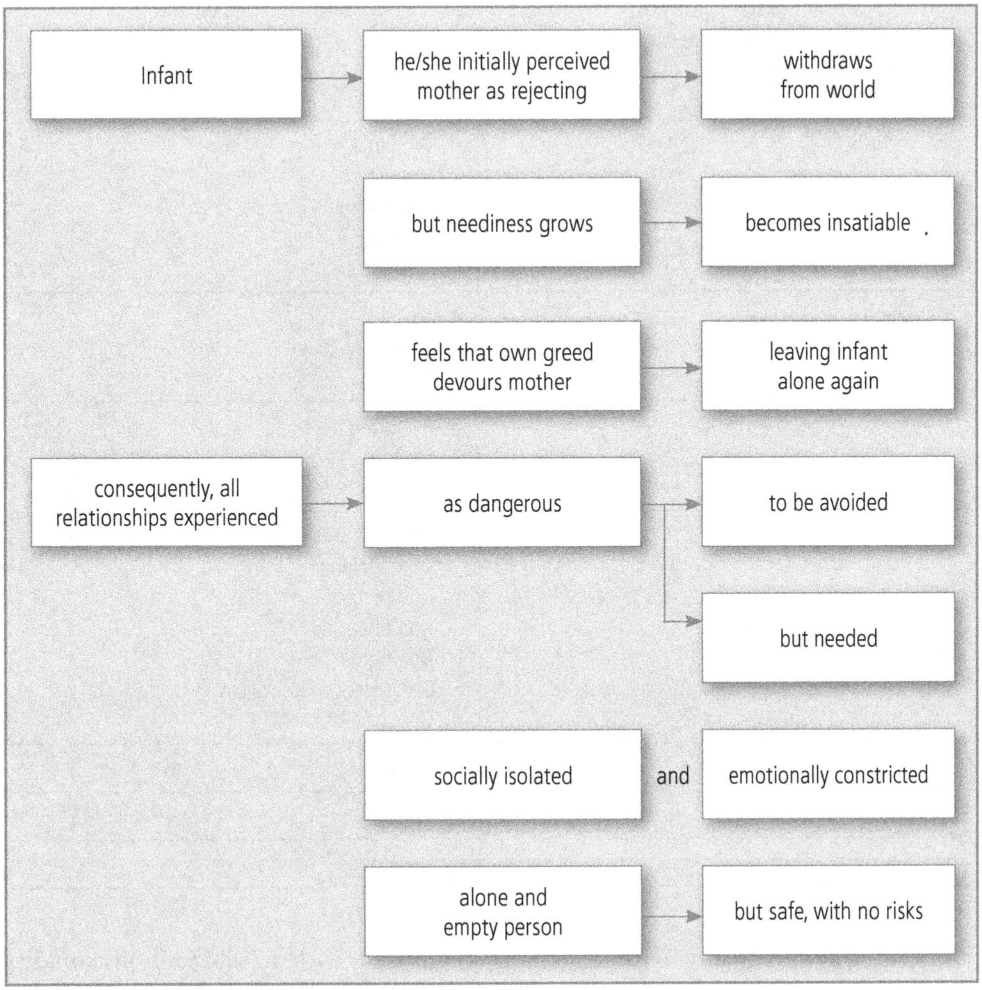

```
┌─────────────────────────────────────────────────────────────────────────┐
│   Infant        →   he/she initially perceived   →   withdraws          │
│                     mother as rejecting              from world         │
│                                                                         │
│                     but neediness grows          →   becomes insatiable │
│                                                                         │
│                     feels that own greed         →   leaving infant     │
│                     devours mother                   alone again        │
│                                                                         │
│   consequently, all →  as dangerous              →   to be avoided      │
│   relationships experienced                                             │
│                                                  →   but needed         │
│                                                                         │
│                     socially isolated   and   emotionally constricted   │
│                                                                         │
│                     alone and                    →   but safe, with     │
│                     empty person                     no risks           │
└─────────────────────────────────────────────────────────────────────────┘
```

Figure 18.11 Experiences and responses to experiences in the person with a schizoid personality disorder

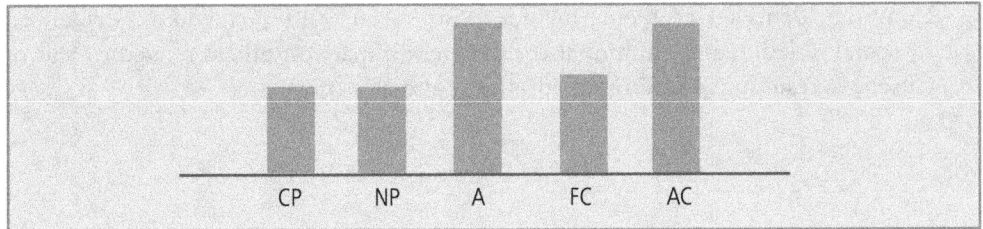

Figure 18.12 Egogram of the schizoid MHCU

Table 18.5 Understanding the MHCU with a schizoid personality disorder within a transactional analysis model

Adaptation	Schizoid
Characteristics	<ul><li>Withdrawn</li><li>Passivity</li><li>Daydreaming</li><li>Avoidance</li><li>Detachment</li></ul>
Description	<ul><li>Shy</li><li>Overly sensitive</li><li>Eccentric</li></ul>
Drivers	<ul><li>Be strong</li><li>Try hard</li><li>Please others</li></ul>
Injunctions	<ul><li>Don't make it</li><li>Don't belong</li><li>Don't enjoy</li><li>Don't be sane</li><li>Don't grow up</li><li>Don't feel (love, sex, joy)</li><li>Don't think</li></ul>
Contact door	<ul><li>Behaviour</li></ul>
Target door	<ul><li>Thinking</li></ul>
Trap door	<ul><li>Feeling</li></ul>

Working therapeutically with a person diagnosed with a schizoid personality disorder

- A major therapeutic goal would be to assist the person in establishing a positive view of social interaction and personal closeness and in reducing negative views of social isolation (educate Adult ego state and replace Parent).
- Common identified problems include poor social skills (behaviour), evidenced by social isolation and emotional constriction; impact on others related to fear of closeness, resulting in feelings of emptiness and aloneness.

The use of individual therapy and group therapy is discussed below.

Individual therapy
- The initial goal would be to motivate the MHCU to see the need for changing their behaviour (contact area) and for engaging with the fear of closeness to others. This would involve exploring the advantages and disadvantages of their social withdrawal and the effect of their behaviour on others.
- The mental health practitioner should educate the MHCU on basic patterns of human interaction and target their thinking.
  - The MHCU typically shows little understanding of interpersonal relationships and may have quite poor social skills, since they have not managed either to observe or to experience such skills.
  - During sessions with the MHCU, the mental health care practitioner may use opportunities to point out the MHCU's characteristic interaction pattern and can provide feedback to the MHCU regarding their impact on others.
  - The MHCU should practise the newly learnt social skills to test these new understandings and skills, both when the mental health practitioner is interacting with the MHCU and during their free time.
- The mental health practitioner should recognise that any change is a slow, painstaking process and that a few, small steps should be taken at a time. There should be a permissive, accepting attitude towards the MHCU's silence.
- The mental health practitioner should remember to monitor their own feelings, as this provides a valuable source of information about the MHCU (that is, their own inner world and defences).
  - If feeling frustrated and rejected by the MHCU, and desiring to give up on them, the mental health practitioner should attempt to understand these feelings rather than to act on them. (The MHCU is probably using the defences of distancing and projective identification and needs more nurturing.)

In this way the mental health practitioner acts as a repository for the MHCU's projections, which helps the MHCU to integrate the good and bad aspects of themselves.

Group therapy
- A person diagnosed with a schizoid personality disorder can benefit from group therapy, since group therapy is oriented towards helping MHCUs with socialisation.
  - It is also a setting in which new parenting can take place, both by the therapists and by other group members (NP).
  - Such MHCUs can benefit a great deal from having regular contact or exposure to others. With time they may experience feelings of acceptance from the group and gradually become more comfortable with people (reinforces the MHCU's FC).

- One difficulty the group therapist may encounter is dealing with other MHCUs who may become resentful towards the MHCU for not sharing in the group as they have. This can result in the group ganging up and trying to force the MHCU to share (another MHCU's CP or RC).
    - Here the therapist must support (NP) the MHCU and help other group members to accept that the MHCU needs to be silent.
- Another difficulty can be that other MHCUs may ignore a withdrawn MHCU and treat the person as if they were not present.
    - Here the therapist's task is to get other members to give feedback to the MHCU regarding the effect of their behaviour on others (only once enough trust has been established in the group).
    - The therapist can also bring the MHCU into the group by pointing out how a pattern that takes place outside the group is now repeating itself inside the group. Point out gently how withdrawn and unreceptive the MHCU is in the group (address MHCU's adult ego).
- It is important to prepare the MHCU emotionally prior to group therapy, since their anxiety will be increased at the very idea of the therapy. A way of doing this is to explore the MHCU's fantasies about what they fear will happen in the group (MHCU's FC).

A combination of individual therapy followed by group therapy is often ideal for many MHCUs in order to increase their positive views of social interaction.

Application by example
An MHCU diagnosed with schizoid personality disorder had been hospitalised following an overdose attempt in relation to his struggle with employment. When he made contact with other people at work he would 'freeze up' with anxiety and withdraw. Instead of working he would sit down and listen to a radio or sleep at his desk. His shyness, withdrawal, detachment and 'living in his own world' were evidence of his withdrawn passivity. The *be strong* driver was evident in the MHCU's lack of emotion. The injunctions *don't feel* and *don't enjoy* were also clearly evident. *Don't grow up* and *don't think* injunctions were apparent from his helplessness and struggle to take responsibility for himself.

Since the MHCU's energy level was so low, the therapist had to devote a great deal of energy to the MHCU's withdrawn passivity, his open door of behaviour, thus entering his world. As therapy progressed, the therapist invited him to his target door of thinking, helping him to move from a passive to an active state, thus making him aware of choices he had made and helping him to take responsibility for his passive behaviour.

Schizotypal personality disorder

The DSM-5 (APA, 2013) diagnostic criteria of schizotypal personality disorder are as follows:

A. A pervasive pattern of social and interpersonal deficits marked by acute discomfort with, and reduced capacity for, close relationships, as well as by cognitive or perceptual distortions and eccentricities of behaviour, beginning by early adulthood and present in a variety of contexts, as indicated by five (or more) of the following:
   1. Ideas of reference (excluding delusions of reference)
   2. Odd beliefs or magical thinking that influence behaviour and are inconsistent with subcultural norms (for example, superstitiousness, belief in clairvoyance, telepathy, or 'sixth sense'; in children and adolescents, bizarre fantasies or preoccupations)
   3. Unusual perceptual experiences, including bodily illusions
   4. Odd thinking and speech (for example, vague, circumstantial, metaphorical, over-elaborate or stereotyped)
   5. Suspiciousness or paranoid ideation
   6. Inappropriate or constricted affect
   7. Behaviour or appearance that is odd, eccentric, or peculiar
   8. Lack of close friends or confidants other than first-degree relatives
   9. Excessive social anxiety that does not diminish with familiarity and tends to be associated with paranoid fears rather than negative judgements about self.
B. Does not occur exclusively during the course of schizophrenia, a mood disorder with psychotic features, another psychotic disorder, or a pervasive developmental disorder.

Note: If criteria are met prior to the onset of schizophrenia, add 'premorbid', for example 'Schizotypal personality disorder (premorbid)'.

(*Reprinted with permission from the* Diagnostic and Statistical Manual of Mental Disorders, Fifth Edition (Copyright ©2013). *American Psychiatric Association. All Rights Reserved.*)

Understanding the psychology of the person diagnosed with a schizotypal personality disorder

At the one end of the continuum, a person diagnosed with a schizotypal personality disorder can present in a very similar way to a person diagnosed with a schizoid personality disorder. At the other end of the continuum, though, there are those MHCUs who are closer in presentation to an MHCU diagnosed with schizophrenia and are even prone to brief psychotic episodes.

Refer to Table 18.5 and the discussion of MHCUs diagnosed with schizoid personality disorder, as this table and discussion applies equally here. More specific injunctions include *don't be sane and don't belong*, resulting in the often-bizarre behaviour characteristics of the MHCU with a schizotypal personality disorder.

Working therapeutically with a person diagnosed with a schizotypal personality disorder
- The principles of individual and group therapy, previously outlined in the management of the MHCU diagnosed with a schizoid personality disorder, also apply to the MHCU diagnosed with a schizotypal personality disorder.
- In addition to the above, a careful assessment needs to be made of the MHCU's ego functioning in terms of their reality testing and judgement. Those MHCUs with better ego functioning will progress more than those with profoundly disturbed ego functioning who may need support with their ability to test reality and with their judgement.
- Social skills training and re-education will help to reduce bizarre behaviours.
- See discussion of the use of psychotropic medication.

Individual therapy may be the preferred modality for treating such an MHCU if their behaviour is too bizarre. Such a person might become a 'scapegoat' in group therapy because they are perceived as being too different from other members.

Paranoid personality disorder

The DSM-5 (APA, 2013) diagnostic criteria of the paranoid personality disorder are as follows:
A. A pervasive distrust and suspiciousness of others such that their motives are interpreted as malevolent, beginning by early adulthood and present in a variety of contexts, as indicated by four (or more) of the following:
   1. Suspects, without sufficient basis, that others are exploiting, harming or deceiving him/her
   2. Is preoccupied with unjustified doubts about the loyalty or trustworthiness of friends or associates
   3. Is reluctant to confide in others because of unwarranted fear that the information will be used maliciously against him/her
   4. Reads hidden demeaning or threatening meanings into benign remarks or events
   5. Persistently bears grudges, that is, is unforgiving of insults, injuries, or slights
   6. Perceives attacks on his/her character or reputation that are not apparent to others and is quick to react angrily or to counterattack
   7. Has recurrent suspicions, without justification, regarding fidelity of spouse or sexual partner.
B. Does not occur exclusively during the course of schizophrenia, a mood disorder with psychotic features, or another psychotic disorder and is not due to the direct physiological effects of a general medical condition.

Note: If criteria are met prior to the onset of schizophrenia, add 'premorbid', for example 'Paranoid personality disorder (premorbid)'.
(*Reprinted with permission from the* Diagnostic and Statistical Manual of Mental Disorders, Fifth Edition (Copyright ©2013). *American Psychiatric Association. All Rights Reserved.*)

Understanding the psychology of the person diagnosed with a paranoid personality disorder

Parenting that is 'good enough' in infancy enables the infant to integrate simultaneously both good and bad aspects of the parent, of the world and within the self. In the paranoid personality disorder, parenting during childhood has involved a predominance of unsatisfying experiences (the good and bad aspects of the parent are kept separate and the outside world and the internal world of the person become just at polarised). The badness within is projected onto outside figures (which themselves became persecuting) to reduce the internal tension between good and bad. Defences used thus include splitting, projection and projective identification.

The MHCU's experience of others is discontinuous; no relationship is perceived as enduring over time. Instead, the MHCU has only the perception of the moment.

Low self-esteem, and feelings of inferiority, often underlie the MHCU's external mask of rigidity and their need for perfection.

Table 18.6 Understanding the MHCU with a paranoid personality disorder in terms of a transactional analysis model

Adaptation	Paranoid
Characteristics	▪ Rigidity of thought ▪ Grandiosity ▪ Projection
Description	▪ Hypersensitive ▪ Suspicious ▪ Jealous ▪ Envious
Drivers	▪ Be strong ▪ Be perfect
Injunctions	▪ Don't be a child ▪ Don't be close ▪ Don't feel ▪ Don't enjoy ▪ Don't trust
Contact door	▪ Thinking
Target door	▪ Feeling
Trap door	▪ Behaviour

The MHCUs are characterised by grandiosity and rigidity, especially in their thinking patterns. Their grandiosity, reflected in unrealistic expectations of themselves (be perfect), is a defence against deep-seated feelings of insecurity and inadequacy. The MHCUs project strongly what they think and feel onto others and are often very accusatory. They operate in a 'move-in and move-out' pattern, making contact with someone one day and then pulling away from them the next.

Very early in life they received messages (injunctions) of *don't trust, don't be a child, don't feel, don't be close* and *don't enjoy*.

Their open door is in *thinking*, which they can do carefully and accurately because of their hypersensitive perception. Their target door or access door is *feeling* and their trap door is *behaviour*.

If their behaviour is criticised, they can become more suspicious and delusional and there is increased projection of the 'bad' onto others.

Working therapeutically with a person diagnosed with a paranoid personality disorder

- A major goal would be to help the MHCU to shift their perception of the origin of their problems from an external source (world and others) to an internal one (the self). Instead of fault finding or blaming, the person moves towards owning their own critical projections.
- Common identified problems include difficulty in trusting others related to frustration with early figures and a predominance of unsatisfying experiences; evidenced by low self-esteem, suspiciousness, a tendency to be guarded and to find fault with others.

Individual therapy is the preferred initial modality of treatment because of the MHCU's mistrust of others. Here the mental health nurse may work in conjunction with a psychologist to achieve the major goal.

Working with the person on an individual basis

- The mental health nurse should build a therapeutic alliance. This process can be extremely challenging because of the MHCU's difficulty in trusting anyone and because of the MHCU's tendency to attack or blame others, including the therapist (projection, projective identification).
    - The mental health nurse must be willing to act as a 'repository' for feelings of hatred, badness, impotence and despair, instead of reacting defensively to attacks from the MHCU.
    - Instead of challenging the MHCU's thinking or construction of events, the nurse should get more detail from the MHCU (contact area). It is also important to empathise with the MHCU's feelings and perceptions of the situation (target area). For example, 'I can see why you might be angry with me if you thought I was criticising you, I don't have any critical thoughts towards you though.'
    - Openness is important when endeavouring to build a relationship of trust with the MHCU.

- The mental health nurse should help the MHCU to identify 'gaps' in their thinking about reality so as to establish a creative doubt about their perceptions of the world.
  - The person with a paranoid personality disorder presents with a 'faulty' perception of the world. The mental health nurse must communicate tactfully with the MHCU in order to bring awareness to their pattern of thinking. Questions must be worded carefully and neutrally so as not to challenge the MHCU's view of the world. For example, 'Did your friend say that she hates you?' If the MHCU responds 'no' to this question it can be used as an opportunity to bring to awareness the limitations of accurately knowing another's feelings. As the MHCU engages more with the work, the mental health care nurse can begin to identify the MHCU's feelings (target door) and help the MHCU to distinguish between emotions and reality.
- Violence can be a real threat when working with MHCUs with this diagnosis because of their constant perception of attack from the world. The following principles are important in this regard:
  - Focus on nurturing and empathising with the MHCU while the relationship of trust is developing.
  - Avoid arousing further suspicion by keeping openness and consistency in interactions.
  - Help the MHCU to maintain a sense of control (communicate respect of their autonomy in order to reduce anxiety).
  - Encourage the MHCU to talk about, rather than to act out, their anger (explore consequences of becoming violent).
  - Give the MHCU plenty of 'breathing space' (in terms of seating arrangements).
  - Be aware and manage one's own feelings when working with the MHCU.
    - If the mental health care nurse feels afraid, avoid situations that might jeopardise one's safety, especially if the MHCU has been physically aggressive in the past.
    - Recognise one's own potential to be destructive and aggressive, instead of seeing these feelings as typical only of such MHCUs.

Application by way of example

A highly sensitive and perceptive young man diagnosed with a paranoid personality disorder had been admitted to the unit following the loss of his brother. The following illustrates how the therapist (X) moved from a thinking to a feeling level in a very gentle and supportive way. The MHCU seemed very guarded at first, sitting quietly, and seeming to invest considerable energy in thinking. The first step taken by the therapist was to invite him to share his thinking aloud and to share the negative feelings he was experiencing, so that these could be dealt with. As the therapist encouraged the MHCU to share his clear thinking regarding how this loss of his brother had affected his life, the co-therapist intervened expertly when he said, 'I imagine you have a lot of feelings about the loss of your brother' and in so doing broke through the MHCUs *be strong* and *don't feel* drivers. As he began to cry and look at the therapist, the therapist moved in and made contact with him on a feeling level.

Although hesitant and hard on himself initially he became more accessible to feeling. His *don't be close* injunction was evident in his fear of closeness and positive feelings. He needed to be 'weaned' into positive feeling and continually reassured that caring about somebody and being close, although scary, would not be destructive.

Cluster B personality disorders

This grouping of personality disorders includes the narcissistic, borderline, antisocial and histrionic personality disorders that share dramatic, impulsive and erratic features.

The histrionic personality disorder

The DSM-5 (APA, 2013) diagnostic criteria for the histrionic personality disorder include the following:

A pervasive pattern of excessive emotionality and attention seeking, beginning by early adulthood and present in a variety of contexts, as indicated by five (or more) of the following:

1. Is uncomfortable in situations in which he or she is not the centre of attention
2. Interaction with others is often characterized by inappropriate sexually seductive or provocative behaviour
3. Displays rapidly shifting and shallow expression of emotions
4. Consistently uses physical appearance to draw attention to self
5. Has a style of speech that is excessively impressionistic and lacking in detail
6. Shows self-dramatisation, theatricality, and exaggerated expression of emotion
7. Is suggestible, that is, easily influenced by others or circumstances
8. Considers relationships to be more intimate than they actually are.

(*Reprinted with permission from the* Diagnostic and Statistical Manual of Mental Disorders, Fifth Edition (Copyright ©2013). *American Psychiatric Association. All Rights Reserved.*)

Understanding the psychology of the person with a histrionic personality disorder
It has been found that persons diagnosed with a histrionic personality disorder have often had significant maternal deprivation as an infant. This lack of maternal nurturance leads to the infant seeking gratification from the father or other caregivers. One of the core unconscious basic beliefs of such persons seems to be 'I am inadequate and unable to handle life on my own, so I'll have to rely on others to take care of me!' In contrast with persons diagnosed with a dependent personality disorder, who get taken care of by emphasising their helplessness and by assuming a passive role, the histrionic person takes the initiative by actively seeking attention and approval from others in an often times child-like manner.

The thinking style of such a person is characteristically global, impressionistic, vivid and interesting, but lacking in detail and focus. Their 'knee-jerk' emotionality is exaggerated, labile and intense and is accompanied by attention-seeking behaviour. Such behaviour can be understood as a defensive system that protects the individual from any genuine feeling states too difficult to experience and is used to manipulate others into taking care of them.

Common defences used by the person with a histrionic personality disorder include:
- denial, repression, idealisation, splitting
- generalisation
- emotionality.

Table 18.7 Understanding the person with a histrionic personality disorder in terms of a transactional analysis model

Adaptation	Hysterical
Characteristics	- Excitability - Emotional instability - Over-reactivity - Dramatic attention seeking - Seductive
Description	- Immature - Self-centred - Vain - Dependent
Drivers	- Please me - Try hard - Hurry up
Injunctions	- Don't grow up - Don't be important - Don't think
Contact door	- Feeling
Target door	- Thinking
Trap door	- Behaviour

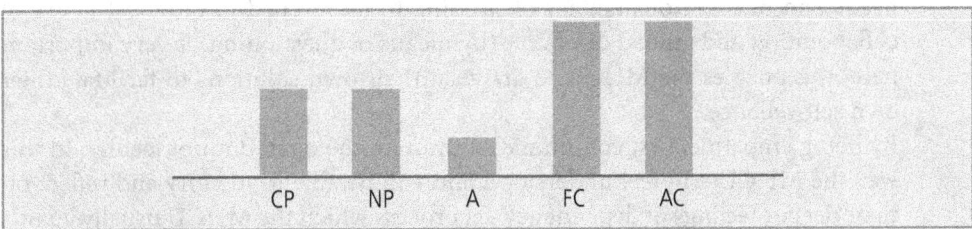

Figure 18.13 Egogram: active dependent style of the histrionic personality

People with histrionic personality characteristics invest their energy for the most part in feeling. They present with excitability, emotional instability and over-reactivity. They are often referred to as attention seeking and dramatic, with behaviour that is experienced by others as immature and self-centred. Although they can be energising to be around, relationships can be difficult. Such persons often attach themselves to others, get close, become dependent and invite conflict within the person they are dependent on.

Their number one driver is *please me* or *please others*, and the messages often come from the parent of the same sex.

In order to make contact with such a person and invite them to change, the mental health practitioner must first communicate and connect with them at a feeling level, which is the level at which their energy is invested (open door). The MHCU can then be invited to change through their target door (that is, their thinking processes); the mental health practitioner must be careful to relate to the MHCU from an equal rather than a 'one-up' position. The trap door to be avoided is the MHCU's behaviour, which usually occurs at an unconscious level.

Working therapeutically with a person diagnosed with a histrionic personality disorder

- A major goal would be to develop the MHCU's (adult) sense of competence and self-reliance, through refining their thinking processes and helping them to experience feelings more deeply, thus enabling the person to communicate their needs more assertively.
- Common identified problems are the struggle to rely on self for care or approval related to relatively early maternal deprivation; evidenced by emotionally dramatic, attention-seeking behaviour, a need for approval from others and impressionistic, global thinking, resulting in problems in relationships with others.

Working with the person with a histrionic personality disorder on an individual basis

Some principles to follow in working with such a person on an individual basis include the following:
- Establish a therapeutic alliance, focusing on specific target problems and goals.
    - The person with histrionic personality disorder readily becomes attached to the mental health care practitioner because of their underlying dependency needs and unconscious fantasy of needing to be rescued to others. The use of collaboration and guided discovery (by means of questioning) is very important here; this enables the MHCU to arrive at their own solutions to facilitate their own self-reliance.
    - By being empathic, first communicate through the open door of feeling. In this way the MHCU will feel understood and will be able to identify and reflect on their deeper feelings of dependency – a process which the MHCU usually guards against.

- Help the MHCU to focus their attention on one issue at a time; this will prevent both the MHCU and the mental health care practitioner from getting lost in all the 'dramatics' of the MHCU's experiences.
- It is important to negotiate clear boundaries with the MHCU by setting limits to demands. Limits must be clear, concrete and immediate (for example, a time limit for individual therapy).
■ Establish the need for detail or specifics with regard to thinking and feeling states.
- Facilitate an awareness of the MHCU's vagueness of perception and superficial impressionistic feelings; explain the consequences of this in terms of their ability to rely on self.
- Help the MHCU to reflect specifically on events and feeling states instead of reporting globally and dramatically on these in a superficial and vague manner.
- As the MHCU reflects on and attends in detail to their internal and external world, they will be able to see the connections between specific thoughts/ideas and specific feelings.
- Reinforce the person's competence and attention to specifics rather than their more commonly reinforced emotionality and tendency for manipulation.
- During individual therapy help the MHCU to develop assertiveness skills – that is, open, honest, direct and specific communication of his/her feelings, thoughts and needs (adult).
- If the MHCU sees the benefit of being more specific and assertive during individual therapy, they may also learn that being assertive and engaging in active problem solving can lead to improved relationships with others in the real world.

Group therapy

Persons diagnosed with a histrionic personality disorder can benefit from group therapy. This is because the group as a whole can:
■ provide a source of nurturing that these MHCUs have often not experienced during childhood
■ provide feedback to individual MHCUs regarding their cognitive style – that is, how they tend to distort their view of themselves and others by omitting details from interactional patterns
■ provide opportunities to exercise their assertiveness and see positive consequences for themselves.

Potential problems that might arise in the group are displays of emotionality, demands to be the centre of attention, blaming of others, appearing to be stuck and pressure from MHCUs to be rescued. The principles outlined under individual therapy can be used here to assist.

When working with the MHCU in both individual and group therapy, the underlying principle is to empower the person by:
■ educating their adult ego state and
■ increasing their capacity to tolerate the 'deeper' feelings contained within the FC.

This can initially be achieved through the therapist's nurturance and later through the group's nurturance and the person's own NP capacity.

Application by example

During an interview with a young female MHCU diagnosed with a histrionic personality disorder, the interviewer was struck by how attractive, and emotionally energetic the MHCU was. As she leaned towards the interviewer, the interviewer made emotional contact by encountering her 'playfully' at a feeling level. The interviewer later commented on her thinking style, upon which the MHCU made a significant and insightful statement: all she needed to do was to think and that was what she needed time and space to do. This statement was reinforced and anchored by the mental health care practitioner. Continuing to talk, the MHCU clearly showed her *please me* driver by using phrases like 'You know' and 'I think so'.

Several times her *hurry up* driver was interrupted by the mental health care practitioner's inviting her to think more clearly. At this point the MHCU expressed anger towards the enmeshed relationships she had with her mother. The mental health care practitioner was then able to intervene here by supporting the MHCU in experiencing the underlying anger and facilitating the continued thinking about adult maturity and the need for separateness from the mother.

The antisocial personality disorder

The DSM-5 (APA, 2013) diagnostic criteria for the antisocial personality disorder include the following:
A. There is a pervasive pattern of disregard for and violation of the rights of others occurring since age 15 years, as indicated by three (or more) of the following:
   1. Failure to conform to social norms with respect to lawful behaviours as indicated by repeatedly performing acts that are grounds for arrest
   2. Deceitfulness, as indicated by repeated lying, use of aliases, or conning others for personal profit or pleasure
   3. Impulsivity or failure to plan ahead
   4. Irritability and aggressiveness, as indicated by repeated physical fights or assaults
   5. Reckless disregard for safety of self or others
   6. Consistent irresponsibility, as indicated by repeated failure to sustain consistent work behaviour or honour financial obligations
   7. Lack of remorse, as indicated by being indifferent to or rationalising having hurt, mistreated, or stolen from another.
B. The individual is at least 18 years old.
C. There is evidence of conduct disorder with onset before the age of 15 years.
D. The occurrence of antisocial behaviour is not exclusively during the course of schizophrenia or a manic episode.

(*Reprinted with permission from the* Diagnostic and Statistical Manual of Mental Disorders, Fifth Edition (Copyright ©2013). *American Psychiatric Association. All Rights Reserved.*)

Understanding the psychology of the person diagnosed with an antisocial personality disorder

Biological factors and problems in the infant–primacy caregiver relationship can on their own or together contribute to the aetiology and pathogenesis of antisocial personality disorders.

Biological factors
- In a number of studies, it has been found that various biological factors, for example genetic, hormonal and neurochemical, as well as organicity and autonomic hyperactivity, can contribute towards antisocial personality disorder (Derefinko & Widiger, 2008).

These biological factors may in turn contribute to early problems in the infant–primary caregiver relationship, making the infant difficult to soothe and comfort and thus creating difficulties of attachment between the infant and primary caregiver.

Infant–primary caregiver relationship
- Antisocial MHCUs often have a history of childhood neglect and or abuse by parental figures, and can be understood within psychodynamic psychological theory as having not achieved the developmental task of object constancy.

Object constancy is the progressive developmental process occurring during the first three years of life. The child develops the capacity for memory and, consistency in distinguishing self from others; and the ability to integrate good and bad experiences of the same person. Lack of basic trust, combined with the absence of loving experiences with a maternal figure, prevents object constancy in the antisocial person.

Common characteristics of antisocial personality disordered persons include the following:
- The persons do not see people as separate individuals with feelings of their own – that is, there is little capacity for empathy.
- They do not usually experience anxiety, depression or guilt in relation to dominance over others.
- Suicide attempts are often in reaction to strong feelings of anger and rage rather than out of hopelessness and depression.
- The persons struggle to manage confrontation or criticism from others effectively, often responding with aggression and behaviour that lacks remorse.

Defences used by the antisocial person include:
- denial

- dissociation from feelings
- displacement
- splitting
- projective identification – of their aggressive introject onto others.

Table 18.8 Understanding the person with an antisocial personality disorder in terms of a transactional analysis model

Adaptation	Antisocial
Characteristics	- Conflict with society - Low frustration tolerance - Need for excitement and drama - Seductive
Description	- Selfishness - Callousness - Irresponsibility
Drivers	- Be strong - Please others
Injunctions	- Don't make it - Don't be close - Don't be a child - Don't feel
Contact door	- Behaviour
Target door	- Feeling
Trap door	- Thinking

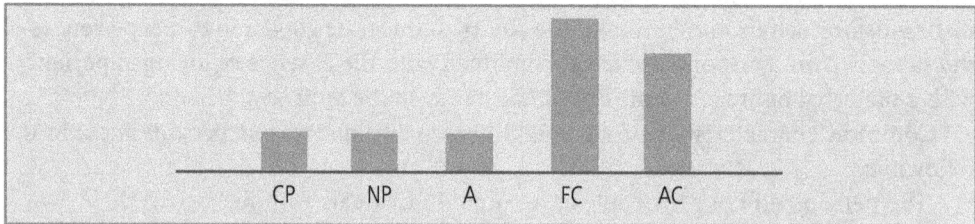

Figure 18.14 Egogram: active independent style of the person with an antisocial personality disorder

Such persons have a low frustration tolerance and experience problems with rules and regulations, which often leads to their being in trouble with the law. They search for excitement and 'drama' as a defence against feelings.

Their number one driver is *be strong*. This enables them to cope with their early emotional deprivation. Their number two driver is *please others* because, if they are able to do this, they can get others to do what they want.

Their injunctions are *don't be a child* and *don't feel* (particularly fear or sadness). A *don't make it* message is also part of their script. *Don't stay close* is also an injunction for antisocial persons because, although they connect quickly with others, relationships do not last long.

The main open door of antisocial persons is their active aggressive behaviour towards themselves or others. The mental health care practitioner starts by confronting this behaviour and then moves to their target door of feeling. Their trap door is their thinking and this should be avoided as this is an area well developed to 'outsmart' others.

Working therapeutically with a person diagnosed with antisocial personality disorder

- A major goal would be to help the MHCU to accept responsibility for their antisocial behaviour in the here and now.
- Common identified problems would include the exercise of power and destructiveness in their relationships with others, related to childhood neglect/abuse; this is evidenced by aggressive acts, impulsivity, lack of remorse, and failure to have empathy for others.

Working with the person with an antisocial personality disorder

It is unlikely that persons diagnosed with an antisocial personality disorder are able to get in touch with their feelings as long as they have the outlet of behaviour to discharge their impulses. It is when they are immobilised in an inpatient setting that they might get in touch with feelings of anxiety and depression. However, these MHCU's disruptive behaviours may interfere with another MHCU's treatment and disrupt the milieu of the inpatient unit. The decision to hospitalise the person must therefore be carefully considered.

Objective criteria must be used as predictors of the possible response to treatment (Gabbard, 1990: 410).

General principles to consider regarding management within the inpatient setting include:

- The treatment of a person with an antisocial personality disorder will be enhanced if the other MHCUs within the unit have a similar pathology. This is because inpatient programmes generally rely heavily on group confrontation by peers who have similar struggles.
- A structured setting with clear and consistently enforced rules, where the consequences for rule breaking are clearly spelt out, will help the MHCU to think before they act.
- Staff members must monitor their own emotional reactions in the unit, both as individuals and in a group context. Three common staff reactions are *disbelief*, *collusion* and *condemnation*.
  - Disbelief may surface as denial of the level of the MHCU's pathology and may cause staff members to deny the presence of psychopathic features; instead, the person may be viewed as depressed or misunderstood.

- Collusion occurs when a relationship of exploitation develops between the MHCU and one or more staff members. Through simulated rather than real feelings regarding states of fearfulness, remorse or sadness, MHCUs can manipulate clinicians into empathising with them.
- Condemnation occurs when staff start state that the antisocial MHCU is untreatable after listening to their history. If this stems from intensive contact with the MHCU, it can be seen as a projective identification with the aggressive introject part of the MHCU.
- Other common reactions include feelings of helplessness in the face of a treatment-resistant MHCU, a desire to be harmful towards the MHCU which grows out of anger, and feelings of invalidity and loss of identity. Fear of assault by the MHCU may cause staff to avoid implementing the firm structure of the unit that is necessary for effective treatment.

- Continual focus on the MHCU's 'faulty' and maladjusted thought processes is a major aspect of their treatment. The staff need to point out repeatedly how the person fails to anticipate the consequences of their behaviour.
- Interventions are based on the here and now. Long-term outpatient treatment is needed for the exploration of past trauma.

Working with the antisocial person on an individual basis

- The mental health nurse needs to be stable, persistent and sure of themselves in order to minimise manipulation within the relationship.
- Repeated appropriate confrontation of the MHCU's denial and minimisation of their antisocial behaviour helps the MHCU to accept responsibility for their actions.
- The mental health nurse needs to help the MHCU to connect their actions with their feelings and think about alternative ways to get their needs in relationships met.
- The mental health nurse should have realistic expectations of the change and improvement the MHCU is capable of implementing.

Application by example

A 20-year-old male diagnosed with an antisocial personality disorder was admitted to the unit with a history of physical violence involving his fiancée. He impressed as both pleasant and charming. The mental health care nurse started by confronting the MHCU's aggressive behaviour and explained the potential consequences of his acting out his angry feelings. The MHCU's *be strong* driver became apparent when he revealed in an emotionless manner how, as a child, he was physically and emotionally abused by his father. The mental health care nurse intervened here when she reflected on how powerless and afraid he must have felt, and for a while saw the sadness in his eyes. However, he moved quickly away from his feelings into the defence of toughness that he had learnt to build around himself in order to survive. The mental health care nurse again confronted his *be strong* driver, this time commenting on how his decision to be tough as a child helped him to cope while he was helpless, but how as an adult he was now better able to protect himself and work through his pain and anger by talking about it and coming to terms with it.

Narcissistic personality disorder

DSM-5 (APA, 2013) diagnostic criteria of narcissistic personality disorder are as follows:

A pervasive pattern of grandiosity (in fantasy or behaviour), need for admiration, and lack of empathy, beginning by early adulthood and present in a variety of contexts, as indicated by five (or more) of the following:

1. Has a grandiose sense of self-importance (for example, exaggerates achievements and talents, expects to be recognised as superior without commensurate achievements)
2. Is preoccupied with fantasies of unlimited success, power, brilliance, beauty, or ideal love
3. Believes that he/she is 'special' and unique and can only be understood by, or should associate with, other special or high-status people (or institutions)
4. Requires excessive admiration
5. Has a sense of entitlement, that is, unreasonable expectations of especially favourable treatment or automatic compliance with his/her expectations
6. Is interpersonally exploitative, that is, takes advantage of others to achieve his/her own ends
7. Lacks empathy, that is, is unwilling to recognize or identify with the feelings and needs of others
8. Is often envious of others or believes that others are envious of him/her
9. Shows arrogant, haughty behaviours or attitudes.

(*Reprinted with permission from the* Diagnostic and Statistical Manual of Mental Disorders, Fifth Edition (Copyright ©2013). *American Psychiatric Association. All Rights Reserved.*)

Understanding the psychology of the person diagnosed with a narcissistic personality disorder

Persons diagnosed with a narcissistic personality disorder impress as self-centred. They often seek praise and constant recognition in order to feel momentarily good about themselves. They do not feel a sense of their own worth or value. In their relationships they tend to be exploitative and insensitive to the needs of others.

In addition, such persons may expect special privileges from those around them without giving anything back in return. They tend to feel easily humiliated or shamed and respond with rage at what they perceive to be criticism or failure of people to react in the way they wish. Such persons can also have elaborate active fantasies about magnificent success in love, sex, beauty, wealth or power.

Common defences used by the person with a narcissistic personality disorder
- primitive
- idealisation/devaluation

- splitting
- projective identification.

Kohut versus Kernberg's understanding of the narcissistic personality disorder

The nature of the narcissistic personality disorder remains a controversial issue, revolving mainly around the models of Kohut (1977) and Kernberg (1984). This is outlined in Table 18.9 and in Figures 18.15 and 18.16.

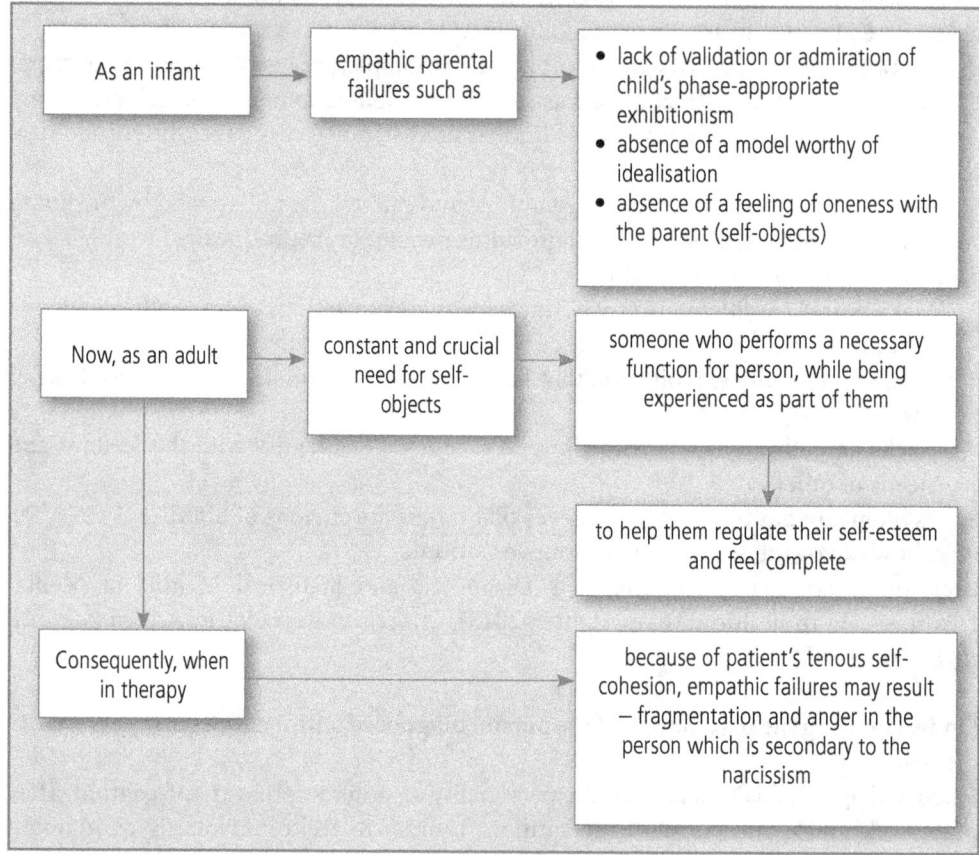

Figure 18.15 Kohut's model of narcissistic personality disorder

Kohut's emphasis is on the internalisation of missing functions, as indicated in Figure 18.15.

Table 18.9 Differences between the models of Kohut and Kernberg

Kohut	Kernberg
1. Theory is based on outpatients who functioned quite well but whose self-esteem was vulnerable to slights	1. Theory is based on a mixture of in- and outpatients who impressed as 'arrogant' and with a haughty grandiosity
2. Differentiates narcissistic from borderline states	2. Defines narcissistic personality as similar to borderline personality, but usually as having better ego functioning in terms of anxiety tolerance, impulse control and reality testing
3. Emphasis is on internalisation of missing functions – no definition of internal object relations	3. Defines primitive defences and object relations typical of borderline personality
4. Defines archaic normal self as one that is developmentally arrested	4. Defines self as a highly pathological structure composed of the fusion of the ideal self, ideal object and real self
5. Accepts idealisation at face value as a normal developmental phase	5. Views idealisation as a defence against rage, envy

Kernberg's emphasis is on the narcissistic person's need for self-sufficiency and pathological internal object relations which allow the MHCU to feel self-sufficient (see Figure 18.16).

Understanding the person with a narcissistic personality disorder in terms of a transactional analysis model

This is illustrated in Table 18.10.

Table 18.10 Understanding the person with a narcissistic personality disorder in terms of a transactional analysis model

Injunctions	- Don't feel - Don't be close
Drivers	- Be strong
Beliefs	- Self: I'm in a class of my own - Others: People are there to be trampled on - Life: Life is a contest already won
Behaviour	- Ignores others' rights
Stroking	- Takes positive strokes; self-strokes
Life position	- I'm okay, you're not okay

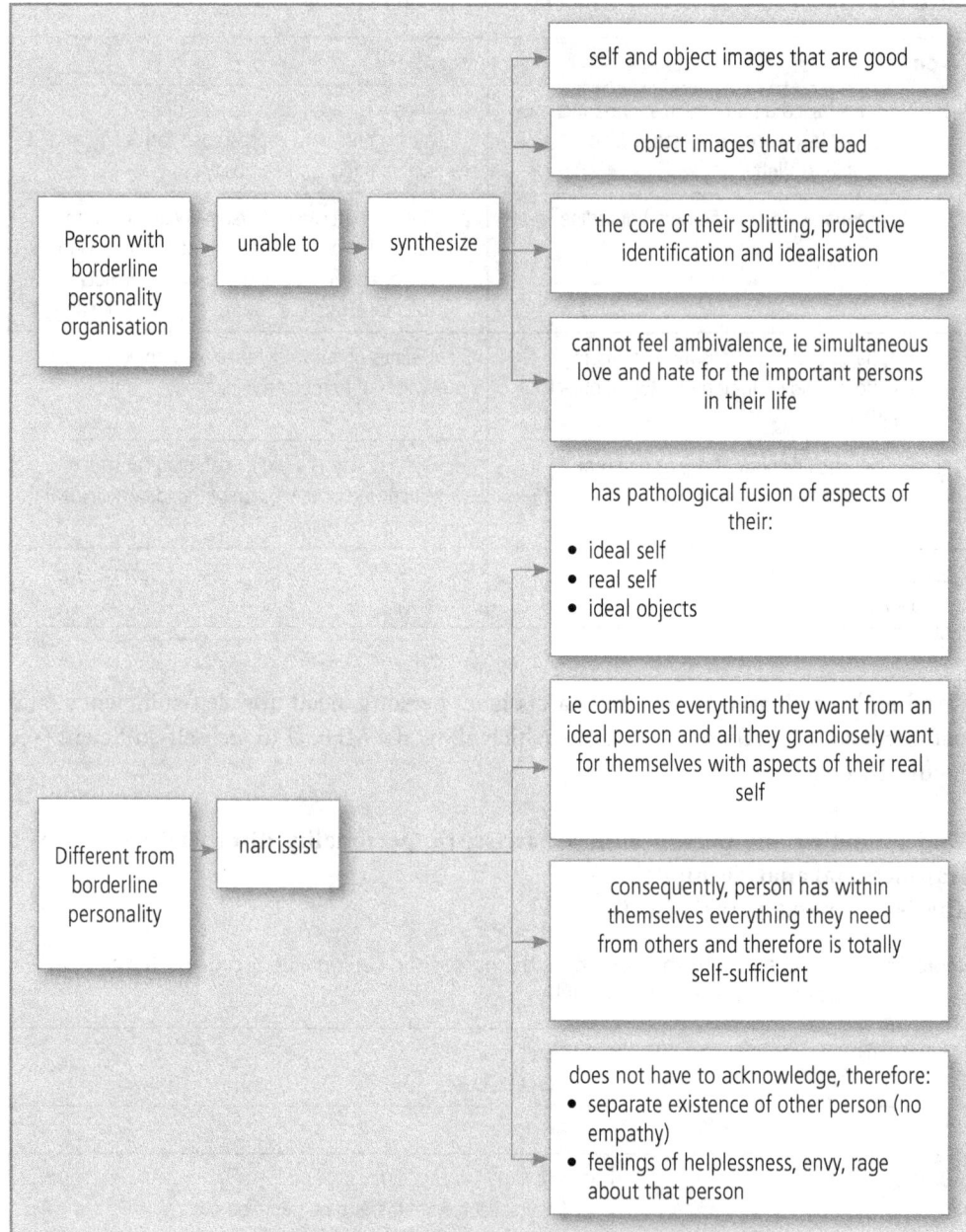

Figure 18.16 Kernberg's model of narcissistic personality disorder

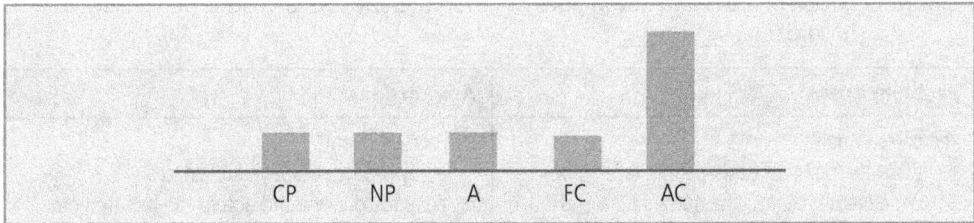

Figure 18.17 Egogram: active independent style of narcissistic personality disorder

Working therapeutically with the MHCU diagnosed with a narcissistic personality disorder

For Kohut, empathy is the cornerstone of the treatment of the person with a narcissistic personality disorder. The mental health nurse needs to:
- actively soothe the person through empathy and try to immerse themselves in the MHCU's internal world; to supportively empathise with MHCU's need for affirmation, for idealisation, or for being like the mental health care nurse (self-object transferences)
- avoid comments that might be viewed as harshly critical and focus rather on the positive side of the person's experience, that is, their progress and
- help the MHCU to identify and seek out appropriate support from others instead of overvaluing separation and autonomy.

Kernberg's approach is more confrontational than that of Kohut. Once an alliance has been established, the MHCU's tendency for intense and selfish desire for something and their demandingness must be confronted and examined from the point of view of their impact on others. Working within this framework the mental health nurse needs to:
- focus in on the MHCU's interpersonal difficulties that prevents them from receiving or acknowledging help
- help the MHCU to develop a concern for others by creating awareness of the ways in which others may be experiencing the MHCU
- act as a 'repository' for the MHCU's rage, idealisation, devaluation and splitting, and projected aspects of themselves.

The mental health nurse also needs to monitor and manage their own negative feelings and use this awareness to identify the defences used by the MHCU.

Group therapy

The problem areas and advantages of group therapy for such persons are summed up in Table 18.11.

Table 18.11 Problem areas and advantages of group therapy for narcissistic personality disorder

Problem areas	Advantages
The person might: - resent the fact that other people take some of the mental health care nurse's time and attention - view group therapy as a situation in which their 'specialness' is overlooked - make observations about other people's problems but deny their own - be 'scape-goated' by the group because of their intense neediness	The person might: - enjoy having a captive audience - have to confront and accept the fact that others have needs and that they cannot be the centre of attention at all times - benefit from feedback from others about the impact of their behaviour on others - benefit from active support from the therapist who can help the others to empathise with the person's need to be recognised and admired

Borderline personality disorder

The DSM-5 (APA, 2013) diagnostic criteria for borderline personality disorder are as follows:

A pervasive pattern of instability of interpersonal relationships, self-image and affects, and marked impulsivity beginning by early adulthood and present in a variety of contexts, as indicated by five (or more) of the following:

1. Frantic efforts to avoid real or imagined abandonment
   Note: Do not include suicidal or self-mutilating behaviour covered in criterion 5.
2. A pattern of unstable and intense interpersonal relationships characterised by alternating between extremes of idealisation and devaluation
3. Identity disturbance: markedly and persistently unstable self-image or sense of self
4. Impulsivity in at least two areas that are potentially self-damaging (for example, spending, sex, substance abuse, reckless driving, binge eating)
   Note: Do not include suicidal or self-mutilating behaviour covered in criterion 5.
5. Recurrent suicidal behaviour, gestures, or threats, or self-mutilating behaviour
6. Affective instability due to a marked reactivity of mood (for example, intense episodic dysphoria, irritability, or anxiety usually lasting a few hours and only rarely more than a few days)
7. Chronic feelings of emptiness
8. Inappropriate, intense anger or difficulty controlling anger (for example, frequent displays of temper, constant anger, recurrent physical fights)
9. Transient, stress-related paranoid ideation or severe dissociative symptoms.

(*Reprinted with permission from the* Diagnostic and Statistical Manual of Mental Disorders, Fifth Edition (Copyright ©2013). *American Psychiatric Association. All Rights Reserved.*)

Understanding the psychology of the person diagnosed with a borderline personality disorder

Understanding and working with persons diagnosed with a borderline personality disorder continues to be one of the biggest challenges both for the novice and the experienced mental health nurse. The struggle that such persons have with the regulation of their affect, sense of self, cognitive processes, impulse control and interpersonal relationships has a pervasive effect on others. There are also often intense and difficult feelings felt between the MHCU and the mental health nurse.

By the age of three most children will have internalised parental figures to such a degree that they are able to experience primary care givers and themselves as whole and separate. Instead of internalising a whole, soothing internal image of primary caregivers that comforts them in times of their physical absence, the person with a borderline personality has a predominance of negative parts internalised which contributes to their intolerance for separation and aloneness. They are overwhelmed by feelings of 'badness' and fear these will destroy any 'goodness' in themselves or in others. Feelings are kept separate through the unconscious defence of splitting. Research findings have shown that many people diagnosed with borderline personality disorder were abused either physically or sexually in early childhood (Cattane et al, 2017) and have had traumatic histories characterised by repeated abandonment and neglect.

Common defences used by a person diagnosed with a borderline personality disorder include:
- splitting
- projective identification
- idealisation and devaluing
- denial.

Working therapeutically with the person with a borderline personality disorder

Major goals in therapy would include:
- Increasing the MHCU's tolerance of their anxiety and anger without impulsively acting it out
- Helping the MHCU (in the long term) to integrate 'good' and 'bad' aspects in themselves and others
- Establishing behavioural strategies with the MHCU to assist their toleration of separations from significant others.

Common identified problems include:
- Intense anger at times evidenced by extreme mood swings, self-damaging acts such as cutting and suicidal behaviour, acting out and argumentativeness
- Intense anxiety at times evidenced by controlling and manipulative behaviour.

Therapeutic principles to consider when working with the MHCU
These principles include the following:
- Establishing a holding, stable treatment environment:
  - Because of the chaotic nature of the MHCU's life, stability needs to be provided by external sources and settings. Such MHCUs benefit from inpatient treatment units with a structured programme.
  - Within such a unit, short frequent contacts help the MHCU to internalise a holding, soothing NP state more effectively. Steadiness, persistence, firmness and a capacity for flexibility are important in tuning in to the MHCU's internal state.
  - The principal healing factor of being a stable repository for the projected aspects of the MHCU's psyche is therapeutic and helps the MHCU to integrate the good and bad aspects within themselves and others.
- Containment of the MHCU's anger:
  - Action is the language of the MHCU – often the person might feel that action is the only option to achieve relief from the intensity of their feeling states.
  - Establish a connection between feelings and actions by helping the MHCU to identify feeling states when confronted with acting-out behaviour.
- Limit setting of those behaviours that threaten the safety of the clinical staff or the MHCU (aggressive outbursts, suicidal gestures):
  - The consequences of acting out need to be clearly spelt out to the MHCU in a non-punitive manner.
  - The therapeutic team needs to decide on consequences and limits for acting-out behaviour, and ensure that these consequences are implemented if the MHCU acts out; for example, if the MHCU is a threat to their own or others' safety, they might need containment in another unit or hospital which is more secure (certification of the MHCU might be required).
- Maintaining a here-and-now focus:
  - Focus on the relationships and difficulties the MHCU is currently experiencing.
- Monitoring of negative staff feelings:
  - Pay ongoing attention to one's own feelings as this prevents acting out by staff members too.
  - Be prepared to share with the team the strong feelings evoked by the MHCU. This provides essential information about the MHCU's internal world.
  - The mental health care nurse needs to be sincere and genuine in dealings with MHCUs. For example, 'I really don't feel I can work with you effectively if you continue to shout at me. I think that it's important for you to work on controlling your anger so that you can express it to me without screaming', expresses the mental health care nurse's own humanness.
  - Progress with MHCUs is often slow, intense and difficult to measure, and repeated inpatient admissions might be required during periods of crisis.
- Administering medication:
  - Lithium can be used to decrease instability and impulsive behaviour.
  - Carbamazepine can also stabilise the MHCU's mood.

- Fluanxol is often used to stabilise the mood and to reduce impulsivity; it is an antipsychotic.
- Dealing with the risk of suicide:
With regard to the risk of suicide in MHCUs suffering from this disorder, refer to the article by M H Stone entitled 'Paradoxes in the management of suicidality in borderline patients' (Stone, 1993: 255–272) or J Paris's review article entitled 'Half in Love with Easeful Death: The Meaning of Chronic Suicidality in Borderline Personality Disorder' (Paris, 2004: 42–48).

Cluster C personality disorders

This grouping of personality disorders includes the obsessive-compulsive, dependent, and avoidant personality disorders that share features of anxiety and fearfulness.

Avoidant personality disorder

The DSM-5 diagnostic criteria for avoidant personality disorder are as follows:

A pervasive pattern of social inhibition, feelings of inadequacy, and hypersensitivity to negative evaluation, beginning by early adulthood and present in a variety of contexts, as indicated by four (or more) of the following:

1. Avoids occupational activities that involve significant interpersonal contact, because of fears of criticism, disapproval, or rejection
2. Is unwilling to get involved with people unless certain of being liked
3. Shows restraint within intimate relationships because of the fear of being shamed or ridiculed
4. Is preoccupied with being criticized or rejected in social situations
5. Is inhibited in new interpersonal situations because of feelings of inadequacy
6. Views self as socially inept, personally unappealing, or inferior to others
7. Is unusually reluctant to take personal risks or to engage in any new activities because they may prove embarrassing.

(*Reprinted with permission from the* Diagnostic and Statistical Manual of Mental Disorders, Fifth Edition (Copyright ©2013). *American Psychiatric Association. All Rights Reserved.*)

Understanding the psychology of the person diagnosed with an avoidant personality disorder

People can be avoidant for a number of reasons, however, the main reason is to defend against feelings of embarrassment, humiliation, rejection and failure. All of these are related to feelings of shame from early developmental experiences.

Persons diagnosed with an avoidant personality disorder have an active, detached style of relating in terms of which they dare not allow themselves to need others for fear of humiliation or rejection; however, unlike schizoid people, they long for close interpersonal relationships.

Table 18.12 Understanding the person with an avoidant personality disorder in terms of a transactional analysis model

Injunctions	▪ Don't need
Driver	▪ Be perfect
Life position	▪ I'm not okay, you're not okay
Beliefs	▪ Self: I'm nothing ▪ Others: Others see through and reject me ▪ Life: Life is a risk, so run away
Behaviour	▪ Withdraws, belittles self
Reinforcing memory	▪ People ignore or reject
Stroking	▪ Hankers after strokes but cannot ask for them

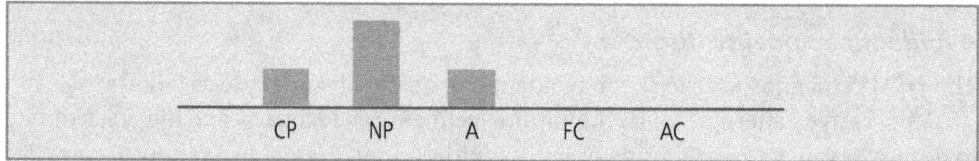

Figure 18.18 Egogram: avoidant personality

Working therapeutically with the person with an avoidant personality disorder

- A main goal would be to help the person to develop a greater trust in themselves and others and to move into a life position of 'I'm okay, you're okay' in order to take more of the risks associated with day-to-day living.
- Common identified problems include active detachment and avoidant behaviour related to fear of shame and humiliation, evidenced by avoidance of specific social situations, symptoms of anxiety, low self-worth, depression, suppressed anger.

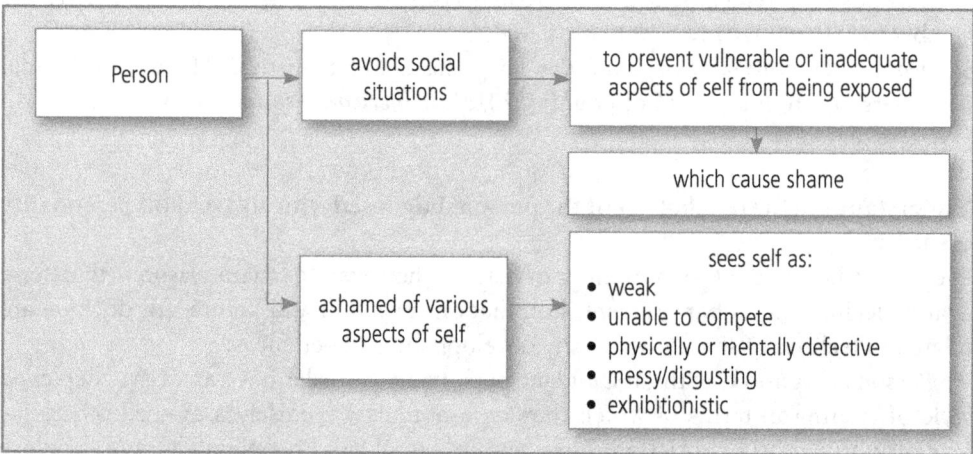

Figure 18.19 Responses of a person with avoidant personality disorder

Therapeutic principles to consider when working with the MHCU

These principles include the following:
- The use of empathic appreciation of the embarrassment and humiliation associated with the feared social situation will increase the MHCU's trust in the mental health care practitioner and engender a sense of feeling soothed and comforted (NP of practitioner).
- Exploring the underlying causes of shame related to early decisions made about the self, and to early developmental experiences, will enable the MHCU to make new decisions (redecision) now as an adult.
- Helping the person to see the value of actively seeking out and experiencing the feared situation will enable them to:
  - desensitise self
  - increase self-worth, trust in self and in others.
- Help the MHCU to express feelings of anger which are often suppressed and connected to the shame experience.
- Group therapy can be of value to the MHCU as it provides them with:
  - an opportunity to expose themselves to the potentially feared social situations
  - an opportunity to receive feedback from others regarding people's perception of them
  - exposure to others' fears and inadequacies that may be similar to their own and provide an opportunity to be nurtured.

Dependent personality disorder

The DSM-5 diagnostic criteria of dependent personality disorder are as follows:

A pervasive and excessive need to be taken care of that leads to submissive and clinging behaviour and fears of separation, beginning by early adulthood and present in a variety of contexts, as indicated by five (or more) of the following:

1. Has difficulty making everyday decisions without an excessive amount of advice and reassurance from others
2. Needs others to assume responsibility for most major areas of his/her life
3. Has difficulty expressing disagreement with others because of fear of loss of support or approval
   Note: Do not include realistic fears of retribution.
4. Has difficulty initiating projects or doing things on his/her own (because of a lack of self-confidence in judgement or abilities rather than a lack of motivation or energy)
5. Goes to excessive lengths to obtain nurturance and support from others, to the point of volunteering to do things that are unpleasant
6. Feels uncomfortable or helpless when alone because of exaggerated fears of being unable to care for themselves
7. Urgently seeks another relationship as a source of care and support when a close relationship ends

8. Is unrealistically preoccupied with fears of being left to take care of themselves.
(*Reprinted with permission from the* Diagnostic and Statistical Manual of Mental Disorders, Fifth Edition (Copyright ©2013). *American Psychiatric Association. All Rights Reserved.*)

Understanding the psychology of the person diagnosed with a dependent personality disorder

Such persons have had a pervasive pattern of parental reinforcement for dependency throughout all phases of development. Dependent characteristics may also mask aggression. Past traumatic separations from significant others can also result in dependent behaviour.

Table 18.13 Understanding the person with a dependent personality disorder in terms of a transactional analysis model

Injunctions	■ Don't grow up ■ Don't think ■ Don't be important
Driver	■ Please me/others
Life position	■ I'm not okay, you're okay
Beliefs	■ I'm unimportant and incompetent ■ Others: Others are important and competent
Behaviour	■ Maximises failures, minimises successes
Reinforcing memory	■ People help out

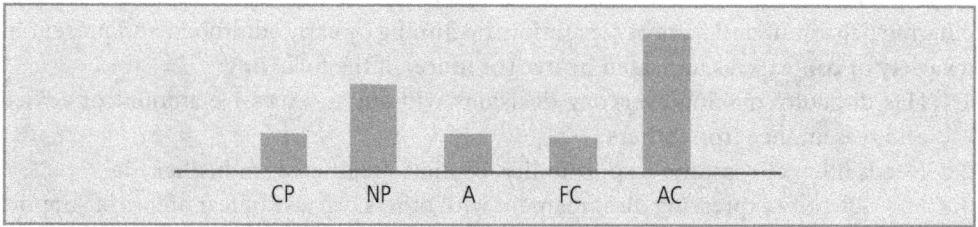

Figure 18.20 Egogram of the dependent personality

People with dependent personality styles include both the histrionic and dependent personality disorders. Both assume an 'I'm not okay, you're okay' position which accounts for their reliance on others for satisfaction of their needs. However, the dependent personality is more passive while the histrionic personality is more active in the search for satisfaction of needs. Both have similar drivers and injunctions.

Working therapeutically with the person with a dependent personality disorder
- The main goal would be to promote independent thinking and caring for self and independent action in the person; that is, develop the MHCU's individual adult and NP.
- Common identified problems include a reliance on others in major areas of their lives, related to past reinforcement of dependent behaviour, previous traumatic separations; evidenced by helplessness, getting others to tell them what to do.

Therapeutic principles to consider
- Help the MHCU to take responsibility for their own decisions, thoughts and actions.
  - This is difficult as the MHCU often presents with feelings of helplessness and asks the mental health care practitioner to direct the process.
  - Discuss this difficulty and explore the consequences of passivity in one's life and the unrealistic expectations the MHCU has of others. In so doing mobilise the MHCU's adult ego state.
- Explore anxieties about separation and loss related to past experiences.
- Positively reinforce the MHCU's independent thinking and decision-making abilities.
- Within a group context, encourage feedback from others regarding the effect of the MHCU's dependency on others. Explain to others, who might attempt to rescue the person, what losses the dependent person could suffer as a result.

Obsessive-compulsive personality disorder

The DSM-5TM diagnostic criteria for obsessive-compulsive personality disorder are as follows:

A pervasive pattern of preoccupation with orderliness, perfectionism, and mental and interpersonal control, at the expense of flexibility, openness and efficiency, beginning by early adulthood and present in a variety of contexts, as indicated by four (or more) of the following:

1. Is preoccupied with details, rules, lists, order, organisation, or schedules to the extent that the major point of the activity is lost
2. Shows perfectionism that interferes with task completion (for example, is unable to complete a project because his/her own overly strict standards are not met)
3. Is excessively devoted to work and productivity to the exclusion of leisure activities and friendships (not accounted for by obvious economic necessity)
4. Is over conscientious, scrupulous, and inflexible about matters of morality, ethics or values (not accounted for by cultural or religious identification)
5. Is unable to discard worn-out or worthless objects even when they have no sentimental value
6. Is reluctant to delegate tasks or to work with others unless they submit exactly to his/her way of doing things

7. Adopts a miserly spending style toward both self and others; money is viewed as something to be hoarded for future catastrophes
8. Shows rigidity and stubbornness.

(*Reprinted with permission from the* Diagnostic and Statistical Manual of Mental Disorders, Fifth Edition (Copyright ©2013). *American Psychiatric Association. All Rights Reserved.*)

Understanding the psychology of the person diagnosed with an obsessive-compulsive personality disorder

These MHCUs often reveal strong unfulfilled dependent yearnings and strong feelings of anger and rage that are out of awareness but are directed at the parents for not being more emotionally available during formative years.

Their quest for perfectionism relates to their belief that, if they can reach a stage of flawlessness, they will receive the parental approval and esteem that they missed as children.

Common defences used by the person with an obsessive-compulsive disorder include:
- isolation of affect
- intellectualisation
- reaction formation
- undoing
- displacement.

Table 18.14 Understanding the person with an obsessive-compulsive personality disorder in terms of a transactional analysis model

Adaptation	Obsessive-compulsive
Characteristics	- Conformity - Conscientiousness
Description	- Tense - Perfectionist - Overly inhibited - Overly conscientious - Overly dutiful
Drivers	- Be strong - Be perfect
Injunctions	- Don't be a child - Don't feel (joy and sex) - Don't be close - Don't enjoy
Contact door	- Thinking
Target door	- Feeling
Trap door	- Behaviour

Perfectionistic, bright and organised, persons diagnosed with an obsessive-compulsive personality disorder devote their energy largely to thinking (their open door). The mental health nurse could first validate the person with something like, 'Gosh, I'm really impressed with the clarity of your thinking. As you were thinking that, what were you feeling?' Moving repeatedly from thinking to feeling and finally to enjoying pleasurable feelings is the main goal of treatment.

Working therapeutically with the person with obsessive-compulsive personality disorder
- A major goal would be to help modify the MHCU's superego (CP), thus helping the MHCU to accept their humanness with all its flaws and imperfections.
- Common identified problems include perfectionistic tendencies and preoccupation with control and order related to early power struggles and lack of emotional availability from parents; evidenced by self-doubt, rigid thinking style, difficulty with dependency and their own anger, and a quest for perfection.

Therapeutic principles to consider when working with the MHCU
- Empathise with the MHCU's fear of loss of control when seeking help in order to establish trust. Work at a pace which the MHCU finds comfortable.
- Move between validating the MHCU's thoughts and encouraging the experiencing of feelings, particularly feelings of anger and dependency on others.
- The use of a non-judgemental, stable neutrality over time helps the MHCU to discover that their perception of the therapist as someone who is critical is related to past relationships.
  - Help the MHCU to recognise their own critical projections onto others.
  - Periodically confront the unrealistic expectations of the MHCU about themselves.
  - The therapist's acceptance of the MHCU helps them to gain increasing self-acceptance.
- Help the MHCU to identify their anger and encourage its expression in order to remove fantasies of its possible destructiveness.
- Group therapy can be useful in that the MHCU gets the opportunity to:
  - experience others' vulnerabilities
  - get feedback from others regarding their rigidity, preoccupation with detail (might accept this feedback without the same power struggle that accompanies feedback from the therapist)
  - see that others are not nearly as critical as they are themselves.

Psychotropic medication and personality disorders
When working therapeutically with a person diagnosed with a personality disorder, the primary focus, as outlined above, is psychotherapeutic. Based on the severity of the symptoms and the level of distress the person is experiencing, psychotropic medication is indicated at times and is able to offer valuable support to other therapeutic

interventions. The medications listed below are used not only during times of crisis and acute admissions, but also to support longer term psychotherapeutic intervention. It should be noted that some medications are related to symptoms that are more characteristic of some personality disorders than others and are therefore more likely to receive such support.

- *Antidepressants.* SSRIs may be used to treat impulsivity, depression, anxiety, mood dysregulation and aggression.
- *Antipsychotics.* Antipsychotics may be used for affective dysregulation, impulsivity, cognitive-perceptual symptoms or aggression. Options include first-generation antipsychotics (for example depot antipsychotics such as flupenthixol) or second-generation antipsychotics (for example risperidone; olanzapine).
- *Anticonvulsants/mood stabilisers.* These may be used for impulsivity, mood lability, aggression or self-injurious behaviour. The most common medications used are sodium valproate and lithium.
- *Benzodiazepines.* These are used only for acute crisis management and as short-term sedative/hypnotic/anxiolytic agents.

CONCLUSION

This chapter has emphasised the difficulty in understanding and working with persons diagnosed with personality disorders. We have looked at the general and specific diagnostic criteria of the current psychiatric classification system, the DSM-5, for personality disorders. In an attempt to facilitate understanding of the persons behind these diagnoses a psychodynamic model, with specific reference to defences used, and a transactional analysis model were discussed in detail. These two models were then applied to personality difficulties more generally and in the final section to the psychology and treatment of specific personality disorders. Common goals, difficulties and treatment options related to each specific personality disorder was then discussed and illustrated by way of example.

This chapter has repeatedly emphasised the importance of self-awareness of the strong emotional reactions that are often evoked within mental health care professionals when working with persons diagnosed with personality disorders. It has also highlighted the importance of considering one's own difficulties, at times, to manage one's emotions and relationships with others and to monitor the tendency to see MHCUs as 'other' and their struggles as somehow unrelated to one's own.

 WEB RESOURCES

http://www.itaa-net.org
> This is the site of the International Transactional Analysis Association. Those interested in getting a better understanding of this therapy approach can access articles, research and training opportunities on this site.

https://sataa.org.za/
This is the site of the South African Transactional Analysis Association.

http://www.sadag.org/
SADAG is Africa's largest mental health support and advocacy group. On this website you will find comprehensive mental health information and resources to help you, a family member or loved one.

http://www.safmh.org.za/
The SA Federation for Mental Health is the largest mental health organisation in South Africa and is often seen as the first place of contact for those in need of mental health information. Their Resource Centre serves as a source of information to the public, MHCUs, the media and mental health professionals in need of information, support or referrals.

http://mentalhealthsa.org.za/
The Mental Health Information Centre of Southern Africa strives to assist the South African public and professionals with up-to-date mental health information as well as an accessible easy-to-use database of mental health professionals.

REFERENCES

American Psychiatric Association (APA). (2013). *Diagnostic and Statistical Manual for Mental Disorders*. 5th edition. American Psychiatric Publishing: Washington, DC.

Berne, E. 1961. *Transactional Analysis in Psychotherapy*. New York: Grove Press Inc.

Cattane, N, Rossi, R, Lanfredi, M and Cattaneo, A. 2017. 'Borderline personality disorder and childhood trauma: exploring the affective biological systems and mechanisms'. *B M C Psychiatry*, 17: 221.

Derefinko, K J and Widiger, T A. 2008. *The medical basis of psychiatry*. 3rd edition. Fatemi, S H and Clayton, P J (eds): 213–226. Totowa, NJ, US: Humana Press 2008. xxii, 799 pp.

Gabbard, G O. 1990. *Psychodynamic Psychiatry in Clinical Practice*. Washington: American Psychiatric Press.

Goulding, M and Goulding, R. 1979. *Redecision Therapy: A Brief Action-oriented Approach*. Northvale, N J: Jason Aronson Inc.

Kernberg, O. 1984. *Severe Personality Disorders*. New Haven: Yale University Press.

Kohut, H. 1977. *The Restoration of the Self*. New York: International Universities Press.

McWilliams, N. 2011. 'The Psychodynamic Diagnostic Manual: An Effort to Compensate for the Limitations of Descriptive Psychiatric Diagnosis'. *Journal of Personality Assessment*, 93 (2): 112–122.

Paris, J. 2004. Half in Love with Easeful Death: The Meaning of Chronic Suicidality in Borderline Personality Disorder. *Harvard Review of Psychiatry*, 12 (1): 42–48.

Stone, M H. 1993. 'Paradoxes in the management of suicidality in borderline patients'. *American Journal of Psychotherapy*, 47 (2): 255–272.

Thunnissen, M. 2010. 'Redecision Therapy with Personality Disorder: How Does It Work and What Are the Result? *Transactional Analysis Journal*', 40 (2): 114–120.

Ware, P. 1983. 'Personality adaptations (doors to therapy)'. *Transactional Analysis Journal*, 13 (1) January: 11–19.

SECTION 4
Care of Special Groups

CHAPTER 19

People who have Experienced Trauma

N Nkosi-Mafutha and M Hlungwani

Learning Outcomes

After studying this chapter, you should be able to:
- understand the use of the term 'trauma' and how it differs from 'crisis'
- understand a normal post-traumatic stress response
- develop skills to assist individuals and families affected by trauma
- develop skills to deal with secondary trauma-related responses, such as vicarious trauma or compassionate fatigue
- develop specialised skills for assisting survivors of particular traumatic experiences such as domestic violence and rape
- develop skills for working with children, families and communities affected by trauma.

Our problems may be great in South Africa, but the spirit and strength of our people is quite extraordinary. Archbishop Emeritus Tutu

INTRODUCTION

The South African context

South Africa is experiencing many political, cultural, technical and social changes. South Africans are confronted with the task of dealing with these changes, many of which have taken place in under twenty years. They are changes that other countries might have undergone over a period of more than hundred years, causing many disturbances because people have been caught unprepared. They have had to adapt to changes that are foreign to South African society, which was characterised for many years by separate development of people based on racial class during the apartheid years. Some of the more important changes are to be found in the area of new ideas and values. The conflicting cultural values and impersonal human relations that exist in the cities have effects that are worsened by the harsh and competitive struggle for survival. South Africa is one of the most unequal societies in the world because of the disparities between the poor and the rich after more than 20 years of democracy. This inequality, coupled with escalating unemployment rates, is the foundation of the poor social cohesion observed in xenophobic attacks, where South Africans are blaming foreign nationals for accepting minimal wages, and the myth is perpetuated that every job given to a foreign national is one less job for South Africans. Moreover, people living in the informal settlements and townships are also discontented because of poor service delivery, leading to what can be called the rebellion of the poor. Such communities resort to blockading of roads, election boycotts, burning of tyres, looting, destruction of buildings, and forced removal of community leaders.

Political violence in the country is slowly ending, apart from in some areas like KwaZulu-Natal. The transition to democracy has been characterised by high levels of crime. Increases in crime in South Africa from 1990 are consistent with experiences of other countries undergoing transition to democracy. It is said that as change proceeds, society and its formal and informal instruments of social control are reshaped. The result is that new areas in crime development, which had been covered up by the legacy of the past, open up. The unfortunate part of this is that South Africa is now said to be one of the most violent countries in the world, and most victims of violence are attacked and murdered in their own homes.

Violence of all forms is rife in South Africa at present. Regarding the crime of rape, all forms of rape are not equally condemned. Society is quick to blame the victim by suggesting that her clothing or behaviour provoked the rape. Research shows that men who rape have experienced childhood trauma. Jewkes et al (2016) indicate that physical and emotional hardships are more common among those who raped. Poverty and childhood ordeals are key factors for some men who rape (Jewkes et al, 2016).

Furthermore, aspects of family violence and dysfunction have been relatively ignored over the past few decades. The harsh reality of child abuse has become a subject of intense research, study and investigation within the last ten years.

The primary characteristic of perpetrators of violence is that they feel powerless. For them violence is a means of reasserting control (Mysyuk et al, 2015). In reasserting his power, the perpetrator also reaffirms his manhood; hence most crimes are perpetrated against women, children and the elderly – many of whom are powerless.

Social change in South Africa is clearly revealed in the breaking down of traditional family values and in the political and social transformation. There is much intolerance regarding change and a lot of anxiety about change. Jewkes et al (2015) describe the 'culture of violence' in South Africa, meaning that as a society we accept and even endorse violence as an acceptable and legitimate means of resolving problems and achieving goals. This culture of violence is a problem for all people living in the country.

DEFINING TRAUMA AND CRISIS

Trauma refers to situations in which a person is rendered powerless and great danger is involved. Trauma in this sense refers to events involving death or injury or the possibility of death and injury. These events must be unusual and out of the ordinary; they are not events that are part of the normal course of life. Trauma encompasses events of such intensity or magnitude of horror that they would overwhelm anybody's usual ability to cope.

Traumatic events are different from crises, in that crises are part of life, even if they may be experienced as traumatic. A crisis is an event that is expected and which will lead to a unstable and dangerous state affecting an individual, group, community or society. For example, although the loss of a job or a parent may change one's life forever, these events are not considered traumas because they are expected life losses.

Table 19.1 List of traumas and crises

Trauma	Crisis
Physical or sexual assault	Poverty
Witnessing death, torture, rape or the beating of another person	Being humiliated
Car accident	Unemployment
Armed robbery	Divorce
Natural catastrophes, eg floods	Disability
Experiences of being a refugee or a survivor of a concentration camp and torture	Illness
Murder of family member or close friend	Loss of possessions
War – combatant	Being neglected by loved ones

Types of traumatic experiences

It is sometimes useful to classify the trauma a person has experienced in order to facilitate decisions about how best to help the trauma survivor.

- *Single traumatic experience*. This is usually a once-off trauma, involving someone unknown to the person. For example, someone who has led a relatively peaceful life and then has to be rescued from a very serious car accident.
- *Multiple trauma*. This term is used when the same person has been exposed to several traumatic experiences. For example, someone may have survived several car accidents, or a car accident and an armed robbery.
- *Continuous trauma*. This term is used when the person is still living in a situation of ongoing danger. For example, during the political violence of the liberation struggle many South Africans lived in continuing danger for several years. Police who work in dangerous situations every day is another example.
- *Complex trauma*. Complex trauma is when the traumatic experiences happen within a relationship, for example domestic violence, where one partner physically abuses the other. A hostage situation may also be called complex trauma, because a relationship usually develops between hostages and perpetrators over time, leading to people adapting their behaviour according to the requirements of the perpetrators. This leads to a situation in which people betray themselves in their efforts to comply with the demands of the perpetrators to avoid further problems.

NORMAL RESPONSE TO TRAUMA

Figure 19.1 shows the normal reactions of a person to trauma. It is important to understand that these responses are completely normal following a traumatic event; almost all survivors of trauma have these reactions. This is called *normal post-traumatic stress response*, which can be described as a normal response to an abnormal event. In fact, it is even more worrying if a person does not show any of these normal reactions.

Trauma survivors have these responses because intense trauma becomes 'stuck' in our bodies and minds. It is as if the trauma has become indelibly imprinted on the person. As one trauma survivor expressed it: 'Every day, all day long, I just keep seeing what happened.'

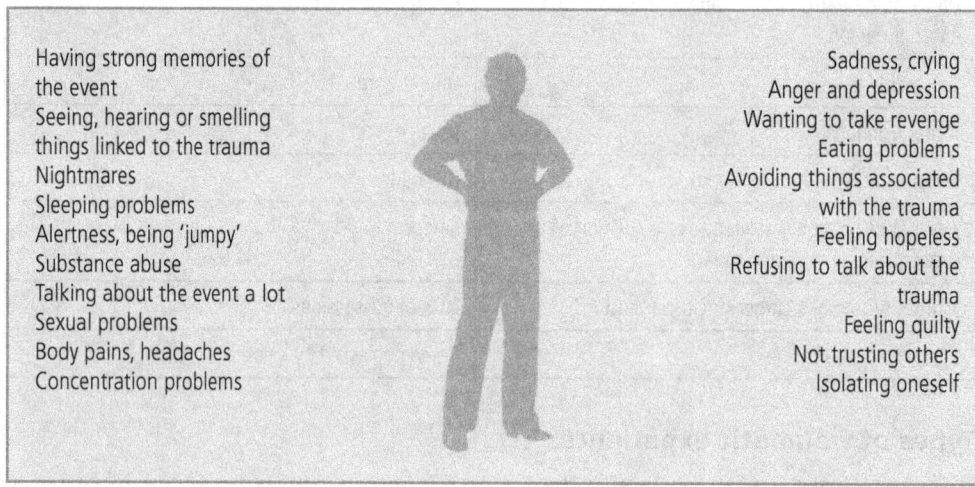

Figure 19.1 Normal post-traumatic response

When trauma is intensely frightening and painful, the person tends to respond in two ways:
1. avoidance and
2. re-experiencing.

Avoidance

One response is to try to avoid what happened. The person tries not to think about the experience and avoids places and things associated with the event; the person refuses to talk about aspects that were particularly awful and may use substances such as alcohol or medicines to block out feelings and memories. Some people even develop loss of some of the senses, such as loss of hearing, or the inability to talk. They avoid the trauma because to think about the event is like 'going back and experiencing it again', which is frightening and painful.

Re-experiencing

At the same time, because the event did happen, it is *part of the memory* and tends to keep coming back into the person's mind. This is when the person experiences nightmares and/or flashbacks or thinks about the event even when they are trying not to. It is as if the memory keeps resurfacing to haunt the person.

The tendency both to avoid the trauma and, at other times, to re-experience it, is normal. It is called the *approach–avoidance conflict*. Most trauma survivors swing between these two responses for some time after the traumatic event. This leads to a third set of symptoms around anxiety or increased arousal which are dealt with in the next section.

DIAGNOSIS OF TRAUMA AND STRESSOR-RELATED DISORDERS

People who have been victims of trauma may develop features of post-traumatic stress. These symptoms can arise, even in people who have had no previous history of psychological difficulties. These symptoms are reactions to an overwhelming external event, or series of events. In general, the development of post-traumatic stress disorder (PTSD) symptoms, and the severity of those symptoms, has more to do with the intensity and duration of the stressful event, than any preexisting personality patterns. In the DSM-5, the listing for PTSD is the only diagnosis for which the origins of the disturbance are related to external events rather than the individual's personality.

When working with people who have been victims of trauma, it is important to be aware that not many people develop full-blown PTSD. More commonly, individuals will develop symptoms of post-traumatic stress and not fit all the criteria for the DSM-5 diagnosis. Symptoms resulting from the exposure to traumas include persistent re-experiencing of the traumatic event, persistent avoidance of stimuli associated with the traumatic event and numbing of general responsiveness, and persistent symptoms of increased arousal. The DSM-5 symptoms of PTSD are outlined below (APA, 2013):

Box 1 DSM-5 symptoms of PTSD for adults, adolescents, and children older than six years

---

DSM-5 PTSD for adults, adolescents, and children older than six years

A. Exposure to actual or threatened death, serious injury, or sexual violence in one (or more) of the following ways:
1. Directly experiencing the traumatic event(s).
2. Witnessing, in person, the event(s) as it occurred to others.
3. Learning that the traumatic event(s) occurred to a close family member or close friend. In cases of actual or threatened death of a family member or friend, the event(s) must have been violent or accidental.
4. Experiencing repeated or extreme exposure to aversive details of the traumatic event(s) (eg, first responders collecting human remains: police officers repeatedly exposed to details of child abuse).
   Note: Criterion A4 does not apply to exposure through electronic media, television, movies, or pictures, unless this exposure is work related.

→

B. Presence of one (or more) of the following intrusion symptoms associated with the traumatic event(s), beginning after the traumatic event(s) occurred:
1. Recurrent, involuntary, and intrusive distressing memories of the traumatic event(s). *Note:* In children older than six years, repetitive play may occur in which themes or aspects of the traumatic event(s) are expressed.
2. Recurrent distressing dreams in which the content and/or affect of the dream are related to the traumatic event(s). *Note:* In children, there may be frightening dreams without recognisable content.
3. Dissociative reactions (eg, flashbacks) in which the individual feels or acts as if the traumatic event(s) were recurring. (Such reactions may occur on a continuum, with the most extreme expression being a complete loss of awareness of present surroundings.) *Note:* In children, trauma-specific reenactment may occur in play.
4. Intense or prolonged psychological distress at exposure to internal or external cues that symbolise or resemble an aspect of the traumatic event(s).
5. Marked physiological reactions to internal or external cues that symbolise or resemble an aspect of the traumatic event(s).

C. Persistent avoidance of stimuli associated with the traumatic event(s), beginning after the traumatic event(s) occurred, as evidenced by one or both of the following:
1. Avoidance of or efforts to avoid distressing memories, thoughts, or feelings about or closely associated with the traumatic event(s).
2. Avoidance of or efforts to avoid external reminders (people, places, conversations, activities, objects, situations) that arouse distressing memories, thoughts, or feelings about or closely associated with the traumatic event(s).

D. Negative alterations in cognitions and mood associated with the traumatic event(s), beginning or worsening after the traumatic event(s) occurred, as evidenced by two (or more) of the following:
1. Inability to remember an important aspect of the traumatic event(s) (typically due to dissociative amnesia and not to other factors such as head injury, alcohol, or drugs).
2. Persistent and exaggerated negative beliefs or expectations about oneself, others, or the world (eg, 'I am bad', 'No one can be trusted', 'The world is completely dangerous', 'My whole nervous system is permanently ruined').
3. Persistent, distorted cognitions about the cause or consequences of the traumatic event(s) that lead the individual to blame himself/herself or others.
4. Persistent negative emotional state (eg, fear, horror, anger, guilt, or shame).
5. Markedly diminished interest or participation in significant activities.
6. Feelings of detachment or estrangement from others.
7. Persistent inability to experience positive emotions (eg, inability to experience happiness, satisfaction, or loving feelings).

E. Marked alterations in arousal and reactivity associated with the traumatic event(s), beginning or worsening after the traumatic event(s) occurred, as evidenced by two (or more) of the following:
1. Irritable behaviour and angry outbursts (with little or no provocation) typically expressed as verbal or physical aggression toward people or objects.
2. Reckless or self-destructive behaviour.
3. Hypervigilance.
4. Exaggerated startle response.
5. Problems with concentration.
6. Sleep disturbance (eg, difficulty falling or staying asleep or restless sleep).

F. Duration of the disturbance (criteria B, C, D, and E) is more than one month.
G. The disturbance causes clinically significant distress or impairment in social, occupational, or other important areas of functioning.
H. The disturbance is not attributable to the physiological effects of a substance (eg, medication, alcohol) or another medical condition.

Specify whether:
With dissociative symptoms: The individual's symptoms meet the criteria for post-traumatic stress disorder, and in addition, in response to the stressor, the individual experiences persistent or recurrent symptoms of either of the following:
1. **Depersonalisation:** Persistent or recurrent experiences of feeling detached from, and as if one were an outside observer of, one's mental processes or body (eg, feeling as though one were in a dream; feeling a sense of unreality of self or body or of time moving slowly).
2. **Derealisation:** Persistent or recurrent experiences of unreality of surroundings (eg, the world around the individual is experienced as unreal, dreamlike, distant, or distorted).

Note: To use this subtype, the dissociative symptoms must not be attributable to the physiological effects of a substance (eg, blackouts, behaviour during alcohol intoxication) or another medical condition (eg, complex partial seizures).

Specify if:
With delayed expression: If the full diagnostic criteria are not met until at least six months after the event (although the onset and expression of some symptoms may be immediate).

Box 2 DSM-5 diagnostic criteria for acute stress disorder

DSM-5 diagnostic criteria for acute stress disorder

A. Exposure to actual or threatened death, serious injury, or sexual violation in one (or more) of the following ways:
1. Directly experiencing the traumatic event(s).
2. Witnessing, in person, the event(s) as it occurred to others.
3. Learning that the event(s) occurred to a close family member or close friend.
   Note: In cases of actual or threatened death of a family member or friend, the event(s) must have been violent or accidental.
4. Experiencing repeated or extreme exposure to aversive details of the traumatic event(s) (eg, first responders collecting human remains, police officers repeatedly exposed to details of child abuse).
   Note: This does not apply to exposure through electronic media, television, movies, or pictures, unless this exposure is work related.
B. Presence of nine (or more) of the following symptoms from any of the five categories of intrusion, negative mood, dissociation, avoidance, and arousal, beginning or worsening after the traumatic event(s) occurred:

Intrusion symptoms
1. Recurrent, involuntary, and intrusive distressing memories of the traumatic event(s). *Note:* In children, repetitive play may occur in which themes or aspects of the traumatic event(s) are expressed.
2. Recurrent distressing dreams in which the content and/or affect of the dream are related to the event(s). *Note:* In children, there may be frightening dreams without recognisable content.

3. Dissociative reactions (eg, flashbacks) in which the individual feels or acts as if the traumatic event(s) were recurring. (Such reactions may occur on a continuum, with the most extreme expression being a complete loss of awareness of present surroundings.)
   Note: In children, trauma-specific reenactment may occur in play.
4. Intense or prolonged psychological distress or marked physiological reactions in response to internal or external cues that symbolize or resemble an aspect of the traumatic event(s).

Negative mood

5. Persistent inability to experience positive emotions (eg, inability to experience happiness, satisfaction, or loving feelings).

Dissociative symptoms

6. An altered sense of the reality of one's surroundings or oneself (eg, seeing oneself from another's perspective, being in a daze, time slowing).
7. Inability to remember an important aspect of the traumatic event(s) (typically due to dissociative amnesia and not to other factors such as head injury, alcohol, or drugs).

Avoidance symptoms

8. Efforts to avoid distressing memories, thoughts, or feelings about or closely associated with the traumatic event(s).
9. Efforts to avoid external reminders (people, places, conversations, activities, objects, situations) that arouse distressing memories, thoughts, or feelings about or closely associated with the traumatic event(s).

Arousal symptoms

10. Sleep disturbance (eg, difficulty falling or staying asleep, restless sleep).
11. Irritable behaviour and angry outbursts (with little or no provocation), typically expressed as verbal or physical aggression toward people or objects.
12. Hypervigilance.
13. Problems with concentration.
14. Exaggerated startle response.

C. Duration of the disturbance (symptoms in criterion B) is three days to one month after trauma exposure. *Note:* Symptoms typically begin immediately after the trauma, but persistence for at least three days and up to a month is needed to meet disorder criteria.
D. The disturbance causes clinically significant distress or impairment in social, occupational, or other important areas of functioning.
E. The disturbance is not attributable to the physiological effects of a substance (eg, medication or alcohol) or another medical condition (eg, mild traumatic brain injury) and is not better explained by brief psychotic disorder.

The symptoms of acute stress disorder are common in the immediate aftermath of the event (the impact phase), when the individual may still be in a state of shock. In the days and weeks that follow (the recoil phase), the post-traumatic features may develop. It is common for symptoms to last between four–six weeks and sometimes up to three months.

Children who witness traumatic events or who are direct victims also develop signs of post-traumatic stress, although the symptom manifestation may be slightly different. See Appendix I for age-related symptoms and information for the parents/guardian on how to manage the child.

Box 3 DSM-5 Diagnostic criteria for adjustment disorder

DSM-5 Diagnostic Criteria for Adjustment Disorder
A. The development of emotional or behavioural symptoms in response to an identifiable stressor(s) occurring within three months of the onset of the stressor(s).
B. These symptoms or behaviours are clinically significant, as evidenced by one or both of the following:
1. Marked distress that is out of proportion to the severity or intensity of the stressor, taking into account the external context and the cultural factors that might influence symptom severity and presentation.
2. Significant impairment in social, occupational, or other important areas of functioning.
C. The stress-related disturbance does not meet the criteria for another mental disorder and is not merely an exacerbation of a preexisting mental disorder.
D. The symptoms do not represent normal bereavement.
E. Once the stressor or its consequences have terminated, the symptoms do not persist for more than an additional 6 months.

Specify whether:
309.0 (F43.21) With depressed mood: Low mood, tearfulness, or feelings of hopelessness are predominant.
309.24 (F43.22) With anxiety: Nervousness, worry, jitteriness, or separation anxiety is predominant.
309.28 (F43.23) With mixed anxiety and depressed mood: A combination of depression and anxiety is predominant.
309.3 (F43.24) With disturbance of conduct: Disturbance of conduct is predominant.
309.4 (F43.25) With mixed disturbance of emotions and conduct: Both emotional symptoms (eg, depression, anxiety) and a disturbance of conduct are predominant.
309.9 (F43.20) Unspecified: For maladaptive reactions that are not classifiable as one of the specific subtypes of adjustment disorder.

Uncommon stress responses

The following symptoms are not considered to be common responses to trauma and if these are presenting problems, referral to the appropriate treatment agency will be required:
- Psychotic episodes
- Clinical depression
- Feeling afraid of things that are not real
- Manic episodes
- Epileptic fits or convulsions
- Excessive use of alcohol, medication or drugs
- Suicide or homicide risk
- Development of phobias.

Continuous traumatic stress

The current diagnostic criteria for post-traumatic stress generally refer to people who are survivors of single traumatic events and for whom the trauma is over. This does not adequately cover people who are continuously exposed to ongoing traumatic events. This is the situation faced by many South Africans, who in the course of their lives face violence all the time and who have been repeatedly traumatised. The term 'continuous traumatic stress' has been developed to describe individuals who have experienced a number of traumatic stressors and who live in situations of ongoing traumatic stress.

Individuals who are living in situations of continuous traumatic stress show symptoms of post-traumatic stress but symptoms tend to be more severe. The individual may have more rigid defence mechanisms and there will be a stronger use of denial and numbing. The counselling approach will have the following goals:

- Aim to reinforce existing coping skills
- Less exploration of feelings – need to keep the mental health care user's (MHCU's) defences intact as this has survival value
- Focus on building self-esteem and reinforce survivor status
- Practical safety issues must be considered – explore safety plans and try to identify some areas in the MHCU's life where they do feel a sense of safety
- Mutual problem solving and forward planning on how to cope if it happens again – to empower the MHCU
- Focus on practical resources
- Explore attributions of meaning and trust issues.

Complex PTSD

The term complex PTSD refers to people who are exposed to prolonged, repeated trauma. Traumatisation occurs within a state of captivity where the victim is unable to flee and is under the control of the perpetrator. Examples of such conditions include prisons, concentration camps, some religious cults and hostage situations. Families in which domestic violence occurs are a significant group at risk for complex PTSD.

The situation of captivity brings the victim into prolonged contact with the perpetrator and creates a special type of relationship which is one of coercive control. In the case of domestic violence and sexual abuse, women and children are rendered captive by a combination of physical, economic, social and psychological means.

Victims of complex PTSD display three broad areas of disturbance which transcend simple PTSD.

1. *Symptom picture.* Symptoms are more complex, diffuse and long lasting. Mental illness symptoms are more common. Somatisation, dissociation and affective changes are common.
2. *Characterological.* Survivors of prolonged abuse develop characteristic identity and personality deformations of relatedness and identity. Isolation and withdrawal are common features and a there is disruption in intimate relationships and mistrust.
3. *Vulnerability.* Victim remains vulnerable to repeated harm, both self-inflicted and at the hands of others.

The treatment of people with complex PTSD is long term and requires intensive psychotherapy. A short-term trauma counselling intervention is not appropriate and referral to a psychotherapist would be necessary.

TRAUMA COUNSELLING AND INTERVENTIONS

The following model of trauma counselling is a short-term counselling intervention that is used with adult survivors of violence. The model (Eagle, 2000) combines principles of cognitive behavioural therapy and psychodynamic therapy. The model has been developed by staff of the Psychology Department at the University of the Witwatersrand and has been used in the Trauma Clinic for the past few years.

The model usually requires four–six sessions. There are five steps to the model which can be used interchangeably within the intervention, depending on the needs of the MHCU and the flow of the session(s). The five components of the model are as follows:

1. Telling/retelling the story
2. Normalising the symptoms
3. Reframing self-blame and survivor guilt
4. Encouraging mastery
5. Facilitating creation of meaning.

It is essential to create the focus of the counselling in the very first meeting with the MHCU, where the MHCU will be informed of the fact that therapy will be conducted over four–six sessions and that the aim is to look at what happened and to work through and learn to cope with the trauma. Some MHCUs may be resistant to talk about what happened and it is therefore important that this focus of the therapy is made clear from the outset.

The five steps are discussed in more detail.

1. Telling/retelling the story

In this phase the counsellor should focus on getting the MHCU to give a detailed description of what happened, eliciting all the factual details, thoughts, feelings and sensations, including sounds, smells and tastes. It is useful also to obtain information about fantasies and imagined aspects of the event. It is important to get as much detailed information as possible and it may be necessary for the story to be retold a few times to fill in all the gaps.

In addition to simply getting the MHCU to relate the story verbally, various other techniques can be used to elicit information. These include using drawings to depict the event, writing the story down and then going through it in a counselling session; using present tense narration; and using the metaphor of watching a film in slow motion.

With some MHCUs who are extremely anxious, it may be necessary to manage the anxiety through relaxation techniques, before commencing the narration. Clients who are highly resistant or mistrustful may need some time to establish a sense of safety and trust with the counsellor before they are able to tell their story. Certain traumas, such as rape, may be more difficult to talk about than others and it may take longer to elicit all the details. The counsellor needs to be gentle and patient in getting the full story.

A useful question to ask in the retelling is: 'What was the worst moment for you?' This provides the MHCU with more information about what was most difficult and frequently relates to thoughts of dying or of being raped or injured. It may also refer to feelings of humiliation.

The purpose of telling/retelling the story is to:
- enable emotional catharsis
- reduce isolation through accompanying the MHCU in their story – as a counsellor, you may be the first person to whom the MHCU has ever told all the details of their story
- provide containment – hearing all the details of the story provides the MHCU with a feeling of safety that someone else can tolerate hearing the full horror of their experience
- reduce anxiety and fear by talking about thoughts and fantasies
- allow the MHCU to access all their feelings, including fear, anger and helplessness
- construct a detailed account of what happened and filling in gaps in memory
- allow the MHCU to feel that someone listens to and believes their story.

2. Normalising the symptoms

In this phase the counsellor reassures the MHCU that their feelings are normal responses to trauma and provides information on post-traumatic stress reactions. It is important not to normalise these reactions too quickly as the MHCU may feel that this minimises their experience. Try and elicit the symptoms from the MHCU and then provide further information about post-traumatic stress. Usually, the MHCU will be suffering from symptoms of post-traumatic stress, without having full-blown PTSD.

The purpose of normalising the symptoms is to:
- reassure the MHCU that their responses are normal reactions to an abnormal event
- educate the MHCU about what symptoms to expect and to help them to understand their symptoms
- reassure MHCU that symptoms will get better with time
- take away the fear that they may be going crazy
- make links between the traumatic experience and symptoms that are experienced.

3. Reframing self-blame and survivor guilt

In this phase the counsellor and MHCU explore feelings of self-blame or survivor guilt. In many cases survivor guilt may not be present, but practically in every case, there are feelings of self-blame. It is suggested that this self-blame presents a wish to 'undo' the trauma retrospectively and to restore a sense of control. However, this self-blame impacts negatively on self-esteem and needs to be addressed.

The counsellor must elicit feelings of guilt and self-blame by asking questions such as:
- Do you think you could have done anything to prevent/change what happened?
- How do you feel you handled the situation?
- Looking back is there anything that you would have done differently?
- Do you in any way feel responsible for what happened?

Blame may relate to the belief that the person could have prevented what happened or could have done something more to stop what happened. Survivor guilt may be present when someone has died in a traumatic incident.

When exploring feelings of guilt, it is essential to go through events very carefully and to explore alternative scenarios and how useful these would have been. Usually, through this process, the MHCU discovers that their guilt is irrational and that under the circumstances they did the best they could.

Case example

Thandi was driving with her brother one evening. They stopped at traffic lights when two armed men attempted to hijack them. During the incident, her brother was shot and the hijackers fled without the car. Thandi had left her brother in the car to try and get help. He died before she returned. She blamed herself for leaving her brother to die alone and she also felt guilty that her brother had even been with her. She had asked him to give her a lift to her home and felt that if she had not asked him to help her, he would not have died.

Through counselling Thandi realised that she had done the right thing in trying to get help for her brother – she was doing the best she could to help him and knew that he needed medical attention. She acknowledged that had she not gone for help, she would have still blamed herself. She also began to see that her request for her brother's help did not cause the hijacking and that this could have happened at any place and at any time – it was a random attack, beyond her control.

There are occasions when a person's actions did cause the situation, for example the drunken driver who knocks over and kills a child. In this situation, the counsellor needs to help the MHCU separate outcome from intent. In this case, the driver was in the wrong for driving while drunk but had not intended to kill a child. Do not offer reassurances when someone has been in the wrong. In this situation, reparations may be useful. In the above instance, the driver may decide, in counselling, to send a letter of apology to the parents or to offer some financial assistance.

The purpose of reframing self-blame and survivor guilt is to:
- reassure the MHCU that they did the best they could under the circumstances
- restore self-esteem through affirming any thoughts, behaviours or strategies that were effective in the situation
- reinforce the fact that their actions facilitated their survival (hence their presence in the room)
- address concerns about how their behaviour may have affected others

- work through alternatives on a cognitive level, that their actions were the most appropriate in the situation
- separate motives from outcome
- explore irrational beliefs that the MHCU may develop after a traumatic incident. For example, a woman who was looking after a friend's child and the child was knocked over by a car may develop an irrational belief of 'I will never be responsible enough to look after a child'.

4. Encouraging mastery

In this phase the counsellor assists the MHCU to carry on with the tasks of daily living and to restore the MHCU to previous levels of coping. It is aimed at counteracting feelings of helplessness.

It is important to let the MHCU know that they will never forget what has happened, but it is how they remember it that is significant and that they should see themselves as survivors.

The purpose of encouraging mastery is to:
- restore the coping capacity of the MHCU
- restore the MHCU's sense of their adult position in the world
- help the MHCU establish and link into support systems
- help MHCU plan and to implement plans
- reduce anxiety.

An most important factor in coping is adequate support and the counsellor must encourage building on and mobilising existing support structures. The client can be provided with various techniques to help with coping. These include relaxation and stress/anxiety management skills; and cognitive techniques such as thought stopping, distraction, time structuring and systematic desensitisation. Goals must be mutually set and 'homework' type tasks set, which are attainable and manageable.

When necessary, the MHCU may need to be referred (see 'Uncommon stress responses'). There may be other difficulties such as marital problems or legal difficulties which will require referral to additional agencies.

5. Facilitating creation of meaning

The final stage of this model is optional and should only be pursued if the MHCU raises meaning as an issue. In many cases, deriving meaning is a long-term process and requires greater distance from the experience. Assisting with establishing meaning usually requires the counsellor to engage with the MHCU's belief system, be this at a cultural, political or existential level. It may involve encouraging the MHCU to consult with other healers such as priests or traditional healers. In some cases, people may want to join activist groups or other communal groups like community-policing forums, or to be involved in training as a rape counsellor. These decisions must come from the MHCU and must not be imposed on them by the counsellor.

The purpose of facilitating creation of meaning is to:
- establish meaning and understanding
- build self-esteem.

DEBRIEFING

Debriefing is a form of crisis intervention which is used when a group of people have been through a traumatic event together. It is a structured group meeting that allows for each group member to ventilate their feelings and reactions to the events.

It is not psychotherapy or psychological counselling. Debriefing does not involved 'curative' interventions and does not prevent reactions from occurring, but it does provide the individual with a framework to contain and understand their reaction and to take further action.

The aim of debriefing

The overall aim of debriefing is to reduce and minimise the occurrence of unnecessary psychological suffering through:
- the ventilation of impressions, reactions and feelings
- developing a clear understanding of the events and reactions, resulting in cognitive organisation
- decreasing tension
- normalising reactions and reducing feelings of isolation and uniqueness
- providing an opportunity for stress reduction education and emotional reassurance
- increasing group support and cohesiveness and mobilising resources within and outside of the group
- preparing participants for emotional reactions and symptoms which may arise
- identifying avenues of further assistance if required.

When debriefing should take place

Debriefings should be offered to a group of people if they have been through a traumatic event (see Table 19.1: List of traumas and crises) and if many individuals in a group appear to be distressed after the event. Groups may come from various sectors such as colleagues, school children, the workplace, etc.

Debriefing is most effective when it is offered after 24 hours and before 72 hours following a traumatic incident. This is not always possible, and debriefings conducted days or weeks later can still help in reducing levels of distress.

A typical debriefing usually lasts about three hours. Ideally it is held in an environment that is perceived to be safe and free of interruptions. Usually a maximum of 15 people would participate.

Pre-debriefing activities

Prior to the debriefing the following must be arranged:
- The debriefing must be announced to all those involved. It is important to try and have present everyone who was involved in the incident.
- The venue must be selected and the time must be set.
- Refreshments should be arranged for the end of the debriefing.

Before the debriefing the debriefing team must familiarise themselves with all the facts related to the incident and any other relevant information. It also helps to have an informal chat with those attending prior to starting the meeting.

The debriefing team

In each group debriefing should be run by two facilitators – one who leads the debriefing, and one who acts as a scribe and writes down the main points raised by the group members. The scribe will also look out for severe emotional reactions in group members.

A model for debriefing

The model for debriefing presented here involves seven phases: the introductory phase, the fact phase, the thought phase, the reaction phase, the symptom phase, the teaching phase and the re-entry phase.

1. The introductory phase

In this phase the group leader introduces the debriefing team and outlines the purpose of the meeting. The leader then sets out certain rules for the debriefing which are designed to minimise the anxieties that the participants may have.
- Initially, group members are reassured that no one has to say anything if they do not want to. The only requirement is that they state their name and their connection with the incident. Group members are specifically asked, however, to listen to what other group members have to say.
- Group members are reassured that everything they say is confidential. They are asked not to repeat what they hear during the session outside of the room and not to take notes or to record the proceedings.
- It should be clearly stated that the meeting is not a tribunal, nor a critique nor a fact-finding mission.
- Group members are asked to talk only for themselves and about their own reactions and not for others.
- Participants are warned that they may feel worse during the session, but that this is normal, as they may be getting in touch with painful feelings. The leader should point out that part of the cost of recovery is to confront painful feelings.

- Group members are advised that the group will continue with no break.
- If participants have to leave, they are requested to do so quietly and to return as quickly as possible. They should be told that if they leave in distress, a member of the team will follow to be with them.
- Group members are then given a brief outline of the structure of the meeting and given the opportunity to ask questions.

2. The fact phase

In this phase each person briefly describes what happened to them during the incident. Participants should describe how they came upon the event, and what the time sequence of events was. The leader may ask brief questions in order to achieve a clear understanding of all the facts. This is necessary because either due to the scope of the incident or due to perceptual narrowing, each person tends to have a restricted view of events.

A complete knowledge of all the events allows the group members to achieve a sense of cognitive organisation, which creates the space for them to think more objectively rather than being overwhelmed. Having a clear picture blocks speculation and reduces anxiety.

3. The thought phase

In this phase the debriefing focuses on decisions and thought processes. An opening question to begin this phase might be: 'What were your first thoughts when it happened, when you arrived on the scene or became involved?' People are often afraid to reveal their first thoughts because they may appear bizarre or reveal disbelief or intense fear.

Further questions that may be asked are: 'What did you do during the incident? Why did you decide on doing what you did?'

At the end of this phase, participants' impressions regarding the scene can be explored. Confronting these memories, and verbalising them, seems to make them less powerful, and they intrude less often.

4. The reaction phase

Questions about thoughts, impressions and actions lead to answers about feelings, and the reaction phase, in which feelings are often explored, is often the longest part of the debriefing. In order for this to be successful, the leaders have to be able to allow people to share feelings, no matter how painful this might be. To cut them off may be very destructive.

It is the process of sharing feelings that establishes similarities and the normality of reactions. Leaders of the debriefing must allow everyone the chance to participate: they must intervene if the ground rules are broken, or if there is destructive criticism.

It is important to watch for those who suffer a lot, who are silent or who have extreme reactions. It may be these people who are most at risk.

5. The symptom phase

During the symptom phase certain reactions are discussed in more detail. Participants are asked to describe symptoms (emotional, cognitive and physical) they experienced at the scene, when the incident was over, when they returned home, during the following days and at the present time. Questions about unusual experiences and difficulties in returning to work, school or routine may be necessary.

The familiar strands of post-traumatic stress (intrusive imagery, avoidance and numbing, hyperarousal), will no doubt appear.

6. The teaching phase

In this phase the scribe will summarise participants' reactions, noting similarities and differences. It is helpful to outline the symptoms of post-traumatic stress in order to normalise the reactions that participants may already be experiencing and to prepare them for future reactions which may occur. Knowledge enables participants to form expectations and to plan coping strategies.

7. The re-entry phase

In the re-entry phase, future planning and coping are discussed, particularly in terms of family and peer group support. One of the main aims is to foster cohesion within the group. It is helpful to explore coping strategies such as relaxation, deep breathing exercises, distraction techniques and anger management. It is also important to discuss at what points participants may need to seek further help and where they could go. Guidelines for knowing when to get help might be: (a) if symptoms do not decrease after about six weeks; (b) if symptoms increase over time; and (c) if workers are unable to function adequately at work or at home.

Follow-up to the debriefing

Participants should be asked if they would like a follow-up session. If so, the follow-up may take place a few weeks after the first debriefing. This meeting will be less structured than the first, and the primary task is to review the group's progress in terms of symptoms and actions taken to deal with them. It may be at this point that some participants are identified as being in need of more extensive help.

Impact on the worker

Debriefing sessions, while involving very powerful interventions, can also be draining on the facilitators. They involve long and emotionally charged interactions. It is important that facilitators are themselves debriefed after a meeting, preferably with a colleague. Self-care tactics are especially important after conducting a group debriefing.

IMPACT OF WORKING WITH VICTIMS OF VIOLENCE AND SELF-CARE

As someone working with victims of violence and trauma, a counsellor may develop secondary traumatic stress disorder. Through hearing the story of their MHCUs, counsellors become witnesses of the trauma. The counsellors' work includes absorbing information about suffering and it often includes absorbing the suffering as well. Various terms have been used to describe secondary traumatic stress disorder. These include compassion fatigue, vicarious traumatisation, secondary victimisation and burnout. The symptoms are very similar to those of post-traumatic stress. Counsellors may develop episodes of sadness and depression, sleeplessness, generalised anxiety and other forms of suffering that are linked to the trauma work.

Working with trauma victims involves empathic connection with people who have experienced traumatic and horrific life events. Vicarious traumatisation is the cumulative impact of victims' stories. It can change your worldview and capacity to deal with life, as well as cause intrusive imagery, somatisation and isolation. If left untreated, it can damage relationships with clients, colleagues and family and can lead to cynicism and despair.

As a counsellor working with trauma, it is essential to monitor one's own behaviours, thoughts and feelings and to recognise when one is suffering from compassion fatigue. One also needs to focus on self-care in order to prevent burnout.

Definition of compassion fatigue

Compassion fatigue can be defined as the natural consequent behaviours and emotions resulting from knowing about a traumatising event experienced by a significant other – the stress resulting from helping or wanting to help a traumatised or suffering person (Sorenson et al, 2016.)

Contributing factors

Various factors contribute to traumatisation that occurs vicariously:

Box 4 Factors contributing to vicarious traumatisation

Factors that contribute to vicarious traumatisation

Nature of stressor present in the trauma and trauma story
- Complexity and type of stressor (natural vs human origin)
- Grotesqueness, death, injury, mutilation and abuse
- Stage in life cycle at exposure
- Role in event
- Moral dilemmas during the event
- Imprisonment by perpetrator
- Duration, severity, frequency of exposure or victimisation
- Degree of community involvement.

→

Personal factors in counsellor
- Personal beliefs, religious values, ideological systems and preconceptions
- Defensive styles and dispositions
- Personal 'historical' data from own life experiences
- Degree of training and experience with trauma and victimisation
- Motivation to work in trauma field
- Theoretical assumptions about personality and life development.

Factors in the MHCU
- Age, race, gender, ethnicity, and cultural dimensions
- Role in traumatic event (perpetrator, victim, witness)
- Personality characteristics
- Defensive and coping styles
- Level of traumatisation and injuries
- Pre-trauma ego strength and coping
- Family dynamics and background factors.

Institutional/organisational factors
- Political context; supportive vs oppositional
- Attitudes towards MHCU population
- Adequacy of resources that help/hinder treatment
- Support available for nurse counsellors.

Source: Adapted from Wilson and Lindy (1994); Peled-Avram (2017)

Signs and symptoms of vicarious traumatisation

Working with trauma can affect the counsellor in various ways and can lead to changes in various aspects of the counsellor's life. The table below outlines some of the reactions that may indicate secondary traumatic stress.

Table 19.2 Signs and symptoms of secondary traumatic stress

Cognitive	Emotional	Behavioural	Spiritual	Interpersonal	Physical
Diminished concentration	Powerlessness	Clingy	Questioning the meaning of life	Withdrawn	Shock
Confusion	Anxiety	Impatient	Loss of purpose	Decreased interest in intimacy or sex	Sweating
Loss of meaning	Guilt	Irritable	Lack of self-satisfaction	Mistrust	Rapid heartbeat
Spaciness	Anger/rage	Withdrawn	Hopelessness	Isolation	Breathing difficulties
Decreased self-esteem	Survivor guilt	Moody	Ennui	Impact on parenting (protectiveness)	Somatic reactions
Preoccupation with trauma	Shutdown	Regression	Anger at God	Concern about aggression	Aches and pains
Trauma Imagery	Numbness	Sleep disturbances	Questioning of prior religious beliefs	Projection of anger or blame	Dizziness
Apathy	Fear	Appetite changes		Intolerance	Impaired immune system
Rigidity	Helplessness	Nightmares		Loneliness	
Disorientation	Sadness	Hyperarousal			
Whirling thoughts	Depression	Elevated startle response			
Thoughts of self-harm or harm towards others	Hypersensitivity				
Self-doubt	Emotional lability				
	Overwhelmed				
	Depleted				

Cognitive	Emotional	Behavioural	Spiritual	Interpersonal	Physical
Perfectionism Minimisation		Use of negative coping (smoking, alcohol or other substance misuse) Accident proneness Losing things Self-harm behaviours			

Management of vicarious traumatisation

An important way of managing vicarious traumatisation is through understanding the principles of self-care. A fundamental principle of self-care is to learn to recognise one's reactions and to take steps to deal with these reactions. When counselling trauma victims, it is important to implement principles of self-care as part of your daily routine. In addition to referring to Orem's model of self-care (Denyes et al, 2001), the following principles in Table 19.3 can also be followed:

Table 19.3 Principles of self-care

Personal	Professional	Societal
Social Support Getting help and talking about feelings Adequate sleep and nutrition Relaxation Exercise Life balance between work and play Contact with nature Humour Creative expression Meditation/spiritual practice Self-awareness Personal therapy	Work balance Realistic work goals Supervision Boundaries/limit setting Getting support/help Professional training and skills development Job commitment Replenishment Adequate leave Supportive management Job commitment Physical setting	Social action Public education strategies Legislative reform Lobbying and advocacy

DOMESTIC VIOLENCE

Legal structures to empower and protect women are in place in South Africa. The Bill of Rights (Constitution of the Republic of South Africa, 108 of 1996) acknowledges the prominence of women in all levels of government and civil society; and the Domestic Violence Act 118 of 1998 addresses violence against women as the criminal offence it is. The Choice on Termination of Pregnancy Amendment Act 38 of 2004 empowered women with reproductive rights. Furthermore, the 16 Days of Activism against Women and Child Abuse has been implemented in the country to bring awareness and to combat violence against women and children around the country (WHO, 2009). In spite of these measures, domestic violence remains high in South Africa.

There are several factors which contribute to domestic violence. In intimate relationships, the frequency of verbal disagreements and high levels of conflict have been associated with physical violence. Violence used as a strategy in conflict might have been learned during childhood. It is also often used to resolve the male's identity crisis. An example of this would be men living in poverty who are unable to live up to their dreams of success. They experience stress and might resort to violence against their partners. Alcohol consumption on its own is associated with interpersonal violence since the effect of alcohol clouds a person's judgement and perception and also reduces inhibitions. Although the relationship between alcohol and violence is a complex matter, excessive intake of alcohol and other related drugs have been reported to be a contributing factor in triggering domestic violence (Collins, 2013; Jewkes et al, 2015; 2016).

Apart from the obvious harm (external signs such as bruises) and the traumatic effect it can have on the family or those who witness it, domestic violence has mental and physical effects. Many people in South Africa, from all economic and cultural backgrounds, suffer repeated physical, emotional and/or sexual abuse from their partners. Domestic violence is an example of complex trauma and is very difficult to deal with because of the personal relationship between the perpetrator and victim.

Cycle of domestic violence

An understanding of the cycle of domestic violence is helpful both to the nurse and to the person involved in the situation. Pointing out this cycle may help to increase the awareness of the person being abused about the ongoing nature of such violence, or at least help them to identify the warning signs in their own situation.

Many people ask what can be done if one becomes aware that someone is caught in this cycle of violence. Usually rational argument is futile. Do not think that one can persuade a person to leave their partner, simply by logically pointing out the patterns. Initially the person may agree to leave the abusive situation, but they usually end up returning soon afterwards. When this happens, people often may not want to return to one for assistance, because of having warned them that the abuse is likely to continue, and now they feel bad or expect to be judged.

Many people wonder what makes it so difficult for someone to leave a situation of abuse, and why so many people return to abusive relationships. The central components of the cycle involve love, hope and fear.

- *Love.* The person knows that their partner has good points and is not 'all bad' as a person. They may choose to focus more on the good, as a way of rationalising the bad. Although it may not seem possible to an objective onlooker, it helps to understand that the abused person often has a genuine and deep love for the partner.

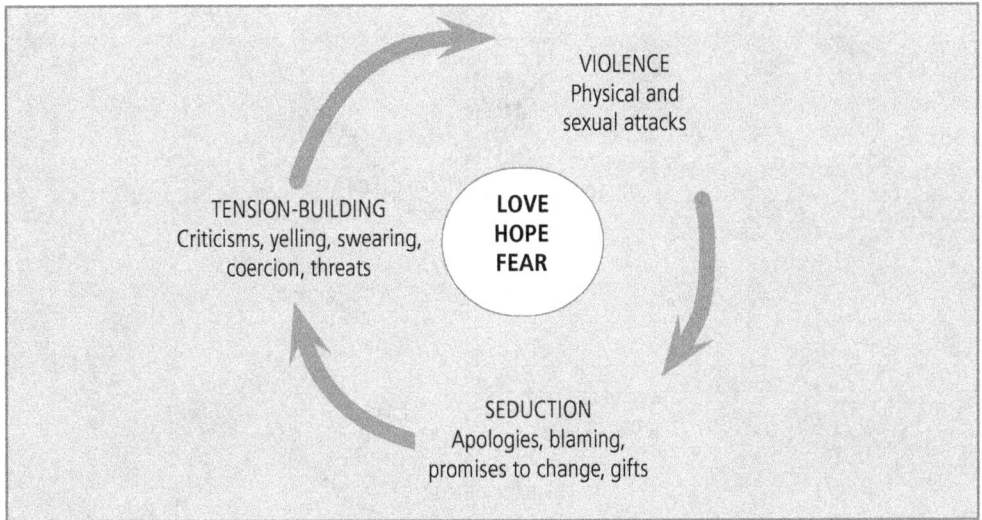

Figure 19.2 The cycle of domestic violence

Source: Adapted from National Centre for Health Research

- *Hope.* Many people hold on to the hope that things will change. They often remember that the relationship started out well, and they believe the abusive partner's promises that they will change and that the violence will stop.
- *Fear.* People are often trapped in relationships by fear. They believe the partner will carry out their threats, for example to kill the person or to harm the children or other family members.

The wheel of domestic violence

Levels of violence usually increase as the abusing partner gains more control over the abused person's life. The wheel's centre, as described in Figure 19.3, is about power and control, and many abusers will try to reduce any control and power the person may have. The abuser uses coercion, threats and intimidation. Repeated verbal attacks from the abuser erode the person's self-esteem and beliefs about self and others who care about the person. Isolation is common; many people describe how their partners gradually restrict their social movements, even cutting them off from family and close friends. Common strategies used by abusers are: minimising the situation, denying that there is a problem, blaming others, and/or using loved ones as leverage against the abused person. Economic control (such as ensuring that the person has no access to money) is often a concrete way of gaining power and limiting options.

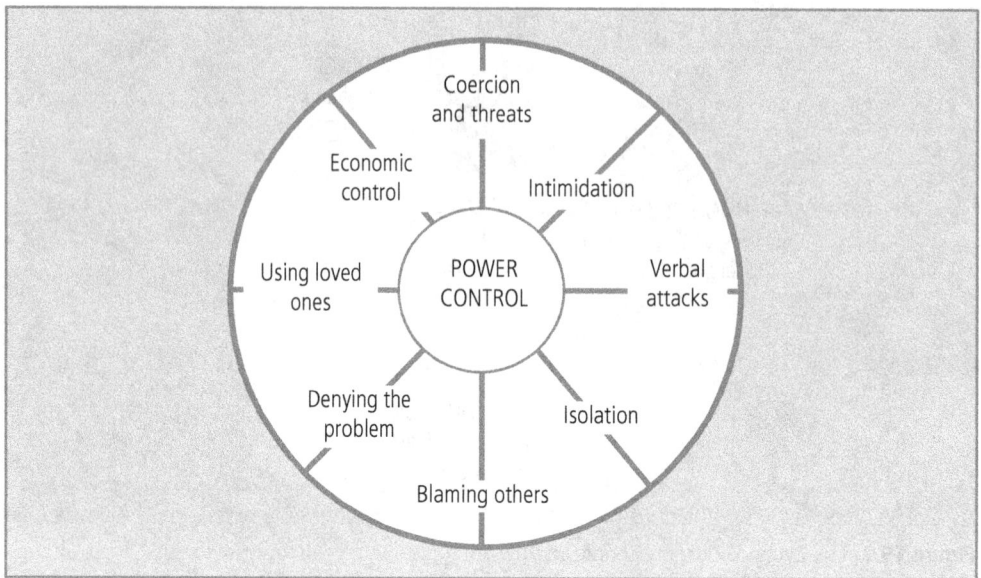

Figure 19.3 The wheel of domestic violence

Source: Adapted from the Duluth Model

The wheel of non-violence

A situation of non-violence relies on equality, including mutual respect, trust and support, honesty, responsibility, economic partnership, fairness and non-threatening behaviour.

Achieving a cycle of non-violence (see Figure 19.4) is a long-term process, which may be facilitated by the following:

- *Support.* One of the most significant and perhaps simplest things that can be done if you suspect someone has been affected by violence or is currently trapped in the cycle of domestic violence, is to offer a supportive relationship. Remember that people do not leave this situation on the basis of logical arguments. Instead, knowing that there is someone out there who knows about the abuse, who cares, and who respects one's decisions, is often what is needed to give a person hope and the courage to change the situation. Gently encouraging them to talk about what is happening, and letting the person know that you respect their decisions, is often the best that can be done. Also essential is to facilitate access to legal support and family support. Often the best people to assist in abusive situations are the family members of the person. With permission, it may be helpful to make contact with the family and to encourage assistance. It may be useful to provide referrals to legal agencies that specialise in this area.
- *Safety plan.* In a situation of high danger and ongoing abuse, it is a good idea to bring up the idea of a safety plan for the person being abused. Identifying times of risk, based on the model of a build up in tension, is essential. This will help the

person to identify danger signs and, with a plan in place, enable them to leave the situation ahead of time, if only until things settle down. In some cases, it is also important to develop an escape plan, to be implemented if violence suddenly erupts. This may mean drawing up a list of friends, family or neighbours to go to for help, or having money available for transport.

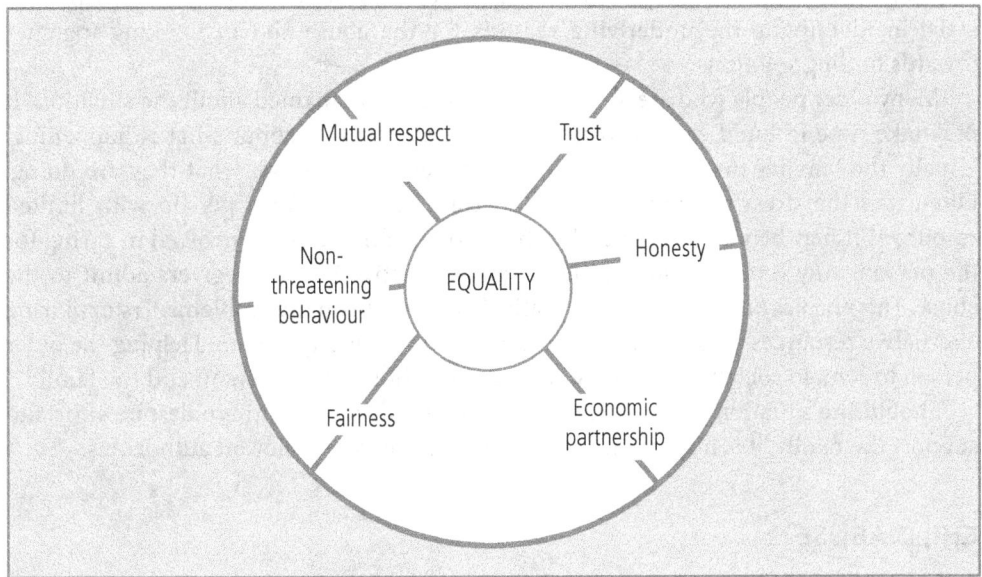

Figure 19.4 The wheel of non-violence

Source: Adapted from the Duluth Model

ABUSE OF THE ELDERLY

Abuse of the elderly has been receiving increased media attention in South Africa. Gray-Vickrey (2000) cautions that we should not only consider physical abuse of the elderly in terms of visible signs of assault, since neglect, financial and emotional abuse are also common. Gray-Vickrey reports that as many as 10 per cent of older adults may be abused and that these cases are seldom reported.

The following factors may contribute to abuse of the elderly:
- The elderly person has an impairment which could be adding to the stress of the caregiving.
- The family has limited resources to look after the older person.
- There have been previous relationship problems with the older person.

History of family violence

The health care practitioner should look out for subtle as well as obvious signs of abuse or neglect. These may include unusual injuries or patterns of injuries. Repeated injuries may be a sign of abuse, as may delays in reporting the injuries. Knowledge of the relationship between caregivers and the older person may also assist with the assessment of the situation.

Because abuse of the elderly tends to be very shocking, many practitioners are tempted to react in an extreme manner. However, it may be more helpful if time is taken to build a trusting relationship with both the caregivers and the older person. This may assist in identifying the underlying reasons for the abuse and in working together towards finding solutions.

Many older people who are abused or neglected feel ashamed about the situation. It may take time to build enough trust for the person to talk about what is happening. Usually the families involved in the abuse feel very guilty about what they are doing. Often it is the stress of their lives or the strain of caring for a person with limited resources. It may help to talk generally about some of the stresses involved in caring for the person. Any intervention will be far more effective if the caregivers admit to the abuse. This enables one to work collaboratively with them on the problems. Try exploring alternative resources for support of the family and the elderly person. Helping the older person to remain socially active may relieve stress, both on the person and the family.

Should the situation seem extreme, or should the abuse continue despite efforts to support the family, it is important to report the abuse to the relevant authorities.

CHILD ABUSE

Although the question relating to a definition of child abuse has been asked across different societies over the last few decades, a specific definition is still quite vague and unclear in most countries.

The Collins English Dictionary defines the word 'abuse' as 'to use incorrectly/ improperly, or misuse'. 'Misuse' in turn, means 'cruel or inhuman or to treat harshly or badly'. When applied to children, abuse therefore suggests any inhuman treatment of children. This implies that child abuse encompasses the physical, sexual or emotional ill treatment or neglect of a child by their parents or other persons responsible for their welfare.

In South Africa, the Child Care Act 38 of 2005 defines a child as any person under the age of eighteen. According to Childline, child abuse occurs when a child receives non-accidental injury for which the parents or guardian (or other adult) is responsible and cannot give a 'reasonable explanation' as to why it happened. As such, child abuse usually involves intentional harm – whether the abuser accepts or admits this or not.

Furthermore, the term 'child abuse' therefore implies the misuse of power by the older person, and the betrayal of the trust the child has in the adult.

There are various types of child abuse. These include physical, emotional, neglect, societal and sexual abuse.

Physical abuse

Physical abuse is any non-accidental injury or pattern of injuries to a child as a result of acts of omission or commission by a parent or care provider that endanger or impair the child's physical or emotional health and development.

Signs of physical abuse are thus more easily recognisable than with other forms of abuse (for example, sexual or emotional) and include bites, bruises, cuts, fractures, scratches, burns, sores, etc.

Although physical abuse of children does occur most commonly among socially deprived families, it is not confined to such families. In South Africa cases have been recorded at every social level of society.

Apart from the physical effects of abuse, children who have been physically abused are left with feelings of worthlessness and unimportance. The child sees themselves as unlovable and are unable to form trusting relationships with others.

Emotional abuse

Emotional abuse involves excessive or unreasonable parental demands that place expectations on a child beyond their capabilities. Examples of emotional abuse include:
- Constant criticism
- Belittling and persistent teasing
- Excessive discipline
- Constant verbal attacks
- Frightening and threatening the child
- Paying little or no attention/affection to the child
- Failure to provide the psychological nurturing necessary for a child's physical growth and emotional growth and development.

There might be acts of omission and commission. Acts of omission may include ignoring or passive rejection of the child or withholding praise and affect, while acts of commission include constant yelling, demeaning remarks, threatening, terrorising and verbal rejection of the child, as well as bizarre and unusual punishment.

Emotional abuse thus covers a range of behaviours, which attack the child's emotional and developmental well-being, and sense of self-worth. As a result of the wide range of parental behaviours involved, emotional abuse is perhaps one of the most difficult forms of abuse to detect. Just as physical injuries can scar a child, emotional cruelty through verbal assaults can cripple or disable a child emotionally, behaviourally and intellectually.

Neglect

Child neglect is continued failure to provide a child with the basic necessities of life. This includes failure to provide the child with adequate food, medical attention, clothing, shelter and adequate supervision needed for the child's optimal growth and development.

This form of abuse is suffered by the largest percentage of abused children in South Africa. Unlike other forms of abuse, neglect is more about what a parent does *not* do rather than that what they *do*. Long-term neglect can result in retarded growth and development – physically, intellectually and emotionally.

Societal abuse

Societal abuse can be defined as ways in which society fails to provide minimal support for citizens. These forms of abuse are less studied but are also quite prevalent in our society and are usually culturally supported. These include:
- Children witnessing family violence
- Social discrimination
- Sexism
- Exposing children to war
- Extreme poverty and homelessness.

Sexual abuse in children

Sexual abuse is defined as the engaging of a child in sexual activities that they do not understand, to which the child cannot give informed consent, or which violate the social taboos of society.

It includes intra-familial (ie abuse within the family – incest), extra-familial (someone outside of the family) and miscellaneous abuse (perpetrated by a person who is neither a family member nor someone known to the child, eg a once-off rape or assault on a child victim).

Another way to view child sexual abuse is to realise that it is exploitation of a child for the sexual pleasure of an adult (or adolescent/older peer) – whether heterosexual or homosexual. It is very important to note that sexual abuse may be with or without the consent of the child. Therefore, even if a twelve-year-old girl agrees to have sexual relations with a twenty-year-old man this is viewed as child sexual abuse – since a child of this age is not in an adequate position to make such a decision.

It is also important to note that child sexual abuse can involve either/both:
1. *Acts of sexual contact.* This includes fondling of genitals (whether the child is clothed or unclothed), frottage, cunnilingus, oral–genital sex, interfemoral intercourse (dry sex), digital penetration, sexual intercourse, sodomy, rape, incest and sexual exploitation (for example, child pornography and child prostitution).
2. *Non-contact sexual abuse.* This involves other forms of sexual abuse in which actual contact is excluded but they are still sexually abusive for the child to experience. This type of sexual abuse includes 'sexy talk' – or inappropriate remarks concerning child pornographic material and involving the child in voyeurism, such as making the child watch sexual acts between adults, etc.

The dynamics involved in child abuse

Child sexual abuse is a process (rather than an event) in which various factors combine to form unique symptoms in each abused child. It is recognised that sexual abuse is almost always *traumatic* and *intrusive*, requiring special coping mechanisms and resulting in *serious harm* to the child' experience of themselves, others and the world.

Unlike other forms of child abuse, sexual abuse represents a distinct form of abuse since it involves both betrayal of trust and physical violation, accompanied by a degree of coercion or deceit.

Their victims know the majority of assailants, and the majority of assaults involve the misuse of authority inherent in age differences and family relationships. It is thus important to remember that child sexual abuse frequently consists of repeated incidents, often starting at an early age (four to six) and recurring continuously, or at intervals, over a period of five to ten years without discovery or being broken off.

Ongoing sexual abuse normally involves less physical force and violence than rape and does not usually begin with intercourse, but rather with fondling of the genitals, masturbation and exhibitionism. These acts then lead to full sexual intercourse over time.

Unlike physical abuse, sexual abuse involves motives, which are mainly 'non-sexual' as the abuser is attempting to express negative feelings, domination, power and control. As a result, various factors (individual, familial and social) are involved in the trauma of child sexual abuse.

The traumagenic dynamics model

The traumagenic dynamics model of child sexual abuse put forward by international experts Finkelhor and Browne (1985) explain four central dynamics involved in child sexual abuse which serve to change the child's mental and emotional orientation to the world and distort the child's self-concept. The four dynamics – betrayal, stigmatisation, powerlessness and traumatic sexualisation – are explained below.

Betrayal
- Children who have been sexually abused experience immense feelings of betrayal when they discover that someone on whom they depend (usually the father in intra-famial abuse), or who is at least respected as an adult authority, has caused them or wishes to cause them harm.
- Betrayal operates in several ways. For some, it occurs at the time of the first abuse, while in others betrayal can be experienced later when the child realises that they were tricked into doing something bad through lies or threats. Abused children often feel immensely betrayed by their mothers (or siblings), especially when the child discovers that their mother is unable or unwilling to believe or protect them.
- Since most youngsters tend to believe that their parents are caring and capable of warding off harm, betrayal in incest cases is severely traumatic. As a result, sexually abused children often experience a lack of trust in adults and a loss of faith in human beings in general.

Stigmatisation

Sexually abused children usually receive negative message from the abuser. As a result, they come to believe that they are evil, worthless and guilty. Abusers often blame or degrade the victim, either directly through threats and pressures for secrecy. Abusers often say things like:
- 'It's all your fault – because you always wear sexy clothes.'
- 'You're bad because you didn't stop me.'
- 'What we're doing isn't wrong – don't you think it feels nice.'
- 'If you tell anyone, they'll know you're very bad.'
- 'If you tell Mom then I will go to jail.'
- 'Secrets are special – this is our special secret.'

Powerlessness

- In child sexual abuse, having one's body space constantly invaded against one's wishes (whether through force or deceit), causes an intense feeling of powerlessness which has a devastating impact on the child's body image.
- These children often feel powerless because their sense of control is repeatedly overruled and frustrated, and they are often forced to deal with threats and secrecy.
- By forcing a child to keep the sexual abuse a 'secret', the victim becomes more and more powerless. In this way the abuser uses their adult power to reinforce the threats and blame which they communicate to the child. In telling the child victim that the abuse is their fault and that it is their 'special secret', the abuser is able to form a bond with the child which keeps the sexually abused victim separate from the outside world – emotionally and psychologically.
- A sense of fear and isolation is often produced by this 'secrecy', causing many sexually abused children to withdraw from their peers.

Traumatic sexualisation

This refers to the way in which sexual abuse shapes a child's sexuality in developmentally inappropriate and dysfunctional ways.
- Child sexual abuse often involves an element of reward, which is offered by offenders for sexual behaviour with the child. It may be something like a special gift, money or simply special attention, which the child does not receive elsewhere. As a result, the relationship between the abused and the abused child becomes highly confusing for the child.
- When the experience is physically pleasant and the reward enticing, the child may have a wish to protect the abuser – in spite of the fear and anger felt towards him. This aspect of reward often teaches these children to use sexual behaviour as a way of manipulating others to meet their needs (hence the high prostitution rate among adult survivors).
- When sexually abused children are treated as 'special' by the abuser, they also become confused about sexual behaviour. The body boundaries of what is 'good

touching' are broken and over sexualised behaviour (like compulsive masturbation) become common – especially in young sexually abused children.
- The confusion about their body boundaries is often expressed by feelings of lack of control over the body and wanting to get rid of something bad from inside. Also, the child's sexuality can become traumatised when frightening and unpleasant memories become associated in the child's mind with sexual activity, resulting in damage to later sexual functioning and intimate relationships.

EFFECTS OF TRAUMA ON CHILDREN

Children are affected by traumatic experiences in the same way as adults. Figure 19.1 is very relevant to children. In addition to the effects described for adults, children may show the following normal responses:
- *Regression.* This is when children go back to behaviour displayed when they were younger, that is, behaviour more common to a younger child. For example, children may start sucking their thumbs again or talk in baby language. Children who stopped wetting their beds may start bedwetting again.
- *Acting out.* The children show anger and have tantrums. They may react sensitively to small things. They may bully other children or misbehave.
- *Fantasy play.* Often traumatic experiences are expressed during the child's play. Games such as 'funerals' are common. The child may also draw pictures of events. This is normal and healthy.
- *Somatic complaints.* Many children will try to get help by complaining about other aches and pains. Examples are complaints about sore arms or legs, stomach-aches, headaches.
- *Avoidance.* The avoidance behaviour is often strong with children. They may refuse to go near the place where the event happened. They may refuse to eat foods that were eaten just before the event took place or refuse to wear the clothing worn on the day it happened.
- *Magical thinking.* Children often make curious links between the event and things that happened just prior to the event. They may believe that something they saw or did caused the event to happen.
- *Self-blame.* Children tend to see themselves as the centre of their world. They often believe they did something to cause the event. For example, if a child had a fight with a brother on the morning of the event, they may believe the fight and the event are connected and that it is their fault that it happened.
- *Fears.* Children affected by trauma may show excessive concerns about safety and fears of violence.
- *Sensitivity to sound.* Traumatised children may be very sensitive to loud noises and unusual sounds.
- *Seductiveness.* Unusually seductive behaviour in young children is an indicator of sexual abuse. This should not be confused with normal emerging sexuality, which is common in all children.

- *Secretiveness.* Sexually abused children may become very secretive about certain behaviours or activities.
- *Complaints about feeling dirty.* Children who have been sexually abused may make comments about being dirty. They may wash themselves often.
- *Complaints about genitals.* Children who have been sexually abused may complain about problems and pain relating to their genital areas.
- *Interest in sexual matters.* Some children who have been sexually abused show excessive interest in things of a sexual nature. For example, they may become very interested in television programmes with a sexual content. This should not be confused with normal developing interest of children and adolescents in sex. Other children may actively avoid anything of a sexual nature.

Once again, these reactions are often completely normal. By helping parents and teachers to understand the child's reaction, they can be helped not to over-react.

Initial (short-term) effects

If a child has been sexually abused, the initial effects may involve the following:
- A child's initial reaction to sexual abuse is shown in changed behaviour. Apart from this however, initial effects of sexual abuse vary and can range from physical, emotional or intellectual to behaviour reactions. (see Section 1.3.4.)
- Studies on the effects of sexual abuse on children of different ages show that sexual abuse may have a different meaning or expression of trauma for children based on their age (Finkelhor & Browne, 1985). Younger children may be less psychologically traumatised at the time of abuse than older children (who may realise sooner that it is wrong), but because younger children do not know the meaning of sexual acts, the physical pain may have a greater impact.
- Younger children may show open and even compulsive sexualised behaviour (as a response to the abuse), or regress to an earlier stage with wetting and soiling. Also, because basic trust develops at an early age and is vitally necessary for later development, one of the outcomes of sexual abuse in very young children is that they often suffer more developmental delays (such as delays in speech, fine and gross motor control, etc) than older children.
- This is important in the school setting, as children who have been classified as intellectually or developmentally 'slow' (even mild or moderately mentally impaired), may very well be suffering the effects of earlier sexual abuse.
- School-age children may show less sexualised behaviour, but may often have problems in school, eating disturbances, lack of self-esteem, difficulty falling asleep and nightmares. The teachers often notice a 'change' in scholastic performance, as the child seems to daydream and lack concentration or interest in the classroom.
- Adolescent victims of sexual abuse often react in a self-destructive way. They may attempt suicide or mutilate their bodies (for example, with razor blades, etc), run away from school or home, become aggressive and promiscuous. All in all, the

adolescent is 'acting out' the trauma, which they have experienced (or still are experiencing) by displaying hatred towards themselves.

Table 19.4 summarises the behavioural signs of a sexually abused child at various stages in life.

Table 19.4 Behavioural signs of a sexually abused child

Pre-school (3–6 years)	Middle childhood (7–12 years)	Adolescent (13–18 years)
Compulsive masturbation Sexualised play – often with younger children Sexualised kissing Regressed behaviours (eg thumb sucking, baby-like behaviours) Excessive clinging Bedwetting/soiling Nightmares	Over sexualised – vocabulary, knowledge and behaviour Public genital display or masturbation Sexual interaction with younger children	Suicide or para-suicide attempts Self-mutilation (cutting self with razor blades, etc) Eating disorders – anorexia nervosa/bulimia/obsessive over-eating Truancy Promiscuity Prostitution Drug and alcohol abuse
Scholastic signs		
	Poor concentration/daydreaming Learning problems Underachievement Truancy Excessive sensitivity about sexual matters Isolates self from peers	Poor scholastic performance Running away from school/skipping classes Isolating self from peers
	Change in temperament or mood Changed appetite Psychosomatic complaints – like untreatable stomach-aches, headaches, etc. Self-induced vomiting Depression/isolation Obsessive/neurotic behaviour Stealing and running away from home Extreme aggression Sleep disturbances/nightmare Nail biting Bedwetting/soiling	Psychosomatic complaints Pregnancy or over-concern about pregnancy. Depression Mental disorders

Long-term effects

The effects of undetected child abuse far outweigh the immediate trauma displayed in child victims, as these generally do not pass with time (after the abuse has ended), resulting in a variety of long-term effects. In general, most child abuse victims carry their 'secret' with them for many years, with the trauma affecting their entire personality and adult years.

The long-term effects of sexual abuse thus show themselves differently from the short-term effects. This is because an adult is able to look back on childhood events from a different psychological perspective in comparison to what a child might do. The most common long-term effects shown in adults who have been abused as children are:
- Low self-esteem
- Interpersonal/relationship problems
- Sexual disturbances
- Anxiety disorders (panic attacks, phobias etc)
- Depression, which is ongoing and severe – seemingly without a 'reason'
- Suicide/suicide attempts
- Substance abuse (alcohol/drugs)
- Psychosomatic problems (continual 'unexplained' illnesses)
- Delinquency (stealing, breaking the law, etc)
- Revictimisation
- Psychiatric conditions (such as schizophrenia, bipolar disorders, personality disorders, etc).

Estimating the long-term effects of sexual abuse is very complex because a variety of factors are involved. These include, for instance, specific aspects of the abuse experiences, the number of incidents, the duration of the abuse and the age when abuse started and ended.

It is important to note that because of the extreme trauma of the sexual abuse experience, many children 'block out' the memory of what has happened to them completely, and may only 'realise/remember' that they were sexually abused when they are in adulthood. Adults who have these abuse memories are extremely disturbed by what they remember, and often start a search for the 'answers' about what really happened, and why nobody helped them as children.

As a result, some mothers of sexually abused children may themselves have been abused as children and only start 'remembering' this when their child discloses that they are being abused. It is therefore vitally important to deal with the mother's pain as well, and to assist her in her discovery process (should this be what she decides). Never ignore an adult who tells you that they were sexually abused as a child, for they are experiencing the same trauma as the child and need therapeutic help. If one ignore the adults who have been sexually abused as children, they may turn to abusing children themselves if they cannot successfully 'overcome' their childhood experiences.

Childhood abuse is thus also important when dealing with the perpetrator (usually the male) and one should carefully investigate the possibility that he has experienced childhood trauma. In this way, one is better able to understand and counsel the abuser – by helping them to overcome their childhood experiences. Table 19.5 describes the myths about sexual abuse in children

Table 19.5 Myths and truths regarding child sexual abuse

Myth	Truth
Incest is not a common phenomenon among civilised people. Drunks and deviants may do it but never families like ours.	It happens in all socioeconomic groups, religions, race, creeds and countries. The saddest thing about incest is that the child is not safe in the one place they should feel safe, and that is home.
The abuser is always a stranger.	Up to 95 per cent of the time the victim knows the abuser.
The child is seductive and causes the adult to be sexually aroused.	It is the adult's responsibility and the adult's confusion regarding nurturance, sex and love.
Many children do not report sexual abuse because they are enjoying it.	Children do not report it because of fear, shame and anxiety. The child is also, very often, sworn to secrecy, threatened, bribed or blamed.
Fathers turn to their daughters sexually when their wives are not satisfying them sexually.	Not all fathers with sexual problems turn to their daughters. Those who do so are affected by role confusion and inadequate personalities/coping with personal stress.
No harm is done by sexual abuse if the child is not physically harmed.	Pregnancy, sexually transmitted diseases and genital trauma are usual results of abuse. However, a child who has been abused always suffers psychological trauma.
My child who was abused seems fine and does not need therapy.	All sexually abused children need to be assessed and treated by professional people. Repressed anxieties cause future problems.
Child sexual abuse never happened and the child is making it up.	Society generally does not want to believe that we do this to our children and therefore prefers to believe that children make it up. The fact that parents/people do not believe them is the most difficult problem children face. Children generally fantasise about positive events and will not use a traumatic event for fantasy.
Child sexual abuse reflects a caring relationship between perpetrator and victim.	It is not so and this is why the child suffers emotional trauma and symptomatic behaviour like aggression, violence, deceit, guilt, etc. The perpetrator only shows caring to entrap the child in an abusive relationship.
There is nothing we can do to stop child abuse. It is as old as mankind.	We can prevent child sexual abuse through education and that is why we have compiled this manual, to help you to do so, too.

Signs and symptoms of an abused child

Considering the various forms of child abuse, one may wonder how to determine whether a child has been abused. What are the signs and symptoms to look out for?

Symptoms of physical abuse
- As physical abuse leaves 'marks', this form of abuse is usually easiest to detect.
- Any injuries that are not consistent with the explanation offered (by the child or adult) should be further investigated. Signs often include continual bruising, cuts or burns.
- Another sign is the presence of several injuries that are in various stages of healing, indicating that they have been inflicted over a period of time.
- Facial injuries in infants and preschool children are also a common sign.
- It is important to remember that many parents will harm the child 'under the clothing' so that other adults (like teachers) will not be able to see the injuries.
- Physically abused children often fear punishment of any form.
- These children often do not want others to touch them at all.
- They may also appear fearful and distrustful most of the time (especially when conflict arises).

Symptoms of emotional abuse
These children have had their self-worth continually broken down. As a result, children who have been emotionally abused may react in many ways. However, reactions of emotionally abused children can often be seen in one of two ways:
1. They may become extremely attention seeking and even disruptive (because they do not receive this attention and affection at home) OR
2. Emotionally abused children may appear extremely withdrawn.

In general, a common symptom is a child with a very low self-esteem and they may seem too eager to please adults.

Symptoms of neglect
Like physical abuse, signs of neglect are quite easy to detect – especially if one knows the family circumstances. These include:
- A child who is continually dirty with 'uncombed' hair, dirt behind the ears, etc
- A child who is suffering from malnutrition – they are stunted in height, disease prone, lack energy, intellectually slow
- A child who has no stable home/guardians to take care of them.

Physical symptoms of sexual abuse

Children who have been sexually abused may or may not exhibit medical signs of abuse. What is definite is that their behaviour will change. These changes are very complex and require the opinion of a trained person or professional (see Table 19.4).

Remember that in two-thirds of children seen for suspected sexual abuse, there will be no physical signs. Only specially trained medical staff may examine sexually abused children.

Physical signs indicating acute sexual abuse

The following physical signs might be present in girls, boys and sodomised children:

Girls:
- vaginal tears and abrasions
- hymenal tears and abnormal dilatation
- presence of sperm or semen.

Boys:
- urethral discharge and bruising.

Sodomised children:
- anal dilatation, bruising and tears
- presence of sperm or semen in anal area.

Physical signs indicating chronic sexual abuse

These include the following:
- signs of venereal diseases namely, discharges, warts or ulcerations
- dilatation of hymenal opening and laxity of muscles surrounding genitals
- scars of hymen or vaginal wall
- poor anal tone, dilatation and scars.

Physical signs mistaken for sexual abuse

A number of physical symptoms might be mistaken for sexual abuse. The following should be taken into consideration to avoid these types of mistakes:
- Accidents, masturbation and the use of tampons are very unlikely to cause injury to the hymen or internal genital structures.
- Tampons do not alter hymenal integrity – studies show no difference in genital examinations of non-abused girls who use, or do not use tampons.
- Natural masturbation in girls is clitoral or labial and does not cause hymenal injury. (It is important to note that hymenal injury is painful.)
- Accidents such as straddle injuries commonly cause injury to anterior or lateral structures and not to the internal vaginal area. The pelvic skeleton and overlaying labia usually protect the hymen from injury. Penetrating injuries result from falls onto a pointed object and it is very rare for the object to penetrate through the hymenal opening into the vagina. In these very rare cases, the hymen is usually not

torn at all and penetration occurs at the lateral margin of the labia minora with the wound entering the vagina through its walls rather than through the hymen.

It is important to note that a violent stretching injury as when a child does a sudden split 'on a slippery surface' can cause midline laceration of genital structures. However, these injuries can also be caused during sexual abuse by violent forced opening of the legs.

The following four points should be taken into consideration:
1. None of the above signs or symptoms can be used on their own to prove child sexual abuse. Usually a child will display a variety of signs and symptoms (some not even behavioural or physical). Also, children who have experienced other emotional trauma (like divorce, witnessing acts of violence, etc) will also display some of these symptoms (especially those related to emotional abused) and may not necessarily have been sexually abused.
2. It is thus vital to explore further any child who is displaying a few of the mentioned symptoms.
3. Early identification of sexual abuse will greatly enhance the healing process.
4. If the abuse has occurred in the past 72 hours, it is considered to be a medical emergency. The child must be seen immediately as delaying the examination will result in the loss of essential information, such as presence of sperm. It is important that when possible the child is not changed, washed or bathed prior to the examination. The clothes that the child was wearing when the abuse happened should be taken with them to the medical personnel.

HANDLING DISCLOSURE ABOUT ABUSE

When a child discloses that they have been or are being abused, special care needs to be taken to handle the disclosure in a calm and sensitive manner. By law the abuse must be reported to the police, but many practitioners make the mistake of doing so in a dramatic and chaotic manner. This leaves the child feeling more out of control and afraid. Care should be taken to deal with the matter in a calm and caring manner. Give the child as much control as possible, even if this is over small decisions such as whom to tell first. But do take important decisions for the child and give the impression that one is a calm and confident adult who is not overwhelmed by the situation. Always keep the child informed; explain to whom one will be talking about the abuse and what one will be saying.

The child's caregivers need to be informed about the matter. Always tell the caregivers without the child present. Parents are likely to react in an emotional manner, which may make the child feel worse. Spend time with the parents to ensure that they are calm before they see the child. You may even discuss with them what they intend saying to the child during the first interaction.

When the mental health nurse reports the matter to the police, ensure the privacy of the child. For example, do not call the police to the clinic or school, or discuss the matter in front of other people. If one of the parents was involved in the abuse, for example, the father, rather have him removed from the home than taking the child away. Placing a frightened child in a strange environment is not helpful at all. If the child needs to be removed from the home, try to take them to a familiar place, such as another family member's house.

HELPING CHILDREN AFFECTED BY TRAUMA

The aims and structure of trauma counselling (see 'Trauma counselling and interventions' in this chapter) can be helpful, although the following should be kept in mind when working with children:

- Children affected by trauma may take much longer to develop trust and to feel safe with an adult. The mental health nurse may need to spend several sessions with the child simply building trust.
- Many children express themselves better through activities such as playing games, drawing pictures and making clay models. Take the time to determine the way in which the child expresses themselves best.
- Once a child is ready to talk about the trauma, they may talk in a stop-and-start manner. This is normal. The child will usually talk in small 'steps' and then not want to talk any more. It is important to be patient and not to push the child into talking about everything at once.
- Because children often feel confused about a traumatic event, time should be spent on helping them to understand what happened. If children are able to organise the event in their memory, they tend to recover better.
- It is important to note that it is unhelpful to expose children to the media about a traumatic event. For example, if they were involved in a train disaster, photographic images in newspapers, radio newscast descriptions, and television footage accompanied by sound have been shown to add to the horror.
- Children's tendency towards magical thinking and self-blame indicates that care must be taken to reassure children that the event was not their fault. First take time to understand exactly why the child thinks it was their fault. Then explain, several times, that the event did not take place because of 'something bad' the child may have done.
- Do not be tempted to provide false explanations. Often one thinks these will make the child feel better, but they may confuse the child more. Also be careful about adding religious connotations to the event, for example saying that 'God meant for this to happen'. Once children are older, they will be in a better position to understand and make sense of what happened and to attach their own meaning to it.
- Safety rituals may be developed. Ask the child what helps them to feel safer. For example, some children like to have a light on at night. Take the child's ideas seriously and never ridicule them, no matter how odd the request.
- It is important to get children back to their normal routine soon after the event. Get children back to school quickly and keep normal bedtimes and other routines. However, if the event occurred at a place to which a child has to return, care should be taken to ensure that the child feels safe.

- Make some allowances for acting out. Expect, and allow for, some tantrums and sensitive behaviour, while retaining some limits. This is a difficult balance to reach. Parents and teachers may need support in giving the child a chance to express feelings while, at the same time, keeping safe boundaries.

The Regional Psychosocial Support Initiative (REPSSI, 2011) have developed a handbook on hero work with children. This means helping them to restructure the trauma story in a way that puts them into the position of a hero who survived the experience.

Counselling children who have been abused usually involves a long-term relationship between the MHCU and counsellor. Consistent caring, safety and support are important. Do not rush the MHCU through any stages of the counselling process. Focus instead on developing a safe space where the MHCU will spontaneously begin to deal with some of the painful past experiences. Children who have been severely physically, emotionally or sexually abused usually benefit from specialised counselling from a psychologist. This may be in the form of play therapy or art therapy for younger children, and verbal therapy for older children.

Bear in mind that one should not only consider the dramatic forms of abuse, that is, sexual abuse and rape. There are many subtle forms of sexual harassment taking place in our society and these also need to be addressed. A health care practitioner is in a position to play a constructive role in the education and empowerment of boys and girls regarding rights and responsibilities. This may prevent further abuse in future.

> *I have learned that it is OK to express my feelings. I was brought up and taught to obey and respect adults, but these days there are people who influence children with bad things, and I know I have the right to say no politely.* (Sinani children's group member)

Holistic management of abused children

Children who have been abused need a holistic form of management. This involves managing physical, emotional, intellectual, social and spiritual dimensions. Consideration should also be paid to the victim's mother. These different dimensions are discussed in the following section.

Physical dimension

When sexual abuse has occurred, it is necessary for the child to obtain antibiotics and post-exposure prophylaxis if penetration took place. Girls who have already reached puberty should receive 'morning-after pills' in the first 72 hours after penetration to prevent pregnancy. Hospital admission is indicated if:
- the child cannot be adequately examined without sedation
- there is a risk of further abuse if the child is sent home
- the child is in need of further investigations or treatment, for example if vaginal bleeding is present.

Emotional dimension

When working with abused children it is important for the helper to:
- respond to victim in a non-judgemental, supportive manner
- reassure the child that they are not to blame for sexual offences
- provide opportunities to experience safe closeness with the potential for interpersonal trust
- encourage the expression of feelings
- encourage the child to interact with groups for victims of incest and sexual abuse. The groups allow victims to confront their fears and anger with support from other victims. They begin to conceptualise themselves as survivors rather than helpless victims
- individual psychotherapy also promotes emotional healing and is usually considered a vital part of the recovery process for abused children. A qualified psychologist or social worker specialising in sexual abuse does this. Teachers, doctors, nurses and other health professionals are *not* qualified to do individual therapy with victims.

Intellectual dimension

In this dimension, a number of preventative measures can be implemented to help avoid future situations of abuse. If the child has been abused, the measures can also assist the child in gaining a cognitive understanding of the abuse.

Preventative measures: early understanding of sexual function

The following sequence of messages should be conveyed by parents and teachers (the language can be adjusted according to the child's age):
- Affection is about caring about family, fellow humans and pets. This involvement evokes warm, pleasant feelings in people of all ages. This affection often involves 'nice' touches. Children should also learn about the negative feelings when being disciplined and feeling lonely, as well as the pleasant feelings of reconciliation.
- Children need to identify unpleasant touches, which are rough and hurt and/or give them a 'bad' feeling. Parents and teachers can help children identify and express what their body is feeling, be it pleasant or unpleasant. Children should be taught that affection is needed by all and occurs between people of all age groups.
- By the age of two or three, children know that boys are different from girls. Often children want to look at one another's bodies to check out the differences – this is normal. They need to be taught that we wear clothes to protect ourselves from the elements (wind, rain, sun, etc) and it is our custom to cover our genitalia/private parts.
- A simple way of showing the young child where their private parts are is by playing a game of crossing the arms over the mouth, chest, groin and buttock.
- As children become a little older, they will want to know about what is inside their body and how their organs work. Teachers/parents need to supply their children with a detailed diagram of the skeleton and bones and how these support the

muscles so our limbs can move. Children should also be told about their lungs and breathing. It can be pointed out how food and liquid pass through the body and how waste is excreted, and the different position males and females use to excrete. It is important to tell children the correct biological names.
- It is also important to explain the sexual function of our body and why the penis is outside the body and how the male seeds are planted inside the female's body where the egg cell is protected through the vaginal opening. (Obviously this discussion is done on different levels depending on the children's age).
- It is best to start talking to children about sexual matters when the child is young and starts questioning. It is important that the child receive the message that sex is and learning about it is a fact of life and not something to fear or be ashamed of. Parents and teachers should continue by explaining the process of falling in love, dating, marriage and conception of children.
- Children should know that a male and female meet and develop a special closeness and trust. This couple expresses these positive feelings by kissing, holding hands and hugging. When couples love each other so much and always want to be together, then they decide to marry.
- Within this union couples express their love by having sex and our anatomy (bodies) makes provision for this. Children should be taught that when couples are ready and by means of this same process, a baby is conceived.
- Children also need to know that the foetus grows inside the mother and after nine months is ready for delivery. It must be explained that the mother is hospitalised and the doctor assists in the delivery. The child must be told that the baby can be born down the birth canal and out of the vagina. They should also be told about breast feeding and bottle feeding, and that bonding takes place because the mother holds the baby and shows affection at feeding times, etc.
- Children should be told about gaining control of their bodily functions and progressing from nappies to a potty and then a toilet. They should also learn about cleanliness and the need to bath.

In this way, children can gain an understanding of the whole body and how they fit into the world. It is important that teachers/parents repeat this educational process until their child has a clear understanding.

Equipping the child with knowledge to prevent sexual abuse
Now that the child has an understanding of their sexual functioning, teachers/parents should start talking to their children about sexual abuse.
- It is important that children are not only given specific rules about strangers in cars or dark alleys with sweets, etc. Children need to be equipped to deal with a broad range of situations.
- By now the children should know about pleasant and unpleasant feelings, and how to express how their body feels and to communicate this to one as a teacher/parent.

- Teachers/parents must encourage children to communicate any unpleasant feeling to them.
- They must also know that they can communicate any unpleasant feeling to anybody. Thus, if a friend is pulling their hair, they have the right not to like it and to tell that person to stop. Children need to be comfortable with saying 'No'.
- Children also need to know that sexual abuse may often evoke pleasant feelings but that it is not to be allowed. They are often lured or tricked into an isolated situation by a friendly and kind adult, which frequently leads to abuse over time.

Safety rules that need to be taught include:
- If I'm in a situation, do I get a pleasant (good) or unpleasant (bad) feeling?
- Does my parent/responsible adult know where I am?
- Can I get help in this situation if I need it?

Children need to be able to answer 'Yes' to all these questions. Should a child get an unpleasant (bad) feeling and a 'No' answer, they must run and tell their parent or responsible adult.

An important aspect of prevention is talking to children about secret keeping. Children must be taught that there are good and bad secrets: Good secrets are like what you and Mom are giving Dad for Christmas. These secrets are fine. Bad secrets are any secrets that make you unhappy or worried at keeping. These secrets must be told to Mom and Dad or a responsible adult immediately.

Children need to know that child abusers often disguise their motives by involving the child in a bad type of game. Bad games involve engaging a child in sexualised play, which involves the child touching, or being touched on their private parts. If children have unpleasant feelings about a game, they have the right to say no.

Children must realise that they have the right to say no to any adult in a difficult situation. They must yell and attract attention to get others to help them.

Social dimension

Suspected or confirmed cases of incest or sexual exploitation should be registered and the family should be investigated by a welfare organisation. Health care providers are in violation with the law if they do not report the cases.

Interventions are designed to assist victims to develop peer relationships and to expand social networks; the caregiver helps them identify activities that may lead to meeting with people of their own age with similar interests, for example participating in community education programmes. The Child Protection Unit (of the South African Police Service) is notified to assist in protecting the victim. Teenagers are encouraged to remain in or return to school.

Spiritual dimension

The mental health nurse assists the victim if necessary, to locate people of various religions in the community who are particularly sensitive to counselling victims with spiritual problems resulting from sexual abuse.

Managing the victim's mother

Whether the sexual abuse has occurred within the family (incest) or not, the mother of the child victim, is one of the most important people in the child's recovery (Bagley & King, 1990). This is because the reaction of the mother and her subsequent support (or lack of support) have a tremendous impact on the child's view of themselves and of the abuse experience. As a result, helping the mother of the child victim becomes essential, for if a mother 'falls apart' and cannot successfully cope with what the child has told her, the child will not have anyone to turn to for family love and support.

Once a disclosure has been made, it is important to get the mother involved (particularly if the abuser is *not* her husband/boyfriend). In cases where the abuser is not the mother's spouse or partner, the teacher may contact the mother and relate to her what the child has said (provided they have the child's permission to do so). However, it is always preferable to get the referring agency to involve the mother directly (for example, a Childline social worker will set up a meeting with the mother). If teachers/community workers do have contact with the mother, it is essential that they remain calm and professional and simply relate the child's symptoms as they are evidenced in the school environment, and provide a factual detailing of the disclosure, while making sure not to 'accuse' or blame the mother for the abuse in any way.

It should be remembered that sometimes (often in cases of incest), the mother has been consciously or unconsciously aware of what has been happening, but has been trying to deny the abuse and refuses to face reality. These mothers are frequently described as 'inadequate' women, because they are often unemployed, cannot provide good care for their children, or suffer from physical or mental illness. They often experience other kinds of problems which have an impact on their self-esteem, such as being battered by their partners, having a substance abuse problem, or being mentally unstable.

Unfortunately, society seems to blame the mother (often more than the abuser) for not protecting the child and for 'colluding' in the abuse, when in fact, several important factors have often made it impossible for her to protect the child or to remove herself and children from the situation. Some of these include economic dependency, cultural traditions and the oppressed position of women in South African society.

By counselling the mother of the abused child, one is often able to 'empower' her to accept her rights as a woman, as a mother and as a wife. In this way, with increased self-esteem, she is better able to support and understand her abused child, and often even becomes a resource for other mothers in the community.

In counselling the mother, similar issues to what the abused child experiences will arise – feelings of helplessness, powerlessness, guilt and shame, anger and loss.

WORKING WITH GROUPS AFFECTED BY TRAUMA

I realised that other people in this group felt the same as me, and we could understand each other. (Member of a Sinani women's group)

Families

Sometimes a whole family may be involved in a traumatic experience together. This is a difficult situation, but if the family is well supported, the experience of what they went through together may even strengthen their relationships with one another.

Be aware of the following dynamics when working with families affected by a traumatic experience:

- Family members may feel responsible for one another. Individuals often feel much guilt for not having been able to protect one another.
- There may also be some blaming, where family members feel betrayed by one another and/or are angry with one another.
- A strong element of shame is often present, where family members feel embarrassed about what they have been through together.
- In some cases, families may feel that their dignity as a family has been damaged by the event.
- Remember that different family members will have different ways of coping with the event. Some may be very avoidant and may not want to deal with the event, while others may want to talk about it openly and confront what happened. Care needs to be taken to make space for these differences within the healing process.

It is usually helpful to see each family member individually. This gives people a chance to talk about their own experiences of the trauma. It is also important to deal with anger and blame towards other family members, so that these are not expressed in a harmful way towards others in the family.

At some stage it may be helpful to see the whole family together, to talk about how the experience has affected them as a group. Very young children should not be included in family sessions, and it may be better to see children and caregivers separately. However, older children and teenagers may be involved in family sessions.

Keep the following in mind during family sessions:

- Carefully structure the sessions so as to make people feel safer. The trauma support workers should be organised and have a clear plan for the session.
- Remember, as the trauma support worker, one is dealing only with the trauma incident. Do not be tempted to deal with other family dynamics that may be of concern at this stage. If other issues arise and need to be dealt with, they should be focused on as a separate process.
- Allow each family member to express their version of what happened. Other family members may find it helpful to hear these different perspectives and to find out about other aspects of the event.

- It is important to deal with feelings of guilt and self-blame. Allow each person to talk about why they feel guilty. Encourage other family members to reassure those who feel guilty that they are not to blame.
- Normalise reactions to the trauma. Talk about different individual styles of coping with trauma and how the family might make space for these.
- Discuss how the family will cope with the event together. Encourage family members to deal openly with the event and not to pretend that it never occurred.

It is always helpful to work together with a colleague when supporting families affected by trauma.

Survivor groups

Group work with survivors of trauma can be one of the most effective forms of support. There are several reasons why groups work well for many trauma survivors:
- Many people feel *safer* working in a group rather than alone.
- In many cultures, it is *more appropriate* to process a major event, such as trauma, together with other people.
- Hearing other people's stories can offer a *sense of relief*.
- Survivors often feel *less alone* when they know others have also been through difficulties.
- Members of the group are able to *support one another*.
- Having your story heard and *accepted* by several people similar to yourself can be a powerful step in the healing process.

However, there are some aspects to bear in mind when working with groups:
- Some people feel less safe in a group and more comfortable talking to just one person. This is often true for people who have been raped or sexually abused. Once again, *never force anyone to share*, but wait until people are ready to share. Encourage group members to talk but allow them the choice not to.
- It may be unhelpful for people to *compare* their traumatic experiences, for example by saying, 'Well, if that is what you went through, my experience wasn't so bad.' Trauma is a personal experience; group members should not rate their traumas in comparison to those of other members.
- Make sure that each person has *enough time* to share their story. Some members may try to block a person's sharing if they become overwhelmed by the story. This may reinforce the idea that the trauma is too terrible to talk about. Also, the possibility of secondary traumatisation by listening to others' stories of victimisation must be considered and managed in the group.
- The initial phase of *establishing safety* is very important and should not be rushed. The issues around confidentiality and trust should be discussed fully. Give group members time to get to know one another properly in the beginning.

Structuring shared experiences

As with individual trauma counselling, sharing experiences should be well structured. The following stages of the counselling model may be applied to groups:

- The idea is to give each group member an opportunity to talk about their experience in detail. Group members should be encouraged to respect individual differences with regard to how much detail the person is willing to share. Be guided by the person telling the story as to how much detail they are ready to share.
- Groups offer a powerful way of normalising trauma responses. Allow group members a chance to talk about how the trauma has affected them. Usually it brings a measure of relief to hear that their responses are normal and that others went through similar reactions.
- Groups also offer a valuable chance to process feelings such as anger and guilt. Having several people acknowledge these feelings is very helpful.
- Sharing ideas about coping is helpful in that it tells people how others are managing under difficult circumstances. This sharing of ideas may assist people in finding better ways of coping themselves, or it may let them know that they are, in fact, doing well.

Supporting communities affected by trauma

Many communities affected by trauma, and especially by violence, have had the normal social fabric of the community unravelled. This means that the usual relationships and social structures have been challenged. The work of reweaving the social fabric involves reconnecting people to one another and rebuilding or repairing structures. It is important for people to participate once again in activities that link them to other people. Re-establishing these links is the main role of the trauma support worker.

The attitude displayed by a trauma support worker towards community members who have been affected by trauma is a most important aspect. Working with communities requires the same principles of respect and trust as those mentioned in relation to individuals. However, long-term commitment is also necessary. Trauma support workers are often tempted to rush in after a community has been affected by a trauma, and certainly their main aim is to help. But many trauma support workers are only able to work with the community for a short space of time. This can actually be more harmful than helpful. Many communities feel abused when people, who rushed into the area during the hype of the trauma, leave again soon afterwards. If one has only a short period of time available, it is better to support the people who will be working in the community for a long time (such as nurses and police). Always check to find out what these people would find helpful or extend an open invitation for them to contact you if they need help at any stage.

Trauma support workers should not see themselves as the ones who are going to make the changes in a community. Instead, they should try to build on what is already happening and empower the community itself. Community members know what is best

for them. They should be encouraged to support one another, rather than relying on the trauma support worker. Trauma support workers should try to:
- Build on resources already present in the community, rather than creating new projects.
- Link different structures, for example if doing training in trauma support work, invite representatives from government departments, churches and traditional healers' associations to attend the training. This promotes connections between community members, which is the main aim of support work in communities affected by violence and other forms of trauma.

Trauma support workers commonly make the mistake of assuming they know what is best for a community. A trauma support worker should take seriously the needs of the community. They should work with expressed needs and support people affected by trauma while working on meeting these needs. For example, it would not be helpful to set up a trauma counselling office when people really need food and shelter. They should take time to find out what the most urgent needs of the community are and offer trauma support at the same time or later, once a trusting relationship has been built.

Violence and trauma tend to affect every person in the community. Where one has sufficient time, it is better to work with different groups within the same community.

Some of the community groups affected by trauma include:
- those in leadership
- service providers (such as nurses, social workers, traditional healers, police)
- adults (both men and women)
- youth (especially ex-combatants where there has been civil conflict)
- children and their caregivers.

Since a trauma support worker usually does not have the resources to work with every member of a community, it is a good idea to look for 'points of leverage'. This means thinking carefully about existing structures within which you can work in order to reach the largest number of people. Examples of community structures – in which one works with a few people, and these people then have an impact on a lot of other community members – include the following:
- leadership structures, such as development committees
- schools and crèches
- support groups, for example burial societies, savings groups
- churches and other religious or spiritual groups
- traditional healers' associations
- government workers, such as doctors, nurses, social workers and police.

It is important to discuss the community's needs with community members and leaders. Trauma support work is much more effective if it happens in response to a request from a community or group.

It should be borne in mind that individual counselling is not necessarily the most effective way to reach people. The trauma support worker should also consider:
- utilising sport and arts activities such as singing and drama
- training others to do trauma support work
- initiating projects to raise awareness and normalise the effects of trauma
- organising income-generating and career-development activities
- organising leadership skills development workshops
- running parenting skills development projects.

Community members should be consulted for advice on the kinds of activities that would be most suitable in the community.

CONCLUSION

This chapter highlights violence as a global public health problem. The mental health consequences experienced by individuals exposed to violence such as physical, sexual, and emotional abuse cannot be over-emphasised. As a mental health nurse, one will have to be skilled and be prepared to interact and manage different people exposed to violence, including those who are part of the vulnerable population.

APPENDIX I
Specific traumas or groups
Rape

One of the most traumatic of experiences is rape. Rape also involves some of the most stressful types of counselling. The normal model of trauma counselling is usually helpful, bearing in mind the following key aspects:
- Avoidance is usually very strong with rape survivors and many fear talking about the rape itself. Most will talk about what happened before and after the act of rape but will avoid mentioning aspects related to the actual time of the rape. The counsellor needs to be very gentle and patient. Be aware that it could take several sessions for the person to build up enough trust to talk in detail about the rape. However, take care not to collude with the avoidance. As a counsellor one usually feels great sympathy and it might seem cruel to 'make' someone talk about such a terrible act. But the person's rate of recovery depends on how soon they are able to begin talking about it.
- Trust in others is usually severely affected. Take time to build this trust, and do not take it personally if the rape survivor seems to take a long time to begin trusting you.
- Be prepared for 'stop-and-start' sessions, where the person talks about some aspects and then does not wish to continue. It is fine to cover the different aspects in stages. The person may also alternate: they may be willing to talk about the rape in one session, but only about general topics in the next session. This is normal. Do not try to rush things.

- Rape survivors almost always blame themselves for what happened. Let the person talk openly about this guilt, before trying to persuade them that it was not their fault. Once the person has expressed the guilt and self-blame, emphasise that no one deserves to go through such an experience. Even if the person placed themselves at risk in some way – for example, by being in a dark area – they did not deserve to be attacked and raped. You may need to repeat this point many times.
- Male counsellors need to be particularly sensitive. Although both male and female counsellors need to proceed with caution, male counsellors in particular should guard against being perceived as 'too interested' in unnecessary details. A person will be hypersensitive to any sign that a counsellor is 'fascinated' by the rape. Exercise caution in the way you introduce the topic and ask questions about the details. Remain totally focused on the person, and on the person's experience and feelings, not on the rapist's actions. Some people believe men should not counsel women who have been raped, because there is a high risk of secondary traumatisation; others believe it may contribute to healing if a male counsellor deals sensitively with a female MHCU. Always allow a woman the choice of speaking to a female counsellor.
- Be sure to discuss ways of feeling safe at home, or in other places, such as at work or while travelling to work. Find out whether there are people with whom the person feels safe and explore ways they can spend more time with these people.
- Encourage the person to be open with a friend or friends about what has happened.
- Always try to speak to the immediate family about the rape (after getting permission from the victim), particularly the partner of the person who has been raped.
- For people in existing partnerships, couples counselling is almost always a good idea after a rape.
- A woman's (male) partner will need to talk about his own distress, which usually includes anger or guilt. Let him talk about this at a session at which the MHCU herself is not present. Once he has had a chance to express his feelings, try to sensitise him to her needs. Emphasise that it may take his partner a long time to recover, and that his patience and care are essential. Encourage him to ask his partner what she would regard as helpful or not helpful in terms of his behaviour towards her.
- Deal with the feelings of family and partners with regard to apportioning blame. They may be angry with the person for placing themselves in a risky situation. Again, emphasise that no one deserves rape or wishes for it to happen. Often, the feeling underlying blame is guilt (being unable to offer protection, etc); try to make space for this guilt to be expressed.
- There are almost always problems with sexuality after a rape. A woman may experience fear during subsequent sexual encounters, even with a trusted partner. Often sexual contact creates strong flashbacks. Alert both partners to this likelihood. Where possible, the woman should initiate sexual contact with the man. He should be prepared for the fact that she may back away several times, even though she initiated the contact. This is completely normal; she should not be rushed, and he should expect her to be 'hot and cold'.

Chapter 19: People who have Experienced Trauma

- On the other hand, if the partner is cautious about approaching the woman sexually, many women feel rejected by the man. They feel the rape has made them unattractive. Alert both to this possibility and talk about how this may be handled, for example, by the man explaining that he still loves her and is still interested, but that he will not initiate sexual contact. If this is clear to both, they may find things somewhat easier and make better progress.
- Obviously, talking openly about what is going on is the best for both partners.
- At times the woman may wish for intimate contact (for example, being held or hugged), without this contact being sexual. It helps if both are aware of this. It helps if she is able to communicate this clearly, and they may even need to develop a shared 'code' to let one another know the intentions.
- Remember that a rape case may reach the courts, so keep notes and make sure you explain the limits of confidentiality to the MHCU.
- Remind yourself that one of the most healing aspects of rape is the fact that the person knows there is someone else who knows and cares.

Case example for a rape case
A mental health nurse, Agnes, had seen a number of MHCUs in the clinic who had been victims of violence. She has been working long and had little support from her management. Recently, her case load had included more and more women who had been traumatised by rape or domestic violence. Over time, she became increasingly nervous when going home after work and when walking alone in her neighbourhood. One of her most recent MHCUs had been brutally raped by a male friend and Agnes found that this MHCU had really upset her. She was of a similar age to Agnes and Agnes found that she could really identify with her MHCU's experience.

Recently, Agnes has become increasingly withdrawn from friends and colleagues, and has begun to avoid late afternoon appointments, so that she would not have to go home in the dark. She has had difficulty sleeping and cannot concentrate at work. Her colleagues have noticed that she is more irritable. She began to refuse to see male clients and the mental health team realised that there was a problem.

The team members asked her if she was getting enough support for her work and encouraged her to talk about her feelings associated with her trauma work. Through discussions with her manager, adjustments were made to her case load and fewer trauma MHCUs were booked for her. It emerged that Agnes herself had been sexually abused as a child and these early memories were intruding on her work. She was encouraged to see a therapist. Agnes also recognised that she was too isolated and her work had become her life. She began to go out more with friends and she joined a gym, which helped her manage her stress. She also found a colleague on her team that she could talk to about the MHCUs that had really upset her and they were available to each other for peer supervision.

Nursing care process

Case example
Janet, a 29-year-old woman who has been raped by a gang of five armed men over a period of four hours, was brought to the psychiatric clinic by her sister, two weeks after the event happened.

Assessment

Physical

Assess physical injuries sustained in the rape. Prioritise life threatening injuries such as bleeding, head injuries, and signs of internal bleeding. Take routine bloods and other specimens. Check gait and the extent of physical functioning. If needed, facilitate hospitalisation immediately.

Clarify where physical signs may be due to emotional states for example tachycardia, sweating and flushing may be due to shock, fear and panic.

As two weeks had elapsed since the rape, the nurse counsellor checked what medical attention Janet had received after the rape. She had not gone for any help, as she felt too ashamed. Therefore, routine investigations were done including a physical examination, routine blood tests and completion of medico-legal forms.

Emotional

Assess emotional expression and themes and appropriateness of affect. Evaluate response patterns. Monitor facial expressions, posture, and emotional expressions and mood.

Janet initially presented as emotionally numb and cut off. After some time with the nurse counsellor, she began to discuss her ordeal. Prominent feelings that emerged were feelings of guilt and shame as well as anger.

Social

Assess the MHCU's self-concept, interpersonal relationships, socialisation, cultural and environmental factors.

Since the incident occurred Janet had become increasingly withdrawn. She had ended her relationship with her boyfriend and had not told him about the rape, as she feared he would blame her. Her sister appeared very supportive but did not know how she could help. Janet said she had difficulty trusting people, especially men, as she had known her attackers.

She had a poor self-esteem and complained of feeling dirty and wanting to wash all the time. She also blamed herself for not doing more during the rape to stop it happening. She was worried about the stigma that would now be attached to her as a rape victim within her cultural community.

Spiritual

Assess the meaning attached to the trauma and the belief in powers greater than oneself. This is particularly significant in that spiritual belief is an important factor that enhances coping with trauma.

Janet belonged to the Zion Christian Church but since the incident had not been to the church and felt angry with God. She also worried that she may be punished because she had not carried out 'tasks' from the church which would serve as a healing ritual.

Intellectual

Observe MHCU's perception, memory, cognition, communication, flexibility and rigidity.

Janet could not remember all the details of the trauma. She had difficulty concentrating and her immediate memory was not good. The nurse counsellor had to repeat questions on occasion. On questioning, she admitted to intrusive memories and flashbacks of the incident. These were not hallucinatory in nature. It was difficult for her to discuss sexual details about the rapes spontaneously. Her knowledge about her rights as a victim were poor and it was difficult to persuade her to report the case to the police.

The nursing diagnosis

Based on the assessment of the above dimensions, a diagnosis will be formulated.
In this case example, Janet was diagnosed as suffering from post-traumatic stress as a result of her trauma.

Table 19.6 The nursing care plan

Problem	Evidence	Objective	Intervention
Physical – vaginal discharge and bruising of genital area, headaches and stomach cramps; scar on forehead	Found on medical examination – Janet had not seen any doctor following the rape	To treat any ailment resulting from the rape and to prevent complications such as sexually transmitted diseases or pregnancy	▪ Medical examination, and then routine blood tests ▪ Treat the discharge. ▪ Send for further tests to exclude for internal injuries ▪ Education on self-care
Emotional – numb, angry, guilt, shame	Janet verbalised these feelings and emotional expression was congruent to what she was expressing	To provide a safe environment for Janet to express her feelings and/or talk about the horror of her experience	▪ Build rapport and follow trauma counselling steps

Social – Janet was withdrawn, mistrustful; sister wanted to help	Janet has not told anybody other than her sister; she does not want to socialise, go to church and has left her boyfriend; her sister confirmed her withdrawal	To increase Janet's social support, as this is the most important factor that aids coping	▪ Explore with Janet available support systems, eg family, friends, church and work ▪ Develop practical steps to link into support structures ▪ Advise sister on ways of supporting Janet ▪ Address Janet's perceived stereotypes of rape and cultural attitudes, which were preventing her from getting support
Spiritual – Janet had not been able to use her spiritual belief as a way of coping	She had not returned to church since the incident and expressed anxiety about not fulfilling necessary healing rituals; she expressed anger at God	For Janet to be able to perform religious rituals for healing	▪ Link her to the church by exploring whom she felt comfortable to talk to within the church ▪ Encourage her to verbalise her anger at God and her fears regarding how the church would respond
Intellectual – poor concentration and memory of the trauma as well as immediate memory; inadequate knowledge about her rights	Unable to remember all the questions during the session and to report all the details of the trauma; had not reported case to the police and delayed seeking help	To restore normal functioning and to empower Janet to effectively pursue her human rights	▪ Check her level of education which may contribute to her understanding ▪ Provide information and education and help her to take things one step at a time ▪ Help her to understand her memory difficulties in the context of PTSD

Implementing the nursing care plan
Implement above steps and arrange for ongoing trauma counselling.

Evaluation
Check each of the above dimensions using information of subjective and objective data. Assess level of improvement in trauma symptoms and deal with any symptoms that have not been resolved through an action plan. Evaluation and planning need to be ongoing.

Janet attended weekly counselling for a period of six weeks at the clinic. She also went for further medical examinations, which were clear. Her vaginal discharge was treated and cleared. Over the course of counselling, there was an improvement in her symptoms and she became less withdrawn. A joint session was held together with her boyfriend during which she told him of what had happened, and he was encouraged to be supportive. She rejoined her church and felt less anxious as she had performed various healing rituals. At the end of counselling, she was motivated to start a support group for other rape survivors.

Janet chose not to report the case to the police, as she feared intimidation within her community. The nursing counsellor tried to work with this but Janet's fear appeared realistic.

APPENDIX II

TABLE #1 Developmental guidelines: Children's reactions to trauma (infancy to 2½ years)

General trauma reactions	Sexual abuse – specific reactions	Memory for trauma	Parental support
■ Disruption of sleeping and toileting ■ Startle responses to loud/unusual noises ■ 'Freezing' (sudden immobility of body) ■ Fussiness, uncharacteristic crying and neediness ■ Loss of acquired speech and motor skills ■ Separation fears and clinging to caretakers ■ Withdrawal, lack of usual responsiveness ■ Avoidance of or alarm response to specific trauma-related reminders involving sights and physical sensations	■ Usual concern/attention to own or others' private parts ■ Demonstration of adult sexual behaviour or knowledge through behaviour ■ Sudden, intense masturbation ■ Inappropriate private touching of others ■ Genital pain, bruising, inflammation, bleeding, discharge or diagnosis of sexually transmitted diseases	■ Memory of trauma may be evident in behaviour or play ■ Snatches of incomplete memory or visual images may remain in memory and be given verbal description by toddlers	■ Maintain child's routine around sleep and eating ■ Avoid unnecessary separations from important caretakers ■ Provide additional soothing activities ■ Maintain calm atmosphere in child's presence ■ Avoid exposing child to reminders of trauma ■ Expect child's temporary regression; do not panic ■ Help verbal child to give simple names to big feelings; talk about event in simple terms during brief chats ■ Give simple play props related to the actual trauma to a child who is trying to play out the frightening situation (a doctor's kit, a toy ambulance, toy doll, etc)

Source: Monahon (1993)

TABLE #2 Developmental guidelines: Children's reactions to trauma (2½–6 years)

General trauma reactions	Sexual abuse – specific reactions	Memory for trauma	Parental support
▪ Repeated retelling of traumatic event ▪ Behavioural, mood and personality changes ▪ Obvious anxiety and fearfulness ▪ Withdrawal and quieting ▪ Specific trauma-related fears; general fearfulness ▪ Post-traumatic play often obvious ▪ Involvement of playmates in trauma-related play at school and day care ▪ Regression to behaviour of younger child ▪ Loss of recently acquired skills (language, toileting, eating, self-care) ▪ Separation anxiety with primary caretakers	▪ Sexualised play with toys or other children ▪ Unusual concern about or attention to own private parts ▪ Uncharacteristic, at times, intense, masturbation ▪ Inappropriate and/or aggressive touching of others or sexualised relating ▪ Sudden, specific fears or mistrust of males, females or particular places	▪ Memory of at least some visual images from traumatic event is likely for the youngest children; many demonstrate recall in words or play ▪ At the older end of this age range, children are more likely to have lasting, accurate verbal and pictorial memory for central events of the trauma	▪ Listen to and tolerate child's retelling of the event ▪ Respect child's fears; give child time to cope with the fears ▪ Protect child from re-exposure to frightening situations and reminders of trauma, including scary TV programmes, movies, stories, and physical or locational reminders of the trauma ▪ Accept and help the child name strong feelings during brief conversations (the child cannot talk about these feelings or the experience for long) ▪ Expect and understand child's regression while maintaining basic household rules ▪ Expect some difficult or uncharacteristic behaviour

→

General trauma reactions	Sexual abuse – specific reactions	Memory for trauma	Parental support
■ Loss of interest in activities ■ Sleep disturbances: nightmares, night terrors, sleep walking, fearfulness of going to sleep and being alone at night ■ Confusion and inadequate understanding of traumatic events most evident in play rather than discussion ■ Unclear understanding of death and the causes of 'bad' events ■ Magical explanations to fill in gaps of understanding ■ Complaints about bodily aches, pains, or illness with no medical explanation ■ Visual images and unpleasant memories of trauma that intrude in child's mind but will seldom be discussed spontaneously	■ Physical indicators: genital pain, bruising, bleeding, inflammation, discharge, diagnosis of sexually transmitted disease		■ Set firm limits on hurtful or scary play and behaviour ■ Avoid non-essential separations from important caretakers with fearful children ■ Maintain household and family routines that comfort the child ■ Avoid introducing new and challenging experiences for the child ■ Provide additional night-time comforts when possible; night-lights, stuffed animals, physical comforting after nightmares ■ Explain to child that nightmares come from the fears a child has inside, that they are not real, and that they will occur less and less over time ■ Provide opportunities and props for trauma-related play

→

General trauma reactions	Sexual abuse – specific reactions	Memory for trauma	Parental support
- Loss of energy and concentration at school - Fear of trauma recurring - Increased need for control - Vulnerable to anniversary reactions set off by seasonal reminders, holidays, and other events			- Use detective skills to discover trigger for sudden fearfulness or regression - Monitor child's coping in school and day care by communicating with teaching staff and expressing concerns - Listen to child's misunderstandings of traumatic event, particularly those that involve self-blame, magical thinking - Gently help child develop realistic understanding of the event - Remain aware of your own reactions to the child's trauma - Provide reassurance to child that feelings will diminish over time - Provide opportunities for child to experience control and make choices in daily activities - Be mindful of the possibility of anniversary reactions

TABLE #3 Developmental guidelines: Children's reactions to trauma (6–11 years)

General trauma reactions	Sexual abuse – specific reactions	Memory for trauma	Parental support
<ul><li>Repeated retelling of traumatic event</li><li>Obvious anxiety and fearfulness</li><li>Specific post-traumatic fears</li><li>Post-traumatic reenactments of traumatic event that may occur secretly and involve siblings or playmates</li><li>Fear of trauma's recurring</li><li>Intrusion of unwanted visual images and traumatic memory that disrupt concentration and create anxiety, often without parents' awareness</li><li>Loss of ability to concentrate and attend at school, with lowering of performance</li><li>'Spacey' or distractible behaviour</li></ul>	<ul><li>Engages in explicit sexual behaviours with other children or attempts to engage older children or adults sexually</li><li>Verbally describes experiences of sexual misuse</li><li>Excessive concern or preoccupation with private parts and adult sexual behaviour</li><li>Sexualised relating to adults</li><li>Hinting about sexual experience</li><li>Sudden specific fear or mistrust of males, females or specific places</li><li>Verbal or behavioural indications of age-inappropriate knowledge of sexual behaviour</li></ul>	<ul><li>Child is likely to have detailed, long-term memory for traumatic event</li><li>Factually accurate memory may be embellished by elements of fear or wish; perception of duration may be distorted</li></ul>	<ul><li>Listen to and tolerate child's retelling of event</li><li>Respect child's fears; give child time to cope with fears</li><li>Increase monitoring and awareness of child's play, which may involve secretive reenactments of trauma with peers and siblings; set limits on scary or hurtful play</li><li>Permit child to try out new ideas to cope with fearfulness at bedtime: extra reading time, radio on, listening to a tape in the middle of the night to undo the residue of fear from a nightmare</li><li>Reassure the older child that feelings, fears or behaviours that feel out of control or babyish are normal after a frightening experience and that the child will feel more like themselves with time</li></ul>

→

General trauma reactions	Sexual abuse – specific reactions	Memory for trauma	Parental support
- Behaviour, mood, or personality changes
- Regression to behaviour of younger child
- Toileting accidents
- Withdrawal and quietening or excesses of aggression and limit setting
- Loss of interest in previously pleasurable activities
- Sleep disturbances: nightmares, sleep walking, night terrors (rare for this age), difficulty falling or staying asleep
- Complaints about bodily aches, pains or illness with no medical explanation
- Concern about personal responsibility for trauma			- Encourage child to talk about confusing feelings, worries, daydreams, mental review of traumatic images, and disruptions of concentration by accepting the feelings, listening carefully, and reminding child that these are normal but difficult reactions following a very scary event
- Maintain communication with school staff and monitor child's coping with demands at school or in community activities
- Expect some time-limited decrease in child's school performance and help the child to accept this as a temporary result of the trauma
- Protect child from re-exposure to frightening situations and reminders of trauma, including scary TV programmes, movies, stories, and physical or locational reminders of trauma

General trauma reactions	Sexual abuse – specific reactions	Memory for trauma	Parental support
- Acute awareness of parental reactions; wish to protect parents from their own distress - Frightened by intensity of their own feelings - Vulnerability to anniversary reactions set off by seasonal reminders, holidays or other events			- Expect and understand child's regression while maintaining basic household rules - Expect some difficult or uncharacteristic behaviour - Listen for the child's misunderstandings of a traumatic event, particularly those that involve self-blame and magical thinking - Gently help child develop a realistic understanding of the event - Remain aware of your own reactions to the child's trauma - Provide reassurance to child that feelings will diminish over time - Provide opportunities for child to experience control and make choices in daily activities - Be mindful of the possibility of anniversary reactions

TABLE #4 Developmental guidelines: Children's reactions to trauma (11–18 years)

General trauma reactions	Sexual abuse – specific reactions	Memory for trauma	Parental support
▪ Trauma-driven acting-out behaviour: sexual acting out or reckless, risk-taking behaviour ▪ Efforts to distance from feelings of shame, guilt and humiliation ▪ Flight into driven activity and involvement with others or retreat from others in order to manage inner turmoil ▪ Accident proneness ▪ Wish for revenge and action-oriented responses to trauma ▪ Increased self-focusing and withdrawal ▪ Sleep and eating disturbances; nightmares ▪ Acute awareness of and distress with intrusive imagery and memories of trauma ▪ Vulnerability to depression, withdrawal, and pessimistic world-view	▪ Sexually exploitive or aggressive interactions with younger children ▪ Sexually promiscuous behaviour or total avoidance of sexual involvement ▪ Running away from home	▪ Acute awareness of and distress with intrusive imagery and memories of trauma ▪ Vulnerability to flashback episodes of recall ▪ May experience acute distress encountering any reminder of the trauma	▪ Encourage younger and older adolescents to talk about traumatic event with family members ▪ Provide opportunities for young person to spend time with friends who are supportive and meaningful ▪ Reassure young person that strong feelings – whether of guilt, shame, embarrassment, or wish for revenge – are normal following a trauma ▪ Help young person find activities that offer opportunities to experience mastery, control and self-esteem ▪ Encourage pleasurable physical activities such as sport and dancing ▪ Address acting out behaviour involving aggression or self-destructive aspects quickly and firmly with limit setting and professional help

→

General trauma reactions	Sexual abuse – specific reactions	Memory for trauma	Parental support
- Personality changes and changes in quality of important relationships evident - Flight into adulthood seen as way of escaping impact and memory of trauma (early marriage, pregnancy, dropping out of school, abandoning peer group for older set of friends) - Fear of growing up and need to stay within family orbit			- Monitor young person's coping at home, school and in peer group - Take signs of depression, accident proneness, recklessness, and persistent personality change seriously by seeking help - Help young person develop a sense of perspective on the impact of the traumatic event and a sense of the importance of time in recovering - Encourage delaying big decisions

REFERENCES

American Psychiatric Association (APA). 2013. *Diagnostic and Statistical Manual of Mental Disorders – DSM-5*. 5th edition. Washington, DC: American Psychiatric Association.

Bagley, C and King, K. 2003. *Child sexual abuse: The search for healing*. Routledge.

Collins, A. 2013. 'Violence is not a crime: The impact of "acceptable" violence on South African society'. *South African Crime Quarterly*, 43: 29–37.

Denyes, M J, Orem, D E and Bekel, G. 2001. 'Self-care: A foundational science'. *Nursing Science Quarterly*, 14 (1): 45–54.

Eagle, G T. 2000. 'The shattering of the stimulus barrier: The case for an integrative approach in short-term treatment of psychological trauma'. *Journal of Psychotherapy Integration*, 10 (3): 301–323.

Finkelhor, D and Browne, A. 1985. 'The traumatic impact of child sexual abuse: A conceptualization'. *American Journal of Orthopsychiatry*, 55 (4): 53–541.

Gray-Vickrey, P. 2000. 'Protecting the older adult'. *Nursing*, 30 (7): 34.

Jewkes, R, Flood, M and Lang, J. 2015. 'From work with men and boys to changes of social norms and reduction of inequities in gender relations: a conceptual shift in prevention of violence against women and girls'. *The Lancet*, 385 (9977): 1580–1589.

Jewkes, R, Nduna, M, Jama-Shai, N, Chirwa, E and Dunkle, K. 2016. Understanding the relationships between gender inequitable behaviours, childhood trauma and socioeconomic status in single and multiple perpetrator rape in rural South Africa: structural equation modelling. *PLoS one, 11* (5): e0154903.

Monahon, C. 1993. *Children and Trauma: A Parent's Guide to Helping Children Heal.* New York: Lexington Books.

Mysyuk, Y, Westendorp, R G and Lindenberg, J. 2016. 'Perspectives on the etiology of violence in later life'. *Journal of interpersonal violence,* 31 (18): 3039–3062.

National Center for Health Research. 'The Cycle of Domestic Violence'. http://www.center4research.org/cycle-domestic-violence/ (Accessed 6 August 2019).

Peled-Avram, M. 2017. 'The role of relational-oriented supervision and personal and work-related factors in the development of vicarious traumatization'. *Clinical Social Work Journal,* 45 (1): 22–32.

Sorenson, C, Bolick, B, Wright, K and Hamilton, R. 2016. 'Understanding compassion fatigue in healthcare providers: A review of current literature'. *Journal of Nursing Scholarship,* 48 (5): 456–465.

The Duluth Model. http://www.theduluthmodel.org/pdf/powerandcontrol.pdf (Accessed 6 August 2019).

The Regional Psychosocial Support Initiative (REPSSI). http://www.repssi.org/Att.aspx?fn=30521fae-65d9-440a-9329-423ba93be935.pdf (Accessed 24 September 2019).

Wilson, J P and Lindy, J D, eds. 1994. *Countertransference in the treatment of PTSD.* Guilford Press.

World Health Organisation (WHO). 2001. *Putting women first: Ethical and safety recommendations for research on domestic violence against women* (No WHO/FCH/GWH/01.1). Geneva: World Health Organisation.

CHAPTER 20

People with a Mental Illness who have Comorbid General Medical Conditions

A A H Smith

Learning Outcomes

After studying this chapter, you should be able to:
- differentiate between the concepts of morbidity, mortality and comorbidity
- discuss the assessment implications of reported bidirectional relationships between physical illnesses and mental disorders
- identify the current common medical comorbidities associated with serious mental illnesses
- differentiate between the risk factors associated with typical/first-generation antipsychotics and atypical or second-generation antipsychotics
- assess the complete risk profile of a mental health care user (MHCU) for diabetes, metabolic syndrome and cardiovascular disease
- implement risk–benefit counselling specifically as it relates to the use of antipsychotic medication and concurrent use of antiretroviral medication
- implement nursing interventions to minimise the risk of developing medical comorbid illness in patients with a serious mental illness
- implement nursing assessment to facilitate primary prevention of mental comorbid illness in patients with physical ill-health.

INTRODUCTION

Over the past 10 years research has increasingly focused on the unmet medical needs of MHCUs, in particular those with serious mental disorders (SMDs). There has also been an increased focus on the bidirectional relationship between mental disorders, specifically SMDs, and physical ill-health (WHO, 2017: 3). It is generally accepted that SMDs include moderate to severe depression, bipolar mood disorder, schizophrenia and other psychotic disorders (WHO, 2018: 4). It is reported that there is a greater prevalence of negative physical health care outcomes in persons with SMDs than there is in the general population (WHO, 2018: 4). A bidirectional relationship refers to one that influences from both sides; in this instance mental disorders influence physical health and physical ill-health influences mental health. We are currently able to know about the existence of this bidirectional relationship as a result of information gained from morbidity, comorbidity and mortality data. Briefly, morbidity refers to having a disease/disorder and a morbidity rate informs us about the number of people who are currently ill with a specific disease or disorder. Comorbidity refers to when one disease or disorder leads to another. Health care statistics are able to report on the number of people with a comorbid disease or disorder and point to the comorbid relationships between the two diseases or disorders. Mortality refers to the number of people who have died. Research mortality rates identify diseases and disorders that result in death.

In 2017, the World Health Organisation (WHO) reported that the mortality rate in people with schizophrenia, referred to as a 'life-shortening disease', is twice as high as that of the general population (WHO, 2017: 7). In 2018 these figures increased from two to three times more than the mortality rate in the general population (WHO, 2018: 4). This essentially suggests that persons with an SMD generally have a life expectancy 10–20 years shorter than that of the general population (WHO, 2018: 4). Mental illness and comorbid general medical conditions have mutually adverse effects on long-term outcomes. This interaction of diseases contributes significantly to the higher-than-expected standard mortality ratios in patients with an SMD.

The Clinical Antipsychotic Trials of Intervention Effectiveness (CATIE) study was one of the first and largest of studies investigating physical health conditions among people with SMDs. The publication of the results of this study were presented in several manuscripts, the first in 2005. Lieberman, Stroup et al (2005) reported that out of the 1 600 participants, those who presented with diabetes (30 per cent) hypertension (62 per cent), and dyslipidaemia (88 per cent) had received no treatment for these physical conditions. In addition, the conclusions of the WHO Europe report, which addressed comorbidity between mental disorders and major non-communicable diseases, concluded there were bidirectional relations between some physical illnesses and mental disorders (WHO, 2017: 3–7). These conclusions, presented in the following section, are startling and point to the importance of integrated, data-driven primary preventive health care to reduce morbidity and comorbidity, and to secondary and tertiary preventive health care to reduce mortality rates.

Another report, the WHO 2016 global report on the increasing risk of type 2 diabetes in persons using psychotropic medicine, builds on the findings of the CATIE study and suggests that there has been little improvement since 2005. The prevalence of type 2 diabetes in the African region has more than doubled between 1980 and 2014, from 3.1 per cent to 7.1 per cent (WHO, 2016: 25; WHO, 2017: 5–8). The severity of the physical health risk in persons with mental disorders, specifically SMDs, is reflected in the evidence-based guidelines released by the WHO on managing of physical conditions in adults with SMDs (WHO, 2018: 4). These guidelines focus on action related to tobacco cessation, weight management, cardiovascular disease and risk, type 2 diabetes, and communicable diseases such as human immunodeficiency virus (HIV)/acquired immunodeficiency syndrome (AIDS), tuberculosis and hepatitis B. The mental health nurse in sub-Saharan Africa needs to be cognisant of the increased metabolic and cardiovascular risk associated with the use of antiretroviral treatment (ART). The ART medication exacerbates metabolic symptom risks that are associated with antipsychotic medication use. This integrated approach to health care is important. Despite this, the data presented earlier in this section indicates limited implementation. Mental health nurses need to consider possible obstacles and address them as best they can in their practice, and in practice areas.

The WHO report that mortality and morbidity rates within the SMD population are compounded by three factors:
1. Mental hospitals in some sub-Saharan African countries lack basic diagnostic equipment and resources, such as medication and well-trained staff with physical health knowledge, that could help in recognising, diagnosing and treating physical illness. The growth in specialised education programmes for health professionals increases the risk of professionals being compartmentalised within their particular disciplinary focus; this in turn may compromise their ability to recognise and/or manage comorbid physical conditions. In many sub-Saharan countries, and definitely in South Africa, undergraduate nursing programs continue to focus on physical health nursing and integrate mental health nursing into this. The choice of specialisation is a function of postgraduate study. This positions the mental health nurse to take the lead in implementing integrated health care within mental health services.
2. Specific demographic factors of persons with an SMD may contribute to morbidity and mortality. Persons with an SMD have a higher incidence of involvement in preventable risk factors such as smoking, addiction, poor diet and lack of exercise (WHO, 2018: 4).
3. The risk of metabolic and cardiovascular disease (CVD) manifesting in changes in body mass index, obesity, hypertension, glucose tolerance and insulin resistance are linked to the long-term use of antipsychotic medication (Lieberman & Hsaio, 2006; WHO, 2017: 5; 2018: 7).

This chapter outlines the increased prevalence of comorbid medical conditions in people with SMDs, contributory and risk factors, and the implications for comprehensive nursing practice.

PREVALENCE OF COMORBID MEDICAL DISORDERS AND SMDs

Just as there is an increased prevalence of comorbid medical disorders within the SMD population in relation to the general population, there may also be multiple comorbid medical disorders in a person with an SMD. Prevalence rates of 66 per cent for a single chronic medical health problem, 50 per cent for two or more chronic medical conditions, 33 per cent for three or more medical conditions and approximately 20 per cent for four or more conditions, have been reported. In addition, medical comorbidities for the different SMDs are very similar. Statistics presented in this section are sourced from two WHO reports (WHO, 2018):

Addressing comorbidity between mental disorders and major non-communicable diseases (WHO, 2017) and *Management of physical health conditions in adults with severe mental disorders, WHO guidelines.*

These and any new WHO publications can be found at www.who.int. For a more comprehensive summary, the WHO (2017) publication, and any later publications, should be read.

Common comorbid conditions

Different research studies within WHO systematic reviews rank health risks related to SMDs differently, and prevalence rates can differ between studies. However, most current studies consistently rank CVD, diabetes, respiratory disease, gastrointestinal disorders associated with substance misuse, and communicable diseases as the comorbid conditions more prevalent in persons with an SMD than in the general population (WHO, 2017: 3–18; 2018: 5–9). In addition, obesity and smoking, both prevalent in persons who have an SMD, are recognised as significant vulnerabilities and predictors of the severity of individual health problems. Age is also a variable that suggests increased risk within the SMD population. Age is associated with an accumulative effect – increased years of smoking and/or other substance misuse, coupled with increased years of psychotropic medication use, specifically antipsychotics, have a potential impact on gastrointestinal, endocrine and cardiovascular systems.

Comorbidities and prevalence rates associated with SMDs

Presented here are medical comorbidities associated with SMDs, and some reported prevalence rates and associations that are the focus of concern and research (WHO 2017; 2018). As awareness of risk increases, the implementation of global and local strategies increases, and hopefully future research studies will indicate change.

Diabetes and SMDs

- The relation between diabetes and depression is bidirectional: people with diabetes are more likely to develop depression, and depression is a risk factor for diabetes.
- Diabetes, specifically type 2 diabetes, is two to three times more common in people with an SMD: moderate to severe depression, bipolar mood disorder, schizophrenia and other psychotic disorders.
- The role of antipsychotic medication in triggering type 2 diabetes should be further evaluated.
- Depression, more common among women (28 per cent) than in men (18 per cent), is two to three times more common in people with diabetes than in those without this disease.
- People with diabetes and a psychotic illness are more likely to die early than people with diabetes alone.
- Adherence to diabetic treatment shows a significant association between depression and non-adherence.
- Diabetes increases the risks for CVD. In a multinational study, 50 per cent of people with diabetes died of CVD (primarily heart disease and stroke).

SMDs and CVD

- People with SMDs die 15–20 years earlier than people from the general population, most commonly from CVD.
- Up to 20 per cent of people with CVD suffer from depression.
- The presence of depression is reported to predict CVD, and depression and/or anxiety are reported to double the risk for a poor outcome after a cardiac event.
- Anxiety disorders are reported to be an independent risk factor for CVD and for adverse events after a myocardial infarction.
- Similarly, depression is reported to increase the risk for CVD by 1.3 times, and the risk of a poor outcome by 1.7 times.
- A person with an SMD has double the risk for a heart attack or a stroke than a member of the general population. In addition, the risk of a long stay as an inpatient is tripled.
- Depression increases the risk for CVD by 1.6–1.9 times over that of the general population and increases the risk for a poor outcome by 2.4 times.
- Depression is associated with a two to three times higher risk of CVD and increased re-hospitalisation rates of patients with CVD.
- Antipsychotic medication influences the electrical current that coordinates each contraction of the heart, placing the heart at greater risk for a fatal irregular rhythm.
- Antipsychotic medication increases the incidence of venous thromboembolism (blood clots in the veins).

Smoking and SMDs

One in three of all cigarettes smoked is smoked by a person with an SMD. While smoking in the general population has fallen by 25 per cent in the past two decades, there has been no similar decrease in smoking among people with SMDs. Smoking within the general population is reported to be between 10–15 per cent while smoking among people with an SMD is reported to be between 70–80 per cent.

It is these figures, and the associated disability adjusted life years (DALYS), that have motivated most health care services, residential and non-residential, to become smoke-free areas.

Pulmonary conditions also show higher prevalence rates (31 per cent). Pulmonary conditions include acute respiratory disorders (33 per cent), chronic obstructive pulmonary disease (11 per cent) and asthma (8 per cent).

While figures vary from country to country, tobacco consumption and excessive alcohol consumption cause about 40 per cent of the total cancer burden, including lung and gastrointestinal cancer.

Communicable diseases and SMDs

People with SMDs are at greater risk for exposure to infectious diseases, including tuberculosis (TB) and chronic hepatitis. Common risk factors include homelessness,

HIV/AIDS positive serology, and alcohol/substance abuse. A person with an SMD is reported to be 4–8 times more likely to die from an infectious disease than someone from the general population.

Sexually transmitted infections such as HIV/AIDS also report a higher prevalence rate (see Chapter 21 on 'Mental Health Nursing in the Context of HIV and TB'). The association between SMDs and HIV/AIDS is complex and bidirectional. Their co-occurrence is frequent; in the United States of America (USA), the median prevalence among persons with an SMD was 1.8 per cent in 2015. This prevalence rate will seem low to the mental health nurse in sub-Saharan Africa. Understanding that SMDs can be precursors to, or consequences of HIV/AIDS, is important. The co-occurrence figure will be proportionate to the local prevalence rate.

VULNERABILITY FACTORS

Why people with an SMD are more likely to have a physical illness than the rest of the population is partially known. Aspects of vulnerability and associated risk can be easily understood. For example, there is a relationship between SMDs and homelessness and communicable diseases. An area of well-known, increased risk is that of weight gain and obesity within the SMD population. Since early 2000, links have been made between the prevalence of metabolic conditions leading to the development of metabolic syndrome and CVD, and the use of antipsychotic medication. The American-funded CATIE study is a seminal study confirming the side effects of psychotropic medication resulting in comorbid medical conditions, specifically the development of more than one comorbidity leading to metabolic syndrome (Lieberman & Hasio, 2006; Lieberman et al, 2005).

Continuing research suggests some antipsychotic medication is less 'risky' in terms of side effects. It is not clear why some antipsychotics seem to produce weight gain, insulin resistance, dyslipidaemia and increased risk of CVD, but it is clear they do. The WHO (2017: 11; 2018: 31) reports that the use of second-generation antipsychotic medication, and some antidepressant medication, is associated with an increased risk of diabetes, progressing to metabolic syndrome which, in nearly all age groups, is a risk reported to be 2–3 times that of the general population. Metabolic syndrome is a term used to describe a number of clinical and biochemical abnormalities that frequently appear together and predict CVD. The abnormalities include insulin resistance, obesity (specifically visceral adiposity), diabetes, hypertension and dyslipidaemia. While tardive dyskinesia (permanent movement issues) was caused by first-generation antipsychotics, now MHCUs using second-generation antipsychotics are at risk of developing metabolic syndrome – CVD and early death. Recent evidence suggests that antidepressant medication might also be having an undesirable effect on weight and metabolic health. A description of metabolic syndrome can be found under 'Metabolic syndrome' in this chapter.

However, the use of psychotropic medication alone may be only part of the answer to medical morbidity, comorbidity and mortality within the SMD population. A number of other contributory factors, aside from those mentioned above, are suggested within various United Nation (UN) publications (UN, 2000; 2015; 2016). These factors are outlined below.

Social determinants of health factors

Social determinants of health, such as poverty and impoverished living circumstances, contribute to the development of physical disease and mental disorders, and they can amplify the bidirectional relationship between physical and mental health. For example, a person struggling with a major depressive disorder has limited financial resources and so buys cheaper high carbohydrate meals that facilitate weight gain. The weight gain may already be occurring because of antidepressant medication and this result exacerbates the depressive disorder.

Accessible, appropriate integrated health care

The integration of mental health care within physical health care in a decentralised health care system varies from country to county and service to service. In many cases, physical and mental health care services remain separate. Skills in physical health care are not evident within mental health services and vice versa. The continued focus by the UN (UN, 2016) and WHO (WHO, 2018) on the importance of accessible and appropriate health care, especially for persons with SMDs, will hopefully improve the nurse's focus on the physical health assessment of persons accessing mental health services, and the mental health of those who are physically ill.

Psychiatric illness-related vulnerability factors

People with SMDs generally pay little attention to their bodies. This inattention extends beyond that of the deterioration in activities of daily living, for example hygiene, associated with the diagnosis of severe mental illness. Some MHCUs are frequently unaware of their bodies as a source of information about their intrinsic well-being. They may therefore accept unpleasant physical sensations as normal or have difficulty, because of cognitive deficits, in recognising physical illness, medical problems, and carrying out required lifestyle changes. A reduction in pain sensitivity is also associated with the use of antipsychotic medication.

Lifestyle factors such as poor diet, inertia and a sedentary lifestyle are often associated with long-term psychiatric disorders and these factors contribute to and exacerbate hypertension and heart disease, glucose regulation abnormalities such as hyperglycaemia, insulin resistance and type 2 diabetes.

High-risk sexual behaviours, such as a lack of condom use, trading sexual favours for commodities like money or drugs, and a reduced knowledge about HIV/AIDS -related issues, increase the risk of sexually transmitted diseases, including HIV/AIDS. (Also read Chapter 21 on 'Mental Health Nursing in the Context of HIV and TB').

The abuse of substances (alcohol and other drugs) resulting in exposure to various health consequences such as hepatitis (through needle-sharing) may also play a role in the increased prevalence of comorbidity in the psychiatric population. Smoking is unusually prevalent among persons with SMDs (88 per cent) and high rates of smoking contribute to asthma, acute respiratory disease, heart disease and lung cancer.

Treatment-related vulnerability factors

A number of medications have adverse physical effects in both the short and long term.

In the first instance, all antipsychotics (second-generation/atypical more than first-generation or typical) increase the propensity to weight gain, hypertension and the development of diabetes. Secondly, hyperlipidaemia is associated with antipsychotic use and can be independent of weight gain. These medical comorbidities are associated with the development of metabolic syndrome, which is linked to CVD and high mortality rates within the seriously mentally ill population. Finally, osteoporosis has also been associated with the use of prolactin-increasing antipsychotics. Gastrointestinal effects such as irritable bowel syndrome and *Helicobacter pylori* infection may be associated with constant medication ingestion and this can be further exacerbated by stress and smoking.

Metabolic syndrome

In 1988, the term Syndrome X was coined by Reaven to describe a cluster of metabolic risk factors that present in an individual MHCU. Reaven (1988) proposed that insulin resistance was central to the cause of type 2 diabetes, high blood pressure and CVD. This cluster of risk factors is now known as metabolic syndrome although there has been some tension over the name and its utility. The specific diagnostic criteria for metabolic syndrome vary from expert to expert, despite all containing the same broad indicators: abdominal adiposity, weight gain, increased blood glucose and cholesterol, and increased blood pressure.

Diagnostic criteria for metabolic syndrome

The following are pertinent diagnostic criteria for sub-Saharan Africa:

An elevated fasting blood glucose or an elevated post-meal glucose with two of the following:
- Abdominal obesity, defined as a waist to hip ratio of > 0.9
- A body mass index (BMI) of a least 30 kg/m^2
- A waist measurement over 93.98 cm (37 inches)
- Cholesterol panel showing:
  - HDL cholesterol lower than 35 mg/dL
  - Blood pressure of 140/90 or above.

NURSING ASSESSMENT, TREATMENT AND MANAGEMENT

Historically, the treatment of the physical and mental health of the MHCU seems to have been split with little sharing of information between the physical and psychiatric practitioners. Even within mental health care facilities there seems to be a determined focus on mental health and minimal or no focus on the physical health of the MHCU. The current primary health care system within the public health model suggests that integration is possible despite the risk of compartmentalisation associated with increasing specialisation. Mental health nurses need to focus attention on how best to integrate medical and psychiatric care within mental health services at hospital and community sites and to guard actively against the idea that 'the other' is attending to the MHCU's physical health needs. These challenges are compounded by the cognitive, social and psychological disabilities of people with serious mental illness that make their participation in the management of their own illness difficult.

The central principle for integrated nursing care is that the more aware nurses are of the potential for psychiatric–physical comorbidity within all the different health populations they serve, the more likely they are to practise comprehensive nursing. Therefore, nurses who recognise that psychiatric–physical comorbidity is as integral to physical health as it is to mental health are more likely to implement specific continuous assessment strategies and treatment protocols that optimise pharmacotherapy, monitor treatment outcomes and identify when immediate medical and/or psychiatric treatment is warranted. For this reason, mental health nurses have a central role in coordinating and integrating the health care of patients with severe mental illness, in helping to timeously diagnose and treat comorbid conditions, and in helping those who are predisposed to them to take preventive measures.

Routine screening and monitoring

A number of different organisations (such as the American Diabetes Association, the American Psychiatric Association, the American Association of Endocrinologists, the North American Association for the Study of Obesity and the WHO) developed recommendations and guidelines on screening and monitoring for persons who have been prescribed high-risk medication. These recommendations are simple and easy to implement, do not require sophisticated resources and are a part of the skill repertoire of every mental health nurse.

Every consumer should have baseline assessments of each of the following with repeated measures:
- A personal and family history of risk factors for CVD, repeated annually
- Weight and height for BMI, then repeated monthly for three months and thereafter quarterly. A person's BMI is calculated as weight in kilograms divided by height in metres squared
- Waist circumference, then repeated annually
- Blood pressure, then quarterly for one year, then annually

- Fasting glucose levels, then quarterly for one year, then annually
- Fasting lipid profile, then quarterly for one year, then every five years.

Evidence-based practice

Read the case study about Amir (WHO, 2017: 6–7):

Amir's story

Presentation. Amir is a 38-year-old man with schizophrenia, who was asked to attend the family doctor by the practice nurse after Amir told her that he felt tired and thirsty all the time. She checked a urine sample and found that it was loaded with glucose. Clinical background: Amir received a diagnosis of schizophrenia when he was 22 years old. Although his clinical records are not entirely clear, as he has moved quite frequently, he appears to be fit and healthy, apart from the schizophrenia. He went to the clinic relatively often for over 18 months to see the practice nurse for a number of self-limiting conditions and other physical health concerns, until five months previously, when he stopped attending. The few consultations before the gap in attendance were characterised by increasing confusion and generally chaotic behaviour, with shouting in the waiting room on several occasions. The clinical record has no family history and does not state whether he smokes or works or whether his weight or blood pressure has been measured in the past 12 months.

The consultation. During the consultation, Amir is quiet, polite and apologetic for his previous behaviour. He explains that he had become increasingly unwell mentally and had been admitted to hospital five months previously. His psychiatrist recently changed his medication to clozapine, and he feels much more settled and comfortable on this new treatment. He has been home for two weeks and noticed that he was much more tired than usual and was drinking all the time. He mentions this to his psychiatrist, who recommended that he see his family doctor. The family doctor focuses on the combination of thirst and tiredness, which are cardinal symptoms of diabetes. Amir tells the doctor that both his father and his mother had type 2 diabetes and that his father died of a heart attack at the age of 55 years. Amir also tells the doctor that he has put on a lot of weight recently, from 91 kg (calculated BMI 33) to over 122 kg (calculated BMI 44). He believes the weight gain is due to his rehabilitation programme; before discharge, he was allowed out to buy meals from take-away restaurants, rather than eating on the ward. He admits that on trips off the ward he took the opportunity to buy cigarettes for his friends and started smoking himself. He currently smokes 20 cigarettes per day.

Clinical issues and implications for practice. This is a complicated picture, with several competing priorities. Confirming the diagnosis of diabetes is central to the consultation but understanding how the diagnosis of schizophrenia can affect the diagnosis and management of diabetes is essential to treating Amir as 'a whole person'.

Management of diabetes
- Confirm diagnosis: The major clinical issue facing the family doctor is to confirm the diagnosis of diabetes. The guidelines from the WHO on the management of diabetes state that HbA1c can be used to diagnose most cases of diabetes but not in a small number of cases when the diabetes is of recent onset, especially if associated with antipsychotic medication, as in the case of Amir. Therefore, it would be inappropriate to use elevated haemoglobin A1c (HbA1c) to diagnose diabetes (a normal value would be considered a 'false negative'). The fasting blood glucose level would be more accurate.
- Diabetes education: Amir should be given information on diabetes and how it is managed. A common misconception is that all patients with diabetes are treated by injections of insulin, while many people with schizophrenia who have been given injections of antipsychotic medication, sometimes against their will, are likely to refuse another injection. It is important to ensure that Amir understands that most patients can be treated by behaviour change and oral medication.
- Behaviour change: The importance of weight loss, diet and exercise cannot be overemphasised at this stage. Every effort should be made to support Amir in losing weight by adopting sensible eating habits and more exercise. Community programmes and access to a dietician and to exercise facilities are necessary to support him as he tries to change his behaviour. The likelihood that Amir is unemployed and depends on state benefits in light of his mental disorder increases the risk that he will find it difficult to adhere to a healthy diet and will resort to cheap, high-calorie meals. The consequence will be poorly controlled diabetes and the development of complications.
- Smoking cessation: Another important aim for Amir is to reduce and then stop smoking. Smoking significantly adversely affects diabetes and increases the risk for complications, such as kidney failure, blindness, impotence, nerve damage and high blood pressure. It is significant that Amir's father died before the age of 60 years of a heart attack, as this is a further independent predictor of CVD. The combination of smoking, diabetes and a family history of CVD make Amir's outlook poor, unless there are significant improvements in his lifestyle. After the consultation, the family doctor will decide how best to inform the psychiatrist of the new diagnosis. Such communication will depend on local circumstances and local agreements.

Supporting medication compliance through knowledge, skill and collaboration

Consider how in this next case study, the basic principles of routine screening and collaboration in supporting medication adherence can be used to address the most common features of comorbidity in the psychiatric population as a routine part of practice.

Risk–benefit medication counselling
Mr Y case study

Mr Y, a 20-year-old man, has been receiving first-generation/typical antipsychotic medication for three weeks. When you review his chart, you discover that he has gained four kilograms in body weight since he started treatment. A full blood count was conducted at the start of his treatment, no abnormalities were noted and no blood tests have been repeated.

When you approach him, you notice that his hands are trembling. He comes immediately when you call and smiles as he greets you. He walks with you to the consulting room and you notice that he holds his arms stiffly by his side and that there is no arm swing.

Mr Y responds to all your questions about his health. He tells you that he is fine, that he has been planning to return to work and has made contact with the company's human resources department. He admits to being nervous about seeing his co-workers again and wonders what they will think, especially as his hands shake now. He tells you that he knows the medication has helped him; he also says he can't wait to stop taking the medication as he constantly feels as if the muscles in his legs are twitching, and he is embarrassed by his shaking hands. He knows that he may need to explain his period of absence to people in the office and why his hands now shake, but he is not sure what to say to them. He had hoped to get a promotion to the administrative office, but he is not sure what will happen now, after his diagnosis and treatment.

Objective
To maintain Mr Y's physical health while promoting medication compliance in order to improve overall quality of life.

Analysis (formulation)
Mr Y is taking antipsychotic medication and has the following physical symptoms: weight gain, extrapyramidal side effects in the form of pseudo-parkinsonism, akathisia and dystonia. From an emotional perspective he is embarrassed about the pseudo-parkinsonism and anxious about the questions he will have to answer in response to people noticing this visible change in his body movements.

The client seems more concerned with his extrapyramidal side effects than with his weight gain. This is not uncommon; a little weight gain may not concern the client as much as the extrapyramidal side effects, which are unusual in the general population and thus represent 'standing out as different from' others. Although the metabolic and cardiovascular changes that can occur may remain subclinical for some time, they represent a greater threat to the client's physical health. The client also makes reference to 'stopping the medication' and this needs to be explored.

What additional data is required (what are the gaps in knowledge)?
Because of the fairly rapid weight gain while taking antipsychotics, it is imperative that the risk for developing metabolic syndrome and CVD be investigated by:

- Taking a family history of the extent of vulnerability – the risk factors – for CVD. This includes asking questions about family members with hypertension, diabetes, hyperlipidaemia (high cholesterol) and cardiac problems including cardiac arrhythmia and myocardial infarction.
- Taking a personal history from the client regarding his physical examination history and any history of hypertension, hyperglycaemia, hyperlipidaemia and hyperglycaemia. The personal history should also focus on any health-promoting behaviour that the client already undertakes, such as involvement in any form of exercise (sport, walking), and dietary awareness and habits (consumption of animal fat, carbohydrates and refined sugar).
- Doing a physical examination. Such investigations include questions about:
  - increase in waist circumference in relation to current weight gain as research indicates that abdominal adiposity increases the risk of type 2 diabetes
  - the calculation of BMI to establish baseline data for body fat and thus the potential impact on blood pressure and cardiac output
  - blood pressure to check for hypertension
  - a fasting blood sugar and fasting lipids to establish baseline and identify any existing areas of risk of metabolic dysfunction
  - the extent of extrapyramidal side effects using a measurement tool such as the Simpson-Angus Scale or the Abnormal Involuntary Movement Scale.

Explore with the client his perceptions of the purpose of medication and his future plans regarding medication use. This allows the caregiver to clarify the client's understanding and identify any misconceptions.

Designing the intervention (what should the content of health education be?)
The following is a list of recommendations:
- Stress the benefits of medication use in relation to reducing psychotic symptoms and improved cognitive functioning. Relate these to Mr Y's employment and ability to function effectively in the work environment.
- It is likely that Mr Y will be taking the medication for a long time, possibly for life. Reducing and stopping the medication is possible for some clients, but this is usually a slow process. Reduction of medication is measured against the re-emergence of any symptoms the client has recently experienced.
- Provide Mr Y with information about the first-generation/typical antipsychotics and the second-generation/atypical antipsychotics.
- Explain to him that there is little difference in therapeutic benefits between the two categories of antipsychotics.
- The extrapyramidal side effects that Mr Y is experiencing are linked to medication use and some are reduced by the use of anticholinergic medication. It is possible to monitor the presence of these side effects and the effectiveness of the anticholinergic

medication. It is also widely accepted that the experience of extrapyramidal side effects is markedly reduced with the use of the second-generation/atypical antipsychotic medication.
- Second-generation/atypical antipsychotic medication has an increased risk of possible weight gain, type 2 diabetes and CVD. Discuss with the client the strategies he can employ to counteract the less desirable metabolic and cardiovascular side effects, for example changing to a low glycaemic index (GI) diet and introducing into his day an exercise programme, such as a daily brisk walk. Explain the monitoring practices that can be employed to help with early detection and treatment of potential metabolic or cardiovascular comorbidities (outlined earlier in this chapter).
- Review the client's personal risk profile with him, making use of data collected from the history (family and personal), the physical examination and laboratory tests.
- Encourage the client to verbalise his perceptions of the current medication side effects that he is experiencing (shaking hands, weight gain, vibration in legs) and his thoughts on the information you have given him.
- Be empathic about his concerns and allow him to think. Provide him with reading material if appropriate or requested.
- Make notes in his records of what you have discussed and ultimately, respect his choice.

CONCLUSION

Despite significant literature easily available about some psychotropic medications and the increased risk of metabolic syndrome, it is not uncommon to find oneself working in a mental health service that has no consistent measures to assess and or to respond adequately to related potential and actual problems. Documented evidence of monitoring practices implemented by mental health practitioners is required in order to motivate for policy development and robust implementation. Policy development should consider standard regular physical examinations of MHCUs and the implementation of monitoring practices at all psychiatric facilities that include, at least:
- personal and family history of CVD and diabetes
- weight and girth measurement
- changes in glucose levels and dyslipidaemia and
- blood pressure.

Such data could assist in the development of a document containing recommendations and protocol for appropriate drug therapy for MHCUs taking into account medical illness, laboratory abnormalities, age, and personal and family history of risk factors.

WEB RESOURCES

http://www.who.int

This site allows free access to global and African research epidemiological data, evidence-based fact sheets, current research, and policy documents and guidelines based on best practice. It is a very valuable and topical site.

https://www.journals.elsevier.com/mental-health-and-prevention
https://www.journals.elsevier.com/archives-of-psychiatric-nursing
http://www.ps.psychiatryonline.org

These sites allow free access to psychiatric and mental health research articles.

http://www.mind.org.uk/

This is a user-driven site, with empowerment and advocacy at its core. It offers excellent information to patients, their families, and mental health care practitioners.

REFERENCES

Lieberman, J and Hsiao, J. 2006. 'Interpreting the results of CATIE', letter to the editor. *Psychiatric Services*, http://www.psychiatryonline.org/cgi/f7/1/139 (Accessed 18 November 2008).

Lieberman, J A, Stroup, T S, McEvoy, J P, Swartz, M S, Rosenheck, R A, Perkins, D O, Keefe, R S, Davis, S M, Davis, C E, Lebowitz, B D, Severe, J and Hsiao, J K. 2005. 'Clinical Antipsychotic Trials of Intervention Effectiveness (CATIE) Investigators. Effectiveness of antipsychotic drugs in patients with chronic schizophrenia'. *New England Journal of Medicine,* 22; 353 (12): 1209–23. https://www.nimh.nih.gov/funding/clinical-research/practical/catie (Accessed 5 May 2019).

Reaven, G M. 1988. 'Role of insulin resistance in human disease'. *Diabetes Journal*, 37 (12): 1595–1607. https://diabetes. diabetesjournals.org/content/37/12/1595.fulltext.pdf (Accessed 9 September 2019).

United Nations (UN). 2000. 'Millennium development goals'. https://www.undp.org/content/undp/en/home/sdgoverview/mdg_goals.html (Accessed May 2019).

United Nations (UN). 2015. 'The millennium development goals report'. https://www.un.org/millenniumgoals/2015 MDG Report/New York (Accessed May 2019).

United Nations (UN). 2016. '2030 Agenda for sustainable development and 17 sustainable development goals'. https://sustainabledevelopment.un.org/sdgs (Accessed May 2019).

World Health Organisation (WHO). 2016. 'Global Report on Diabetes'. http://www.who.int/publications/ (Accessed January 2017).

World Health Organisation (WHO). 2017. 'Addressing comorbidity between mental disorders and major non-communicable diseases'. http://www.who.int/publications/Geneva (Accessed December 2017).

World Health Organisation. 2018. 'Management of physical health conditions in adults with severe mental disorders, WHO guidelines'. http://www.who.int/publications/ (Accessed March 2019).

CHAPTER 21

Mental Health Nursing in the Context of Human Immunodeficiency Virus and Tuberculosis

J R Naidoo

Learning Outcomes

After studying this chapter, you should be able to:
- describe how the co-infection of human immunodeficiency virus (HIV) and tuberculosis (TB) relates to common mental health disorders
- identify the psychological problems among people living with HIV/TB
- therapeutically manage mental health problems associated with HIV and TB.

INTRODUCTION

Within a changing health care context in South Africa, it is crucial for all nurses to have a sound knowledge of the management of mental illness in its relationship to chronic and comorbid illnesses. This is especially imperative in light of the significant comorbidity of HIV and TB in South Africa, where an estimated two thirds of individuals diagnosed with HIV and TB are living with a mental health disorder (UNAIDS, 2018; Gupta et al, 2015).

It is well known that South Africa is the epicentre of the HIV epidemic. The country contributes to less than 1 per cent of the world population but is estimated to account for 30 per cent of the global incidence of HIV and TB co-infection. The most common presenting illness among people living with HIV is TB, and it is the major cause of HIV-related deaths (UNAIDS, 2018). People living with HIV are 16–27 times more likely to develop TB, in comparison to persons without HIV. Sub-Saharan Africa bears the brunt of the dual epidemic, accounting for approximately 86 per cent of all deaths from HIV associated with TB in 2016 (Venter, 2018; WHO, 2016; Manda et al, 2013).

The HIV epidemic is referred to as a psychiatric epidemic, in light of the complex bidirectional relationship of neurological disorders associated with HIV and TB. This is further reflected in Table 12.1. Moreover, mental health disorders can arise as a side effect of antiretroviral treatment (ART), or as a result of the stigma, psychological distress and socioeconomic determinants related to the diseases of HIV and TB, and the treatment processes. Furthermore, depression and substance abuse, which are commonly found among 25 per cent of the South African adult population, are known to increase the likelihood of high-risk behaviours that can contribute to the transmission of HIV (Bongongo et al, 2013). It is also true that depression is strongly associated with substance abuse (Saban et al, 2014).

The risk factors for mental illness among people living with HIV and TB are complex. There are higher rates of mental health disorders among people living with HIV and TB, which impact on health outcomes, specifically treatment adherence, retention in care and mortality. A recent study in Ethiopia found that people living with HIV and TB have significantly poor mental health outcomes and poor quality of life (Duko et al, 2015).

The complexity and nature of HIV/TB, and the pathophysiological influence of these diseases on various systems, challenge health care providers in terms of management and treatment strategies. These varied challenges impact directly on the well-being of an individual and on the stressors which are inherent in the illnesses and in their treatment and management, threatening the equilibrium of a person's functioning. The impact and burden of HIV/TB are strongly associated with the increase in mental disorders and this is especially significant in low- and middle-income countries (such as South Africa). It is against this backdrop that there has been a need for an integrated approach towards managing mental health, HIV and other related comorbid illnesses.

Table 21.1 The interrelationship between HIV and mental health disorders

1. *Risk taking and HIV.* A pre-existing, undiagnosed and untreated mental illness is related to high HIV/AIDS-risk behaviours, which may lead to an individual's contracting HIV.
2. *Biological.* The effect of the neurotoxicity of HIV on the central nervous system (CNS) causes mental illness. Cognitive impairment and dementia are serious consequences of HIV on the subcortical region of the CNS. Depressive and anxiety disorders, which occur due to HIV infection in the CNS, often co-exist with cognitive impairment.
3. *Psychological.* The emotional and psychological consequences of living with HIV, and the impact of HIV-related stigma and discrimination, cause adjustment disorder and major depression. Furthermore, research findings reveal that there is an increase in depression among people living with HIV during stages 3 and 4 of the disease-progression of HIV (Nanni et al, 2015; Kinyanda et al, 2017; Ayano et al, 2018). The stigma and discrimination arising from living with HIV may give rise to mental health problems which may attract further stigma and discrimination.
4. *Side effects of medication.* The side effects and interaction of ART and psychotherapeutic medication cause changes and even an increase in body mass, sedation, insomnia and sexual dysfunction. The interaction of ART and selective serotonin reuptake inhibitors (SSRIs) – antidepressants – can result in agitation and weight loss.
5. *Primary psychiatric disorder.* Some people living with HIV may already have a pre-existing diagnosis of mental illness and this, compounded by the stress of their HIV diagnosis, may further precipitate depression or anxiety disorders.

THE RELATIONSHIP BETWEEN HIV/TB CO-INFECTION AND MENTAL ILLNESS

The World Health Organisation (WHO) advocates that 'there is no health without mental health' (WHO, 2013), and researchers suggest that there will be a growing emphasis on mental health in the next two decades, with depression estimated to be a leading burden of the disability-adjusted life years (DALYs). Currently more than a quarter of depression prevalence occurs in low- and middle-income countries (such as South Africa), where HIV and TB are prevalent.

South Africa currently has an estimated 7.1 million people living with HIV, which equates to 19 per cent of the total adult population. There is also a disproportionate risk of HIV transmission and infection among women, partly due to physiological factors, but also largely due to gender-based violence and social determinants such as intergenerational and transactional sex (Dellar et al, 2015). The latest South African statistics show that rates of new HIV infection among women aged 15–24 years are four times greater than that of men in the same age category (Maughan-Brown et al, 2018). Adding further to the burden of HIV on the health care system and to the person living with HIV, is the dual infection of TB and HIV. It is known that HIV is driving the TB epidemic in South Africa, with a TB and HIV co-infection rate of up to 60 per cent.

The presence of a mental disorder is noted as a significant predisposing risk to individuals engaging in high-risk behaviours such as substance abuse and high-risk sexual behaviour. These are major risk factors for HIV infection and transmission. This is especially true in the context of South Africa, with high levels of alcohol and substance abuse, such as the use of crystal methamphetamine (tik), which is known to increase high-risk sexual behaviour, and to cause depression, mania and is even associated with psychosis. On the other hand, HIV is known to have a direct physiological effect on the CNS, directly resulting in depression, mania or other cognitive disorders. There is also the psychological trauma of being diagnosed and living with a chronic illness. In addition, opportunistic infections because of HIV and ART, specifically efavirenz, can also contribute to the development of mental disorders. There is a complex interaction between HIV/TB and mental disorder co-infection which can negatively impact on a person's quality of life. Further to this, while there is still a paucity of evidence on the long-term impact of HIV/TB and mental disorder co-infection, some evidence suggests that while the advent of ART significantly decreased HIV-associated dementia, there are recent reports of a rise in HIV encephalopathy (Stoloff & Josoka, 2015; Duko et al, 2015).

In a South African study, it was reported that more than 50 per cent of the population of people living with the dual diagnoses of HIV and TB presented with a common mental disorder, specifically depression, in comparison to people with HIV only (Manda et al, 2013). Regardless of the aetiology, living with HIV and mental illness, and especially living with a co-infection of HIV/TB and mental illness, creates significant challenges for nursing care. All three diseases – HIV, TB and mental illness – are diseases associated with stigmatisation and this poses greater barriers to care for individuals living with HIV, TB and mental illness. Denial, social isolation, stigma and discrimination, fear, and disease or treatment misunderstanding can contribute to medication non-compliance. Another major challenge to the care of people living with HIV, TB and mental illness, is pharmacological management, due to potential drug interactions. Within this context of the dual epidemic of HIV and TB, it is imperative that nurses at all levels of care routinely screen, monitor and integrate mental health nursing care and interventions.

PSYCHOLOGICAL CONDITIONS ASSOCIATED WITH HIV/AIDS AND TB

A number of psychological conditions are associated with HIV and TB. These include anxiety, post-traumatic stress disorder (PTSD); mood disorders and cognitive impairment. Substance abuse will also be discussed in relation to people living with HIV and TB.

Anxiety and PTSD

As previously stated, research has demonstrated that common mental disorders, in particular depression and anxiety, are twice as likely to occur among people living with HIV. While HIV and TB do not directly cause anxiety-related disorders, research estimates that there is a significantly higher prevalence of anxiety-related disorders (16 per cent) among people living with HIV in comparison to people not infected with HIV, where the estimated prevalence is 3 per cent (Tesfaw et al, 2016). Anxiety is normal, especially when one experiences a chronic illness like HIV. However, concern should be noted when patients demonstrate prolonged and exaggerated anxiety, as this can negatively interfere with treatment adherence. Anxiety among people living with HIV and TB is mostly due to social stigma, self-blame, judgement, and among women, anxiety and worry related to reproductive health issues.

It is estimated that PTSD is significantly higher among people living with HIV than in the general population, with there being an estimated 42 per cent prevalence of PTSD among people living with HIV (Tesfaw et al, 2016). A diagnosis of HIV can bring on PTSD. This happens when people living with HIV feel that their lives are being threatened or they fear of loss of life, due to various social and personal triggers such as stigma, discrimination and even a fear of abuse and violence. Untreated PTSD can lead to many negative health consequences, such as comorbid major depression and substance-use disorders, problems with treatment adherence, and poor quality of life. A recent systematic review on the management of PTSD among people living with HIV found that group therapies focusing on coping with HIV, trauma, sexual risk reduction and stress were found to be more significant than group therapies aligned only to the disease management of living with HIV (McLean & Fitzgerald, 2017).

Mood disorders

In this section, depression, psychosis and mania are examined in relation to people living with HIV and TB.

Depression

Anyone can become depressed, but people with serious illnesses such as HIV and TB are at greater risk. It is imperative that nurses screen and consider depression when dealing with people living with HIV and TB, especially considering that within a general population there is an estimated 10 per cent prevalence of depression, in comparison to an almost 50 per cent prevalence of depression among people living with HIV and TB. Furthermore, depression has a lifetime prevalence estimate ranging from 10–60 per cent. This means that 10–60 per cent of all people living with HIV and TB will become depressed at some time during their illness. Depression is associated with increased HIV mortality and, if left untreated, is associated with an increased viral load and a decline in CD4 lymphocytes, thus speeding up the progression of HIV to AIDS-defining illnesses and mortality. It is also reported that ARTs like efavirenz can cause depressive symptoms. This medication is associated with side effects such as nightmares, confusion, concentration difficulties, loss of memory hallucinations, delusions, suicidal ideation, paranoia and mania.

Diagnosis may be complicated by the fact that depression and HIV manifest with similar somatic or affective symptoms. Fatigue, lethargy, low libido, low appetite and weight loss may be manifestations of either HIV-related illnesses or depressive disorder. In contrast, cognitive and affective symptoms – such as feeling sad, losing interest in formerly enjoyable activities, guilt and irritability – are components of only depression. It is important to assess how a person living with HIV will respond to treatment for depression in order to establish whether they are presenting with depression or other opportunistic conditions associated with HIV.

Nurses need to be mindful that when assessing people living with HIV/TB, minor types of depression can also present as mood and cognitive symptoms (such as negative thoughts and flight of thoughts), as opposed to neuro-vegetative symptoms like sleep and/or appetite disturbances. The use of depression rating scales such as the Hamilton Depression Rating Scale (HDRS) have proven to be effective in making a conclusive diagnosis. Such evaluations, assessing for the potential comorbid illness of depression, should be conducted in all health care facilities. If a positive diagnosis of depression is made among people living with HIV and TB, the nurse should establish whether such patients have had or are having any thoughts of suicidal ideation. This is in spite of the fact that recent studies report a lower incidence of suicide among people living with HIV and TB. Suicide has decreased especially since the advent of ART. However, it still remains very important for nurses to discuss suicidal ideation with patients, especially during times of diagnosis, deterioration of physical health and following losses of friends and significant others due to an HIV-defining illness or TB.

Given that depression among people living with HIV and TB is multi-faceted, it follows that the care and treatment needs to be holistic with a combination of treatment approaches to yield the best results. Antidepressants and psychotherapy have proved to be effective forms of treatment. The initiation of antidepressants is a based on a stepwise process, starting low and going slowly. The use of SSRIs have been shown to be effective in the management and treatment of depression among people living with HIV and are the most widely prescribed medication for depression. The use of SSRIs is especially effective as they pass through the P450 system, which assists in significantly interacting with HIV-related medication and therefore improving the efficacy of managing cognitive symptoms.

In addition to the pharmacological treatment of depression among people living with HIV, several non-pharmacological interventions are effective. These include psychotherapy modalities such as cognitive behavioural therapy (CBT), which has been shown to contribute to a significant decrease in depressive symptoms among people living with HIV. The use of CBT involves structured interventions that teach and facilitate skills development to help patients modify thought processes and behaviours related to depression. This form of psychotherapy also assists patients with coping strategies that help them to deal with the diagnosis of HIV, as well as exercises that assist them in positively reframing their approach towards living positively with HIV as a chronic illness.

Symptoms of depressive disorders among people living with HIV and TB
When assessing and diagnosing a patient, it is important for the nurse to note that a major depressive disorder may be characterised by five or more of the following symptoms occurring in a two-week period.
- Depressed mood almost all day, every day **OR**
- Loss of interest or enjoyment of usually pleasurable activities for most of the day **AND**
- Significant weight loss in the absence of dieting or medial illness or weight gain of more than 5 per cent of body weight in one month or decreased/increased appetite
- Insomnia or hypersomnia
- Psychomotor agitation or retardation (observable by others, not only subjective feelings, feelings of restlessness or of being slowed down)
- Fatigue or loss of energy
- Feelings of worthlessness or excessive or inappropriate guilt (may be delusional)
- Diminished ability to think or concentrate or indecisiveness
- Recurrent thoughts of death, dying or of ending one's own life, with or without a specific plan.

(Jonsson et al, 2013; Chuah et al, 2017; APA, 2013.)

Psychosis and mania

While psychosis and mania are less common among people living with HIV and TB, (the prevalence is less than 6 per cent), it is still important to for nursing practitioners to consider and manage these conditions. Even though most cases of psychosis develop in advanced HIV disease (specifically stages 3 and 4) and seem to be associated with the presence of cognitive impairment, psychosis and mania can also occur as a result of substance abuse among individuals with chronic mental illness. Patients who present with HIV-related psychosis will also present with features of cognitive impairment, which can lead to HIV-related dementia if left untreated.

Signs and symptoms of psychosis or mania experienced by people living with HIV and TB
Mania is characterised by abnormally and persistently elevated (high) mood or irritability accompanied by at least three of the following symptoms:

1. Overly inflated self-esteem
2. Decreased need for sleep
3. Increased talkativeness
4. Racing thoughts
5. Distractibility
6. Increase in goal-directed activity such as shopping
7. Physical agitation
8. Excessive involvement in risky behaviours or activities.

(Jonsson, 2014; Stoloff & Joska, 2015)

Use of ART with people experiencing mental disorders

It is important to note that the use of ART as per the South African National ART guideline is safe (Department of Health, 2014; 2019). In particular, there has been evidence demonstrating the safety of efavirenz use among patients with a severe mental disorder. Thus, avoiding efavirenz to avoid worsening psychosis or depression is not warranted.

Cognitive impairment

A consequence of the HIV replication on the brain is what is known as an HIV-associated neurocognitive disorder (HAND). Cognitive difficulties may be caused by HIV, including HIV-associated dementia (HAD). Dementia is defined as a 'loss of intellectual abilities of sufficient severity to interfere with social or occupational functioning' (Zhou & Saksena, 2013).

The following observations can be made about these neurocognitive disorders associated with HIV:

- Less commonly used terms like HIV encephalopathy and AIDS-dementia complex also refer to HAD.
- The decline in cognitive function in HAND is characterised by memory loss, cognitive slowing (withdrawal can be prominent), and gait disturbances (loss of balance, stumbling).
- A spectrum of cognitive disorders is represented by HAND. Asymptomatic neurocognitive impairment (ANI) and mild neurocognitive disorder (MND) are the milder forms of HAND (APA, 2013).

These types of neurological disorders are often classified according to the extent of neurological and functional impairment, MNDs and HAD.

In South Africa, the prevalence of HAND prior to the ART-era was 42 per cent in people living with HIV but this was reduced to a prevalence of 25 per cent when ART became effective.

Dementia and HIV

Dementia is one of the most common and clinically important CNS complications of late HIV-1 infection. It is a source of great morbidity and, when severe, is associated with limited survival. Although the severity and the signs and symptoms may vary among patients, the general characteristics of HAD involve three functional domains, namely cognitive deficits, behavioural changes and motor involvement. The clinical presentation of dementia varies. Patients may develop ambulation or gait problems, mania, panic, psychosis, social isolation or anxiety.

A significant increase in overall morbidity is associated with HAD. This results from a combination of factors, including a greater number of hospitalisations, longer hospital stays, and decreased life expectancy. Patients with cognitive difficulties have problems with compliance and adherence to their medication regimen. The most important implication of a neuropsychological impairment involves the quality of life: this relates to increased risk-taking behaviour, difficulties of functioning in a work environment and impaired visuospatial functions, especially motor vehicle driving.

Criteria for the diagnosis of HAD include cognitive deficits in two or more cognitive domains causing impairment in activities of daily living (ADL) and an abnormality in either motor or neurobehavioral function. In the early stage, findings from the mental state examination (MSE) and the general neurologic examination are normal, but later the patient exhibits inattention, impaired concentration, memory loss, slowed verbal responses and a blunted affect. During a history-taking interview the following complaints may be common:

- Impairment in memory (short term and long term), abstract thinking, judgement, and higher cortical functioning
- Personality changes that interfere with relationships
- Inability to carry out normal social or occupational functions
- Experience in some patients of only minor forgetfulness and diminished visual or motor skills.

The treatment and management of HAD is aligned to the management of HIV, specifically to the maintenance of high levels of CD4 lymphocytes.

Substance abuse

Substance abuse among people living with HIV/TB poses a complex challenge for mental health care practitioners, as it compromises the immune system, but also serves as an unhealthy coping mechanism. In the South African context, alcohol and substance abuse, especially that of cannabis, heroin and crystal methamphetamine (tik) has plagued many communities. Those who are particularly affected are lower socioeconomic communities. The effect of substance abuse among people living with HIV/ TB is especially detrimental. It is widely known that substance abuse is an inhibitory factor towards ART adherence, and that forms of substance abuse – alcohol and especially methamphetamine – can have a toxic effect on the immune system by hindering immune reconstitution in someone who is on ART. Nursing practitioners should be aware that substance abuse among people living with HIV/TB is often indicative of another underlying problem like depression and needs further assessment and treatment.

PSYCHOTROPIC DRUG INTERACTIONS WITH HIV/TB

Given the significant numbers of people who experience co-infection of HIV, TB and related mental health issues within South Africa, it is imperative that nursing practitioners are aware of the potential drug interactions between the drugs used in the treatment of TB, ART and psychotropic medication.

As the need for holistic care of patients at a primary health care level becomes more emphasised especially in the context of managing HIV, TB and mental illness, it is important for the nursing practitioner to be aware of the potential interactions. This is in order to minimise side effects, which may hamper treatment adherence in the spectrum of care of all three illnesses (HIV, TB and mental disorders). Table 21.2 provides an overview of the commonly used drugs in South Africa to treat HIV, TB and common mental disorders.

Table 21.2 Commonly used drugs for treating HIV and TB

	Drug	Potential side effects	
		Neuropsychiatric	**Other**
Anti-TB medications	Isoniazid	Neuropathy; seizures; psychosis; movement disorders	GIT disturbances; liver damage; haematological effects
	Ethambutol	Neuropathy; delirium (with or without psychosis)	Ocular toxicity; gout; renal damage
	Rifampicin	Sedation; weakness; delirium (with or without psychosis)	GIT disturbances; liver damage; dizziness
	Aminoglycosides (eg streptomycin; kanamycin)	Muscle weakness; tremor; vertigo	Ototoxicity; renal damage
	Quinolones (eg ciprofloxacin; ofloxacin; levofloxacin; moxifloxacin)	Headache; delirium (with or without psychosis); hallucinations; seizures	GIT disturbances; dizziness
	Cycloserine & teridazone	Anxiety; delirium; mood disturbances; psychosis; headaches; tremor; seizures; sedation	GIT disturbances; dizziness

	Drug	Potential side effects	
		Neuropsychiatric	Other
Anti-TB medications (continued)	Ethionomaide	Anxiety; delirium; mood disturbances; psychosis; headaches; seizures; sedation	GIT disturbances
Antiretroviral medications	Efavirenz	Abnormal dreams; headaches; inattention; insomnia; depression; psychosis	Skin rashes; dizziness
	Lamivudine (3TC)	Depression; insomnia; peripheral neuropathy;	GIT disturbances; skin rashes; pancreatitis
	Emtricitabine	Insomnia; abnormal dreams; depression	Dizziness
	Tenofivir	Delirium	GIT disturbances; renal damage
	Zidovudine	Headaches; myalgia; insomnia; delirium; modd disturbances	GIT disturbances; haematological effects
	Atazanavir	Insomnia; depression	GIT disturbances; dizziness
	Ritonavir	Sedation	GIT disturbances; dizziness; metabolic abnormalities; syncope
	Nevirapine	Headache	Skin rash; fever

Source: Stender (2013)

CONCLUSION

The WHO's statement, 'there is no health without mental health' can be extended to the role of the nurse. At a 2017 conference convened by the Association of Nurses in AIDS Care (ANAC), it was stated that 'all nurses are mental health nurses'. In a low- and middle-income country such as South Africa, which is challenged by a number of socioeconomic factors, the triple burden of HIV, TB and mental health disorders is especially rife. This illuminates the role of the nurse as one of an integrated primary health care provider, with the skills to assess and provide holistic nursing care for clients with a potential co-infection of HIV, TB and mental health disorders. Regarding the treatment of mental health conditions related to HIV, it is especially important to mitigate poor treatment adherence to improve health outcomes and the quality of life for people living with HIV, TB and mental disorders.

REFERENCES

American Psychiatric Association (APA). 2013. *Diagnostic and Statistical Manual of Mental Disorders*. 5th edition. Washington, DC: American Psychiatric Association.

American Psychological Association. 'Pharmacologic interventions for HIV-associated neurocognitive disorders'. https://www.apa.org/pi/aids/resources/exchange/2013/01/pharmacologic-interventions.aspx (Accessed November 2018).

Ayano, G, Solomon, M and Abraha, M. 2018. 'A systematic review and meta-analysis of epidemiology of depression in people living with HIV in east Africa'. *BMC: Psychiatry*, 18: 254. doi: 10.1186/s12888-018-1835-3.

Bongongo, T, Tumbo, J and Govender, I. 2013. 'Depressive features among adult patients receiving antiretroviral therapy for HIV in Rustenburg district, SA'. *South African Journal of Psychiatry*, 19 (2): 31–34. doi: 10.7196/SAJP.418.

Chuah, F L H, Haldane, V E Cervero-Liceras, F, Ong, S E, Sigfrid, L A, Murphy, G, Watt, N, Balabanova, B, Hogarth, S, Maimaris, W, Otero, L, Buse, K, McKee, M, Piot, P, Pablo, P and Helena Legido-Quigley, H. 2017. 'Interventions and approaches to integrating HIV and mental health services: a systematic review'. *Health Policy and Planning*. doi: 10.1093/heapol/czw169

Dellar, R, Waxman, A and Abdool Karim, Q. 2015. 'Understanding and responding to HIV risk in young South African women: Clinical perspectives'. *South African Medical Journal*. 105 (11): 952. doi: 10.7196/SAMJ.2015.v105i11.10099.

Department of Health. 2014. *National Consolidated Guidelines for the Prevention of Mother to Child Transmission of HIV (PMTCT), and the Management of HIV in Children, Adolescents and Adults*. Republic of South Africa: National Department of Health: Pretoria.

Department of Health. 2019. *2019 ART clinical guidelines for the management of HIV in adults, pregnancy, adolescents, children, infants and neonates*. Republic of South Africa: National Department of Health: Pretoria.

Duko, B, Gebeyehu, A and Ayano, G. 2015. 'Prevalence and correlates of depression and anxiety among patients with tuberculosis at Wolaita Sodo University Hospital and Sodo Health Center, Wolaita Sodo, South Ethiopia, Cross sectional study'. *BMC: Psychiatry*, 15: 214 doi: 10.1186/s12888-015-0598-3.

Gupta, A, Wood, R, Kaplan, R, Bekker, L G and Lawn, S D. 2015. 'Tuberculosis incidence rates during 8 years of follow-up on an antiretroviral treatment cohort in South Africa: Comparison with rates in the community'. *PLoS ONE*. 7 (3): e34156. doi: 10.1371/journal.pone.0034156.

Jonsson, G. 2014. 'An approach to assessing mental health disorders in the general HIV clinic'. *HIV Nursing Matters*. 5 (3): 22–27.

Kinyanda, E, Weiss, H A, Levin, J, Nakasujja, N, Birabwa, H, Nakku, J and Mpang, R. 2017. 'Incidence and Persistence of Major Depressive Disorder among People Living with HIV in Uganda'. *AIDS and Behaviour*. 21: 1641–1654. doi: 10.1007/s10461-016-1575-7.

Manda, S O, Masenyetse, L J, Lancaster, J L and Van der Walt, M L. 2013. 'Risk of death among HIV co-infected multidrug resistant Tuberculosis Patients Compared to Mortality in the General Population of South Africa'. *Journal of AIDS and Clinical Research*, 2: 3–7.

Maughan-Brown, B, George, G, Beckett, S, Evans, M, Lewis, L, Cawood, C, Khanyile, D and Kharsany, A. 2018. 'HIV Risk among Adolescent Girls and Young Women in Age-Disparate Partnerships'. *AIDS Journal of Acquired Immune Deficiency Syndromes*, 78 (2): 155–162. doi: 10.1097/QAI.0000000000001656.

McLean, C P and Fitzgerald, H. 2017. 'Treating post-traumatic stress symptoms among people living with HIV: A critical review of intervention trials'. *Current Psychiatry Reports*, 18 (9). doi: 10.1007/s11920-016-0724-z.

Nanni, M G, Caruso, R, Mitchell, AJ, Meggiolaro, E and Grassi, L. 2015. 'Depression in HIV-infected Patients: A Review'. *Current Psychiatry Reports*, 17: 530. doi: 10.1007/s11920-014-0530-4.

Saban, A, Flisher, A J, Grimsrud, A, Morojele, N, London, L, Williams, D R and Stein, D J. 2014. 'The association between substance use and common mental disorders in young adults: results from the South African Stress and Health (SASH) survey'. *PAN African Medical Journal*, 17 (1): 11. doi: 10.11694/pamj.supp.2014.17.1.3328 .

Stender, S C. 2013. 'Complexities in managing patients with co-morbidities: understanding the potential side effects of mental health and HIV/TB medications'. *HIV Nursing Matters*, 5 (3): 34–35.

Stoloff, K and Joska, J. 2015. 'HIV/AIDS and mental health'. In: *Primary Care Psychiatry: A practical guide for southern Africa*. 2nd edition. Juta: Cape Town: South Africa.

The Joint United Nations Programme on HIV/AIDS (UNAIDS). 2018. 'Ending tuberculosis and AIDS: a joint response in the era of Sustainable Development Goals-country submissions'. *UNAIDS*. Geneva: Switzerland.

Tesfaw, G, Ayano, G, Awoke, T, Assefa, D, Birhanu, Z, Miheretie, G and Abebe, G. 2016. 'Prevalence and correlates of depression and anxiety among patients with HIV on follow up at Alert Hospital, Addis Ababa, Ethiopia'. *BMC: Psychiatry*, 16: 36. doi: 10.1186/s12888-016-1037-9.

Venter, W D F. (2018). 'HIV and Tuberculosis prevention and control in South Africa: An overview'. *South African Journal of Public Health*. 2 (3): 52-54. doi: 10.7196/SHS.2018.v2.i3.61.

World Health Organisation (WHO). 2013. 'Comprehensive Mental Health Action Plan for 2013–2020'. *WHO*. Geneva: Switzerland.

World Health Organisation (WHO). 2016. 'Global Tuberculosis Report 2016'. *WHO*. Geneva: Switzerland.

Zhou, L and Saksena, N K. 2013. 'HIV-associated neurocognitive disorders'. *Infectious disease report*, 6 (5): e8. doi: 10.4081/idr.2013.s1.e8.

CHAPTER 22

Mental Health Nursing of Children and Adolescents

L van Rhyn

Learning Outcomes

After studying this chapter, you should be able to:
- differentiate between the most common psychiatric disorders of childhood and adolescence
- access the mental health and functioning of children, adolescents and their families
- implement basic nursing interventions for children and adolescents.

INTRODUCTION

Children under 18 are legal minors in the context of South Africa and account for about one third of the South African population of approximately 56.5 million people (Statistics South Africa, 2017). The worldwide prevalence of children and adolescents suffering from a mental disorder is 13.4 per cent (Polanczyk et al, 2015: 345). It is difficult to determine the prevalence in South Africa as recent statistics on mental disorders in children have not been published. A study conducted in the Western Cape in 2006 indicated a prevalence of 17 per cent. Epidemiological studies in high-, middle- and low-income countries show that approximately one in five children suffer from a mental disorder.

Despite significant gains in tackling the major causes of child mortality and evidence of an urgent need for child and adolescent mental health services (CAMHS), resource-poor countries continue to lag behind in CAMHS development. Some of the obstacles in the development of adequate mental health services are the magnitude of child mental health problems that remain invisible to policy makers, an absence of child mental health policies to guide the process of service development, and overburdened professionals working in child mental health. Criminal and domestic violence towards children and adolescents has become a major public issue and the number of cases of physical and sexual abuse seen in a variety of settings has escalated alarmingly. The majority of these children and youth are from disadvantaged backgrounds and many fall under the category of 'children with special needs'. These children grow up in poverty, are subjected to physical, emotional and/or sexual abuse, have experienced or witnessed various forms of violence in their families and communities, and some are addicted to alcohol and other substances. Such children are at risk for various mental health problems, which include anxiety states, attention-deficit/hyperactivity disorder

(ADHD), post-traumatic stress disorder, behavioural and antisocial disorders, and depression resulting in suicide (Flisher et al, 2010).

Unmanageable caseloads and ineffective judicial procedures mean that survivors and their families often remain unsupported and at risk.

There is a need to provide primary health care workers with mental health skills and thus integrate child and adolescent mental health care into the primary health care structure. Such a move could make mental health accessible to all children.

Mental health nurses generally have limited exposure to child psychiatry during their basic training. The South African Nursing Council (SANC) has introduced an advanced diploma in child psychiatric nursing, but specialised training for this diploma is at present offered at only one tertiary education centre in the country. The number of nurses involved in the care of children with psychiatric problems is therefore extremely limited. It is an urgent priority to train more mental health nurses in child and adolescent psychiatry and to develop systems in which their expertise can be utilised to the maximum. The country also needs many more therapists who can counsel children and families in their mother tongue, especially African languages.

MENTAL DISORDERS IN CHILDREN AND ADOLESCENTS

A meta-analysis completed by Polanczyk et al (2015: 345) on the worldwide prevalence of child and adolescent mental disorders indicated that the most common disorders are anxiety (6.5 per cent), depressive (2.6 per cent), attention-deficit/hyperactivity (3.4 per cent) and disruptive (5.7 per cent) disorders.

This chapter will focus only on the most common disorders diagnosed in children and adolescents.

The DSM-5 does not have a separate classification for child and adolescent mental disorders as was the case in the past (APA, 2013). Any diagnoses can be made in children if they meet the diagnostic criteria.

Specific learning disorders

Learning disorders are neurodevelopmental disorders caused by the interaction between heritable and environmental factors. They are characterised by persistent difficulty relating to learning academic skills in reading, written expression or mathematics. A learning disorder starts in early childhood and is inconsistent with the overall intellectual ability of the child. These children find it difficult to keep up with their peers in certain academic subjects, whereas they may excel in others. The disorder results in underachievement. This is unexpected because of the child's potential and the opportunity the child would have had to have engaged in the learning opportunities available.

The main treatment for these disorders is remedial scholastic strategies and emotional support. Nurses are mostly involved in supporting and counselling these children to help them cope with their emotions and possible issues with their self-image

Autism spectrum disorders

Prior to the development of the DSM-5, autism spectrum disorder was conceptualised as five discrete disorders, namely autistic disorder, Asperger's disorder, Rett's disorder, childhood disintegrative disorder, and pervasive development disorder not otherwise specified. Recent clinical consensus has shifted the conceptualisation of autism spectrum disorder towards a continuum model (Grinker et al, 2012).

The core diagnostic impairments are divided into two domains: deficits in social communication and restricted repetitive behaviour. Aberrant language development and usage is no longer considered a core feature of autism spectrum disorder. Approximately one-third of children meeting the current DSM-5 diagnosis of autism spectrum disorder exhibit intellectual disability.

The global prevalence of this disorder is approximately 1 per cent and it is diagnosed four times more often in boys than in girls. A combination of psychosocial and psychopharmacological interventions is the choice of treatment (Bakare & Munir, 2011).

Attention-deficit/hyperactivity disorder (ADHD)

Rates for ADHD have been reported to be 7–8 per cent in prepubertal elementary school children. Epidemiological studies suggest that ADHD occurs in about 5 per cent of youth including children and adolescents. A review of the epidemiology of ADHD symptoms among African school children indicated that the prevalence is between 5.4 per cent and 8.7 per cent (Bakare, 2012). The South African studies documented a prevalence of about 5 per cent which concurred with the worldwide prevalence as reported by Polanczyk et al (2015).

A debate exists as to whether ADHD might be a cultural construct. The opinion that geographical location may have some influence on the epidemiology of ADHD remains, despite a few studies having concluded that culture and geographical location may have little or no influence on the epidemiology worldwide (Bakare, 2012).

Aetiology of ADHD

The current consensus is that the aetiology of ADHD involves complex interactions of neuroanatomical and neurochemical systems. The suggested contributing factors include prenatal toxic exposures, prematurity and prenatal mechanical insult to the foetal nervous system. Food additives, colourings, preservatives and sugar have also been suggested as possible causes of hyperactive behaviour. No scientific evidence indicates that these factors cause ADHD. There is also no evidence that omega-3 fatty acids are beneficial in the treatment of ADHD.

There is evidence of a genetic basis for the disorder. Siblings of hyperactive children have about twice the risk of having the disorder as children in the general population. When ADHD coexists with conduct disorder in the child, alcohol-use disorders and antisocial personality disorders are more common in the parents than in the general population (American Academy of Pediatrics, 2011).

Minimal, subtle and subclinical brain damage may be responsible for the genesis of ADHD. Soft neurological signs are frequent. They are subtle neurological abnormalities and involve impairment in the ability to perform several motor and sensory tests. Symptoms are rigidity, gait imbalance and tremors. No clear-cut evidence implicates a single neurotransmitter in the development of ADHD, but many neurotransmitters may be involved in the process.

The human brain normally undergoes major growth spurts at different stages of development. Some children have a maturational delay in the growth sequence and then manifest with symptoms of ADHD that appear to be temporary. Some children with ADHD have abnormal electroencephalograph (EEG) patterns.

Children in institutions are frequently overactive and have poor attention spans. These signs result from prolonged emotional deprivation and they disappear when deprivational factors are removed, such as when the child is adopted or placed in a foster home. Stressful emotional events, severe chronic abuse, maltreatment and neglect are associated with certain behavioural symptoms that overlap with ADHD. These include poor attention and poor impulse control. Predisposing factors may include the child's temperament, genetic-familial factors and the demands of society to adhere to a routinised way of behaving and performing. Socioeconomic status does not seem to be a predisposing factor.

Clinical features

ADHD is rarely recognised until a child is at least toddler age. The most cited characteristics in children with ADHD in order of frequency are (Sadock et al, 2015):

- Hyperactivity
- Attention deficit (short attention span, distractibility, perseveration, failure to finish tasks, inattention and poor concentration)
- Impulsivity (action before thought, abrupt shifts in activity, lack of organisation and jumping up in class)
- Memory and thinking deficits
- Learning disabilities
- Speech and hearing deficits.

Associated features often include perceptual motor impairment and emotional lability.

A significant percentage of children with ADHD show behavioural symptoms of aggression and defiance. School difficulties often exist.

The DSM-5 has made several changes to the diagnostic criteria of ADHD in youth. In the past, ADHD symptoms had to be present by the age of seven years but according to the DSM-5, several inattentive and hyperactive-impulsive impulses must be present by the age of 12 years. Previously there were two subtypes of ADHD, namely the inattentive; and hyperactive/impulsive. In the DSM-5, the subtypes have been replaced by the following three specifiers, which essentially denote the same groups: (1) combined presentation; (2) predominantly inattentive presentation; and (3) predominantly hyperactive/impulsive presentation. Additional changes in the DSM-5 include the provision for a comorbid ADHD and autism spectrum diagnosis. A further change is the DSM-5's requirement of only five rather than six symptoms of either inattention, or hyperactivity and impulsivity in adolescents 17 years and older.

Intervention

The following are some of the strategies that can be implemented when intervening in children and adolescents with ADHD.

Pharmacotherapy

Pharmacotherapy is considered the first line of treatment and includes the following different types of medication:
- Central nervous system stimulants are the first choice of agents in that they have been shown to have the greatest efficacy with generally mild and tolerable side effects, for example Ritalin (in children six years and older), Concerta and Dexedrine (in children three years and older).
- Second-line agents with evidence of efficacy include Strattera, a norepinephrine uptake inhibitor.
- Examples of antidepressants are Wellbutrin and Effexor.

Psychosocial interventions

Medication alone is often not sufficient to satisfy the comprehensive therapeutic needs of children with ADHD and is usually one facet of a multimodal regimen that involves (Sadock et al, 2015: 1178):
- psycho-education
- academic skills remediation
- cognitive behavioural therapy (CBT)
- social skills groups
- behavioural techniques at home and in the classroom
- evaluation and treatment of coexisting learning disorders or additional psychiatric disorders
- education to children and parents about the purpose of medication
- opportunities to talk about their feelings regarding the medication
- structuring of the environment
- keeping children responsible for meeting reasonable expectations
- group therapy to increase self-esteem and the sense of success.

Oppositional defiant disorder

The DSM-5 criteria for oppositional defiant disorder are as follows (APA, 2013):

A. A pattern of angry/irritable mood, argumentative/defiant behavior, or vindictiveness lasting at least 6 months as evidenced by at least four symptoms from any of the following categories, and exhibited during interaction with at least one individual who is not a sibling.

   Angry/Irritable Mood
   1. Often loses temper.
   2. Is often touchy or easily annoyed.
   3. Is often angry and resentful.

   Argumentative/Defiant Behavior
   4. Often argues with authority figures or, for children and adolescents, with adults.
   5. Often actively defies or refuses to comply with requests from authority figures or with rules.
   6. Often deliberately annoys others.
   7. Often blames others for his or her mistakes or misbehavior.

   Vindictiveness
   8. Has been spiteful or vindictive at least twice within the past 6 months.

   Note: The persistence and frequency of these behaviors should be used to distinguish a behavior that is within normal limits from a behavior that is symptomatic. For children younger than 5 years, the behavior should occur on most days for a period of at least 6 months unless otherwise noted (Criterion A8). For individuals 5 years or older, the behavior should occur at least once per week for at least 6 months, unless othenwise noted (Criterion AS). While these frequency criteria provide guidance on a minimal level of frequency to define symptoms, other factors should also be considered, such as whether the frequency and intensity of the behaviors are outside a range that is normative for the individual's developmental level, gender, and culture.

B. The disturbance in behavior is associated with distress in the individual or others in his or her immediate social context (e.g., family, peer group, work colleagues), or it impacts negatively on social, educational, occupational, or other important areas of functioning.

C. The behaviors do not occur exclusively during the course of a psychotic, substance use, depressive, or bipolar disorder. Also, the criteria are not met for disruptive mood dysregulation disorder.

Specify current severity:

   Mild: Symptoms are confined to only one setting (e.g., at home, at school, at work, with peers).
   Moderate: Some symptoms are present in at least two settings.
   Severe: Some symptoms are present in three or more settings.

Conduct disorder

The aetiology, clinical features and intervention strategies are dealt with in relation to this disorder.

Aetiology

No single factor can fully account for a child's antisocial behaviour and conduct disorder. Many biopsychosocial factors contribute to the development of the disorder.

Some parental attitudes and faulty child-rearing practices influence the development of children's maladaptive behaviours. Harsh, punitive parenting characterised by severe physical and verbal aggression is associated with the development of children's maladaptive aggressive behaviours. Chaotic home conditions are associated with conduct disorder. Broken homes per se are not causatively significant; it is the strife between the parents that contributes to conduct disorder. Parental psychopathology, child abuse and negligence often contribute to this disorder. Sociopathy, alcohol dependence, psychosis and substance abuse in the parents are associated with conduct disorder in their children. Psychodynamic hypotheses suggest that children with conduct disorder unconsciously act out their parent's antisocial wishes.

Current theories suggest that socioeconomically deprived children are at a higher risk for developing the disorder. Unemployed parents, lack of a supportive social network and poor participation in community activities seem to predict conduct disorder. Alcohol use among adolescents is associated with increased delinquent and aggressive behaviour. Drug intoxication can aggravate the symptoms.

Conduct disorder and ADHD often coexist. Studies indicate decreased noradrenergic functioning and blood serotonin is increased (Sadock et al, 2015).

Children who are exposed to violence for long periods, especially those who endure physically abusive treatment, often behave in aggressive ways. ADHD, central nervous system (CNS) dysfunction or damage, and early extremes of temperament can predispose a child to conduct disorder.

Clinical features

Conduct disorder does not develop overnight. Many symptoms evolve over time until a consistent pattern develops that involves violating the rights of others. The average age of onset is younger in boys than in girls. Boys most commonly meet the diagnostic criteria by 10 to 12 years of age, whereas girls often reach 14 to 16 years of age before the criteria are met.

Children who meet the diagnostic criteria for conduct disorder express their overt, aggressive behaviour in various forms. Aggressive antisocial behaviour can take the form of bullying, physical aggression and cruel behaviour towards peers. Children may be hostile, verbally abusive, defiant and negativistic towards adults. Persistent lying, frequent truancy and vandalism are common. In severe cases, destructiveness, stealing and physical violence often occur. Sexual behaviour and regular use of tobacco, alcohol and illegal psychoactive substances begin usually early in the life of these children and adolescents. Suicidal thoughts, gestures and acts are frequent in children with this disorder who are in conflict with peers, family members and the law. They are unable to solve their difficulties.

Intervention

Milder forms of these conditions should be addressed by working with parents/caregivers to help them in the therapeutic handling of the children. Parent-teaching programmes such as systematic training in effective parenting (STEP) can assist parents in being consistent and using behaviour modification approaches to handle the children's behaviour (Zisser & Eyberg, 2010). Direct training of parents in child management skills and careful assessment of family interactions are suggested.

Treatment strategies for young children that focus on increasing social behaviour and social competence are believed to reduce aggressive behaviour. An environmental structure that provides support along with consistent rules and expected consequences can help control a variety of problem behaviours.

In more serious conditions much more robust approaches are needed, and even then, prognosis is often poor. First, comorbid disorders in the family should be addressed to reduce the level of stress and dysfunction in the family. This could mean treatment for substance abuse or other psychiatric conditions for parents, or family therapy to assist the family in dealing with interpersonal conflict. Secondly, a network approach to dealing with the behaviour of the child is indicated. This means that all those adults working with the child should meet to decide on a coherent approach. This ensures that they do not undermine each other's efforts nor does it allow the child to manipulate conflict between them. Teachers, parents, social workers, adult siblings and other interested adults should be included. The plan the group draws up should be based on behaviour modification principles, but aversive conditioning should be limited and firm, consistent limit setting within a warm and caring environment used as far as possible.

When a family is abusive or chaotic, a child may have to be removed from the home to benefit from a consistent and structured environment.

Elimination disorders

These disorders include enuresis and encopresis.

Enuresis: aetiology

Psychiatric disorders are present in only about 20 per cent of enuretic children and are most common in enuretic girls, in children with symptoms during the day and the night, and in children who maintain the symptoms into older childhood. Although most children with enuresis do not have a comorbid psychiatric disorder they are at higher risk for the development of another psychiatric disorder. A spontaneous resolution of nocturnal enuresis occurs in about 15 per cent of children per year. Nocturnal enuresis is 50 per cent more common in boys and accounts for 80 per cent of children with enuresis.

Difficulties in the child's neuromuscular and cognitive development, socio-emotional factors and toilet training may delay urinary continence. In a longitudinal study of child development, those children who were enuretic were about twice as likely to have concomitant developmental delays as were dry children. Although there may be a genetic basis for enuresis, much can be accounted for by tolerance for enuresis in those families.

A child with enuresis has a functionally small bladder so that the child feels an urge to void with little urine in the bladder. Some studies report that nocturnal enuresis occurs when the bladder is full because of lower than expected levels of the night-time antidiuretic hormone. Those factors allow for a higher than usual urine output. Enuresis does not appear to be related to a specific stage of sleep or time of the night. Little evidence indicates that enuretic children sleep more soundly than do other children.

Psychosocial stressors appear to precipitate some cases of enuresis. In young children the disorder has been particularly associated with the birth of a sibling, the start of school, hospitalisation between the ages of two and four, the break-up of a family because of divorce or death and a move to a new environment.

Enuresis: Clinical features

Enuresis is the repeated voiding of urine in the child's clothes or bed. The voiding may be involuntary or intentional. The child must exhibit a developmental or chronological age of at least 5 years. According to the DSM-5 the behaviour must occur twice a week for at least three months or must cause distress or impairment in functioning to meet the diagnostic criteria. It is diagnosed only if the behaviour is not caused by a medical condition. Children with enuresis are at a higher risk for ADHD compared to the general population.

Enuresis: Intervention

A treatment plan can be developed after medical causes of urinary dysfunction have been ruled out.

An assessment must be made; the family is the logical source of information about toilet training and the prevalence of enuresis. Information about the age at which toilet training was commenced and the technique used supplies clues regarding the family's expectations and the effectiveness of their toilet-training methods. Record keeping is helpful in determining a baseline; following the child's progress may itself be a reinforcer.

Appropriate toilet training with parental reinforcement can be helpful. Look out for stressors that may cause the behaviour. One of the therapeutic objectives of the nurse is to help the family to re-establish physical and psychological security and to offer this to the child.

Methods which may prove effective are to leave a night-light on, to allow the child to sleep with a favourite toy, to restrict fluids in the evening and to take the child to the toilet regularly.

Behaviour therapy can also be successfully implemented. Nocturnal enuresis often clears up spontaneously if it is ignored. Children are rewarded after passing urine in the toilet. Fluids are encouraged to provide a reason for frequent reinforcement. Star charts are particularly helpful. Children are taught a structured procedure for elimination, that is, to go to the toilet, remove clothes, void, maintain hygiene and dress again. They are also rewarded for periods of keeping dry. Accidents are not punished and no special attention is paid to them. Personal hygiene should be maintained.

Another conditioning technique is the enuresis alarm, which consists of a urine-sensitive pillow connected to an alarm system. As soon as the pillow becomes wet, the alarm goes off because the urine acts as an electrolyte and completes an electric circuit. This wakes the child, which means that they must get up, pass urine, change pyjamas and bed linen and reset the alarm. The child is taught by this means to inhibit urination to avoid the unpleasant experience. Dryness results in more than 50 per cent of cases. Difficulties may include child and family non-compliance, improper use of the apparatus and relapse.

Bladder (interval) training is another technique that may be attempted. Children with nocturnal enuresis pass very little urine during the day and it is possible that they have not yet learned to interpret the sensation of a full bladder. A few days are chosen during which there is no pressure and no interruptions and large amounts of fluids (about 400 ml) are given every half hour. The child is encouraged to try and lengthen the intervals between urination. Every time the sensation to void is experienced, the urine must be held back a little longer.

Another basic intervention for children with enuresis and bowel dysfunction is to assess whether chronic constipation is contributing to urinary dysfunction. Dietary fibre should be increased in the diets of these cases.

Nurses must realise that parents are often very anxious and must be reassured and supported. The child must be taught to pay particular attention to hygiene, as unpleasant odours may lead to teasing and rejection by peers. The nurse must support the child without being judgemental. Drugs should rarely be used to treat enuresis and then only as a last resort in intractable cases causing socio-emotional difficulties for the child. Tofranil has been used successfully, but the success does not often last as tolerance often develops after six weeks of therapy. This second-line medication, imipramine (Tofranil) is typically reserved for when other therapies fail. It is not known exactly how imipramine exerts its action to prevent nocturnal enuresis, but prevention is believed to be linked to the drug's ability to block acetylcholine receptors (Scheffel et al, 2017).

Encopresis: Aetiology

The lack of appropriate toilet training or inadequate training may delay the child's attainment of continence. Evidence indicates that encopretic children suffer from lifelong ineffective sphincter control leading to infrequent defecation, withholding of bowel movements and avoidance of defecation. Children may avoid the pain of having a bowel movement, which then causes impaction and overflow soiling. The resulting chronic rectal distension from large, hard faecal masses may cause loss of tone in the rectal wall and desensitisation to pressure. Many children become unaware of the need to defecate and overflow encopresis occurs, usually with relatively small amounts of liquid or soft stool leaking out.

In about 5–10 per cent of cases faecal incontinence is caused by a medical condition like spinal cord damage.

Sexual abuse can predispose a child to encopresis, but it is not a specific indicator of sexual abuse.

A power struggle between the parent and the child over issues of autonomy and control can cause the disorder. Such battles frequently cause behavioural problems. Psychiatric difficulties may be present.

Encopresis may be associated with neuro-developmental problems, including easy distractibility, short attention span, low frustration tolerance, hyperactivity and poor coordination. Encopresis may also be precipitated by life events, such as the birth of a sibling or a move to a new home. Occasionally, the child has a special fear of using the toilet. Encopresis sometimes appears to be a regression after such stresses as a parental separation or the start of school.

Encopresis is not as common as enuresis but its prognosis is poorer.

Encopresis: Clinical features

Encopresis is the passing of faeces into inappropriate places at least once a month for three months

To receive a diagnosis of encopresis a child must have a developmental or chronological age of at least four years. The DSM-5 includes two specifiers to encopresis, namely encopresis *with* constipation and overflow incontinence and encopresis *without* constipation and overflow incontinence. If the faecal incontinence is directly related to a medical condition the diagnosis cannot be made.

Encopresis: Intervention

The treatment plan for encopresis cannot be established until a medical assessment of bowel function, as well as a full psychiatric evaluation, is completed.

One first has to distinguish between encopresis with constipation and overflow incontinence, and encopresis as a result of anxiety or inability to control the bowel. Retention encopresis is generally treated with laxatives, stool softeners and enemas until the bowel is empty, after which routine elimination is taught. Nurses must be sensitive and supportive and show empathy when using these measures, as both the symptom and the treatment are concerned with the same part of the body. Star charts and CBT can be used.

The nurse must ensure that the child feels secure by reducing anxiety during toilet training and by teaching the parents to foster this security through ensuring that toilet behaviour is a desirable and rewarding experience for the child. The child's feelings of anxiety and guilt about the encopresis are best managed by making use of play. Relatively structured play allows the child to express concerns and serves as a non-threatening way of sharing feelings with others. The nurse should win the child's confidence in order to address the emotional subject of elimination. School nurses can support children by ensuring privacy for regular changing of soiled clothes to avoid teasing and rejection by peers. Learning bladder and bowel control is an important step in enabling children to take part in normal daily life.

Family tension regarding the symptom must be reduced and a non-punitive atmosphere must be created. Interactive parent–child family guidance and counselling is useful for easing family tension, for treating encopretic children's reactions to their symptoms (such as low self-esteem and social isolation), and for treating those cases of encopresis after a long period of faecal continence that are reactions to psychological stressors.

Anxiety disorders

Anxiety disorders are among the most common disorders in youth. Anxiety disorders are characterised by recurrent emotional and physiological arousal in response to excessive perceptions of perceived threat or danger.

Separation anxiety disorder, generalised anxiety disorder and social anxiety disorder in children are often considered together in the evaluation process and differential diagnosis. They are also considered together in the development of treatment strategies because they are highly comorbid and have overlapping symptoms. A child with one of these three disorders has a 60 per cent chance of having at least one of the other two disorders as well.

Aetiology

Evidence for the influences of parental psychopathology and parenting styles on the emergence of anxiety disorders in children has been found in multiple investigations. Parental overprotection has been associated with an increased risk of the development of anxiety disorders in children. Insecure parent–child attachment is associated with higher than expected rates of anxiety disorders in childhood. It is also a well-known observation that maternal depression and anxiety have led to an increased risk for anxiety and depression in children. The temperamental traits of shyness and withdrawal in unfamiliar situations can increase the risk for the development of an anxiety disorder in childhood and adolescence.

Young children, who are immature and dependent on a mothering figure, are particularly prone to anxiety related to separation. The disorder occurs when the child has a disproportionate fear of mother loss. The character structure pattern in many children with separation anxiety disorder includes conscientiousness, eagerness to please and a tendency towards conformity. Families tend to be close-knit and the children often seem to be spoiled or the objects of parental over-concern.

External life stresses often coincide with the development of the disorder. The death of a relative, illness in the child, a change in the child's environment or a new school are frequently noted in the histories of these children.

Anxiety may be communicated from parents to children by direct modelling. Some parents appear to teach their children to be anxious by overprotecting them from expected dangers or by exaggerating the dangers. For example, a parent who cringes in a room during a lightning storm teaches the child to do the same. A parent, on the other hand, who becomes angry with a child when the child expresses fear of a given situation may promote a phobic concern in the child by exposing the child to the intensity of the anger expressed by the parent. Social learning factors in the development of anxiety reactions are magnified when parents have anxiety disorders themselves.

Genetic studies suggest that genes account for at least one-third of the variance in the development of anxiety disorders (Cortina et al, 2012). Heritability for anxiety disorders in children and adolescence ranges between 36 and 65 per cent, with the highest estimates found in younger children. Family studies have shown that the offspring of adults with anxiety disorders are at an increased risk of having an anxiety disorder themselves. Separation anxiety disorder and depression in children overlap.

Clinical features

The clinical features of separation anxiety disorder, generalised anxiety disorder and social anxiety disorder will be examined separately.

Separation anxiety disorder

This disorder is diagnosed when developmentally inappropriate and excessive anxiety emerges related to separation from the major attachment figure. According to the DSM-5, separation anxiety disorder is characterised by a level of fear or anxiety regarding separation from parents or a primary caregiver which is beyond developmental expectations. There may be a pervasive worry that harm will come to a parent upon separation which leads to extreme distress and sometimes nightmares related to separation issues. The DSM-5 requires the presence of at least three symptoms related to excessive worry about separation for a period of at least four weeks. The worries often take the form of refusal to go to school, fears and distress on separation, repeated complaints of physical symptoms such as headaches and stomach-aches when separation is anticipated.

Generalised anxiety disorder

Children with this disorder have significant distress in activities of daily life. It is focused on the child's fears of incompetence in many areas including school performance and in social settings. According to the DSM-5 (2013: 222), children with this disorder experience at least one of the following symptoms:
- restlessness
- being easily fatigued
- irritability
- muscle tension
- sleep disturbance
- 'mind going blank'.

They tend to feel fearful in multiple settings and expect more negative outcomes when faced with academic or social challenges compared with peers. Children and adolescents with this disorder tend to be overly concerned about potential natural disasters such as earthquakes or floods. These worries can interfere with their daily activities. These children are continuously worried about the quality of their performance in academics and sports and often seek excessive reassurance about their performance.

Social anxiety disorder (social phobia)

This diagnosis is made when children experience intense discomfort and distress in social situations and are impaired by their fear of scrutiny or humiliation. Their distress may be expressed in the form of crying, tantrums, avoidance, freezing or even becoming mute. According to the DSM-5, this disorder is characterised by consistent anxiety and distress in almost all social situations. Children must experience the anxiety in the presence of peers and not only with adults.

Intervention for anxiety disorders

The treatment of all three of these anxiety disorders in children is often considered together because of the frequent comorbidity and overlapping of symptomatology between them.

A multimodal comprehensive treatment approach usually includes CBT (James et al, 2013), family education, family psychosocial intervention and pharmacology. Refusing to go to school associated with separation anxiety can be viewed as a psychiatric emergency. A comprehensive treatment plan involves the child, parents, the child's peers and school. Firm encouragement to attend school is maintained while appropriate support is also provided. When a return to a full school day is overwhelming for the child, a programme should be arranged so that the child can progressively increase the time spent at school. Behaviour modification in the form of graded contact with an object of anxiety can be useful in the treatment of anxiety disorders.

Evidence-based research has shown that the combination of selective serotonin reuptake inhibitors (SSRIs) and CBT is safe and effective in the treatment of anxiety disorders in children (Silverman & Field, 2011).

Major depressive disorder

The DSM-5 utilises the same criteria for major depressive disorder in youth as in adults except that for children and adolescents an irritable mood may replace a depressed mood in the diagnostic criteria. The clinical presentation is strongly influenced by the developmental level of the child or adolescent.

Aetiology

The following observations can me made regarding the aetiology of major depressive disorder:
- Children's moods are especially vulnerable to the influences of severe social stressors such as chronic family discord, abuse and neglect, and academic failure.
- Parental mental illness and substance abuse or poverty are factors.
- Learning problems and underachievement can cause depression in a child.
- There is a genetic basis for major depressive disorder – it tends to cluster in the same families. Having one depressed parent probably doubles the risk for the offspring. Having both parents depressed probably quadruples the risk of a child having a mood disorder before age 18 when compared with the risk for children with two unaffected parents (De Vries et al, 2013).
- Boys whose fathers died before they were 13 years old are more likely to have depression than boys whose parents did not die before they were 13.
- Prepubertal children in an episode of a major depressive disorder secrete significantly more growth hormone during sleep than do normal children.
- Hypoglycaemia is suggested in some studies as a cause of depression in children.
- Separation or loss can be a cause. The loss may be real (for example, parental divorce) or symbolic.

Hospitalisation and depressive symptoms

A South African study was conducted among black children during hospitalisation for orthopaedic procedures (Hall & Sambu, 2016). A significant correlation between hospitalisation and depressive symptomatology was found. According to a recent review, at least 20 per cent of children admitted into hospital display some degree of behavioural or emotional disturbance (Polanczyk et al, 2015).

In hospital, children are separated from parents, siblings, peers and familiar environments. This separation deprives them of the psychological and social support necessary for adaptation to the strange surroundings and events, and sometimes also to pain and discomfort. It has been suggested that surgery, in particular, poses a significant risk for the child. Maternal separation often elicits depressive-like symptoms.

It is probable that illness and hospitalisation have different meanings for and effects on children from different cultural and social groups. An increased risk of problem behaviours in response to hospitalisation has been found to be associated with coming from a deprived and disadvantaged home. The difficult circumstances of many black South African children may have a negative effect on their experience of hospitalisation.

Socioeconomic conditions, as well as long distances to urban health services, make it difficult for parents to pay regular visits to their children in hospital. The ability of parents to visit their children has been found in some studies to influence the child's experience of hospitalisation.

Clinical features

According to the DSM-5 the diagnostic criteria for a major depressive episode consist of at least five symptoms for a period of two weeks including either a depressed or irritable mood or a loss interest or pleasure.

Additional features of depression in children

There are a number of additional features of depression in children, which include:
- A failure to make expected weight gains
- Daily insomnia or hypersomnia
- Psychomotor agitation or retardation
- Daily fatigue or loss of energy
- Feelings of worthlessness or inappropriate guilt
- Diminished ability to think or concentrate
- Recurrent thoughts of death
- Somatic complaints like abdominal pain, headaches and dizziness
- Social withdrawal and sad appearance
- Mood-congruent hallucinations
- A poor self-esteem
- Anhedonia and ambivalence
- A sense of hopelessness, loneliness and boredom
- Declining academic performance
- Aggressive behaviour and violent outbursts
- Enuresis
- Failure to thrive
- Bad dreams
- Negativistic behaviour
- Feelings of restlessness, grouchiness, sulkiness and a reluctance to cooperate in family ventures
- Inattention to personal appearance
- Increased emotionality

- Sensitivity to rejection in love relationships
- Poor peer relationships
- Delusions which centre on themes of guilt, physical disease, death, nihilism, deserved punishment, personal inadequacy and sometimes persecution, especially in adolescents
- A description of feelings as follows: sad, empty, low, down, blue, very unhappy, crying, or having a bad feeling inside that is there most of the time.

Intervention

To prevent this disorder as a result of hospitalisation, all efforts to reduce anxiety in hospitalised children should be made. Parents should be allowed to stay with their children, play activities to support the child emotionally should be implemented, and procedures should be explained. The child must be prepared regarding the consequences of certain nursing and medical interventions. For example, when a child has to go to the operating theatre, dolls can be used to explain this to the child beforehand.

Other interventions that apply to major depressive disorder include family counselling and education, as well as individual counselling of the child. However, these forms of counselling have to be structured and directed. The child can be taught social and problem-solving skills through modelling and role-playing techniques.

Group therapy for children and adolescents with chronic mood disorders functions best when integrated with a variety of individuals from other diagnostic realms. Relaxation techniques can also be implemented. Medication (antidepressants) is often used and therapeutic and side effects should be monitored.

Another form of therapy, CBT, is widely recognised as an efficacious intervention for the treatment of moderately severe depression in children and adolescents. This form of therapy aims to challenge maladaptive beliefs and enhance problem-solving abilities and social competence. The best evidence-based treatment seems to be a combination of Prozac with CBT (Sadock et al, 2015). There is evidence that fluoxetine (Prozac) leads to greater and faster improvement than placebos or psychotherapy in adolescents. Considering both the high response to non-specific interventions and safety concerns, antidepressants should be used cautiously in youth, and limited to patients with moderate-to-severe depression for whom psychosocial interventions are either ineffective or not feasible (Vitiello & Ordonez, 2016).

Suicide in adolescents

Mood disorders do increase the risk of suicide and so any suicidal behaviour associated with depressed mood is a matter of serious concern. Although completed suicide is relatively rare in children, the incidence of suicide attempts reaches a peak during the mid-adolescent years. Mortality from suicide, which increases steadily through the teens, is the third leading cause of death at that age.

Child abuse, domestic violence, sexual abuse, eating disorders or substance abuse (by family members or the child themselves) may be important comorbidities that can be missed if not specifically sought.

Warning signs of potential adolescent suicide

These are the warning signs of potential suicide in adolescents:
- Drastic changes in behaviour, for example sudden withdrawal in an otherwise socially active person
- Stated feelings of sadness, loneliness, hopelessness or despair
- Increased impulsive risk-taking behaviours, for example disregard for safety
- Alienating behaviours, for example withdrawal or aggression
- Giving away possessions, especially those with special meaning
- Preoccupation with death and dying
- Sudden changes in personal appearance and hygiene
- Previous suicide attempt or gesture
- Direct suicidal comments such as 'I wish I were dead'.

Risk factors for adolescent suicide

The risk factors for suicide in adolescents include:
- Loss of significant relationship with friend, family member or pet
- Suicide of a friend, relative or public figure
- Homophobic response of family members to an adolescent's sexual preference, for example rejection
- Divorce of parents
- Break-up with girlfriend or boyfriend
- Non-attainment of a significant goal, such as acceptance at a particular college
- Dropping out of school
- Only child in the family
- Previous conduct disorder
- Previous suicide attempt.

Nursing interventions for the suicidal adolescent

The nurse can intervene when an adolescent is suicidal in these ways:
- Always take seriously the expression of a wish to die.
- Provide a safe environment.
- Obtain a verbal contract that the individual will not do anything to harm themselves. without talking to a responsible adult.
- Check on the adolescent's feelings of safety and control at frequent intervals.

Post-traumatic stress disorder (PTSD)

The most common stressors for PTSD in children are violence, rape, physical and sexual abuse. Although there are no reliable epidemiological statistics available for the sexual abuse of children, it is commonly diagnosed. Nurses in child psychiatric units in South Africa report that approximately 60–70 per cent of girls seen in these units have been sexually abused (Mathews et al, 2013). Sexual abuse is not a psychiatric diagnosis, but it causes severe emotional distress in children.

Aetiology

Risk factors in children for developing PTSD include pre-existing anxiety and depressive disorders. Suggestions are that a genetic predisposition for anxiety disorders as well as a family history indicating increased risk of depressive disorders may predispose a trauma-exposed child to develop PTSD. Symptoms of PTSD can be modelled to children by parents, for example during natural disasters.

Family support and reactions to traumatic events may play a significant role in the development of PTSD. Adverse parental emotional reactions to a child's abuse may increase the child's risk of developing PTSD. Lack of parental support and psychopathology among parents (especially maternal depression) have been identified as risk factors in the development of PTSD after a child has been exposed to a traumatic event.

Clinical features

PTSD is characterised by a set of symptoms including intrusive memories of the trauma, persistent avoidance of stimuli that are reminders of the traumatic event, persistent negative alterations in cognition and mood and alterations in arousal, mainly seen as hyperarousal and irritability following a traumatic event. In the DSM-5, the traumatic event criterion is defined as exposure to actual threatened death, serious injury or sexual violence. This exposure can occur directly, by witnessing it; learning of a traumatic event to a family member; or experiencing repeated exposure to trauma precipitated by social or natural disasters. Exposure to trauma through electronic media, movies, television or photographs is excluded from the criteria. If PTSD is diagnosed in children under six years of age, it falls under the preschool subtype.

Developmental factors strongly influence the manifestation of the symptoms of PTSD. In children and adolescents, re-experiencing of a traumatic event is observed through play, recurrent nightmares without recall of the traumatic events and behaviour that re-enacts the traumatic situation along with agitation, fear and disorganisation.

Intervention

The registered nurse should refer the patient to a professional nurse qualified in advanced child and adolescent psychiatric nursing or to a psychologist. However, if these professionals are not available, the following approaches can be used (Hermenau et al, 2011):

- Encourage desensitisation by allowing the child to speak about the incident in a supportive environment, or to express feelings through drawing or playing
- Help the child to assert themselves in threatening situations by teaching assertiveness skills
- Building self-confidence can help the child to cope with the aftermath of trauma
- Implement psycho-education regarding the nature of typical emotional and psychological reactions to traumatic events
- Guide the use of muscle relaxation and focused breathing
- Apply the principles of crisis intervention and debriefing.

Adolescent substance abuse

Many risk and protective factors influence the age of onset and severity of substance use among adolescents. Psychosocial risk factors mediating the development of substance-use disorders include parental modelling of substance use, family conflict, lack of parental supervision, peer relationships and individual life events. Other risk factors include leisure boredom, lack of anger control in families, maternal passivity, comorbid psychiatric disorders such as conduct disorder and depression, impulsivity and early onset of cigarette smoking (Peltzer, 2010).

Protective factors that mitigate substance use among adolescents include variables such as a stable family life, a strong parent–child bond, consistent parental supervision, investment in academic achievement and a peer group that models prosocial family and school behaviours.

Studies on alcoholism demonstrated a greater prevalence among biological children of alcoholics than among adopted youth, which suggests a genetic contribution towards the development of alcoholism.

The greater the number of risk factors, the more likely it is that an adolescent will be a substance user (Myers et al, 2010).

ASSESSMENT OF CHILDREN WITH MENTAL HEALTH DISORDERS

A comprehensive evaluation of a child includes clinical interviews with the parents, the child and the family. Clinical interviews allow for the most flexibility in understanding the evolution of problems over time and in establishing the role of environmental stressors.

Sources often disagree about a variety of symptoms and behaviours during a comprehensive assessment of a child. When faced with contradictory information, the nurse must realise that those differences may reflect an accurate picture of the child's presentation in different settings.

Interviewing the child

The four general reasons for interviewing children include:
1. Making a psychiatric diagnosis, such as a major depressive episode
2. Obtaining information about physical or sexual abuse
3. Encouraging children to talk about their understanding of traumatic events which they may have witnessed or in which they may have been involved
4. Getting the child's perspective on why they have been brought for an interview and how they understand their present problems.

Five possible objectives for the assessment of the mental health of children are to (Merrel, 2011):
1. Determine in which areas and to what extent the child differs from other children of the same age group.
2. Determine the chronicity of the problem.
3. Identify the areas of strength of the child and the family from the viewpoint of the family and the nurse.
4. Formulate hypotheses about previous and current contributing factors, and the interaction between the factors.
5. Plan priorities for intervention.

The success of an interview with a child depends on prior preparation. Children are an excellent source of information about their own symptomatology, but they often have difficulty with the chronology of symptoms; they are sometimes unwilling to talk about behaviours that have got them into trouble; and they may have difficulty in verbally expressing their feelings and experiences. Information from the family, the school and any community agencies involved may help to explain the reasons for the referral and to plan the process and content of the interview.

The process of the child interview

A number of factors may influence the process of the interview. These include the developmental abilities of the child, factors within the interviewer, factors within the child and, finally, the way in which the interviewer interacts with the child.

The developmental abilities of the child

The order in which these clinical interviews take place is influenced to some extent by the developmental age of the child. For example, some authors believe that adolescents should be interviewed before their parents. One of the major developmental tasks of the adolescent is to establish their own identity as a person, separate from those of the parents. It is therefore important for adolescents to feel that the interviewer's impressions of them have not been biased in any way by prior in-depth contact with the parents.

On the other hand, interviews with young children usually begin with the parents

present, since very young children may be frightened by the interview situation. Having the parents present also provides an opportunity for the nurse to assess the parent–child interaction. At some point in the interview process the child should be seen without the parents present. There are two major reasons for this:
1. The child might not feel free to talk openly for fear of eliciting a critical or undermining response from the parent(s).
2. Children might minimise their problems and anxieties through fear of the parents' response, or to protect the parents.

Knowing the developmental norms associated with the age of the child to be interviewed helps the nurse to match the content and process of the interview with the child's developmental abilities. For example, fear of imaginary dangers such as ghosts or monsters is a feature of children aged two to five. The nurse could use this knowledge as a basis for enquiring about the nature of any fears the child might have:
Nurse: Do you see monsters? What do the monsters want to do to you?

The level of confidentiality in a child assessment is correlated with the age of the child – that is, just about all specific information is shared with the parents of a very young child and more privacy is reasonable with an adolescent. School-age and older children may be told that if the nurse becomes concerned that they are a danger to themselves or to others, that information will have to be shared with other adults. However, the nurse must determine whether a child is safe in their environment and make clinical judgements about whether the child is a victim of abuse or neglect.

Factors within the interviewer
Many people may feel the need to rescue the child from the situation or problem that they are facing. In instances where the professional's attempt to engage with the child elicits negative or angry responses from the child, the professional may become angry and/or demoralised.

Four factors within the interviewer that may interfere with the process of the interview are:
1. There may be overidentification with the child because of the way the interviewer was treated as a child.
2. The interviewer may experience emotional residue from old conflicts in response to certain behaviours in the child.
3. Racial, religious and political prejudices within the interviewer may influence their interactions with the child.
4. The interviewer may feel threatened by sexually attractive children and adolescents and concentrate more than is necessary on sexual aspects of development or ignore these aspects altogether.

The interviewer may also overidentify with the parents' struggles with the child, because of their own experiences as a parent.

Factors within the child
Children are first and foremost members of a family system, which provides them with a sense of identity. Because of this, children are often ambivalent about sharing their problems and feelings, even if the problem involves them and other members of the family. They may feel ashamed to talk about things that they have been punished for doing. They may feel guilty about disclosing a family secret such as parental conflict but, at the same time, they want the behaviour to stop.

Children sometimes feel responsible for family problems, particularly sexual abuse. Professionals are often confused about why a child who initially claimed that they were a victim of sexual abuse later withdraws their statement. This is because the consequences of the claim may be far worse for the child than the abuse itself. Examples of what these consequences could be are: the loss of a family member such as the father; fear of being harmed by an avenging family member; economic hardship for the rest of the family through loss of a breadwinner; feeling responsible and guilty for sending a loved one to jail.

An adolescent may approach an interview with apprehension or outright hostility but open up when the nurse is neither punitive nor judgemental. Nurses must be aware of their own responses to an adolescent's behaviour (countertransference), so as to remain therapeutic, even in the face of a defiant, angry or difficult adolescent. Nurses should set appropriate limits and should postpone or discontinue the interview if they feel threatened or if patients become destructive to property or to themselves.

The interview should always include an exploration of suicidal thoughts, assaultive behaviour, psychotic phenomena, substance use and sexual relationships. Once a rapport has been established, many adolescents appreciate the opportunity to tell their side of the story and may reveal things that have not been disclosed to anyone else.

Guidelines to facilitate the process of the interview
The following guidelines could facilitate interaction with children of any age (Red Cross War Memorial Children's Hospital, nd):
- A child may find offices or clinics very intimidating. A short walk may ease the tension and allow the child to see you as a non-threatening, friendly person.
- Conduct the interview in a spirit of fun, exploration and enthusiasm. Be friendly and relaxed. Avoid a serious, rushed and super-professional attitude – it is quite acceptable to sit on the floor with the child. Show interest, give feedback and reassurance, and do not express either positive or negative judgements about what the child says.
- Use action-oriented tools. Play materials are used for young children and a game is played, or something is made in the case of older children. Examples of toys in an interview room include paper, pencils, paint, a writing board, clay, a sandpit, cars, dolls, puppets, storybooks, building blocks and various games, for example card and board games.
- Allow the child to take the lead. The self-concept and developmental functioning of children are reflected in their perception of life events. Do not offer suggestions,

answers or solutions to problems unless they fit the child's explanation. However, it is essential to guide a child who cannot take the lead.
- There are two levels to all communication: the process and the content. Look and listen carefully. The conduct of children is just as important as what they say, and all observations are relevant data. For example, the response of a child to your touch may be an indication of their ability to relate to adults.
- Direct questions can be very threatening. Children respond more easily to examples and fantasy and speak more readily about other children than about themselves. The following are examples of questions that could be asked: 'Tell me about good (bad) mothers and fathers you have seen on television or whom you have read about in storybooks. Do you know someone like that?' or 'If trees could talk, what would they say to you?'
- Use the child's language and frame of reference when following up themes that have touched a chord ('I wonder what makes them do that?').
- Take the child's side and show empathy in times of stress. Give feedback in a manner that will not be viewed as judgemental or as criticism. A monologue works well when sensitive areas such as the child's problem behaviour are being discussed. Tell a story and watch carefully for non-verbal responses.
- Do not limit the assessment to one session. Additional contact adds validity to a database.

The content of the child interview

Guidelines regarding the content of the child interview are set out in Table 22.1.

Obviously, most children will be unable to give an account of their own developmental history; part of the family interview will thus be used to obtain this information.

Table 22.1 Child psychiatric interview (CPI)

Child psychiatric interview (CPI)
The child psychiatric interview is intended as a guide for the process of interviewing children. It is not a checklist and it is not intended to be all-inclusive. Where specific information is required, for example with abused, depressed, psychotic or autistic children, reference to more specialised interviews is indicated.
A. Introduction and interviewing 1. Escort child to and from waiting room. 2. Welcome child and set at ease. 3. Initially with younger child, use play and observation, then move into verbal communication. 4. Reassure that confidence will not be betrayed unless the information has to be revealed, such as in a report for court, in which case an explanation to the child is necessary. 5. Discuss reason for referral. What do you call this place? Do you know why children come here? 6. Useful materials: drawing materials, construction toys (eg Lego, blocks) and family of dolls. As far as possible the remaining part of the room should be free of toys or other distracting objects.

→

Child psychiatric interview (CPI)

B. General questions

This includes general topics and conversation about recent events and activities.
1. What they like doing on weekends.
2. What television they watch.
3. What their hobbies/interests are and what games are played.
4. Ambitions and aspirations. What they would like to be when grown up.
5. Three wishes.
6. Island companion.
7. Free drawing – eg ask the child to draw whatever they like and to tell a story about the drawing on completion.

C. Structure and specific questions

1. School: How are you getting on there? Any homework? Who helps? What do you like best and least? Why? Likes or dislikes the teacher – specify. Likes or dislikes subjects – specify. Likes or dislikes activities – specify.
2. Peers: Do you have one special friend? Enquire about teasing, bullying or anxieties. Specify peer contacts and child's popularity or isolation. Do you ever feel lonely?
3. Appetite: Do you like eating? Enquire about eating patterns. Enquire about weight loss or gain.
4. Sleep: Some children do not like getting up in the morning. How about you? What about going to sleep at night? Enquire about sleep problems.
5. Dreams: Everyone dreams; what do you dream about? Do you have bad, nasty, scary, etc, dreams? How often? Do you wake up? Who comes to comfort you?
6. Worries: Most people worry about something. What kinds of things do you worry about? Does thinking about unpleasant or nasty things ever stop you from getting to sleep? Do you ever get nasty/unhappy/worrying thoughts? What is your biggest worry?
7. Depression: Do you ever cry? Do you feel really unhappy sometimes? Do you sometimes feel sad for no reason?
8. Fears: Many children have things they are afraid of, such as snakes or spiders. Enquire about fears of shadows, dark, ghosts, cats, dogs, etc. Are these fears in the past, or present? What do you do when you meet whatever things you are afraid of? Are you afraid of things happening to you or your family? What kind of things?
9. Anger: Everyone gets angry sometimes – what gets you angry? What do you do when you are angry? Do you get into fights sometimes? Do you like fighting? Are they 'friendly' or 'real' fights? Who do you fight with? How often? What makes you stop being angry?
10. Home: Who lives there? What is father's/mother's work? Do you have your own bedroom? Who do you get on best with? Do you have any brothers or sisters? We all have fights with siblings – do you fight often? Are they real or friendly fights?
11. By now the presenting problem should have been dealt with – if not, it should be actively dealt with at this stage. Enquire about frequency, severity and duration of problem(s). Ask for examples, for instance in the case of sexual abuse, enquire about the room or house in which the abuse occurred, who was present, how often it occurred and where the parent was.

Mental status examination

This section of the interview is generally obtained through observation of the patient during the specific questioning period.

→

Child psychiatric interview (CPI)

A. General appearance
Note the child's general physical appearance, body posture, dress and grooming. Do they appear neglected? Do they appear small/large for age? Note facial expression. Also note waiting room behaviour, separation and reunion.

B. Interview reaction
Note the child's general reaction to interviewer. The following factors may be noted:
eye contact; preoccupation with anxiety or depressive lapses; reserve or expansiveness; self-confidence and esteem; spontaneous remarks; rapport with interviewer – capacity to engage; response to interviewer – friendly, open, teasing, hostile, negativistic, shy, sullen, ingratiating, precocious or familiar; cooperation and compliance.

C. Cognition
Note the child's: level of general information; attention span; distractibility; persistence; impulsivity; curiosity; memory. Note general impression of intellectual level.

D. Motor reaction
Note the child's: hyperactivity; fidgetiness; muscle tension; coordination – fine/gross; clumsiness; tics; involuntary movements.

E. Affect
Specify whether the child appears: sad; tearful; depressed; sullen; withdrawn; anxious; hostile; angry; negative; oppositional.
Note whether there is any: oddness/flatness/incongruity; guilt feelings; suicidal thinking.
Also note the child's emotional expressiveness and range.

F. Speech
Note if any of the following are present: stammer/stutter; lisp; articulatory defects; indistinct expression; aphasia.
Also note comprehension and use of language.

G. Thought content
Note whether there is any impairment of cognition manifested in the following: inappropriate behaviour or speech; irrelevant answers to questions; repeated words or phrases; tendency to drift away from topic; lack of coherence; delusions or false beliefs; illogical thought patterns; irrational or strange behaviours; hallucinations – sight, sound, touch, taste or hearing; mood swings; lack of insight; bizarre behaviours.

H. Summary
1. Diagnosis – Preliminary
2. Formulation – Hypothesis of relation of disorder to presenting problem and current or antecedent events.

Interviewing the family

A family interview may involve a number of interviews, each with a different constellation of family members. A family interview is important because the symptoms with which children present are often a reflection of the functioning of their families.

Sometimes an interview with the entire family, including the parents' other children, can be enlightening. The purpose is to observe the attitudes of the parents towards the patient and the affective responses of the children to their parents. The nurse's job is to maintain a non-threatening atmosphere in which each member of the family may speak freely without feeling that the nurse is taking sides with any particular member.

The nurse must validate each family member's feelings in the setting, because a lack of communication within the family often contributes to their problems. The parents may be interviewed together, without other family members present. Here, the objectives would be to get a chronological account of the child's growth and development, the parents' perspective on family dynamics, their marital history, their beliefs about the cause and nature of the child's problems, and their expectations of professional intervention.

An example of a family assessment format

Introduction

Name
Record the name of the index patient and the names of all the other family members present. Indicate reasons for the absence of significant members.

Orientation
Orient the family by clarifying what each member expects of the interview and what each hope to get out of it. Give feedback by explaining what you, the therapist, plan and hope to achieve with the interview, and explain why the whole family must be present.

Presenting problems
Each individual member of the family describes the problem or problems that brought the family for assessment. Record the problems, their duration and possible precipitating factors.

Family functioning

Problem solving
This is the ability of the family to solve instrumental and affective problems at a level that maintains effective family functioning.

Communication
There are a number of ways in which information is transmitted within the family:
- instrumental (goal directed, task directed and without emotion)
- affective (emotion laden and person directed)

- direct or indirect
- clear or masked.

Roles in the family
Who does what? Are the roles complementary? Is there mutual acceptance of roles? What constitutes the mother role, father role and child role?

Affective responsiveness
How freely are negative and positive emotions shown? Who shows them? To whom are they shown?

Affective involvement
The degree to which the family as a whole takes an interest in and respects the interests and activities of individual members.

Behaviour control
There are different patterns that the family adopts for coping with three types of situations:
1. Physically dangerous situations, for example a child playing with fire
2. Meeting and expressing psychobiological needs, for example reaching adolescence and entering into relationships with partners
3. Interpersonal socialising behaviour – within and outside the family, for example joining new groups.

There are four styles of behaviour control, namely rigid, flexible, laissez-faire and chaotic. Identify the one used by the family.

Parent assessment
- Physical health
- Personality
- Psychiatric disorders:
    - current emotional condition
    - history of previous disorders
    - duration
    - treatment
- Alcohol/substance abuse:
    - quantities
    - duration
    - effects
- Violence:
    - towards spouse, peers or children.

Marital relationship
- Previous marriages:
  - father
  - mother
- Marital status:
  - father
  - mother
- Courting and marriage
- Relationship (including sexual aspect).

Social circumstances
Circle of friends, use of free time, community involvement

Families of origin
- Paternal/maternal families (including step-grandparents)
- Ages
- Education
- Occupation
- Religion
- Physical health
- Personality
- Psychiatric disorders
- Alcohol/substance abuse
- Violence (criminal record)
- Marital relationship
- Parent–child relationship
- Siblings
- Familial illnesses.

This assessment may take longer than one session. A genogram can be compiled on completion of the assessment. The family is referred to a therapist for family therapy if there are serious problems.

Individual child assessment
This is the assessment of the child based on information about the child obtained from parents/caregivers.

Development history
This may be taken in the presence of the whole or part of the family.

Birth order
Age difference between index child and previous child/pregnancy.

Pregnancy as related to this child
- Planned
- Conceived out of wedlock (be very tactful in obtaining this information if it is not volunteered spontaneously)
- Physical health
- Emotional health
- Significant events (this refers to emotionally significant events during pregnancy and includes the death of a parent and desertion by the father of the child).

Birth
- Labour
- Delivery:
  - full term
- Normal vertex delivery
- Forceps delivery
- Breech delivery
- Caesarean section delivery:
  - birth weight
  - sex preference
  - postpartum
- Mother: any physical or psychological problems
- Child: first six weeks after birth, for example prolonged incubation.

Early development
- Mother and child relationship
  - Feeding
  - Sleeping
  - Crying
  - Restlessness/irritability
  - Role of father.

Milestones
- Motor activities:
  - sitting
  - crawling
  - standing
  - walking
- Language:
  - babbling
  - using words

- constructing sentences
- comprehending
▪ Bladder control:
  - day
  - night
▪ Bowel control.

Physical health
▪ Illnesses
▪ Seizures
▪ Operations
▪ Injuries
▪ Hospitalisations.

Separations
▪ Details about periods of separation during early childhood:
  - Age of child
  - Length of separation
  - Nature of alternative care
  - Reaction of child

Facilities for care
Whether the mother is absent or works.

School history
▪ Schools attended by the child and reasons for changing schools
▪ Scholastic ability
▪ Adjustment
▪ Refer to the child's conduct and general and social adjustment with peers and teachers
▪ Request permission to obtain a report from the school.

Interests and activities
Self-help: the child's ability to perform age-appropriate self-help activities.

Physical health and functioning
▪ Eating
▪ Sleeping
▪ Seeing
▪ Hearing
▪ Bladder and bowel control
▪ Sexual behaviour and knowledge
▪ Psychophysiological symptoms
▪ Record any problems in the areas mentioned.

Children's drawings

Having children draw pictures of themselves and of their family provides important assessment data. When asked to draw a picture of themselves and their family, children project specific fears, anxieties and concerns. In addition to viewing drawings within the child's developmental context, it is important to ask the child about the drawings, because artwork can easily be misinterpreted. Although the child's drawings are a rich source of assessment data, they need to be examined within the context of other assessment data for verification.

The child's drawings of human figures provide an index of the child's body image. Drawings of a three- to four-year-old child usually depict large heads and eyes, with arms and legs as appendages of the head. Gradually the trunk appears, with arms and legs as stick appendages. The child's overemphasis or omissions of body parts gives clues to the child's body image. Excessively large hands may indicate aggression, small arms and hands withdrawal and denial. Clearly defined body boundaries indicate a balance of body parts of the person on the drawing paper and are signs of a positive body image.

Children's drawings rarely include genitals. When the child draws genitals or stylised sexual figures, the nurse must realise that the child's drawing may be in response to rape, trauma or sexual abuse.

Often children draw what they cannot say.

Principles for assessing the behaviour of children

These four principles can be applied when assessing the behaviour of children:
1. Behaviour should be evaluated in terms of standard development characteristics and age-appropriate competencies.
2. Behaviour should be gauged against the background of the developmental problems of a specific stage that could make children vulnerable to stress and anxiety. An example would be loss and separation situations, such as divorce and death, which may be viewed by children as punishment or desertion because of egocentric thoughts. Such misunderstandings can cause serious emotional problems.
3. The unique patterns of children must be considered. For example, a child who appears to be aloof and shy may have a good friend. Such conduct should not be summarily dubbed as disturbed.
4. Children may function poorly in one or two areas while performing well in others. A problem must be identified when the balance is disturbed.

If special investigations are available and the nurse deems them necessary when assessing a child, the child may be referred. Special investigations include psychometry, audiometry, neurological investigations and occupational therapy evaluation.

MANAGING EMOTIONALLY AND BEHAVIOURALLY DISTURBED CHILDREN

There are some basic strategies that can be used by nurses to manage emotionally and behaviourally disturbed children. These strategies should be adapted to take the child's unique difficulties into account. Management also involves cooperation between the parents, health professionals and teachers, because home and school are major aspects of the child's life.

Communication principles

There are a number of communication strategies that can be applied:
- Be consistent and firm, but gentle.
- Give clear and simple instructions, repeat these three to four times if necessary, and maintain eye contact while doing so.
- Instructions or information should be exact, without qualifiers. Break down the information into small, easily assimilated sections.
- Give one task at a time and, if necessary, break it down into small, achievable steps.
- Help the child to perform/complete a task instead of criticising them for failing to attempt it. Overt and implied pressure can increase the child's anxiety and resistance to the intervention.

Fantasy control

Children may retreat into fantasy when they feel threatened or if they are left alone. If this happens:
- Gently remind the child where they are and who you are
- Do not join in with the child's fantasy or wait for them to finish the theme.

Structure

The child's inner world may be chaotic and, because of this, they may perceive the real world as a dangerous and strange place. It is therefore important to create some kind of order for the child.

External rules and limit setting can help, and the following guidelines can be implemented:
- Establish and maintain a predictable environment. Maintain regular routines of eating, sleeping, playing and discipline.
- Maintain a calm and simple environment to promote attention and subsequent learning. For example, the child should sit as near as possible to the teacher to reduce the possibility of being distracted by other children.
- Create a positive environment in which the child's needs, abilities and self-esteem can be nurtured.

- Tell the child about any changes to the environment before they are made, including what they are, when they will happen and where they will happen.

Limit setting

This helps to provide structure and, consequently, helps the child to feel safe because of the boundaries that are provided. Children may have difficulty with understanding the need for limits. Avoid lectures; simply state the rules and back them up. Use as few words as possible and keep instructions simple, focusing on one thing at a time. The goal is for the child to develop self-control and, with it, self-respect.

Behaviour control and physical restraint

When children become increasingly anxious, their behaviour may become more chaotic. When this happens, the following procedures may be beneficial:
- Physical containment with gentle and persistent reminders of reality may be necessary. For example, holding children gently while softly reminding them where they are, who they are and what is happening is far more anxiety reducing than shouting or slapping a child.
- If the child bolts, it is better to run with the child in as calm a manner as possible, rather than to chase them. If the child feels that they are being chased, fears about the possibility of being harmed will be reinforced.
- Ask the child what they think. This will make them feel safer. If possible, implement the measures suggested by the child. This may help to increase the child's self-esteem and problem-solving skills.

Other therapies

Children with communication disorders may need speech therapy, those with motor skill disorders may need physiotherapy, and those with learning disorders may need some form of remedial education. However, these facilities are not always available; if they are, a referral should be made. Occupational therapy is helpful for many children as it provides opportunities for learning new skills, developing coordination and is a form of constructive distraction. Special schools are not readily available to the majority of the population of this country. If these are available, they can play a therapeutic role in the life of the child.

Family involvement

Family involvement is important at all levels of intervention. The family needs to know about the disorder, and also needs to work on the issues within the family and within the marital relationship that may be contributing to the child's behaviour and individual members' distress. The following may prove advantageous:

- Education about the disorder, medical treatments and symptom management techniques
- Techniques to manage tension in the home, for example communication and conflict resolution skills
- Parenting skills
- Methods and styles of discipline
- Family therapy or couple counselling may be useful in dealing with marital and family issues
- Support groups may be helpful for parents and the other children in the family. Parents often feel frustrated because they have worked so hard and yet their child continues to have problems. Communicating with other parents struggling with similar problems can help to relieve the burden that family members may experience.

CONCLUSION

The vast majority of children in South Africa are exposed to environmental conditions which are known to be detrimental to mental health, namely social disadvantage and family stress. Social disadvantages include poverty, malnutrition, disease, lack of educational opportunities and inaccessible health and welfare facilities. Probably the most important factor in the causation of childhood mental health problems is the exposure of young children in the intimacy of family life to damaged parents.

Two other major circumstances contribute to social disadvantage and family stress within the South African context. The first is the structural violence inherent in our society. The second circumstance is associated with developments in southern Africa generally, namely urbanisation; the breakdown of traditional ways of life, including the extended family system; the abuse of substances by the young, and their unguarded sexual activity.

Current psychiatric services for children in South Africa include the following:
- Child and family units that is part of the government psychiatric hospitals
- Child guidance clinics
- The private sector
- Psychiatric community services
- Consultation services and information centres
- Day care centres
- Trauma counselling clinics like the Tygerbear Foundation for Traumatised Children and their Families in the Western Cape, and Teddy Bear Foundation's Medico-legal Clinic in Johannesburg.

The drawbacks of these services are that they are geographically poorly distributed and concentrated mainly in the cities. The bottleneck that prevents the development of child psychiatric services is situated at the administrative and not at the legislative level. The organisation of existing services is such that children and their parents go from one specialist (educational, health and social work) to another in search of expert advice.

The valuable time of experts, who are in short supply, is thus taken up unnecessarily. Furthermore, the available services of the health, social and educational authorities are not sufficiently coordinated.

Other problems include the following:
- Information about available services and problems regarding psychiatric disorders in children is not sufficiently available and accessible.
- The essential services of a coordinated professional team are not available in all cases.
- Services cannot be effectively extended before the required staff has been trained, yet there is a shortage of training facilities.
- There are no coordinated figures regarding the extent of psychiatric disorders in children in South Africa. Existing statistics are not collected in a simple manner and a comprehensive view therefore cannot be obtained.

It seems that a monumental task awaits us if we are to provide for the mental health needs of children.

WEB RESOURCES

saacapap.org.za

This is the website for the South African Association for Child and Adolescent Psychiatry and Allied Health professions. Get information on this website about the conference held by the Association. All members have access to the SAACAPAP's journal namely the Journal of Child and Adolescent Mental Health. This is the only African Journal of its type.

www.health.gov.za

The website contains policy guidelines on child and adolescent mental health from the National Department of Health.

www.health.uct.ac.za

This is the website of the Children's Institute, a multidisciplinary institute aiming to contribute to policies, laws and interventions that promote equality and realise the rights and improve the conditions of all children in South Africa.

https://www.savethechildren.org.za.

This is a website where one can learn all about the rights of children in South Africa.

REFERENCES

American Academy of Pediatrics. 2011. 'ADHD: Clinical Practice Guidelines for the Diagnosis, Evaluation and Treatment of Attention-Deficit/Hyperactivity Disorder in Children and Adolescents'. *Pediatrics,* 128 (5). doi: 10. 1542/peds.2011–2654.

American Psychiatric Association (APA). 2013. *Desk reference to the diagnostic criteria from DSM-5.* Arlington, VA: American Psychiatric Association.

Bakare, M O. 2012. 'Attention deficit hyperactivity symptoms and disorder (ADHD) among African children: a review of epidemiology and co-morbidities'. *African Journal of Psychiatry,* 15: 358–361.

Bakare, M O and Munir, K M. 2011. 'Autism spectrum disorders (ASD) in Africa: a perspective. *African Journal of Psychiatry'*, 14: 2018–2210.

Cortina, M A, Sodha, A, Fazel, M and Ramchandani, P G. 2012. 'Prevalence of child mental health problems in sub-Saharan Africa; A systematic review'. *Archives of Pediatric Adolescent Medicine*, 166 (3): 276–281.

De Vries, K M, Mak, J Y, Bacchus, L J, Child, J C, Falder, G, Petzold, M, Astbury, J and Watts, C H. 2013. 'Intimate partner violence and incident depressive symptoms and suicide attempts: A systematic review of longitudinal studies'. *PLOS Medicine,* 10 (5). doi: 10.1371/journal.pmed.1001439.

Flisher, A J, Townsend, L, Chikobvu, P, Lombard, C F and King, G. 2010. 'Substance use and psychosocial predictors of high school dropout in Cape Town, South Africa'. *Journal of Research and Adolescence*, 20 (1): 237–255.

Grinker, R R, Chambers, N, Njongwe, N, Lagman, A E, Guthrie, W, Stronach, S, Richard, B O, et al. 2012. '"Communities" in Community Engagement: Lessons learned from autism research in South Korea and South Africa'. *Autism Research,* 5 (3): 201–210.

Hall, K and Sambu, W. 2016. 'Demography of South Africa's children'. *South African Child Gauge*, Children's Institute, University of Cape Town, South Africa.

Hermenau, K, Hecker, T, Ruf, M, Schauer, E, Elbert, T and Schauer, M. 2011. 'Childhood adversity, mental ill-health and aggressive behavior in an African orphanage: Changes in response to trauma-focused therapy and the implementation of a new instructional system'. *Child and Adolescent Psychiatry and Mental Health*, 5 (29): doi: 10.1186/1753-2000-5-29.

James, A C, James, G, Cowdrey, F A, Soler, A and Choke, A. 2013. *Cognitive behavioural therapy for anxiety disorders in children and adolescents (Review).* The Cochrane Collaboration: Wiley.

Mathews, S, Abrahams, N and Jewkes, R. 2013. 'Exploring mental health adjustment of children post sexual assault in South Africa'. *Journal of Child Sexual Abuse*, 22 (6): 639–657.

Merrel, K W. 2011. *Behavioral, social and emotional assessment of children and adolescents.* 3rd edition. New York: Routledge.

Myers, B J, Louw, J and Pasche, S C. 2010. 'Inequitable access to substance abuse treatment services in Cape Town, South Africa'. *Substance Abuse Treatment, Prevention and Policy*, 5 (28): doi: 10.1186/1747-597X-5-28.

Peltzer, K. 2010. Leisure time physical activity and sedentary behaviour and substance abuse among in-school adolescents in eight African countries. *International Journal of Behavioral Medicine*, 17 (4): 271–278.

Polanczyk, G V, Salum, G A, Sugaya, L S, Caye, A and Rohde, L A. 2015. 'Annual Research Review; A meta-analysis of the worldwide prevalence of mental disorders in children and adolescents'. *Journal of Child Psychology and Psychiatry*, 56 (3): 345–365.

Red Cross War Memorial Children's Hospital, Psychiatric Outpatient Unit. nd. *Diagnostic Assessment of the Child and Family.*

Sadock, B J, Sadock, V A and Ruiz, P. 2015. *Kaplan and Sadock's Synopsis of Psychiatry.* 11th edition. Philadelphia: Wolters Kluwer.

Scheffel, E C, De Simone, E M and Davidian, M H. 2017. Bed-wetting: Approaches to Nocturnal Enuresis in children. *US Pharmacist,* 42 (5): 32–25.

Silverman, W K and Field, A P. 2011. *Anxiety disorders in children and adolescents.* 2nd edition. New York: Cambridge University Press.

Statistics South Africa. 2017. Department of Health, South Africa. www.statssa.gov.za (Accessed 15 June 2019).

Vitiello, B and Ordonez, A E. 2016. 'Pharmacological treatment of children and adolescents'. doi: 10.1080/14656566.2016.1244530.

Zisser, A and Eyberg, S M. 2010. 'Parent–child interaction therapy and treatment of disruptive behaviour disorders' in Weisz, J R and Kazdin, A E (eds). *Evidence-based psychotherapies for children and adolescents.* New York: Guilford Press.

CHAPTER 23

Nursing Forensic Mental Health Care Users

L R Uys and T Bock

> **Learning Outcomes**
>
> After studying this chapter, you should be able to:
> - explain the concepts 'fitness to stand trial' and 'criminal responsibility'
> - distinguish between different types of forensic mental health care users (MHCUs)
> - discuss the role of the psychiatric nurse in the observation unit and the security unit
> - discuss the problems in the forensic psychiatric system.

INTRODUCTION

The word 'forensic' means pertaining to the law or the courts of law. Forensic psychiatry refers primarily to dealings with mentally ill offenders, but other aspects of contact between the mental health system and the justice system are also included, such as assessment of a mental health care user (MHCU) regarding their contractual and testamentary capacity (Kaliski, 2006: 85). Testamentary capacity refers to the ability of a person to draw up a testament (will): whether they understand what they are saying. Contractual capacity refers to the ability of a person to understand the terms of and to appreciate the implication of the contract.

When forensic psychiatry is mentioned the common understanding is that it deals with the MHCU who allegedly committed a crime while being mentally ill. The definition of forensic psychiatry also includes the term 'psycholegal', as explained by Kaliski (2006: 2). In mental health care, psycholegal work is performed by health practitioners like psychiatrists or psychologists in private practice or mental health care practitioners in large psychiatric institutions dedicated to conducting psycholegal assessments. This definition is further expanded on by Sukeri et al (2016: 1) through explaining that forensic psychiatric services entail the assessment, management and treatment of mentally disordered persons or prisoners who are in conflict with the law and who require a psychiatric assessment.

The recognition that the justice system cannot deal with crimes committed by those suffering from a mental disorder in the same way as it deals with crimes committed by other lawbreakers, is not new (Dorrell, 1991). Perhaps the famous Pinel, who loosened the chains of the criminally insane and transferred them to care facilities, can be regarded as the first health worker to identify the inability of the justice system to manage the criminally insane effectively. MacPhail and Verdun-Jones (2013: 1) emphasise that although there is a link between mental illness and violence, incarceration cannot be the only strategy to deal with the mentally ill offender. The focus should rather shift towards prevention, through addressing the alleged offender's environment and social support, along with a reduction of environmental stressors.

Criminal law involves the punishment of crimes by the authorities. A crime consists of two elements:
- *actus reus*: a wrongful physical act or omission
- *mens rea*: a guilty mental state.

With regard to the mentally ill person, it is their *mens rea* that is usually questioned. Questioning the *mens rea* implies the state, through the court, needs to prove beyond any reasonable doubt that the accused committed an unlawful act (*actus reus*) accompanied by a simultaneous fault (*mens rea*), either intentionally or through negligence and that the accused had the criminal capacity to do such an unlawful act (Louw, 1993).

There is a legal presumption that states that 'every person is presumed to be sane, and therefore the onus of proving mental illness rests on the accused' (Sithole, 2007: 5). However, under the Criminal Procedure Act 51 of 1977, section 78 reads:

> *If it is alleged at criminal proceedings that the accused is by reason of mental illness or mental defect or for any other reason not criminally responsible for the offence charged, or if it appears to the court at criminal proceedings that the accused might for such a reason not be so responsible, the court shall in the case of an allegation or appearance of mental illness or mental defect, and may, in any other case, direct that the matter be enquired into and be reported on in accordance with the provisions of section 79.*

HISTORICAL BACKGROUND

Ancient law held people responsible for what they did, virtually without exception. The Code of Hammurabi is a good example: insanity is not mentioned at all, nor is infant criminality and capacity considered (Hallevey, 2015: 108). In Roman law it was recognised that children and the insane (the *furiosus*) could not be held liable for murder. This was also accepted in Roman–Dutch law, with the *Constitutio Criminalis Caroli* of 1532 stating that sanity is a prerequisite for punishment (Hallevey, 2015: 108). Hallevey is echoed by Swanepoel (2015: 3238) who asserts it still holds true that mentally ill persons cannot be blamed and punished for their behaviour while they are actively mentally ill.

There are many indications of the informal acceptance that insanity exempted a person from punishment under English law (Finkleman, 2013: 814). The system of King's Pardon, by which an insane person found guilty of murder would automatically be brought before the monarch for pardoning, was in effect until the time of Queen Victoria. When she ascended the throne at the age of 18, the system was changed so that the death sentence in such cases would be recorded, but not pronounced by the judge.

In 1843, Danile M'Naghten was tried in England for shooting Drummond, who was the secretary of the Prime Minister, Sir Robert Peel. M'Naghten thought that Drummond was the Prime Minister himself. He was found to be suffering from paranoia and the criteria established during this case, which became known as the M'Naghten Rule, read as follows (Finkleman, 2013: 814):

> *To establish a defence on the ground of insanity, it must be clearly proved that, at the time of the committing of the act, the accused was labouring under such a defect of reason, from disease of the mind, as not to know the nature and quality of the act he was doing, or, if he did know it, that he did not know he was doing what was wrong.*

In South Africa, the first concession to the mentally ill in criminal law was the 'special verdict' instituted in 1891. This meant that the person was found guilty as charged but declared to have been insane at the time of committing the crime. The court then had the discretion to order detention in any suitable place. In 1953, a case against Koortz led to the equivalent of the M'Naghten Rule being formulated for South Africa. It read (Kruger 1980: 156):

> *A person is not punishable for conduct which would in ordinary circumstances have been criminal if, at the time, through disease of the mind or mental defect –*
> *(a) he was prevented from knowing the nature and quality of the conduct, or that it was wrong; or*
> *(b) he was the subject of an irresistible impulse which prevented him from controlling such conduct.*

In 1967, after the assassination of Prime Minister H F Verwoerd in Parliament by a mentally ill man, the Rumpff Commission of Inquiry into Criminal Responsibility of Mentally Disordered Persons and Related Matters recommended a new formulation, which was incorporated into the Criminal Procedure Act 51 of 1977. Section 78 of this Act reads:

> *A person who commits an act which constitutes an offence and who at the time of such commission suffers from a mental illness or mental defect which makes him incapable –*
> *(a) of appreciating the wrongfulness of his act or*
> *(b) of acting in accordance with an appreciation of the wrongfulness of his act, shall not be criminally responsible for such an act.*

Kruger (1980: 155) states that the M'Naghten Rule was reviewed by the Rumpff commission and now states that, if the accused of an alleged offence does not understand the wrongfulness of their act due to mental illness, they shall not be held responsible. Table 23.1 explains the difference between mental illness versus mental defect.

Table 23.1 Mental illness versus mental defect

Mental defect	Mental illness
Condition which manifests with low-level intellectual ability	Those who suffer from a mental illness
Neurocognitive or neurodevelopmental disorders	Mental illness manifesting with illusions, delusions and hallucinations rendering a person incapable of insight into their actions

CURRENT LEGAL PROVISIONS IN SOUTH AFRICA

A person's fitness to stand trial and their criminal intent or capacity are issues that are often dealt with in the courts and have a bearing on mentally ill persons facing trial. Table 23.2 sums up these central concerns.

Table 23.2 Fitness to stand trial versus criminal capacity

Fitness to stand trial	Criminal intent/capacity
Does a person's mental state allow them to understand the court proceedings and allow them to make a proper defence?	Can a person be held accountable or responsible for any offences allegedly committed? Does the person understand the wrongfulness of their acts?

Fitness to stand trial

The fitness of the accused to stand trial may be questioned at any time during the criminal proceedings, either by the accused, the defence, the prosecution or the court. Fitness to stand trial refers to the question of whether or not the person's mental state allows them to understand the proceedings well enough to make a proper defence.

There are different procedures to be followed if at any stage the accused's capacity to understand the proceedings in a court of law is questioned. In order to determine the fitness to stand trial it is necessary that the accused be evaluated by a panel of experts. Kaliski (2006: 42) explains that the criminal law in South Africa is based on the ability of an accused being able to understand the trial proceedings in a court of law.

If there is any concern that the accused may not be able to understand the proceedings, the questionability of the accused's understanding must be investigated.

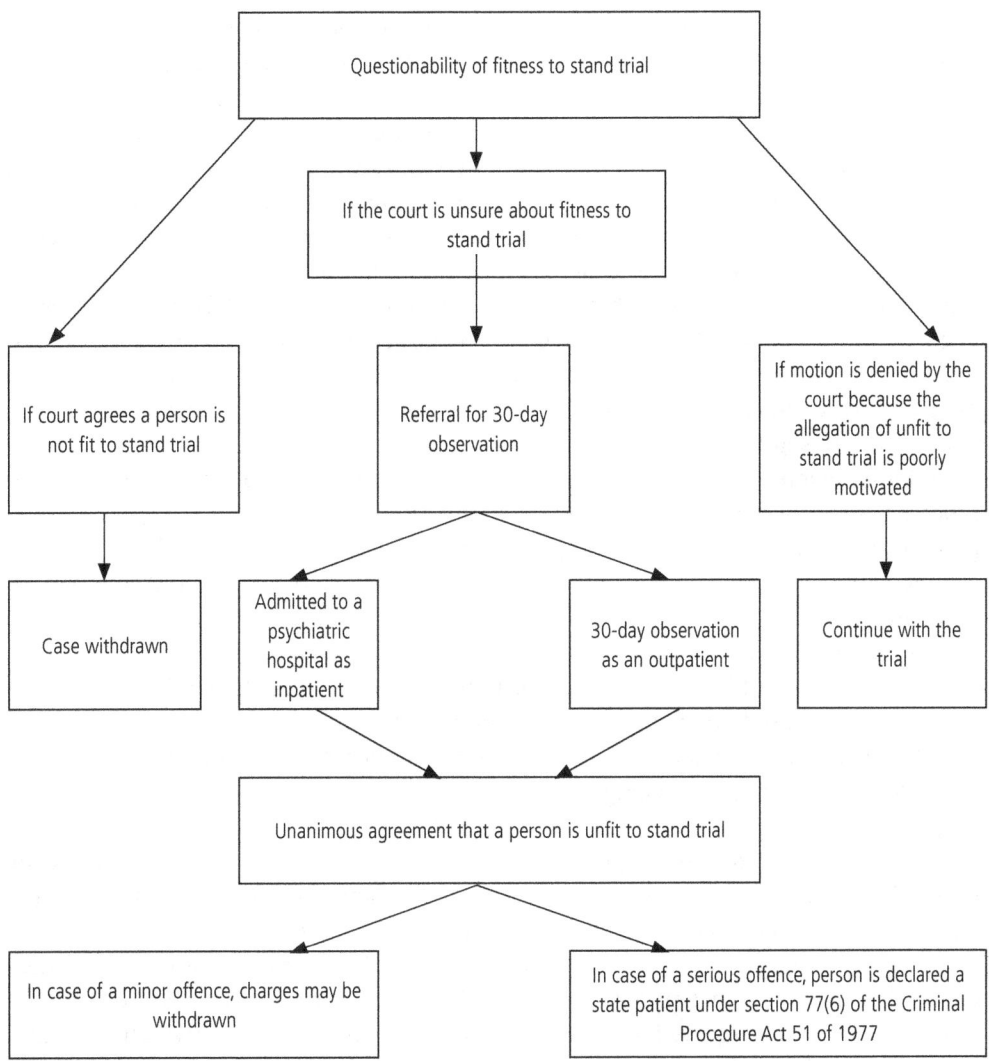

Figure 23.1 Flow diagram if the fitness to stand trial is questioned (Bock, 2018)

In the past, if the MHCU who was admitted for observation was accused of a serious offence for which the death penalty (which was abolished on 6 June 1995) could be imposed, three psychiatrists could be involved in the decision, namely the superintendent of the psychiatric hospital, a state-appointed psychiatrist and one appointed by the defence. In South Africa mental health care nurses are at present sometimes involved in the decision about an accused's fitness to stand trial because of the shortage of psychiatrists and beds in observation units.

Recent developments within the South African law system, as are evident in *S vs Pistorius*, make it clear that forensic mental health examinations may be conducted on an 'outpatient' basis (Pillay, 2014: 377). The case of *S vs Pretorius* entailed a situation where the accused was accused of homicide in that he shot and killed his girlfriend. The defence had reason to believe that the accused suffered from a mental illness and that this precondition could impact on his ability to testify in a court of law. Subsequently the judge issued an order for the accused to be evaluated for a mental illness. As the accused was not known to have previously offended, and there was no evidence of a previous mental illness, the court allowed a concession for outpatient evaluation rather than hospitalisation. This day visit, as opposed to detaining an accused for 30 days in a forensic mental health facility, albeit uncommon, is nothing new as this has been practised at several mental health care facilities throughout South Africa where there is a scarcity of mental health resources. A study conducted in Limpopo Province showed that 85 per cent of persons under observation could be assessed on an outpatient basis by a multidisciplinary team (Sukeri et al, 2016). However, unfortunately outpatient observation was not granted at that time. Outpatient observation is also recommended for minors, where detainment in an observation centre could be traumatic for such a person, thus the persons under observation will be under the supervision of their parents or guardian and will be brought to the outpatient facility on a daily basis.

The multidisciplinary team must make a psychiatric diagnosis and answer the following questions:
- Does the accused know what the charge involves?
- Does the accused know what it means to be tried in a court of law?
- Does the accused understand the proceedings in court?
- Does the accused understand that the court must decide on their guilt or innocence with regard to a specific charge?

It must be remembered that a person might be mentally ill and still understand the proceedings well enough to stand trial. Fitness to stand trial is not the same as the criteria for an involuntary admission for 72-hour observation.

If the accused is found to be unfit to stand trial, the charge may be withdrawn, or they can be declared a state patient under section 77(6) of the Criminal Procedure Act 51 of 1977. This provision of the South African Criminal Procedure Act (which is similar to the Criminal Law Act of 1967 in the United Kingdom), has been criticised because it does not allow the facts of the case to be fully investigated. A person in the same circumstances as Demetrio Tsafendas, who was accused of murdering Dr Verwoerd, could be found unfit to stand trial and declared a state patient, which then means that the murder would never be investigated in an open court. This may prejudice the MHCU, because they will be considered a state patient involved in a serious crime for the rest of their lives, without their guilt ever having been established. If they were not implicated in the crime, it would be unfair to make them a state patient as opposed to treating them under the provisions of the Mental Health Care Act 17 of 2002.

Criminal responsibility/capacity

In South Africa, the question of whether or not an accused can be held responsible for a criminal act or omission on the grounds of insanity can be raised by the defence or the prosecution, and evidence may be led in this regard. The state is required to prove that an accused has the psychological capacity to be held responsible for their conduct (Kaliski, 2006: 39). Criminal capacity is defined as 'Being of sufficiently sound mind so that one may be found guilty of committing a crime, such as being of a certain age and having sufficient mental faculties to understand the difference between right and wrong' (TheLaw.com, nd). In such cases, the judge makes the final decision. If the defence raises the issue of criminal responsibility/capacity, it forms part of a plea of not guilty.

The South African, American and German definitions of criminal responsibility are very similar. They combine the right–wrong criterion (unable to appreciate the wrongfulness of the act) with the ability to conform to the requirements of the law (unable to act in accordance with such an appreciation).

The following aspects of criminal responsibility in the South African context should be kept in mind:

- The definition of mental illness or mental defect in the Criminal Procedure Act 51 of 1977 is not the same as that in the Mental Health Care Act 17 of 2002. For example, psychopathic disorders, also known as antisocial disorders and antisocial personality disorders, are included in the Mental Health Care Act, while these are specifically excluded from the Criminal Procedure Act.
- Alcoholism as such does not lead to non-responsibility unless it incorporates a mental illness. However, it may be taken into account during sentencing.
- Emotional distress or stress in itself is not acceptable as a defence on the grounds of insanity.
- Witchcraft or the belief in witchcraft is not regarded as a mental illness.
- The result of a hearing to establish responsibility can be one of the following:
  - The MHCU may be found not responsible and declared a state patient under section 78(6) of the Criminal Procedure Act 51 of 1977. In this case they can be kept in a psychiatric hospital for an undetermined time.
  - The MHCU may be found not responsible and acquitted. An example of this is a case in which an offence was committed as the person awoke from a nightmare. He was found not responsible and acquitted.
  - The person may be found to have diminished responsibility, in which case this fact can be used as extenuating circumstance.
  - The person may be found responsible, and the trial and sentencing proceeds.

The Mental Health Care Act 17 of 2002 has addressed much of the criticism levelled against the previous Mental Health Act 18 of 1973 for not sufficiently safeguarding the rights of the accused. Some of the criticisms and the changes in this regard are as follows:
1. *State patients have no right of appeal to anybody to enquire why they are still being detained.* In terms of section 20 of the Mental Health Care Act, MHCUs may apply for an enquiry into the grounds for their continued detention. This is not possible

in the case of state patients. In 1956 a full bench of the Supreme Court ruled against such an enquiry in the case of *Khan vs the Commissioner of Mental Health*, and in 1978 a decision that the court cannot be involved was made in the case of *Jurgens vs the Attorney-General*.

In the United Kingdom a patient detained in a similar manner can apply for a review of the case by a Mental Health Review Tribunal, although the tribunal can only make a recommendation and not order a release (Whitehead 1982).

In South Africa, anybody, including the state patient, a spouse or associate or a 'person authorised to act on behalf of a state patient' may apply for discharge of the MHCU according to article 47 of the Act. In essence, this protects the rights of the person in the same way as an appeal would have done.

2. *In the case of a state patient, the curator ad litem and the prosecutor are the same person.* The *curator ad litem* is a person appointed to act as a curator in issues of litigation, on behalf of a person who is a minor or mentally or physically incapacitated to act on their own behalf (Abrahams & Gross, 2017). An MHCU admitted under the Mental Health Care Act has a *curator ad litem* from a different system than from the one in which they are detained, in the form of the Attorney-General of the area. In the case of a state patient, however, the Attorney-General is both the prosecutor and curator – this is an untenable position. In the Mental Health Care Act section 4(b) states that the judge must specifically consider whether a conflict of interest exists and appoint another legal practitioner to act on behalf of the MHCU in such a case.

3. *The detention order of the state patient amounts to an indefinite sentence, the length of which is dependent on extremely subjective criteria.* Although Kruger (1980) is at pains to point out that a declaration as state patient does not amount to punishment of a guilty person and that there can therefore not be a direct relationship between the offence and the 'measure' of detaining the state patient, it is clear that the length of detention is often based on the characteristics of the crime and not on the condition of the state patient (Henning, 1983). In this way the psychiatric treatment system has been co-opted into the service of the Department of Correctional Services, serving as agents of social control rather than as agents of therapy (Stone, in Webster et al, 1985).

In the UK, the detention of an MHCU under similar conditions may be for a specific time only, after which they are subject to the conditions laid down by the Mental Health Act 2007 in that country. Therefore, in essence, the Mental Health Care Act in South Africa does not allow a judge to incarcerate a person for a period of time after which a sentence is completed and a person may be discharged. Discharge is entirely dependent on the mental health status of the MHCU.

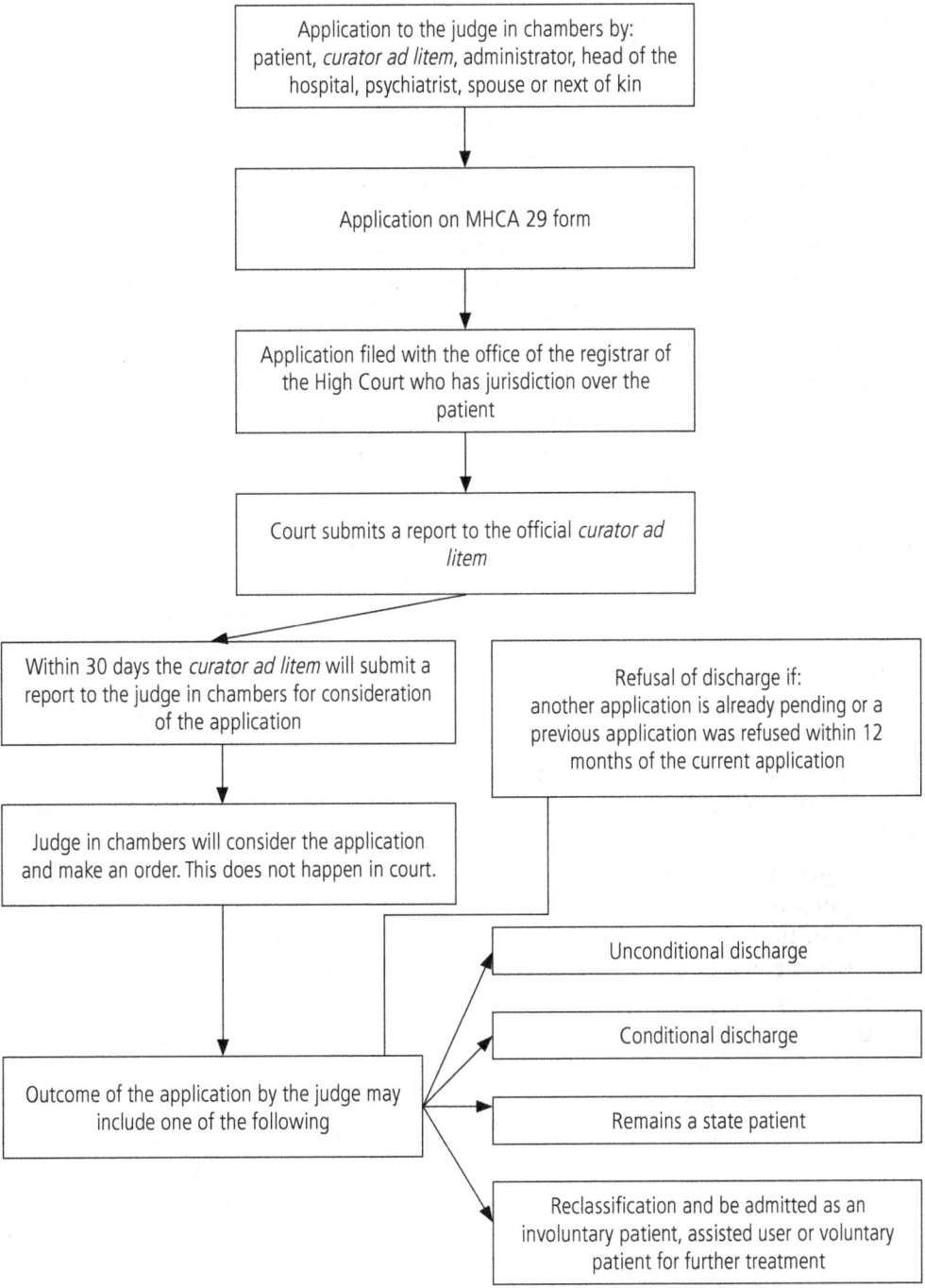

Figure 23.2 Discharge of a state patient (Bock, 2018)

The release of a state patient is often dependent on a prediction about whether the state patient is still potentially dangerous. The problem in this regard is the risk associated with assessing and declaring that a person no longer has a potential for violence or committing a crime. Prediction becomes a guessing game. Roffey and Kaliski (2012: 229) report that actuarial tools, such as the structured professional judgement tool (SPJ), are quite helpful in short-term predictions of the propensity of a person for violence. However, they caution that such tools cannot provide a prediction of 100 per cent probability. In similar fashion, Hvidhjelm et al (2014: 536) agree that short-term predictions of violence are more accurate than long-term predictions when they used the Brøset Violence Checklist as a predictor of violence. Their statements concur with Zabow (1989) who cautions that the penalty for a wrongful discharge is high. The clinician who makes the prediction, and who then discharges an MHCU with a low propensity for violence, is held liable for such a discharge where the MHCU commits a deed. Because of this, it is understandable why there is such a low rate of discharge of state patients in South Africa.

Unlike a person who has been declared fit to stand trial and then receives a prison sentence, the person who is declared unfit to stand trial, and who becomes a state patient, is classified indefinitely and may be admitted to a psychiatric hospital for many years without discharge. Statistics reported by Kaliski (2013) confirm the long stay of forensic psychiatric MHCUs: it is reported that there are at least 50 MHCUs admitted to forensic wards annually but only approximately five discharges per annum. The indefiniteness of the MHCU's sentence causes enormous suffering to them and their families. Coleman (1984) graphically describes the despair caused by the repeated applications for release, the hopeful waiting, and the disappointment at refusal. He believes that even a long sentence, but a specific one, is easier to bear than the recurrent disappointments of an indefinite sentence.

Coleman (1984) also refers to the effect of this system on the treatment process by pointing out that when the length of hospitalisation depends so much on the good opinion of the staff, it might be difficult for MHCUs to share negative thoughts and feelings in therapy. Since anything that they say may be used against them, they say only what might be acceptable.

Although this problem is not directly addressed in the Mental Health Care Act, the new procedures in the Act might in reality address this issue.

Thomson et al (2016: 155) emphasise that the outcome relating to the discharge of a state patient is so much better if there is a multi-agency approach for the aftercare of state patients, as followed in the UK. The authors quote a decrease of 15 per cent down to 6 per cent in violent acts among recently discharged state patients where the multi-agency approach is followed. The approach involves halfway houses for discharged patients, and the use of social services, correctional services and police officers where the state patient is discharged on probation. Measures which improved the reincorporation of the state patient back into society included educating the community, the creation of employment services and the receipt of social grants. Similar programmes are implemented throughout Europe. Often due to the long hospitalisation of state patients in forensic units, there is no direct family they can be discharged to, and they often feel destitute and rely heavily on the availability of state resources for their basic needs.

SERVICES PROVIDED FOR A MENTALLY ILL OFFENDER

Provision for a mentally ill offender varies from one country to the next. An important factor in determining the form of the service is the state's policy regarding which sector should render the service.

In the UK, prison health care falls under the ambit of the National Health Services (NHS) and according to the Sainsbury Centre for Mental Health (nd), approximately 80 per cent of the UK prison population suffers from a form of mental illness. There are, however, still three high-security hospitals – Broadmoor, Ashworth and Rampton – previously known as prisons for the criminally insane. They are institutions dealing with mentally ill persons who committed serious crimes while suffering from a serious mental illness. According to the West London NHS Trust (nd), these hospitals are now no longer referred to as prisons but as hospitals that provide specialist services such as assessment, treatment and care in conditions of high security for mentally ill persons.

Mentally ill offenders in Japan are cared for in prison hospitals within the justice system (Sakuta, 1991). Nakatani (2011) explained this is because of the steadily increasing number of crimes committed by mentally ill offenders and because Japan has two different systems in dealing with mentally ill patients and mentally ill prisoners. The separation of mentally ill patients from mentally ill offenders is directly linked to the increase in mentally ill offenders.

In the United States of America (USA), persons awaiting trial are kept in 'jail' and criminals who have already been sentenced are kept in 'prison'. From these facilities persons can be referred to special security hospitals in the prison service (or back). If necessary, the special security hospital can refer the person to a civil mental hospital. Mentally ill offenders in the USA therefore usually find their way into the health system, either to a special security hospital, or to a civil mental hospital.

In South Africa, mentally ill offenders are dealt with in psychiatric hospitals, although they can be held in prison or in prison hospitals. In most psychiatric hospitals there are special units for these MHCUs, where medium to low security is available (security unit). In one hospital, a maximum-security unit exists (built specifically for this purpose). The Mental Health Care Act (section 41) stipulates that the head of the national Department of Health, in concurrence with the heads of the different provincial departments of health, may designate health establishments which may admit, care for and treat state patients.

It is important to note that a state patient is a detainee and not a convicted and sentenced prisoner (Landman & Landman, 2014: 169). Landman and Landman (2014: 169) further explain that a convicted offender is punished and receives a finite sentence in relation to the crime committed. However, the state patient who is detained does not receive a sentence as they are not morally responsible for the criminal act. Therefore, detention is only valid once the state patient fully recovers from a mental illness or is stable and well controlled on treatment to the extent where they are no longer a threat to self or society. The low rate of discharge from forensic units and the comorbid increase in the number of annual admissions of forensic MHCUs have placed an immense burden on the availability of resources for forensic MHCUs. The increase in the number of forensic MHCUs from 2005 in 1997 to 8 000 in 2013, and an admission rate of 50 state patients annually with a discharge of only five patients per annum, is evidence of the fact that there is a severe shortage of forensic psychiatric beds and services (Kaliski, 2013: 13). Kaliski (2013: 13) further reports that there is a correlation between the increase in the number of forensic MHCUs and the deinstitutionalisation of long-term MHCUs, as 80 per cent of current forensic MHCUs had contact with psychiatric services prior to the alleged offences for which they are currently detained (Kaliski, 2013: 15). Similar findings are confirmed by Marais and Subramaney (2015: 86).

The burden on forensic psychiatric services is reportedly compounded by the utilisation of forensic mental health services to provide long-term hospitalisation for people with serious mental illness who cannot be contained in the community (Kaliski, 2013: 15).

CLASSIFICATION OF FORENSIC PSYCHIATRIC PATIENTS
Classification according to legal status

Steadman and Cocozza (1974) from the USA provide the following classification of patients in forensic psychiatric units according to their legal status:

- *Mentally ill inmates.* According to the authors, this group accounts for about 40 per cent of the patients in forensic units in the USA. These are offenders who were arrested, convicted and sentenced, and who became mentally ill while serving time in prison. They are then transferred to a psychiatric hospital. In South Africa legal provision is made for these patients in Chapter 4 of the Mental Health Care Act.
- *Defendants incompetent to stand trial.* In the USA, this group accounts for about 40 per cent of forensic psychiatric patients. In South Africa they are called state patients.
- *Not guilty by reason of insanity.* Also called state patients in South Africa, this group accounts for about 4 per cent of the forensic patients in the USA.
- *Dangerous mentally ill.* This group is quite different from the previous three. In this case patients were civilly committed to a psychiatric hospital, but because of their behaviour and condition, they are deemed dangerous and are therefore held in a high-security unit.

Classification according to type of problem

From the literature it would seem that the following types of patients can be expected in forensic units:

- *Inadequate functioning.* This group needs greater supervision because of poor intellectual functioning, inadequate social skills and other handicaps. They may be inclined to clash repeatedly with the law, and even in the institution find it difficult to keep to rules and routines. They need long-term supervision. In a study by Marais and Subramaney (2015: 88) reportedly 29 per cent of state patients fall within this category in South Africa.
- *Personality disorders.* This group has specific personality disorders, especially antisocial and borderline personality disorders, and need a therapeutic community-type treatment setting. In this kind of setting the patient can explore and acknowledge their pattern of behaviour, understand the motives underlying it, and modify their behaviour in the longer term.
- *Seriously violent.* The outstanding characteristic of this group is the propensity for serious violence. Marais and Subramaney (2015: 88) report that as many as 68 per cent of state patients in South Africa fall within this category of seriously violent offenders.
- *Substance abuse.* Substance abuse plays an important role in a large proportion of forensic psychiatric cases. Marais and Subramaney (2015: 88) report that in South Africa, the incidence of alcohol and substance abuse was much higher in the forensic population than in the general population. This confirms the need for treatment programmes to address the problem of substance abuse.

THE NURSE IN THE OBSERVATION UNIT

Persons are sent for observation either before or during their trial to establish their fitness to stand trial or their criminal responsibility, or (during their prison term) to establish whether they are mentally ill and need treatment. In some hospitals the observation and security MHCUs are in the same unit. Landman and Landman (2014: 169) refer to a person under observation as an observanda (singular) or observandi (plural), because this person is neither a prisoner nor a detainee at this point.

The observation unit is a specialised ward where people who are being evaluated for fitness to stand trial are accommodated. There is no therapeutic ward programme in these units as the accused is not yet a hospital patient. There is no therapeutic treatment modality nor is there a possibility of administering psychotropics, as the aim of this unit is to assist with the objective observation of the patient in order to present the state with a comprehensive report of their findings. The objectives of an observation unit are to:
- prevent the escape of an accused or sentenced person
- observe the inmate systematically in order to establish their psychiatric condition, and identify observandi who are malingering
- protect the human rights of the observanda
- ensure the safety of the staff and observanda.

From these objectives it is clear that the staff in this case do not have a treatment function. They only have diagnostic and custodial functions. This might be difficult for the staff, and is probably not the kind of setting that every nurse will be interested in working in. It should be noted that article 46-3 of the Mental Health Care Act states that if the person is ill to such a degree that there is a danger to self or others, treatment should commence immediately. Landman and Landman (2014: 173) confirm that even though there is no provision for a state patient to be treated and medicated without consent, the Mental Health Care Act allows for treatment to commence under section 32 if the observanda holds a threat to the safety to self or others. In such cases it is often necessary to commence with treatment even before the finalisation of reports with regard to whether the observanda can stand trial.

In order to prevent the escape of these observandi, it is important that this kind of unit should provide for maximum security. The Mental Health Care Act makes provision for MHCUs who cannot be contained in an ordinary mental hospital to be transferred to a maximum-security unit (article 22-1). The Mental Health Care Act also makes provision for such a transfer to be assisted by the police (article 27).

Systematic observation is dependent on the nurses having a clear understanding of the following:
- *The reason for why the person has been sent for observation.* Is it to establish their fitness to stand trial or criminal responsibility, or is only the mental illness of the prisoner at issue?
- *The alleged crime and the possible psychiatric diagnoses.* Unless the nurse is aware of the issues involved, their observations cannot be planned systematically. The nurse should revise their knowledge of the psychiatric diagnoses involved and make sure that they know what the critical points are.

The nurse working in the observation unit must constantly guard against judging the observanda based on alleged crimes; to stay non-judgemental might be difficult when working in a high-security unit that in itself seems like a prison environment with high levels of security and strict rules. Devnick (2010: 23) made a similar observation about the nurse's attitude and the forensic mental health care work environment.

In an observation unit, nurses should report on the mental status of every observanda every day. During the day nurses gather data on every aspect of the mental status examination, such as attention, concentration, mood and intelligence, and record this in their daily report at the end of each day. Any incidents that occur such as aggression or altercations with fellow observandi could also be slotted in under the appropriate heading of the mental status examination, as feedback must be provided regarding such incidents. Special opportunities for observation can be created, so that all aspects are observed in different situations. For example, attention, concentration, memory and intelligence can be observed during an interview with the nurse, but also while playing board games or completing ward tasks.

The observanda may also be sent to another facility, such as a hospital, for special tests, but not for a period longer than eight hours (Mental Health Care Act, article 47-4).

The regulations of the Mental Health Care Act set out as follows the information the court will require from the mental health system:

1. A review of the medical and psychiatric history
2. Clinical findings during the time of observation
3. A summary of the relevant facts and circumstances of the offence as supplied by the prosecutor
4. The estimated (where possible psychologically assessed) intelligence level of such a person
5. The psychiatric diagnosis (if any)
6. An assessment of whether the person can cooperate in their own defence
7. An assessment of whether the person at the time of the offence would have been disturbed to the extent that from a psychiatric point of view they were not responsible for their acts
8. An assessment of the type of treatment (if any) considered to be fairest to such a person and safest for the community.

It is also important to have orientation groups in observation units in which inmates are oriented to the legal process that has brought them to the unit, and the implications of the findings of that process. According to the Mental Health Care Act, the observanda has to be informed that a mental status report will be submitted by a mental health practitioner to a court of law, and that they are under no obligation to divulge information (article 46–1). Criminals sometimes think that they will get away with a lighter sentence if they are found to be insane. This used to hold truth in the case of crimes carrying the death penalty but in most other cases state patients are in fact incarcerated a great deal longer than prisoners serving specific prison sentences, due to the difficulty in risk assessment for future violence in the long term. Giving appropriate information about the legal system might help observandi with real psychiatric problems to understand their situations and might discourage malingering.

Nurses might also sometimes be asked to undertake observation in a prison setting, especially when there is a shortage of medical practitioners. This situation is undesirable as in South Africa there is no accredited training course for a psychiatric forensic nurse. Nedopil et al (2015: 80) make a valid point in stating how extensive the knowledge of the practitioner should be in dealing with forensic MHCUs. Nedopil et al (2015: 82) further conclude that in order for the mental health care provider to make any valuable contribution, training is essential.

THE NURSE IN THE SECURITY UNIT

The MHCUs in security units remain in hospital for between five and nine years on average (Wool, 1991). This long-term stay is also referred to Marais and Subramaney (2015: 86). This means that these units are long-term treatment and rehabilitation units. Steadman and Cocozza (1974) state that three general themes run through the research literature about these units: detention, lack of treatment, and a strong psychiatric conservatism regarding the release of these MHCUs.

In general, the objectives of these units are to:
- treat the MHCU for their psychiatric condition and achieve remission as soon as possible
- decrease the potential for future violence
- improve the chances of successful reintegration into society
- monitor the condition of the state patient and propose leave of absence and discharge appropriately.

Treating the MHCU and achieving remission as soon as possible

To achieve the first of these objectives, the programme in the forensic unit does not have to be very different from that in an ordinary psychiatric unit. The MHCUs are probably acutely or chronically ill and the usual physical and psychosocial treatment methods would be used. However, in the orientation of these MHCUs, the reality of the legal conditions under which they have been admitted must be included. In ordinary circumstances MHCUs know that when they are stable, they will be discharged. In this case it is not that simple, especially if the crime involved serious violence. From the outset, they have to understand the length of the average stay in the unit, and that their discharge depends on some assurance regarding the safety of the community. They should understand the chain of decision making involved in discharge and that their stay will probably be a long one. Another aspect that needs special attention is substance abuse, since it plays a role in so many of these cases.

> Let me get this statement out of the way right at the start: psychologists are pretty bad at predicting the potential for violent behaviour. – Maximillian Wachtel, PhD

Decreasing the potential for future violence

To decrease the potential for future violence, this aspect must be addressed directly in the treatment programme. Mattiuzzi (2008) categorises the typology of violent offenders as listed below. This typology will assist mental health care providers to understand and categorise violence in order to manage it.

Chronically aggressive individuals

Chronically aggressive individuals are people who display the following characteristics:
- They are easily frustrated, limited or poor impulse control.
- They frequently express anger or hostility.
- They resent authority and are defiant with supervisors.
- They may express hostility through 'passive-aggressive' behaviour.
- They believe violence and/or aggression are legitimate responses to various interpersonal problems in life (for example, if someone provokes you, you fight

back). Although they might never admit it, pleasure or reinforcement is derived from the expression of anger (for example, it feels good to blow someone off; it makes you feel alive; it gives you a sense of power).
- They often display the characteristics of a 'stimulus seeker' – they engage in bold, fearless, or reckless behaviour and are prone to substance abuse.
- Most typically, violence occurs in a situational context: an offence, fight, or disagreement.
- Sometimes they just get carried away in a particular situation (domestic violence, child battering).
- They are less likely to engage in acts of unexpected 'explosive' violence.

The over-controlled hostility type
The over-controlled hostility type of violent offender displays these characteristics:
- They rarely display or express anger – they do not cuss or yell and may be offended by such actions.
- They are emotionally rigid and inflexible: they appear to be polite, serious, and sober, rarely 'loose' or jocular; they are cognitively rigid and inflexible: very strict about interpreting rules; they usually go for the letter, rather than the spirit of the law.
- They are morally righteous and upstanding: see themselves as 'good people'.
- They are often judgemental: they see others as 'not such good people'.
- They are non-assertive or passive; their passivity causes others to take advantage of them.
- Anger builds up like in a pressure cooker, before they explode.
- After the violence, people say that they never expected it, 'he always seemed like such a nice guy; he was always so quiet'.

The hurt and resentful
The violent offenders who fall into this typology have these characteristics:
- They feel that people walk over them and that they are never treated fairly.
- When they are passed over, there is always someone else to blame.
- Things are easier for everyone else: other people get more and have more advantages.
- They do not accept criticism well.
- In response to reprimands, they develop grudges, which are sometimes deeply held.
- They are often whiners and complainers, as a matter of attitude.
- They wallow in their victimisation and are psychologically impotent.
- Violence occurs because they hold grudges and are 'impotent' to deal with their anger in other ways.

The traumatised

The traumatised type of violent offender displays the following characteristics:
- Aggression occurs in response to a single, massive assault on their identity.
- Something happens that is potently offensive, absolutely intolerable, and which strips them of all sense of personal power.
- The essence of their existence (or their manhood) will be destroyed if they do not respond.
- Violence is predictable and preventable.

The obsessive

This type of violent offender has these characteristics:
- They are immature and narcissistic individuals who demand or crave attention and affection.
- They absolutely cannot stand to be deprived of desired gratifications, like a baby who cries because mother removes the breast.
- When deprived of love, they continue crying; they might make repeated phone calls, pursuing the object of their obsession.
- As frustration continues, their actions escalate; aggression is displayed in overt fashion such as sending 'dead flowers', causing punctured tires, suicide gestures.
- There is violence because of jealousy and possessiveness: 'if I can't have her, nobody can' or 'if she won't have me, she won't have anything'.

The paranoid

The paranoid violent offender exhibits these characteristics:
- As a jealous type, they delusionally believe their lover is unfaithful.
- As a persecuted type, they delusionally believe that people are out to get them.
- They typically engage in behaviours which make their paranoid beliefs come true.
- Their delusions may reach the point at which the person is grossly out of contact with reality (may be insane).

The insane

The insane violent offender has these characteristics:
- They rarely do not understand the nature and quality of their actions.
- More typically, they have fundamental misperceptions of reality; they are incapable of rational behaviour; their delusional beliefs deprive them of the ability to know that their behaviour is wrong; their beliefs and perceptions are incongruent with reality.
- They have twisted, psychotic beliefs about what is right, what is wrong, and what is necessary.

The just plain bad and angry

These violent offenders display the following characteristics:
- They show a combination of most of the mentioned characteristics (except for insane): they are angry, hostile, jealous, resentful, impotent, and disturbed individuals, who are socially isolated, socially inadequate, and who feel worthless.
- They may be seeking attention.
- They may be seeking revenge.

Dealing with aggression and violence in a treatment programme

In order to deal with aggression and violence in a therapeutic programme, a detailed history of each MHCU's violence should be taken, and not only the incident that led to the admission. The situational, social, victimisation and cultural aspects should be fully explored. Furthermore, corroboration of the MHCU's account of the violence should be obtained from family, friends, court records and any other available source so that the extent, intensity and situational factors can be accurately identified (Dietz, in Webster et al, 1985). Nurses should also keep detailed records of all incidents of aggression in the ward, both physical and verbal, so that the MHCU's progress can be evaluated.

Treatment approaches used in the management of aggression and violence include the following:
- *Individual counselling* to explore the MHCU's reflection and perception of the violence.
- *Group therapy*, which focuses on an exploration of feelings and appropriate expression, as well as teaching mature coping mechanisms, including problem solving. Dutton (in Webster et al, 1985) shows that husbands who assault their wives display a very poor ability to identify their own feelings and express these appropriately. The use of anger diaries and the teaching of alternative ways of satisfying power motivation are advocated.
- *Family therapy and/or marital therapy* in the case of sexual violence in the family, in which feelings about the crime, the disclosure of the crime and the aftermath of the criminal proceedings are explored. The patterns of interaction in families of origin and the present family are also explored. MacInnes et al (2013: 532) echo the importance of family involvement and the need for families to be involved in the hospitalisation of the forensic MHCU, as ultimately the MHCU might be discharged back to the family as primary care giver.
- *Management of aggression and violence on ward level* to equip mental health care workers. Bock (2015) proposes that all staff working with MHCUs should undergo training in the management of aggression and violence. It is evident in her study that mental health care workers feel under-equipped to deal with MHCU-related aggression and violence.

Exposure to the nature of the offence committed by the forensic MHCU might lead to countertransference in the therapeutic relationship between the mental health care provider and the user. Exposure to the MHCU's aggression and violence may influence the mental health care provider's judgement, as the experience with the MHCU becomes part of the experience of the mental health care provider. Experiences lead to the formation of attitudes; therefore, it is possible that the mental health care provider's experience might add to enduring attitudes, a deduction also confirmed by Cacioppo and Berntson (1994: 401). Resonating with this, the attributional theory postulates that the inference the health care provider makes about the cause of the user's behaviour might directly influence their attitude towards the user. Bock (2015) observes that attitudinal changes caused by experience to violence often entails a harsher application of rules, or out of fear, a lack of applying any rules.

Bock (2015) proposes that training of care givers and the community should include recognition of and prediction of violence and aggression, de-escalation techniques, dignified break-away techniques, cultural awareness, safety and the creation of a therapeutic environment. All of these will assist in the rehabilitation and reintegration of the MHCU back into the community.

Successful reintegration in society

To reach the objective of successful reintegration into society, it is important that social and other role relationships should be maintained during the MHCU's hospitalisation. Relationships damaged during the court proceedings should be re-established as soon as possible. This might be a fairly difficult task. In a survey of state patients in one South African psychiatric hospital, it was found that 36 per cent had no contact with their families and no way of contacting them (Ngubane & Uys, 1994). The usual route for making contact with families is to use the services of social workers in outlying districts. Community nurses may also be of help in this regard. Integration of psychiatric care in the primary health care system should enhance this aspect of care. Once families have been contacted, they should be fully involved in the assessment, treatment and rehabilitation of the MHCU.

Another way in which reintegration can be reached is through improving the life and job skills of MHCU. This may include teaching them life skills such as parenting, assertiveness and better use of recreational time, as well as job-related skills like literacy, training in bricklaying, carpentry or roofing. According to the Mental Health Care Act (article 50), the Department of Education is responsible for the establishment of educational programmes for learners in the compulsory age group or those entitled to basic adult education programmes. The Department of Correctional Services maintains an extensive training system, and forensic psychiatric MHCUs could be incorporated into this system. This would mean that a state patient applies for a specific training course and is then transferred to the prison for the duration of that course. It is important that state patients be occupied in a meaningful way for the period in which they have to stay in a psychiatric hospital. The rendering of pure custodial care with no meaningful programmes will lead to institutional neurosis at worst, and very poor work habits at best.

Discharge of the forensic MHCU/state patient

A final objective for mental health care workers in security units has to do with decisions about discharging the MHCU. This is one of the most problematic issues in forensic units. Perhaps one of the most important ways of improving discharge rates is to ensure that there is a scientifically based and progressive treatment programme. If it can be shown that the MHCU has received all possible treatment and has completed the treatment and rehabilitation successfully, this should form some rational basis for discharge.

However, the prediction of future violence will always come into the decision and should be addressed directly.

Fazel et al (2012: 4) performed a systematic review to examine the predictive validity of different assessment tools on 73 samples involving 24 847 individuals in 13 different countries. The outcome of this study showed that the predictability of future violence depends on the type of tool used by the evaluator. It is clear that it is indeed a great risk to attempt to evaluate the risk associated with discharging the mentally ill offender. This sentiment is echoed by Dolan and Doyle (2000) who reiterated that predicting violence is an inexact science, thus adding to views that psychiatrists should be over-cautious about predicting violence. Coid et al (2013: 388) and Wachtel (2012) cautioned that the use of instruments is more accurate when performed on MHCUs in a health care setting, as opposed to the general population, and when MHCUs are discharged into their communities.

Dietz (1985) in Weisstub (1987: 174) listed first-rank predictor variables. These first-rank predictors remain relevant especially for the cautious practitioner who must formulate an educated prediction of the probability of a mentally ill offender to re-offend. The presence of one of the criteria is enough to predict that violence will be repeated. This therefore decreases the likelihood of discharge and reintegration into society. These variables are:

1. One murder with mutilation of the corpse
2. One murder with vampirism or cannibalism
3. One murder with antemortem sexual sadism
4. One contract murder
5. One sniper murder of a stranger
6. One abduction with torture of the victim
7. Three forcible rapes of strangers
8. One arson episode with sexual arousal
9. Two arson episodes for profit
10. One kidnapping for ransom
11. One bombing of an occupied building
12. Two bombings of motor vehicles
13. One forcible rape with torture of the victim
14. Two episodes in which a child under 12 was forcibly raped or tortured
15. One instance of insertion of the penis in a body orifice of an infant
16. Three batteries of an individual child under 12

17. Three batteries of a spouse within one year
18. Three or more felonious assaults within one year with escalating degrees of violence
19. Two unprovoked attacks with a lethal weapon on strangers
20. Five violent offences of any kind
21. Threats to kill another named person uttered three or more times, at least two of which included no display of anger, and extending over a period of at least three months
22. Preoccupation with a casual acquaintance or stranger lasting more than three months with at least one attempt at direct communication with the other person and at least one potentially injurious action directed at the other person or a surrogate, or association, effigy or symbol of the other person
23. A plan to commit an intolerable crime that the person says they fully intend to carry out, and a history of any violent felony
24. Delusional beliefs not acknowledged as such by the person that, if true, would justify an intolerable crime; a history of violent felony and a history of stopping medication against medical advice.

Coid et al (2013: 387) reiterate that all the instruments used to predict the probability of future violence are merely moderately accurate. The authors caution that this holds true especially for persons diagnosed with a personality disorder, and more specifically an antisocial personality where the predictability of the actuarial tools used ranged between poor to none.

The creative use of the leave of absence option may assist the team in making the discharge decision. This means giving the MHCU leave to visit specified family or friends, or even spend a trial period in a halfway house. During this period responsible persons in that situation could observe the MHCU and report back to the team on their behaviour and adjustment.

The decision to discharge forensic psychiatric MHCUs is made easier if comprehensive community services such as halfway homes, accessible clinics, staff who do regular home visits, a crisis service, and day-hospitals are available. Since all these services are under-developed in South Africa, it can be expected that hospitalisation in South Africa would be longer than in other western countries.

THE CONFLICTING ROLE OF THE MENTAL HEALTH NURSE IN A FORENSIC UNIT

Worldwide, there is much confusion about the role of the nurse in a forensic unit. Debates continue as to whether the forensic mental health nurse is a specialist (Devnick, 2010: 5). The mental health care nurse enters into a therapeutic relationship with the MHCU as highlighted by Uys and Middleton (2010: 184). Allen and Jones (2002: 458) warn that mental health care nurses often enter into custodial relationships as opposed to care relationships with MHCUs. This is even more so in observation units where a mental health care nurse often has to act as a second health professional in the assessment of an

MHCU sent for an observation period. These nurses experience conflict between their roles as carers versus custodians (Fishwick et al, 2001: 188).

The Mental Health Care Act has clear guidelines and stipulations which must be followed when dealing with state patients. Use is made of terms like 'monitoring a patient' which sounds more like custodial care than care in its true essence. The nature of care in high-risk units and knowledge of the reason why a particular MHCU is declared a state patient and under compulsory care are catalysts in MHCUs potentially viewing the mental health care nurse as a custodian rather than a care giver. This statement is reiterated by Devnick (2010: 21) where she cites Kettles and Walker (2007) who observe that the role of the forensic mental health nurse is a power dynamic where the nurse renders care in a strict environment filled with 'rules, security and constraints', while having to negotiate therapeutic encounters with MHCUs.

The author herself also experienced these perceptions from MHCUs when they were referred for 30-day observations and they requested to go for weekend leave or to be discharged. The nursing staff had to inform them that according to hospital policy and the Mental Health Care Act they could not be discharged due to the court referral. The MHCUs would often claim that the hospital was a prison and they were deprived of their rights as the nurses were prison wardens.

The role of the nurse as custodian rather than care giver is further exacerbated by the mere fact that during ward rounds, they need to give feedback on the behaviour of the MHCUs. This adds to the perception of the nurse in the forensic ward as a custodial care giver as opposed to a therapist.

Devnick (2010: 21) cites Holmes (2005) who reported that nurses, who were deployed in forensic units to render mental health care, experienced a 'culture shock' when they were faced with the secure setting, heavy control and the high levels of constant direct observations in the forensic unit. The forensic nurse therefore often finds themselves confronted with two opposing philosophies, namely rendering care and preventing risk. The nurse needs to create a caring environment within the secure constraints of a closed forensic unit.

Adding to the conflicting role of the forensic nurse is a situation well known to the author. This is when empathic nursing responses, in attempting to create a therapeutic environment, may be seen by the MHCU with a personality disorder as an opportunity to manipulate the nurses to bend rules. This is a situation that can compromise the security in the ward. The conflict between duty and care for the observandi is cited to be the central cause of conflict for mental health nurses with regard to their profession. This is described by Devnick (2010: 33) who cites Austin et al, 2003; Burrow, 1993a; Fisher, 2007; Peternejl-Taylor, 1999 and Walsh, 2009.

THE FORENSIC NURSE

The South African Nursing Council (SANC) defines a forensic nurse as a professional nurse with an additional qualification in forensic nursing, specialising in the application of forensic science and clinical nursing practice, who is registered as such by the SANC

(SANC, 2014). There is no such category as a psychiatric forensic nurse specialist, nor is there any training for such a category of nurse. Devnick (2010: 19) echoes this concern in stating that there are limited training opportunities and skills development of nurses working in the forensic units in Canada. In similar fashion, Kaliski (2006: 2) reported that the professional who conducts psychological assessment and who testifies in court does not have the requisite qualifications or the expertise to do so. There are no formal training programmes or examinations in forensic mental health in South Africa. This status quo ensures that the nurse practising in a forensic mental health unit renders custodial care. It is essential that the nurse who practices in an area of specialisation such as forensic mental health be equipped with the skills to render care in these areas.

The author of this chapter concurs with Nedopil et al (2015: 82) and Devnick (2010: 51) in stating that a clear distinction must be made between a psychiatric nurse and a forensic psychiatric nurse, and if there is indeed a difference then the training of this category of nurse should also be distinguished from that of the ordinary psychiatric nurse.

CONCLUSION

Throughout the world, forensic MHCUs are detained far longer than is preferable due to the difficulty in predicting their future behaviour a ral onus which rests on the shoulders of the forensic psychiatric team in safeguarding the community.

Two systems meet in the forensic unit, namely the judicial system and the mental health care system. This complicates the work of the team, since it is not always a comfortable mix. The judicial system is designed to punish and rehabilitate criminals; the health system is designed to treat and rehabilitate MHCUs. While the judicial system deals mainly with the safety of the community, the health system deals chiefly with the safety of the MHCU. In the judicial system, criminals have limited choice and control, while in the health system the aim is to give them maximum choice and control. In the judicial system the relationship between workers and criminals is adversarial; in the health system it is a helping relationship.

In forensic psychiatry these systems overlap, with resultant grey areas and a confusion of roles and philosophies. Nurses who specialise in this area of psychiatric nursing should understand their dual role and develop a philosophy in the unit that would accommodate the dual role of the nurse, namely that of caregiver first and making custodial care secondary to the caring role. It is imperative that the necessary training be provided to nurses working in the forensic psychiatry system, in order to allow for nurses to render care as opposed to an emphasis on custodial care alone. Clarity on these conflicting issues will greatly assist unit staff to find fulfilment in this very interesting and challenging area of specialisation.

WEB RESOURCES

http://www.priory.com/psych.htm
> This is the website of *Priory Medical Journals*, which has a section dedicated to forensic psychiatry. Full articles can be accessed. Click on Psychiatry On-Line and then on Forensic Psychiatry On-line.

www.justice.gov.za/legislation/acts/acts_full.html
> This website provides full copies of all the South African laws, as well as the amendments. It is a useful site to check what is actually stated in the Acts.

REFERENCES

Abrahams and Gross. 2017. Curatorship – what does it entail? www.abgross.co.za/curatorship-what-does-it-entail/ (Accessed 9 June 2019).

Allen, C and Jones, J. 2002. 'Acute wards: problems and solutions. Nursing matters in Acute Care'. *Psychiatric Bulletin*, (26): 458–458.

Anon. nd. 'The Constitutional Court abolishes the death penalty', From South African History Online, [online] www.sahistory.org.za (Accessed 9 July 2017).

Bock, T M. 2015. 'The culturally safe management of aggression and violence in mental health care institutions'. Thesis in the Fulfilment of the Degree of Doctor of Philosophy. North West University: Mahikeng.

Bock, T M. 2018. *Flowchart of the discharge of a State Patient*. Unpublished. Western Cape College of Nursing: Metro East, Bellville.

Cacioppo, J T and Berntson, G G. 1994. Relationship between attitudes and evaluative space: A critical review with emphasis on separability of positive and negative substrates. *Psychological Bulletin*, 115 (3): 402–423.

Coid, J W, Ullrich, S and Kallis, C. 2013. 'Predicting future violence among individuals with psychopathy'. *The British Journal of Psychiatry*, 203: 387–388.

Coleman, L. 1984. *The Reign of Error. Psychiatry, Authority and Law*. Boston: Beacon Press.

Devnick, B R. 2010. 'The Forensic Mental Health Nurse: Confusion, illusion or specialization? A scoping literature review'. Thesis in the partial fulfilment of the Degree of Master of Nursing. University of Victoria. http://dspace.library.uvic.ca:8080/bitstream/handle/1828/4092/Devnick_Betty_MN_2010.pdf?sequence=1&isAllowed=y (Accessed 24 February 2018).

Dietz, P E. 1985. 'Hypothetical criteria for the prediction of individual criminality'. In: C D Webster, M H Ben-Aron and S J Hucker (eds). *Dangerousness: Probability and prediction, psychiatry and public policy*: (87–02). New York: Cambridge University. Press.

Dolan, M and Doyle, M. 2000. 'Violence risk prediction: Clinical and actuarial measures and the role of the Psychopathy Checklist'. *The British Journal of Psychiatry*, 177 (4): 303–311.

Dorrell, S. 1991. 'Crime and mental illness'. *Journal of the Royal Society of Health*, June: 114–117.

Fazel, S, Singh, J P, Doll, H and Grann, M. 2012. 'Use of risk assessment instruments to predict violence and antisocial behaviour in 73 samples involving 24 827 people: systematic review and meta-analysis'. *British Medical Journal (BMJ)*: 345.

Finkleman, P. 2014. *Encyclopaedia of American Civil Liberties.* (Volume 1, A to F). New York: Routladge, Taylor & Francis Group, https://books.google.co.za/books?id=TXoKAgAAQBAJ&pg=PA814&lpg=PA814&dq=King's+pardon+for+mentally+ill&source=bl&ots=GPnY9IXgBC&sig=hJ97HBGH9waDFWgDTTGd-o3p5kE&hl=en&sa=X&ved=0ahUKEwi_o4jPrvPYAhUECcAKHWriCkkQ6AEIKDAA#v=onepage&q=King's%20pardon%20for%20mentally%20ill&f=false (Accessed 25 January 2018).

Fishwick, M, Tait, B and O' Brien, A J. 2001. 'Unearthing the conflicts between carer and custodian: implications for participation in Section16 hearings under the Mental Health Compulsory Assessment and Treatment Act (1992)'. *Australian, N Z Journal of Mental Health Nursing.* Sept, 10 (3): 187–194.

Henning, P H. 1983. 'Beleid ten opsigte van die ontslag van presidentspasiënte'. *Tydskrif vir Regswetenskap,* 8 (2): 132–142.

Hallevey, G. 2015. *The matrix of Insanity in Modern Criminal Law.* Switzerland: Springer. https://books.google.co.za/books?id=t0EPCgAAQBAJ&pg=PA108&lpg=PA108&dq=The+Code+of+Hammurabi+is+a+good+example:+insanity+is+not+mentioned&source=bl&ots=PrW04enqFW&sig=mvAffrjty55lWg03qWtIH2vUjCw&hl=en&sa=X&ved=0ahUKEwjRsfawsfPYAhWrJsAKHYHhDz0Q6AEIKjAB#v=onepage&q=The%20Code%20of%20Hammurabi%20is%20a%20good%20example%3A%20insanity%20is%20not%20mentioned&f=false (Accessed 25 January 2018).

Hvidhjelm, J, Sestoft, D, Skovgaard, L T and Bjorner, J B. 2014. 'Sensitivity and specificity of the Brøset Violence Checklist as a predictor of violence in forensic psychiatry'. *Nordic Journal of Psychiatry*, 68: 536–542.

Kaliski, S (ed). 2006. *Psycholegal assessment in South Africa.* Cape Town: Oxford University Press.

Kaliski, S. 2013. 'Reinstitutionalisation by stealth: The Forensic Mental Health Service is the new chronic system'. *African Journal of Psychiatry.* 16: 13–17.

Kruger, A. 1980. *Mental Health Law in South Africa.* Durban: Butterworth.

Landman, A A and Landman, W J. 2014. *A Practitioner's Guide to the Mental Health Care Act.* Cape Town: Juta.

Louw, R. 1993. Criminal negligence and mens rea: is the reasonable man test an unreasonable one? Dissertation Master's Degree. University of Cape Town: Cape Town. http://hdl.handle.net//11427/17317 (Accessed 10 June 2019).

Marais, B and Subramaney, U. 2015. 'Forensic state patients at Sterkfontein Hospital: A 3-year follow-up study'. *South African Journal of Psychiatry.* 21 (3): 86–92.

MacInnes, D, Beer, D, Reynolds, K and Kinane, C. 2013. 'Carers of forensic mental health in-patients: What factors influence their satisfaction with services?'. *Journal of Mental Health,* 22 (6): 528–535.

MacPhail, A and Verdun-Jones, S. 2013. 'Mental Illness and The Criminal Justice System Prepared for Re-Inventing Criminal Justice: The Fifth National Symposium'. Montreal QC, Canada: January 2013.

Mattiuzzi, P G. 2008. 'Why do people kill? A Typology of Violent Offenders'. *Everyday Psychology,* http://www.everydaypsychology.com/2008/07/why-do-people-kill-typology-of-violent.html#.WmoDEkxuLoo (Accessed 25 January 2018).

Nakatani, Y. 2011. 'Treatment of offenders with mental disorders: focusing on prison psychiatry'. *Seishin Shinkeiqaku Zasshi,* 113 (5): 458–67.

Nedopil, N, Taylor, P and Gunn, J. 2015. 'Forensic psychiatry in Europe: The perspective of the Ghent Group'. *International Journal of Psychiatric Clinical Practice,* 19: 80–83.

Ngubane, V G and Uys, L R. 1994. 'Social support networks for black psychiatric inpatients'. *Curationis,* 17 (2): 6–9.

Pillay, A P. 2014. 'Could *S v Pistorius* influence reform in the traditional forensic mental health evaluation format?'. *South African Journal of Psychology,* 44 (4): 377–380.

Roffey, M and Kaliski, S Z. 2012. '"To predict or not to predict-that is the question" An exploration of risk assessment in the context of South African forensic psychiatry'. *African Journal of Psychiatry.* 15: 227–233.

Sainsbury Centre for Mental Health. nd. *Briefing. Mental Health Care and the Criminal Justice System.* http://www.ohrn.nhs.uk/resource/policy/SCMHMHandtheCJS.pdf (Accessed 25 January 2018).

Sakuta, T. 1991. 'Prison psychiatry in Japan'. *Medicine and Law,* 10: 275–284.

Sithole, S E. 2007. 'A comparative analysis of mental illness as defence in criminal law'. Magister Legum thesis. Port Elizabeth: Nelson Mandela Metropolitan University.

South Africa. 1977. *Criminal Procedure Act, No 51, as amended by section 14 of Act no.105 of 1982.* Pretoria: Government Printer.

South Africa. 2002. *Mental Health Care Act No 17 of 2002.* Pretoria: Government Printer.

South African Nursing Council (SANC). 2014. 'Competencies – Forensic Nurse: May 2014'. SA Nursing Council. Pretoria: Government Printer.

Steadman, H J and Cocozza, J J. 1974. *Careers of the Criminally Insane.* Lexington: Lexington Books.

Sukeri, K, Betancourt, O A, Emsley, R E, Nagdee, M and Erlacher, H. 2016. 'Forensic mental health services: Current service provision and planning for a prison mental health service in the Eastern Cape'. *South African Journal of Psychiatry,* 22 (1): 1–8.

Swanepoel, M. 2015. 'Legal aspects with regard to mentally ill offenders in South Africa'. *PER: Potchefstroomse Elektroniese Regsblad,* 18 (1).

TheLaw.com. nd. 'Law Dictionary & Black's Law Dictionary. 2nd edition, s.v. criminal capacity. https://dictionary.thelaw.com/criminal-capacity/ (Accessed 10 June 2017).

Thomson, L D G, Goethals, K and Nedopil, N. 2016. 'Multiagency working in forensic psychiatry: Theory and Practice in Europe'. *Criminal Behaviour and Mental Health,* 26: 153–160.

Uys, L and Middleton L. 2010. *Mental Health Nursing: A South African perspective.* 6th edition. Cape Town: Juta.

Wachtel, M. 2012. 'Risk assessment: How psychologists predict future violent behaviour'. *PsychLaw Journal.* http://www.psychlawjournal.com/2012/08/risk-assessment-how-psychologists.html (Accessed 25 January 2018).

Webster, C D, Ben-Aron, M H and Hucker, S J. 1985. *Dangerousness: Probability and Prediction, Psychiatry and Public Policy.* Cambridge: Cambridge University Press

Weisstub, D N (ed). 1987. *Law and Mental Health: International perspectives.* New York: Pergamon Press.

West London NHS Trust. nd. 'Broadmoor Hospital'. http://www.wlmht.nhs.uk/bm/broadmoor-hospital/ (Accessed 25 January 2018).

Whitehead, T. 1982. *Mental Illness and the Law.* Oxford: Basil Blackwell.

Wool, R. 1991. 'The present and future handling of the mentally disturbed offender'. *Journal of the Royal Society for Health,* Part I (October): 203–205; part II (December): 248–251.

Zabow, T. 1989. 'Psychiatric evidence in extenuation: assessment and testimony in homicide defendants'. *Medicine and Law,* 8: 631–639.

SECTION 5
Appendices

APPENDIX ONE

INPATIENT EVALUATION SCALE

This evaluation scale was drawn up to:
1. assist the nursing staff to gather basic information about patients in an orderly, thorough and scientific manner
2. assist the nursing staff to obtain the information they require for the day-to-day and long-term planning of nursing care
3. assist the nursing staff to see in which areas the patients are making progress and in which they are making no progress
4. serve as a research instrument.

The scale consists of two sections.

Section 1
Section 1 consists of 20 items in the form of a questionnaire that the nurse fills in with the patient on admission. It covers the patient's general background and expectations.

Section 2
Section 2 takes the form of a rating scale, each item being rated on a 5-point scale as follows: a scale point of 1 represents seriously abnormal conduct, while a scale point of 5 represents normal conduct. Scale points 2, 3 and 4 represent various successive behavioural conditions on this continuum.

It can be schematically represented as follows:

Scale points	1	2	3	4	5
	Seriously abnormal		Continuum		Normal conduct

This section is completed by the nurse within the first week of admission and at regular intervals thereafter.

The following points are important to remember when evaluating a patient:
1. Every scale is drawn up in such a way that it measures the entire spectrum of possible behavioural intensity. Do not be afraid to use the extremes, ie 1 or 5. Some patients' conduct often justifies this. The most common mistake in the use of evaluation scales is always to remain 'in the middle'.
2. Take enough time to complete the scale, otherwise it will be less valid. If you are not sure of an item's point value, make sure by observation before completing the item. You may allow yourself to be influenced by the observations of other team members but only in the case of first-hand observations that the members personally share with you.

3. Date your evaluation and sign it in the appropriate column.
4. Do not omit items. Fill them all in, even if it is difficult to decide where the patient fits in. Use the remarks column to describe your problems with the evaluation or important symptoms for which there are no points on the scale.
5. Give a point based only on the patient's conduct during the period of evaluation and not on previous conduct.
6. It sometimes seems as though a patient could be classified on more than one point on the scale. Choose the point best suited to the patient.
7. If the patient's conduct is changeable or episodic, record the most pathological conduct during the prescribed period.

INPATIENT EVALUATION SCALE
Part 1: Evaluation scale
Section 1
1. Name: .... Age: ....
2. Reg. no.:
3. Ward:
4. Sex:
5. Religion:
6. Home language:
7. Diagnosis:
8. Educational standard:
9. Occupation:
10. Address:
11. Name and address of next-of-kin:
12. What problems or complaints brought you to the hospital/clinic today?
13. Has something like this happened to your family before?
14. What do you think caused it?
15. What helps it or makes it worse?
16. What effect do the problems have on your and your family's daily life?
17. Is there anything about which you are worried, such as the care of your children or your work?
18. What do you expect of the treatment and/or the hospital?
19. Have you ever been visited by a social worker?
20. What are your hobbies? How do you spend your free time?

	1	2	3	4	5	Date	Remarks
1. Physical							
1.1 Bath	Totally dependent on nursing care	Needs help, supervision and training by nurses	Needs supervision by nurses	Manages with help of family or others	Independent		
1.2 Wash	"	"	"	"	"		
1.3 Dress	"	"	"	"	"		
1.4 Hair and/or beard	"	"	"	"	"		
1.5 Teeth	"	"	"	"	"		
1.6 Pressure parts	"	"	"	"	"		
1.7 Nails	"	"	"	"	"		
1.8 Appetite	Does not eat, refuses to eat or eats too much, over- or underweight	Eats too much or too little more than 50 % of time, is obviously over- or underweight	Episodes of eating too much or too little, eg during stress, or weight changes	Occasionally too much or too little	Normal		
1.9 Table manners	Poor or must be fed	Eats with minimum cutlery, must be fed at times	Eats very untidily with normal cutlery	Not very good, for example speed	Normal		
1.10 Supervision required for own and others' safety	Is totally dependent on nurses, always	Needs supervision more than 50 % of time	Needs supervision for long periods	Needs supervision occasionally for short periods	Independent		

→

	1	2	3	4	5	Date	Remarks
1.11 Sleep	Cannot fall asleep for hours every night, very restless, sleeps more than 12 hours/24 or wakes very early	Has definite sleep disturbances (as described in 1) more than 50 % of time	Has many sleep disturbances for long periods	Happens occasionally for one or two nights or days	Normal		
1.12 Urine	Incontinent or has indwelling catheter	Has control with much supervision and encouragement by nurses	Usually has control, but has long periods of incontinence during physical or psychological setbacks	Occasionally has a single incident of incontinence	Normal		
1.13 Faeces	"	"	"	"	"		
2. Social							
2.1 Contact with family	Patient or family refuses contact	Contact from one side only or very unsatisfactory	Sometimes letters and/or visits that satisfy	Goes to family for leave	Can be discharged to family; satisfactory		
2.2 Contact with patients	No real contact	Alone more than 50 % of time or makes superficial contact if approached	Good contact with one or two	Extends good contact to more than one or two	Good contact with most patients		
2.3 Social activities	No participation	Can be persuaded to participate	Evidently enjoys going, does not participate	Sometimes takes limited part	Normal participation		

→

	1	2	3	4	5	Date	Remarks
2.4 Social conduct	Unacceptable	Unacceptable more than 50 % of time	Episodes of unacceptable conduct	Will be accepted to some extent in some social circles	Will be accepted in most social circles		
2.5 Contact with staff	No real contact	Alone more than 50 % of time or makes superficial contact if approached	Makes good contact with one or two	Extends good contact to more than one or two	Good contact with staff		
3. Orientation							
3.1 Time	No concept of time	Reacts to certain learnt stimuli, eg bell for meals	Usually does all routines on time	Can do simple planning for use of time	Can plan day sensibly, not unsettled by busy programme		
3.2 Own abilities	No concept of own abilities	Completely out of proportion, too much or too little	Seeks outside judgement	Judgement according to premorbid performance	Realistic		
3.3 Routine	Must always be told to follow routine	Follows ward routine passively, sleeps when not guided in activities	Can learn more complicated routines, does routine work	Can deviate from routine if initiative comes from outside, flexible	Takes initiative to changes in routine but can keep to set routine		
3.4 Money matters	No management	Asks only for requirements, not money	Interested only in pocket money	Reliable with small amounts, eg to buy clothes	Manages own business well		

→

	1	2	3	4	5	Date	Remarks
3.5 Instructions	No reaction	Usually reacts to simple instructions	Usually reacts to more complicated instructions	Can use own discretion to a limited extent	Can be trusted to carry out instructions but also to use discretion to act differently		
3.6 Perseverance	Cannot complete simplest tasks, play and work impossible	Can focus attention on one thing for only a few minutes	Can focus attention on pleasant things or short tasks	Can work for a few hours a day	Normal workday, relaxation and problem solving possible		
3.7 Own faults	No concept of exactly what own faults are	Takes all blame or puts it all on others	Realises faults but makes excuses	Can acknowledge faults privately	Can acknowledge faults realistically in a group		
3.8 Sense of responsibility	Takes no responsibility	Takes responsibility for little self-care with supervision and encouragement	Takes responsibility satisfactorily for own care	Takes responsibility for self and own work	Takes responsibility for self, own work and others		
3.9 Setting of limits necessary	Locking up or transfer to closed ward essential, as well as large doses of strong sedatives	Large doses of strong sedatives enough	Firm, clear verbal control	Ward rules and good supervision necessary, takes chances if supervision is relaxed	Acts within ward rules even without supervision		

→

	1	2	3	4	5	Date	Remarks
3.10 Taking of decisions	Takes no decisions	Asks others to take decisions	Always takes irresponsible decisions or very ambivalent	Occasionally takes irresponsible decisions and sometimes ambivalent	Seeks advice, takes own decisions and bears consequences		
3.11 Medication (do 3.12 if none prescribed)	Refuses to take or does not swallow	Takes only under strict supervision or if forced	Takes if proferred	Fetches own medication, usually on time	Knows own medication, fetches it regularly and on time		
3.12 General reliability regarding own therapy	Refuses all cooperation	Comes to therapy only under very good supervision or if forced	Comes to therapy of own accord but is very passive and takes part only superficially	Participates actively and enthusiastically in some therapy	Uses all forms of therapy enthusiastically		
4. Psychopathology							
4.1 Depression	Severe, uninterrupted and intense feeling of sadness, thoughts morbid, negative about self, not able to do anything	Constantly but not very intense, talks about it but can continue with routine	Sometimes sad, but not too bad, talks about it if asked	No signs of depression			
4.2 Suicide	Constant thoughts, has a definite practical plan, previous serious attempts	Less serious attempts, plans unformed or impractical	More passive wish, no attempt so far	Admits old thoughts of suicide, denies now	No signs		

→

	1	2	3	4	5	Date	Remarks
4.3 Anxiety or fear	Constantly seeks reassurance, anxiety/fear so bad that routine not followed, sometimes looks frightened, starts, trembles	Anxious more than 50 % of time, but sometimes lighter	Talks of anxiety/ fear but continues with routine	Transient, mentions only if asked	No signs of anxiety		
4.4 Rage or aggression	Extremely physical or verbal, difficult or impossible for staff to control	Noisy, threatening, rude, sarcastic more than 50 % of time	General attitude, outbursts of rage	Sometimes brief outbursts of rage	No signs of aggression or rage		
4.5 Motor restlessness	Generally intense, uncontrollable, does not sit still for a moment, even has trouble finishing meals	Restlessness so bad for long periods that gets very little done, yet constantly busy	Restlessness for short periods, a few days	Sometimes restless for short periods at night or during the day	No signs of restlessness		
4.6 Motor retardation	Very bad, can do little, stuporous, very dependent on nursing care	Movements noticeably slow more than 50 % of time, gets little done	Long periods of retardation or some short, acute episodes	Just observable retardation of movements	No signs of retardation		
4.7 Delusions	Established, general basis of most conduct	Very loose system, leaves out, adds, yet influences conduct	Ideas and thoughts at times, no system	Ideas can be questioned at times	No signs of delusions		

→

	1	2	3	4	5	Date	Remarks
4.8 Hallucinations[4]	Constantly hallucinates, basis of most conduct, not at all influenced by presence of staff, no contact	Starts hallucinating in presence of staff, yet has contact	Talks about it without being asked, present for long periods	Looks as though is hallucinating	No signs of hallucination		
4.9 Thought disturbance	Word salad or just impossible to understand	Very difficult to follow	Many loose associations, woolly	Ambiguous at times	No signs of thought disturbance		
4.10 Elation	Extreme euphoria and elation in facial expression, attitude and speech constant	Euphoric, noisy more than 50 % of time or a few very acute episodes	Constantly in high spirits, not too bad, signs such as flamboyant dress	Occasional signs of elation for one day or part of a day	No signs of elation		
4.11 Memory	General amnesia, cannot function	Medium- and/or short-term memory seriously disturbed	Short-term memory disturbance	Value signs of memory disturbance	No signs of memory disturbance		
4.12 Verbal productivity	Total mutism (aphasia), never says a word	Very low verbal productivity, questions must usually be repeated	Only answers questions but does not expand	Answers questions completely but seldom begins a conversation or subject	Normal verbal productivity		

APPENDIX TWO

UNIVERSITY OF NATAL FUNCTIONAL ASSESSMENT SCALE (UNFAS)

First contact date

Use the following key when filling in the scale:
- Criterion fully met — 2
- Criterion partially met — 1
- Criterion not met — 0
- Not observed or not applicable — –

1. Interpersonal status
1.1 Has a friendship relationship with at least one person
1.2 Shows acceptable social habits and behaviour
1.3 Relationship with family stable and satisfactory
1.4 Engages in simple conversation about concrete subjects
1.5 Is generally satisfied with their life

2. Self-care status
2.1 Appears clean and neat
2.2 Dresses appropriately
2.3 Copes with situations that are moderately stressful
2.4 Alcohol and/or drug intake not a problem

3. Treatment and mental status
3.1 Has attended clinic regularly over the last year
3.2 Takes prescribed medication regularly without assistance
3.3 Behaviour free from positive signs of mental illness
3.4 Is oriented to time, place and person
3.5 Has remained out of the hospital for the last two years
3.6 Short-term memory is normal
3.7 Shows insight in own situation
3.8 Shows good judgement in everyday situations

4. Community adjustment status
4.1 Handles own finances effectively
4.2 Uses appropriate community services effectively
    4.2.1 Medical facilities
    4.2.2 Recreational facilities
    4.2.3 Transport
    4.2.4 Church
    4.2.5 Shops

The following two aspects of functioning are addressed by choosing the appropriate category for the patient to get the score for that section.

5. Employment status
Category
0   Unemployed, little or no evidence that patient takes responsibility for any jobs at home
1   Unemployed but works consistently on jobs around the house. Takes responsibility for these
2   Unemployed, but does voluntary work outside the home, or is working in protected workshop
3   Works in sheltered employment, or is retired due to age
4   Takes full responsibility for housework (housewife), studies or works in the open labour market, not necessarily in a full-time capacity

6. Living status
Category
0   Unstable living conditions
1   Living with family of origin or other relatives
2   Living in a sheltered environment, such as a half-way house or special home
3   Lives in boarding establishment with minimal supervision
4   Lives independently with own spouse and children, or alone, or with friends without supervision

TOTAL: [54]

Percentage: $\frac{Total}{Possible\ total} \times 100 =$

Assessment done by: Date:

PSYCHIATRIC OUTPATIENT: FUNCTIONAL ASSESSMENT GUIDELINES
1. Interpersonal status
- Items 1.1 and 1.3 need to be assessed with the input of the family and a home visit will probably be necessary.
- Items 1.2 and 1.4 can be assessed in an interview with the patient.
- Item 1.2 refers to whether the patient will stand out in a crowd because of behaviour, or whether they behave quite acceptably.

2. Self-care status
- Items 2.1 and 2.2 can be assessed in an interview with the patient, while the other items need the input of family.
- Item 2.3 refers to everyday situations like having to deal with household appliances that break, or toothache, or a visit by family. It does not refer to highly stressful

events such as major loss. On the Social Phobia Scale (SPS) scale in the DSM-5, the stress should not rate higher than 2 (mild).
- Item 2.4 is scored as 1 if the person has a history of abuse, but there is no current evidence of abuse.

3. Treatment and mental status
- Items 3.1 and 3.5 can be assessed by studying the patient's record.
- Item 3.3 may need some input from the family. The other items can be assessed during an interview with the patient.
- Positive signs of mental illness refer to the presence of abnormal behaviour, thought, perception, and not the absence of motivation or friendships or social interaction.
- 3.1 Regular attendance means that the patient has not missed more than three appointments over the last year.
- 3.2 If the patient gets assistance from the family, mark 1.

4. Community adjustments status
This whole section can be assessed during an interview.

5. Employment status
This section has to be assessed with the help of the family.

6. Living status
This section can be assessed during an interview with the patient.
Dear Parent/Relative/Friend
Please read the following questions carefully and provide us with answers concerning …'s behaviour at home, and if possible, give us more details on each answer that might be helpful to us in our joint effort to help them to continue to get better.

Question 1
Do they have friends or at least a friend with whom they are intimate enough to share secrets or whom they approach for certain problems?

Answer

_____

_____

Question 2
Are they able to maintain good interpersonal relationships with family members, for example when they are in need of help do they consult other family members or do members also ask for help from them as a family member?

Answer

_____
_____

Question 3
Do they cope well with moderate stress at home, for example when they are worried about any event such as losing valuable articles in the house or when there is misunderstanding in the home or when they feel bodily pain or are in trouble?

Answer

_____
_____

Question 4
Do they have any history of alcohol abuse and if so, do they have problems when they have taken liquor, for example fighting with others or any other abnormal behaviour?

Answer

_____
_____

Question 5
How is their general behaviour at home? Do they show any positive signs of mental illness – if so, what do they do that you see as abnormal?

Answer

_____
_____

Question 6
If they are not employed, do they take any responsibility for jobs at home or not, for example gardening, cleaning, cooking, etc?

Answer

_____
_____

Question 7
Do they consistently do jobs around and outside the home and take full responsibility for these as indicated above?

Answer
_____
_____

Question 8
Do they do voluntary jobs outside the home, for example help neighbours with a job to be done, such as preparing for a party, cleaning the yard, painting, etc?

Answer
_____
_____

Question 9
Do they take full responsibility for the housework (housewives), for example ironing, cleaning, cooking, without being urged to do these tasks, and do they use their discretion about jobs to be carried out or doing private study, or do they work in the open labour market as a part-time or full-time worker?

Answer
_____
_____

Thank you
Signature
NB These questions should be translated into the language of the family.

(Dube, B E. 1989. *Developing and Testing of an Instrument for Functional Assessment of Psychiatric Outpatients.* Durban: University of Natal.)

APPENDIX THREE

EXAMPLES OF QUESTIONS USED IN A PSYCHIATRIC HISTORY

HALLUCINATIONS

Did you hear voices or sounds that could not be heard by other people when you were sick? If yes:
- What did you hear?
- When did these voices first start? (If the patient cannot remember, ask: How old were you when the voices started? Was it winter/summer/nearly winter/nearly summer?)
- Did the voices give a running commentary on your behaviour or thoughts?
- How many voices did you hear? Did they talk to each other or to you?
- Did you ever see things that other people could not see? If yes, what did you see? (Visual hallucinations)
- Did you have strange feelings in your body or did it feel as if there were things crawling on your skin? When? (Tactile hallucinations)
- Did you smell things others could not smell? (Olfactory hallucinations)
- Did you have strange tastes in your mouth? (Gustatory hallucinations)

DELUSIONS
- Have parts of your body changed or stopped functioning?
- Has there been an outside force controlling your thoughts and actions? Have thoughts been taken out of your head/put into your head?
- Are there people who want to harm you, speak badly about you or take too much notice of you? Who are these people? Why do you think they do this? Compared to other people, do you see yourself as better than most people or are you the same as others?
- Are you a prominent, rich, strong or clever person?
- Are you especially close to God/Christ? (Name the patient's specific religious deity.) In what way?
- Do you have any special powers or abilities?
- Are there people or forces out to get you? Who?

(Traditionally, illness or misfortune may be attributed to bewitchment by others, including family members, therefore it is not delusional unless it includes many people or hospital/clinic staff or other patients.)

Affect or mood
- Did you feel so good or happy that other people thought you were not yourself? When did this start?

- Do you feel more irritable than usual, or get into fights?
- Have you felt especially full of energy or full of exciting ideas (at work, with friends, at home)?
- Have you felt very sad or depressed nearly every day for two weeks?
- Are you becoming disenchanted with the things you used to enjoy (frequency, duration)?
- Has your appetite changed? How? Was there a change in the fit of your clothes?
- How were you sleeping? Did you have trouble falling asleep, waking often in the night, waking up too early while others were asleep? Did you sleep too much, even in daytime?
- Did you feel worthless about things you had done or not done? Did you feel tense inside your body?
- Were you more tired than usual every day?

Psychomotor activity
- Were you so fidgety and restless that you were unable to sit still? Or did you talk or move more slowly?

Thought disturbances
- Do you have trouble thinking or concentrating?
- Do you feel as if your thoughts are racing away and you can't control them? Have you been thinking a lot about death or wanting to kill yourself?
- How are you going to kill yourself? Have you worked out a plan?
- Were you more talkative than usual?

Orientation
- Do you know where you are? Where?
- What is the time now? If not sure: Is it morning, midday, afternoon, night-time, middle of the night?
- Who brought you to the hospital/clinic?

Intellectual ability
- How did you do at school?
- If below Grade 4 and mental disability is suspected, ask: How many legs does one cow/dog have? Two cows? Three cows?
- Did you go to college/university?

PRECIPITATING FACTORS
- Just before you became ill, did you have any stresses at home/work/with a loved one? What happened? How did you feel about yourself? What did you do to get rid of the stressful feelings?

- Did you stop taking your medication before you became ill? Can you remember what made you stop taking your medication?
- Have you been in an accident where you were hit on the head?
- Just before you became ill, were you taking too much alcohol/dagga/other drugs? If yes: How much each day and for how long? Did you become ill after you stopped taking alcohol, etc?
- If the person is female and of child-bearing age, ask: How old is your last-born child?

APPENDIX FOUR

EVALUATION OF GROUP WORK

Nurse: _____

Evaluator: _____

Date: _____

Instructions to the evaluator
Mark each criterion with a cross on a scale of one to five as you believe it applies to the nurse.
1 = ineffective
5 = exceptionally effective
(For office use only)
Questionnaire no: (1–3)

Evaluation criteria	Interval scale
1. Did the nurse decide on an objective for the group beforehand?	1 2 3 4 5 (4)
2. Has the nurse set criteria for the inclusion of members?	1 2 3 4 5 (5)
3. Is the chosen activity appropriate for the achievement of the objective of the group work?	1 2 3 4 5 (6)
4. Were individual interviews conducted with prospective members?	1 2 3 4 5 (7)
5. Do members comply with the criteria set for inclusion in the group?	1 2 3 4 5 (8)
6. Is the number of members suitable for the particular group work?	1 2 3 4 5 (9)
7. Is the nurse sensitive to the physical set-up of the group?	1 2 3 4 5 (10)
8. Does the nurse provide opportunities for introduction to the group?	1 2 3 4 5 (11)
9. Is the goal of the group work discussed?	1 2 3 4 5 (12)
10. Are rules made and accepted by the group?	1 2 3 4 5 (13)
11. Does the nurse come up to the expectations of the group?	1 2 3 4 5 (14)
12. Are activities introduced to the group in a stimulating and concrete way?	1 2 3 4 5 (15)
13. Is group activity linked to the normal functioning of the members?	1 2 3 4 5 (16)
14. Does the nurse apply techniques to encourage group interaction?	1 2 3 4 5 (17)
15. Does the nurse succeed in activating the group here and now?	1 2 3 4 5 (18)

→

16. Does the nurse cope with obstacles during the group process?	1	2	3	4	5	(19)
17. Does the nurse succeed in maintaining a balance between the various leadership functions?	1	2	3	4	5	(20)
18. Does the nurse succeed in identifying dynamics during the group process and in responding appropriately?	1	2	3	4	5	(21)
19. Does the nurse use summaries during group work?	1	2	3	4	5	(22)
20. Does the nurse apply mental health nursing skills to initiate and maintain the group process?	1	2	3	4	5	(23)
21. Does the nurse succeed in keeping individual interactions goal directed?	1	2	3	4	5	(24)
22. Does the nurse succeed in getting all the members involved?	1	2	3	4	5	(25)
23. Does the nurse succeed in keeping the group process goal directed?	1	2	3	4	5	(26)
24. Does the nurse follow the cues given by individual members and the tempo of the group process?	1	2	3	4	5	(27)
25. Does the nurse succeed in balancing group leadership and group participation?	1	2	3	4	5	(28)
26. Does the nurse avoid the use of his/her own frame of reference in group work?	1	2	3	4	5	(29)
27. Does the nurse offer members an opportunity to verbalise their experience of the group process?	1	2	3	4	5	(30)
28. Are the group-work goals evaluated and achieved?	1	2	3	4	5	(31)
29. Is the group work summarised succinctly and in a concrete manner at the end of the session?	1	2	3	4	5	(32)
30. Is an opportunity for follow-up presented?	1	2	3	4	5	(33)
31. Does the nurse keep to the structure and process of group work?	1	2	3	4	5	(34)
32. Does the duration of the group work correlate with the identified objective?	1	2	3	4	5	(35)

Evaluation of the nurse's ability to analyse group dynamics

To what extent does the nurse:

33. describe and analyse group interaction?	1	2	3	4	5	(36)
34. describe and analyse the group atmosphere?	1	2	3	4	5	(37)
35. identify and motivate the roles of the members?	1	2	3	4	5	(38)
36. identify, explain and motivate the style of leadership used?	1	2	3	4	5	(39)

→

37. identify less-than-effective aspects of the way in which the group is handled?	1 2 3 4 5	(40)
38. identify positive aspects of the way in which the group is handled?	1 2 3 4 5	(41)
39. identify problem areas in the way in which the group is handled?	1 2 3 4 5	(42)

Remarks: _____

Average mark: _____

42–55	=	Ineffective	=	0–26 %
56–82	=	Less than effective	=	27–39 %
83–107	=	Below average	=	40–51 %
108–135	=	Average	=	52–64 %
136–160	=	Above average	=	65–76 %
161–187	=	Effective	=	77–89 %
188–210	=	Exceptionally effective	=	90–100 %

APPENDIX FIVE

EVALUATION OF MENTAL HEALTH EDUCATION

Student: _____

Evaluator: _____

Date: _____

Instructions to the evaluator
Mark each criterion with a cross on a scale of one to five as you believe it applies to the nurse.
1 = ineffective
5 = exceptionally effective
(For office use only)

Questionnaire no: (1–3)

1. To what extent did the nurse assess the target group or person?	1	2	3	4	5	(4)
2. To what extent were objectives set for the mental health tuition?	1	2	3	4	5	(5)
3. To what extent did the nurse make use of teaching media and aids?	1	2	3	4	5	(6)
4. How effectively did the nurse create learning opportunities for the target group?	1	2	3	4	5	(7)
5. How appropriate was the content of the mental health tuition?	1	2	3	4	5	(8)
6. To what extent did the nurse make use of interpersonal skills in the teaching process?	1	2	3	4	5	(9)
7. To what extent did the nurse encourage participation of the group or person in the teaching process?	1	2	3	4	5	(10)
8. To what extent were the objectives of the mental health tuition achieved?	1	2	3	4	5	(11)
9. To what extent were opportunities for follow-up offered?	1	2	3	4	5	(12)

Remarks: _____

Average mark: _____
9–17	=	Ineffective	=	0–29 %
18–23	=	Less than effective	=	30–39 %
24–29	=	Below average	=	40–49 %
30–36	=	Average	=	50–60 %

37–44	=	Above average	=	61–74 %
45–51	=	Effective	=	75–85 %
52 and more	=	Exceptionally effective	=	86–100 %

APPENDIX SIX

TIME-EVENT CHART FOR A PATIENT WITH ANXIETY SYMPTOMS

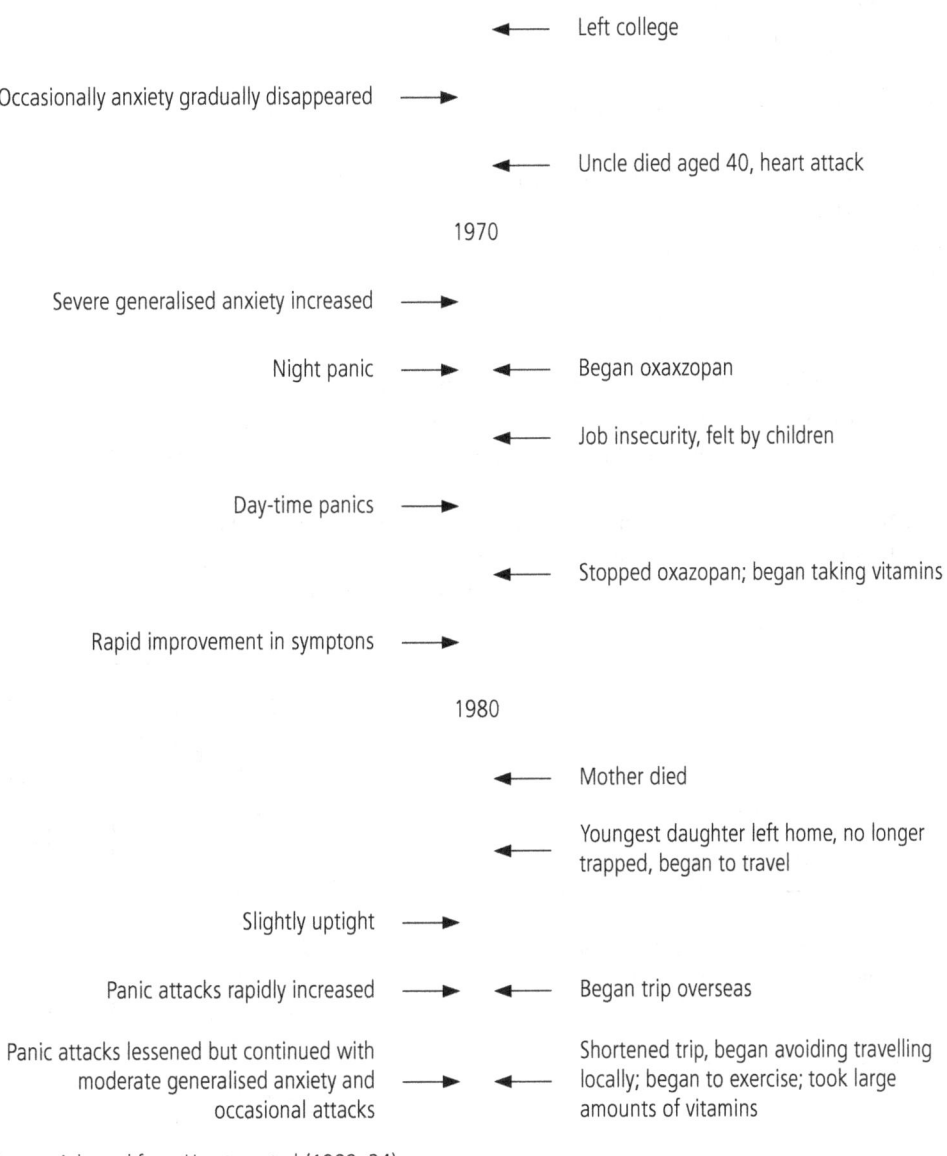

Source: Adapted from Hawton et al (1989: 24)

APPENDIX SEVEN

HAMILTON ANXIETY RATING SCALE (HAM-A)

This scale is in the public domain:
https://dcf.psychiatry.ufl.edu/files/2011/05/HAMILTON-ANXIETY.pdf

The main purpose of this scale is to assess the severity of anxiety symptoms. The scale consists of 14 items (phrases that describe feelings people have).

Each item is scored on a scale of 0 (not present) to 4 (severe), with a total score range of 0–56, where a total score of:

Less than 17 = Mild severity
18–24 = Mild to moderate severity
25–30 = Moderate to severe

The scale can be used with children, adolescents and adults.

With the patient, find the answer from 0–4 that best describes the extent to which they have these symptoms and then work out the total score and severity rating.

0 Not present –
1 Mild – Occurs irregularly and for short periods
2 Moderate – Occurs more constantly and for longer periods
3 Severe – Continuous and dominates patient's life
4 Very severe – Incapacitating

	0 Not present	1 Mild	2 Moderate	3 Severe	4 Very severe
1. Anxiety Worries, anticipation of the worst, fearful anticipation, irritability					
2. Tension Feelings of tension, fatigue, moved to tears easily, trembling feelings of restlessness, startle response, inability to relax					
3. Fears Of dark, of strangers, of being left alone, of animals, of traffic, of crowds					
4. Insomnia Difficulty in falling asleep, night terrors, unsatisfying sleep, fatigue on waking, dreams, nightmares					
5. Intellectual (cognition) Difficulty in concentration, poor memory					

→

	0 Not present	1 Mild	2 Moderate	3 Severe	4 Very severe
6. Depression Loss of interest, lack of pleasure in hobbies, depression, early waking, diurnal swing					
7. Somatic (muscular) Pains and aches, twitchings, stiffness, myoclonic jerks, grinding of teeth, unsteady voice, increased muscle tone					
8. Somatic Tinnitus, blurring of vision, hot and cold flushes, feelings of weakness, prickling sensation					
9. Cardiovascular symptoms Tachycardia, palpitations, pain in chest, throbbing of vessels, feeling faint, missed beat					
10. Respiratory symptoms Pressure or constriction in chest, choking feelings, sighing, dyspnoea					
11. Gastrointestinal symptoms Difficulty in swallowing, wind, burning sensations, abdominal pain, nausea, vomiting, looseness of bowels, loss of weight, constipation					
12. Genitourinary Frequency and urgency of urination, amenorrhoea, menorrhagia, frigidity, loss of libido, impotence, premature ejaculation					
13. Autonomic symptoms Dry mouth, flushing, pallor, sweating, giddiness, tension headache					
14. Behaviour at interview Fidgeting, restlessness or pacing, tremor, furrowed brow, strained face, sighing or rapid respiration, facial pallor, swallowing, belching					
TOTAL					

STANFORD PANIC APPRAISAL INVENTORY

Listed below are 20 statements reflecting some common feelings and thoughts that people report during sudden attacks of panic or extreme anxiety. Read each item carefully and then choose the number from the scale that best describes the degree to which you are troubled by the feeling or thought. Then write the number on the line opposite each statement.

0	1	2	3	4	5	6	7	8	9	10
Not at all troubling		Mildly troubling		Moderately troubling			Markedly troubling		Extremely troubling	

1. I may faint. ....

2. People will stare at me. ....

3. I may become hysterical. ....

4. I may have a heart attack. ....

5. I may drive off the road and crash. ....

6. I may do something uncontrollable like jump out of a window. ....

7. I may scream. ....

8. I may not be able to move from one spot. ....

9. I may be put into a mental hospital. ....

10. I may get sick to my stomach. ....

11. People will laugh at me. ....

12. I may lose my balance and fall. ....

13. I may suffocate. ....

14. I will be an embarrassment to my family and friends. ....

15. I may die. ....

16. I may go insane. ....

17. I may lose control of my bowels. ....

18. I will be trapped. ....

19. Others will think I am weird. ....

20. I may have a brain tumour. ....

FEAR QUESTIONNAIRE

Choose a number from the scale below to show to what extent you would avoid each of the situations listed below because of fear or other unpleasant feelings. Then write the number you have chosen on the line opposite each situation.

0	1	2	3	4	5	6	7	8	9	10
Would not avoid it		Slightly avoid it			Definitely avoid it		Markedly avoid it			Always avoid it

Leave this area blank

Situation		
Main phobia you want treated (describe in your own words)	....	
Eating or drinking with other people	....	
Being watched or stared at	....	
Talking to people in authority	....	
Being criticised	....	
Speaking or acting before an audience	....	Soc
Travelling alone by bus or coach	....	
Walking alone in busy streets	....	
Going into crowded shops	....	
Going far from home alone	....	
Large open spaces	....	AG
Injections or minor surgery	....	
Hospitals	....	
Sight of blood	....	
Thought of injury or illness	....	
Going to the dentist	....	Bl

Section 2

1. Have you ever had attacks of extreme anxiety or panic that seem to come on suddenly in situations or places that pose no real danger? Yes/No
2. If yes, please check each of the symptoms below that you experienced during your last bad panic attack.
   - Shortness of breath
   - Choking or smothering sensations
   - Palpitations (heart racing or pounding)
   - Chest pain, pressure, tightness or discomfort
   - Sweating
   - Feeling faint (does not mean you actually have to faint)
   - Dizziness or unsteadiness
   - Nausea or abdominal distress
   - Depersonalisation or derealisation (things seem unreal or you feel detached from your body)
   - Numbness or tingling in any part of your body
   - Hot or cold flushes
   - Trembling or shaking
   - Fear of dying
   - Fear of going crazy or doing something uncontrolled
   - Other (please describe)
3. How many panic attacks (including milder ones) have you had in the last seven days?
4. How many panic attacks (including milder ones) have you had in the last month?
5. Do some of your panic attacks occur out of the blue in safe situations, such as when you are at home? Yes/No

Section 3

1. Are you bothered by many different symptoms?
2. Do you find that you are often aware of various things happening in your body?
3. If a disease is brought to your attention through the radio, television, newspaper or someone you know, do you worry about getting it yourself?
4. Is it easy for you to forget about yourself and think about all sorts of other things?
5. Do you think that you worry about your health more than most people?
6. Are you afraid of illness?
7. Is it hard for you to believe the doctor when he tells you there is nothing for you to worry about?
8. Do you get the feeling that people are not taking your illness seriously enough?
9. Have you always had one thing or another wrong with your health?
10. Have others told you that you spend too much time talking about your health?
11. Do you think something is wrong with your health that the doctors have not been able to find?

12. Do you find yourself worrying about your health?
13. Do you feel you need to see your physician even though you are not always able to?

Section 4
1. Have you been depressed or down or without interest in most things every day for the past two weeks?
2. Do you have a poor appetite or significant weight loss?
3. Have you had trouble falling asleep, waking frequently, staying asleep, waking too early or sleeping too much?
4. Have you lost interest or pleasure in your usual activities?
5. Have you been having trouble thinking or concentrating?
6. Have you been thinking about death or hurting yourself?
7. Have you had some kind of pain in your body nearly every day for the last six months?

Section 5
Below is a list of problems and complaints that people sometimes have. Check one of the spaces to the right that best describes how much that problem bothered or distressed you during the last week, including today.

	Not at all	A little bit	Moderately	Quite a bit	Extremely
Nervousness or shakiness inside					
Trembling					
Suddenly scared for no reason					
Feeling fearful					
Heart pounding or racing					
Feeling tense or keyed up					
Spells of terror or panic					
Feeling so restless you could not sit still					
The feeling that something bad is going to happen to you					
Thoughts and images of a frightening nature					

Section 6
Circle a number that best describes your situation now.

Work
Because of my problems my work is impaired.

0	1	2	3	4	5	6	7	8	9	10
Not at all			Mildly		Moderately		Markedly		Very severely (cannot work)	

Social life/leisure activities
(With other people at parties, socialising, visiting, dating, outings, clubs and entertaining)

Because of my problems my social life/leisure is impaired.

0	1	2	3	4	5	6	7	8	9	10
Not at all			Mildly		Moderately		Markedly		Very severely (I never do these)	

Family life/home responsibilities
(For example, relating to family members, paying bills, managing home, shopping and cleaning)

Because of my problems my family life/home responsibilities are impaired.

0	1	2	3	4	5	6	7	8	9	10
Not at all			Mildly		Moderately		Markedly		Very severely (I never do these)	

APPENDIX EIGHT

GLOSSARY OF PSYCHIATRIC TERMS

Abstract thinking: Ability to understand the meaning of events, experiences and communications. The person can also use and understand metaphoric speech appropriately, for example the proverb 'a rolling stone gathers no moss' is correctly interpreted to mean that people who move around a great deal seldom put down roots.

Active phase: The second stage of schizophrenia, during which the patient begins showing prominent psychotic features such as delusions, hallucinations, incoherence or marked loosening of associations, catatonic behaviour, flat or grossly inappropriate affect.

Affect: A person's observable emotional responses, seen in the person's non-verbal behaviours such as facial expression, posture, gestures and tone of voice. Affect is what the examiner sees; it is the outward manifestation of emotion. Affect may be referred to as inappropriate, flat or blunt, depending on the degree of apathy. A disturbance in affect is common in schizophrenia but may also be found in severe depression.

- *Blunt affect.* A mood disorder in which the person shows little emotional response, regardless of what they are saying or what is going on around them, for example Didi is talking about the recent death of her cousin Jamie in a car accident; there is some evidence of emotion in her non-verbal behaviour, such as evidence of tears in her eyes, but her voice is flat and her face is expressionless.
- *Flat affect.* A mood disorder in which the person shows no emotion; the face remains expressionless and the voice tone is monotonous, regardless of what the person is saying or what is going on around them. For example, Mimi talks about the loss of her child; she sits immobile, her face shows no expression, her voice is monotonous. There is no evidence of any emotion in her non-verbal behaviour, even though the experience she is talking about is tragic.
- *Inappropriate affect.* A mood disorder in which the person's emotional responses are totally unsuited to what they are saying or what is going on around them, for example Sally laughs when talking about her father's abuse of her as a child.

Aggression: Forceful goal-directed action that may be verbal or physical. It is the behavioural part of the emotion of rage, hostility or anger, for example Prudence is feeling angry; she shouts at the nurse and slams the door.

Ambivalence: Simultaneous conflicting feelings, attitudes or thoughts in a person towards another person, object or event, for example Israel desperately wants to get married, but at the same time he is terrified of committing himself to one person for the rest of his life.

Anxiety: A term used to describe feelings of uncertainty, uneasiness, apprehension or tension that a person experiences in response to an unknown object or situation.

Apathy: Lack of feeling, concern, interest or emotion. The person seems detached from the environment and totally indifferent to it.

Bipolar mood disorder: A type of mood disorder involving both manic and depressive episodes. This disorder usually appears first in the form of a manic episode. The subsequent episodes may appear in a variety of patterns:
- Manic episode alternating with a depressive episode, with a normal period of functioning between the two, that is, an initial manic episode, then a normal period, depressive episode, normal period, manic episode and so forth
- Manic episode followed immediately by a depressive episode followed by a period of normal functioning, that is, a manic episode, depressive episode, normal period, manic episode, depressive episode, normal period and so forth
- In rare cases the mood may shuttle back and forth between mania and depression with no intervals of normal functioning (cycling type) OR depressive and manic symptoms may occur at the same time (mixed type).

Catatonia: A disturbance in psychomotor behaviour that can either take the form of stupor, rigidity, excitement or waxy flexibility. Catatonia is most commonly related to schizophrenia but is not often seen any more. It is regarded as one of the positive and active signs of schizophrenia.
- *Catatonic excitement.* The person shows agitated, purposeless motor activity which is influenced by external stimuli.
- *Catatonic rigidity.* The person may hold a rigid posture for hours and resist efforts to be moved.
- *Catatonic stupor.* Motor activity is markedly slow and the person seems unaware of the environment.
- *Waxy flexibility.* The person can be 'moulded' into positions which are then maintained. When the examiner moves the limbs, they feel as if they are made of wax.

Cognition: Mental processes such as thought, memory, attention, perception and interpretation.

Concrete thinking: An inability to find the meaning of events, communications and experiences. Communications are taken literally, for example the proverb 'a rolling stone gathers no moss' is interpreted to mean that stones which roll do not gather moss because they are moving all the time.

Content of thought: Refers to the information conveyed in a sentence. Delusions, overvalued ideas and concrete thinking are the common symptoms of disturbed content of thought.

Conversion: see Somatoform disorders.

Delusion: An irrational belief which has no basis in reality but which cannot be changed by logic or argument. These are among the most common schizophrenic thought disorders. There are many different types of delusions.

Delusions of control (also called delusions of influence): The belief that other people, forces or perhaps extraterrestrial beings are controlling one's thoughts, feelings and actions, often by means of electronic devices which send signals directly to one's brain. The common delusions of control are thought broadcasting, thought insertion and thought withdrawal.

- *Thought broadcasting.* The belief that one's thoughts are being broadcast to the outside world, for example, by radio, television or any electronic device, so that others can hear them. For example, Nonhlana says the security police are broadcasting her political beliefs over the radio.
- *Thought insertion.* The belief that others are inserting thoughts, especially obscene ones, into one's head, usually by means of electronic devices or mental telepathy, for example Mary claims that the TV announcer is telling her that her psychologist wants to have sex with her.
- *Thought withdrawal.* The belief that other people are removing thoughts from one's head, for example Simon says his neighbours are drawing out his thoughts from his head with a vacuum cleaner.

Delusions of grandeur: The belief that one is an extremely famous, powerful and important person, for example God. Common in schizophrenia and manic disorders.

Delusions of hypochondriasis (hypochondriacal delusions): The unfounded belief that one is suffering from a hideous physical disease or a bizarre physical affliction, for example Patience claims her liver is being carried away in pieces.

Delusions of nihilism (nihilistic delusions): The belief that one, others or the whole world has/have ceased to exist, for example Mdu claims he is a spirit returned from the dead.

Delusions of persecution (often called paranoid delusions): The belief that one is being plotted against, spied upon, threatened, interfered with or otherwise mistreated, particularly by a number of parties joined in a conspiracy, for example Nonhlana believes that the security police are spying on her and watching her every move.

Delusions of reference: The belief that events or stimuli unrelated to the individual are actually referring to the patient, for example while watching a TV programme on wildlife, Jenny thinks her life is being depicted on TV.

Delusions of sin and guilt: The belief that one has committed a terrible sin or inflicted great harm on others, for example Harold claims he has killed his children and can never be forgiven.

Depersonal isolation: A subjective sense of being unreal, strange or unfamiliar to oneself, for example James says he feels as if he is not really present in his daily life, as though he is walking in his sleep.

Depression: A mood state characterised by a feeling of sadness, dejection, despair, discouragement or hopelessness. Depression is thought to be precipitated by a loss of some kind, real or imagined, such as self-esteem, a love object, independence, freedom, physical integrity, autonomy, youth, material possessions, for example Zacharia became depressed when his crop was lost during a severe drought.

Derealisation: A subjective sense that the environment has changed in some way or is strange and unreal, for example John walks into his office and feels as if it is a stranger's office and he is a visitor.

Distractibility: Rapid shift of attention from one stimulus to another, for example while talking to his mother, Madoom notices a magazine lying on the couch and abruptly turns his attention to it. As he picks it up, he notices someone passing by and runs to the window to have a look. A person who is distractible seldom focuses their attention on something for more than a few seconds or minutes at a time.

Echolalia: Pathological repetition of the words or phrases of one person by another; tends to be repetitive and persistent, and may be spoken with mocking or staccato intonation.

Echopraxia: Pathological imitations of the movements of one person by another.

Form of thought: The way in which words are put together so that ideas, feelings and thoughts are expressed in sentences that make little sense. The most common forms of thought disorders are:

- *Circumstantiality.* A pattern of speech in which the person starts talking about something and gives a great deal of unnecessary detail before eventually coming back to the topic.
- *Clanging.* A characteristic speech pattern of schizophrenia in which a series of words are used together because they rhyme or sound similar, without regard to logic. 'Sister Lee is a flea, she pees in a tree'.
- *Flight of ideas.* Rapid, continuous verbalisations or a play on words produces constant shifts from one idea to another; the ideas tend to be connected and in less severe forms can be followed by the listener. Common in a manic episode. Example. 'I went to the shop and what a flop did you know that she flipped her lid when I left her driving on the left side of the road is a real pain I nearly had an accident and the last time I had a pain was when I had my tonsils out.'
- *Incoherence.* Pattern of speech that is generally not understandable. Thoughts and words run into each other with no logical or grammatical connection.
- *Loosening of associations.* Form of thought in which ideas shift from one to another in an indirectly related way or in a completely unrelated way. When the problem is severe, speech may be completely incoherent. This is characteristic of schizophrenic speech patterns.
- *Neologisms.* A schizophrenic speech pattern in which new words are made up by combining parts of other words or in which common words are used in a unique fashion. It is sometimes possible to understand this form of communication, for example a nurse asks a patient why she is not eating supper. The patient replies. 'No, I had a belly bad luck and brutal and outrageous.' (I have a stomach-ache and I don't feel well).
- *Tangentiality.* A pattern of speech in which the person starts talking about something, wanders off the point and never returns to it.
- *Thought blocking.* An abrupt interruption in the train of thinking, before a thought or idea is finished; the person indicates no recall of what was being said or was going to be said.

- *Word salad.* A schizophrenic speech pattern in which words or phrases are combined in a disorganised fashion, seemingly devoid of logic and meaning. It is generally not possible to understand this form of communication, for example a patient says, 'rapid is falling and too much mayonnaise ice in the cinema'.

Hallucination: A sensory perception that occurs in the absence of any appropriate external stimuli. May occur in any of the five senses. Hallucinations may be mood-congruent or mood incongruent.

- *Auditory hallucinations.* False perceptions of sound, usually voices but also various noises such as music, etc. In depressive disorders auditory hallucinations involve themes such as guilt, deserved punishment, inadequacy and worthlessness. In manic disorders auditory hallucinations involve themes of inflated worth and power. When auditory hallucinations first start, the person often regards them as friendly because their content is friendly. As they become established, the content (what the voices are saying) becomes more threatening and the person becomes more frightened by them. The content of the voices that schizophrenics hear is usually derogatory and hostile towards the hearer. More than one voice may be heard at a time, and the voices might talk directly to the person or to each other about the person, for example Moses hears three voices talking to one another about what an evil person Moses is.
- *Gustatory hallucinations.* False perceptions of taste, such as unpleasant tastes. Often associated with temporal lobe epilepsy.
- *Olfactory hallucinations.* False perceptions of smell.
- *Somatic hallucinations.* False sensations of things occurring in or on the body, for example, snakes crawling inside the stomach.
- *Tactile hallucinations.* False perceptions of touch or surface sensations, as from an amputated limb (phantom limb) or a crawling sensation on or under the skin.
- *Visual hallucinations.* False perceptions of sight involving formed images, for example people, and unformed images, for example flashes of light.

Hyperactivity: Increased activity and restlessness; activity is usually goal directed, unlike psychomotor agitation. Hyperactivity is common in a manic episode and usually accompanies an expansive mood.

Hypochondriasis: see Somatoform disorders.

Ideas of reference: A belief that one is being talked about by others or that events in the environment somehow refer to oneself, even though there is no objective evidence for this. An idea of reference is similar to a delusion of reference but is less firmly held than a delusion.

Illusion: A false interpretation or perception of a real environmental stimulus that may involve any of the five senses, for example a person mistakes a belt for a snake. Visual and auditory illusions are the most common.

Insight: The ability to analyse a situation and understand the true meaning of an experience, for example Vani hears voices; she knows that hearing voices is not normal and realises she needs help. Insight can be impaired, for example Alpheus forgets to phone his girlfriend for a week; when he sees her again, she is angry with him and he cannot understand why. His insight is impaired; he is unable to recognise that his behaviour has offended his girlfriend.

Judgement: The ability to assess a situation correctly and act appropriately within that situation. Insight and judgement often go hand in hand, that is, if insight is impaired, judgement might also be impaired. Judgement may be normal or impaired.

- *Impaired judgement.* A decreased ability to assess a situation correctly and act appropriately in that situation, for example a patient walks naked in the street; a person swears and shouts at a stranger for dropping litter on the pavement.

Magical thinking: The belief that one's thoughts, words or actions can cause or prevent events, for example Princess believes that if she says the word 'help', God will come down out of the sky to help her.

Major depression: A type of mood disorder characterised by major depressive episodes occurring without intervening manic episodes. Onset is usually gradual, occurring over a period of several weeks to several months; the mood disorder lasts longer than a manic episode and ends slowly and gradually. The prominent features are: depressed mood; loss of pleasure or interest in usual activities; disturbance of appetite; sleep disturbance; psychomotor retardation or agitation; loss of energy; feelings of worthlessness and guilt; difficulties in thinking; recurrent thoughts of death or suicide. A severely depressed person may show psychotic features, for example delusions of guilt, nihilistic delusions, auditory hallucinations of worthlessness and guilt.

Mania: An emotional state characterised by intense and unrealistic feelings of elation. A manic episode begins suddenly over the course of a few days. It may last from several days to several months and usually ends as abruptly as it began. The prominent features are: elated, expansive or irritable mood; hyperactivity; talkativeness; flight of ideas; inflated self-esteem; sleeplessness; distractibility; reckless behaviour. A person in a manic phase may show thought disorders similar to those of schizophrenia, for example illogical thinking, incoherence, loosening of associations and grandiose delusions.

Mannerisms: Stereotyped involuntary movements, for example Harold continually wrings his hands.

Memory: The ability to recall stored information.

- *Immediate retention and recall.* The ability to recall information immediately after it was presented, for example an examiner gives a patient five words and then one minute later asks them to recall the five words.
- *Recent.* The ability to recall information about events of the past few days.
- *Recent past.* The ability to recall information about events of the past few months.
- *Remote memory.* The ability to recall information about childhood and important events known to have occurred when the person was younger.

Mental disorder: A clinically significant behavioural or psychological syndrome or pattern that occurs within a person and is associated with distress or disability. It is not an expectable response to a particular event or experience. The term mental disorder is used instead of mental illness. Mental illness is too vague a term and implies that people who do not meet the criteria for mental health are therefore mentally ill.

Mental health: A state of being in which a person is simultaneously successful at working, loving and resolving conflicts by coping and adjusting to the recurrent stresses of everyday living. This does not mean that a mentally healthy person has no problems. They might at certain times experience severe distress but is generally able to cope with the distress.

Mood: A prolonged, sustained emotion subjectively reported by the patient. A mood refers to an emotion that the person experiences most of the time and one that colours the person's whole life. A mood may be expansive, irritable, elevated, euphoric, labile, depressed, sad, anxious or happy.

- *Elevated.* Air of confidence and enjoyment; a mood more cheerful than normal but not necessarily pathological.
- *Euphoric.* An exaggerated sense of physical and emotional well-being inconsistent with reality. People in a euphoric mood have limitless enthusiasm for whatever they are doing or plan to do and feel they can accomplish anything.
- *Expansive.* Expression of one's feelings without restraint, frequently with an overestimation of one's significance or importance. Generally considered pathological.
- *Irritable.* The person is easily annoyed and provoked to anger, especially when someone tries to interfere with their behaviour, for example Simon becomes intensely annoyed when the nurse reminds him to take his medication or asks him to stop banging on the door.
- *Labile.* Unstable, rapidly shifting mood, usually shifting between sadness, anxiety, euphoria, in a very short space of time.

Mood-congruent hallucinations and delusions: Hallucinations and delusions the content of which is appropriate to the mood, for example a depressed person hears voices telling them they are bad, and a manic person hears voices telling them they have god-like powers (mood-congruent auditory hallucinations); a depressed person believes they have committed a terrible sin for which not even God can forgive them, and a manic person believes that they are the incarnation of God (mood-congruent delusions).

Mood-incongruent hallucinations and delusions: Delusions and hallucinations the content of which is not consistent with the mood, for example a depressed person hears voices telling them they are a fantastic person; a manic person hears voices telling them they are worthless.

Mood disorder: A disturbance of mood in which feelings of sadness or elation become intense and unrealistic. Previously called affective disorders. The mood disorders are major depression, mania, bipolar mood disorder.

Negative symptoms: In schizophrenia the absence of something, for example poverty of speech, flat affect, withdrawal, inattention.

Non-verbal communication: Communication between two or more people without the use of words. Facial expressions, body posture, gestures and tone of voice are examples.
Orientation: A level of consciousness in which a person is aware of the position of self in relation to time, surroundings or other people. Disorientation is common in people with an organic brain disorder. Sometimes depressed people can seem disoriented but this is more because they lack the energy to think about the question that was asked.
- *Orientation to person.* The ability to know who one is and who other people are.
- *Orientation to place.* The ability to know where one is, that is, name of town, city, country, hospital.
- *Orientation to time.* The ability to know what year it is, what day it is, what date it is, the season of the year. To be disoriented to time, the person must be more than one day off the correct day of the week and more than several days off the correct date.

Overvalued ideas: Unreasonable, sustained false beliefs maintained less firmly than a delusion. The person values his/her ideas too much and is reluctant to change them, even if presented with alternative information. Overvalued ideas do not seem as bizarre as delusions. Overvalued ideas include suspicious ideas, suicidal ideas, ideas of reference and ideas of inference. Overvalued ideas are a disturbance in content of thought.
- *Suicidal ideas.* Recurring thoughts of wanting to kill oneself and/or preoccupation with methods of suicide.
- *Suspicious ideas (sometimes called suspicious ideation).* Suspicious ideas are a less severe form of paranoia where the person seems mistrustful of the intentions of others, is often hostile and guarded.

Panic: Acute, episodic, intense attack of anxiety associated with feelings of dread and unbearable autonomic arousal, for example increased respiration and pulse rate. Patients sometimes feel as if they are having a heart attack.
Perceptual processes: The experience of sensing, interpreting and comprehending the world. It is the mental process by which sensory stimuli are brought into awareness. Hallucinations affecting the five senses, and illusions, are the most common perceptual disturbances.
Positive symptoms: In schizophrenia the presence of something, including hallucinations, delusions, bizarre behaviour and incoherent thought patterns.
Post-traumatic stress disorder (PTSD): The term PTSD is used to signify a disorder or illness (as opposed to a normal post-traumatic stress response). PTSD is diagnosed when symptoms are severe enough to interfere with the person's normal living, symptoms are present for at least one month after the trauma and include avoidance, re-experiencing and increased arousal (anxiety).
Poverty of content of thought: The result of loosened associations is that the language of the psychotic person conveys very little information. The person might use many words, all grammatically correct, but communicate poorly.
Poverty of speech: There is a restriction in the amount of speech used. Replies may be monosyllabic.

Premorbid functioning: The level of social, occupational, self-care and interpersonal functioning before the onset of the disorder.

Pressured speech: Rapid speech that is increased in amount and difficult to interrupt. This is commonly associated with a manic disorder.

Prodromal phase: The initial stage of schizophrenia, during which the person generally becomes withdrawn and socially isolated. Blunted or flat affect is common, speech may be rambling and hygiene poor. Behaviour is often strange, for example talking to oneself in public or collecting garbage. Role functioning, for example as wage earner or homemaker, is impaired. The person may have unusual perceptual experiences, for example recurrent illusions, sensing the presence of a force or person not actually present and odd ideas, for example overvalued ideas, ideas of reference or ideas of inference.

Psychiatric nursing: A speciality within the nursing profession in which the nurse directs efforts towards the promotion of mental health, the prevention of mental disturbances, early identification of and intervention in emotional problems, and follow-up care to minimise long-term effects of mental disturbance.

Psycho-education: An approach used with patients and family caregivers which emphasizes the goals of (1) decreased client vulnerability to environmental stimulation through educated psychopharmacology; (2) increasing family stability by increasing both knowledge and coping strategies.

Psychomotor agitation: Excessive overactivity, usually non-productive and in response to inner tension.

Psychomotor retardation: Decreased activity, visible slowing of thought, speech and movements.

Psychosis: A state in which a person's mental capacity to recognise reality, to remember, think, communicate with others, respond emotionally and behave appropriately is impaired, thus interfering with the person's capacity to deal with life's demands. Examples include schizophrenia, bipolar depression and paranoia.

Residual phase: The third phase of schizophrenia, during which behaviour is similar to that seen in the prodromal phase.

Schizophrenic disorders: Serious psychiatric disorders characterised by impaired communication and a loss of contact with reality (see 'Psychosis'), a deterioration from a previous level of functioning in work, social relations and self-care, and a duration of at least six months.

Slow speech: Slow, hesitant speech. The person may take a long time to answer questions. May be accompanied by thought blocking.

Social withdrawal: A lack of attention to or interest in the goings-on of the external world, accompanied by emotional detachment. This is an early sign of schizophrenia. Preoccupied with their own thoughts, schizophrenics gradually withdraw from involvement with other people and the environment. Social withdrawal is also found in a major depressive episode.

Somatoform disorders: The primary feature of these disorders is that psychological conflicts take a somatic or physical form. Some patients complain of physical discomfort, for example stomach pains and headaches. Others show an actual loss of or disturbance in some normal physiological function, for example, suddenly being unable to see or to move a limb. In either case there is no organic evidence to explain the symptom while there is evidence from the person's history that the symptom is linked to psychological factors. The three main forms of somatoform disorder are hypochondriasis, somatisation disorder and conversion disorder.

- *Conversion disorder.* In conversion disorder there is an actual disability – the loss or impairment of some motor or sensory function. Conversion symptoms vary considerably but among the most common are blindness, deafness, paralysis and loss of sensation. There is no organic evidence for these symptoms, but they are not faked. They are involuntary responses not under the person's conscious control. The DSM-5 regards this disorder as an expression of psychological conflict or need. These symptoms serve two important psychological purposes. First, they block the person's awareness of internal conflict (primary gain) and, secondly, they excuse the person from responsibilities and attract sympathy and attention (secondary gain). Many people with this disorder are undisturbed by their symptoms and are eager to discuss them but not to part with them. With conversion disorder, differential diagnosis is important and difficult. Malingering (conscious faking of symptoms in order to avoid some responsibility) must be excluded and this is often hard to do. Sometimes symptoms are very similar to those of true organic disorders. There are three signs that differentiate organic disorders from conversion disorders:
  1. Rapid appearance of symptoms, especially after some psychological trauma. Organic symptoms tend to emerge more slowly.
  2. Indifference to their symptoms – patients with organic symptoms are more likely to be upset by their symptoms.
  3. Selective symptoms – if paralysed legs move during sleep, the cause is generally not organic.
- *Hypochondriasis.* The primary feature of this disorder is a terrible, enduring fear of a specific disease, for example cancer. This fear is maintained by constant misinterpretation of physical signs and sensations as abnormal. The person has no real disability but is convinced that a disability is about to appear and so spends each day waiting for the signs to emerge. When a sign emerges, for example a new body pain, the person becomes convinced that a disease process is at work throughout their body. The person is usually an avid reader of medical journals and related literature, so by the time they arrive at the doctor, they have already diagnosed their illness. The person generally disbelieves the results of medical tests and examinations and will often try to cure themselves through strenuous medical regimes or by dosing themselves with pills, for example vitamins. The person does not fake the symptoms but genuinely believes they are ill and suffers terribly as a result. This disorder affects men and women equally.
- *Somatisation disorder.* This disorder is characterised by many and recurrent physical complaints that have persisted for several years and have caused the person to seek medical help. Like hypochondriasis there is no organic base for the symptoms. This disorder differs from hypochondriasis in that the person is preoccupied with

the symptoms rather than with a fear of disease. A second difference is the way the two groups approach their symptoms. Whereas the hypochondriac may try to be scientific about their symptoms, for example measuring their blood pressure five times a day, the person with a somatisation disorder usually describes their symptoms in a vague, dramatic and exaggerated way. A third difference is that the hypochondriac usually fears a single disease and his/her complaints tend to be fairly specific. In somatisation disorder, on the other hand, the complaints are many and varied. This disorder is more common in women than in men but is still rare, affecting only two or three women per thousand.

Stereotypy: Repetitive, purposeless actions that may be carried out for hours at a time, for example head-rubbing or pacing.

Trauma: An emotionally painful and damaging event. While many experiences are painful, not all can be called traumatic. Traumatic experiences are sudden and shocking, involve high danger and intense feelings of fear, helplessness or horror. The distinction between traumatic and painful events is made in reference to the specialised ways of assisting the person's recovery. Classifications of traumatic experiences:

- *Single traumatic experience.* Usually a once-off trauma involving a stranger, for example a violent mugging.
- *Multiple trauma.* When the same person has been exposed to several traumatic experiences. For example, someone may have survived several car accidents, or someone is abducted during a vehicle robbery, subjected to a terrifying high-speed car chase and then injured in a car accident.
- *Continuous trauma.* The person is living in a situation of ongoing danger, for example police officers working in dangerous situations.
- *Complex trauma.* The traumatic experiences happen within a particular relationship, for example domestic violence, which leads to people adapting their behaviour according to the requirements of the perpetrator in order to avoid further danger or harm.

REFERENCES

American Psychiatric Association (APA). 1994. *Diagnostic and Statistical Manual of Mental Disorders.* 4th edition. Washington, DC: American Psychiatric Association.

Bootzin, R and Acocela, J R. 1988. *Abnormal Psychology: Current Perspectives.* 5th edition. New York: Random House.

Kaplan, H and Sadock, B. 1988. *Synopsis of Psychology.* 5th edition. Baltimore: Williams & Williams.

Shriver, L R. 1990. *Basic Concepts of Psychiatric-mental Health Nursing.* 2nd edition. Philadelphia: J B Lippincott.

Index

Please note page numbers in *italics* refer to tables and figures.

1CCSM (Level 1 Cross Cutting Symptom Measure) 186
9-delta-tetrahydrocannabinol (THC) 440

A
abortion *see* termination of pregnancy
absconding of MHCUs 123, 126, 550–552
absorbing activities 308
abuse
    of children 110, 638–656, *645*, *647*
    disclosure of 110, 134
    of elderly 467, 637–638
    Mental Health Care Act 107–109
    see also trauma
accessibility of mental health facilities 68, 347, 684
accommodation *see* housing
Accutane (isotretinoin) 329
acetylcholinesterase inhibitors 488
acquiescent behaviour vs assertive behaviour *168–169*
ACT *see* assertive community treatment
act-deontologists 130
acting out 261, 643, 652
act-utilitarianism 129
acute dystonic reaction 405
acute stress disorder 619–620
Addison's disease 387
ADHD *see* attention-deficit/hyperactivity disorder
ad hoc planning 51
adjustment disorder 621, *694*
adolescents *see* children and adolescents
Adult Primary Care Guidelines 361
advertisements for alcohol 423
advocacy by consumers 95–96
affect, definition of 185
aggression
    acquiescent behaviour vs *168–169*

    assertive behaviour vs *168–169*
    definition of 261
    in forensic mental health care users 761–762
    management of 91–92, 260–274, *263*, *265*, *268–271*, 550–552, 761–762
    in persons with intellectual disabilities 550–552
    see also anger; violence
agitation 261, 471
agnosia 471
agoraphobia 297
AIDS *see* HIV/AIDS
akathisia 405
Al-Anon family groups 438–439
albumin in urine 434
alcohol-related disorders 418–439
    in adolescents 724
    anxiety disorders and 283
    approach to patients 427
    assessment 427–432, *427–431*, *432*
    classification of *411*
    comorbidity 685
    dependence 420
    diagnostic criteria *417*
    domestic violence and 634
    education of patients 434–436, *435*
    employee assistance programmes (EAPs) 439
    families of persons with 436–439
    forensic mental health care users 749
    HIV/AIDS and 700–701
    intoxication 421, 432–433
    mood disorders and 330
    nursing interventions 425–427, 432–434
    prevalence of 410, 418–419
    prevention of 421–425
    stages of alcoholism 420–421
    tuberculosis and 700–701
    withdrawal 421, 433–434

alpha-blocker augmentation *320*
alternative healing practices 8
Alzheimer's disease 460–461, 469, 470, 471
aminoglycosides *701*
amnesia 354–355, 461
amok 158
amphetamines *412–413*, *444*, 445, 446
anabolic-androgenic steroids *413*
ancestors 152–153
anger 260–274, *263*, *265*, *268–271*
    see also aggression; violence
ANI *see* asymptomatic neurocognitive
    impairment
animal-assisted therapy 480
anticipatory guidance *see* life skills approach
anticonvulsants *319*, 387, 552, 608
antidepressants
    anxiety disorders *318–320*
    attention-deficit/hyperactivity disorder
        (ADHD) 709
    comorbid medical conditions 683
    history of 7
    HIV/AIDS *694*, 697
    intellectual disabilities 552
    major depressive disorder 721
    personality disorders 608
antimalarial medications 387
antipsychotic medication
    anxiety disorders *318–320*
    comorbidity 681–685
    intellectual disabilities 551
    personality disorders 608
    schizophrenia 389–390, 400–407, *402–404*
    side effects *402–404*
antiretroviral treatment (ART)
    commonly used types *702*
    comorbidity 679
    mental disorders and *694*, 695, 697, 699, *702*
    mood disorders 329
    schizophrenia 387
antisocial personality disorders 588–593, *590*,
    707, 755, 764
antispasmodics 447

anxiety disorders 283–325
    agoraphobia 297
    anxiety as phenomenon 287–289
    anxiety response 284–287, *284*, *285–286*
    assessment of 303–307, *305*, 796–802
    in children and adolescents 706, 716–719
    cognitive behavioural perspective 289–292,
        290, *291*
    definition of anxiety 288–289
    diagnostic criteria 293, *293*
    generalised anxiety disorder 298, *318*
    HIV/AIDS and *694*, 696
    interacting with anxious MHCUs 301–303
    levels of anxiety 289
    medication for 317–323, *318–321*, *322*
    neurocognitive disorders and 469
    normal vs pathological anxiety 292–301
    nursing interventions 307–317, *311*, *314*
    obsessive-compulsive disorders 293, *293*,
        298–301, *299–300*, *320–321*
    panic disorders 283, 295–297, *318–319*
    phobias 293–294
    prevalence of 283
    social anxiety disorder 295, *319*
    substance-related disorders and 418
    time-event charts 795
    tuberculosis and 696
anxiolytics *412*, *417*
apartheid 11–12, 18, 613
apathy 471
approach–avoidance conflict 617
apraxia 471
Aristotle 131
ART *see* antiretroviral treatment
'ASKED' 154
assertive behaviour 167–169, *168–169*
assertive community treatment (ACT) 256
assessment 179–213
    aims of 180
    clinical formulations 206–207, *207*
    context for 181–184, 201, *201–202*
    diagnosis 207–208, *208*
    examples of questions used 787–789
    fear questionnaire 799–802

of groups 208–211, *209–211*
Hamilton Anxiety Rating Scale (HAM-A) 796–797
healthy lifestyle functioning 200–201
holistic view of 180–181
Inpatient Evaluation Scale 773–781
interviews 186–195, *188–195*
of mental status 196, *196–198*
monitoring troublesome symptoms 205–206, *206*
of physical condition 199–200, *199*
process of 184–185
for psychiatric diagnosis 185–186
specific 202–206, *203*, *205*, *206*
Stanford Panic Appraisal Inventory 797–798
time–event–symptom charts 204–205, *205*
time-to-event charts 204
University of Natal Functional Assessment Scale (UNFAS) 782–786
assisted mental health care users 114–116
asthma 682, 685
'asylums', use of term 4
asymptomatic neurocognitive impairment (ANI) 699
ataxia 471
atazanavir *702*
atenolol 329
attention behaviour 551
attention-deficit/hyperactivity disorder (ADHD) 706, 707–709, 713
attitudes, of mental health care nurses 84, 166–167, *166*, 244
attributional theory 762
atypical antipsychotics *318*, *319*, *320*
autism spectrum disorders 707
autistic thinking 395
autonomy 132–133, 138
avoidance 616, 643
avoidant personality disorder 601–603, *602*

B

'Band Aid' response 230
Batho Pele principles 143
BDI-II *see* Beck Depression Inventory

Beck, A T 291
Beck Depression Inventory (BDI-II) 331
Beck's Suicide Intent Scale 363, 378–380
Beers, Clifford 7
behaviourally disturbed children 737–739
behaviour management 90–92, 550–552, 738
behaviour modification 397, 482, *482*
beneficence 133, 138
benzedrine *413*
benzodiazepines
    anxiety disorders 296, *318–320*, 321, *322*
    mood disorders 329
    personality disorders 608
    schizophrenia 401
Berne, Eric 562
beta-blockers *318–319*, 321, *322*
betrayal 641
Bill of Rights 633
binge drinking 419
biological needs 347–350, *349*, 369
biological variation and culture 153
biomedical model 181
biopsychosocial model 181
bipolar mood disorders 327–328, 366–371
birth injuries 500
Block, Peter 335
body mass index (BMI) 685, 686
borderline personality disorder 598–601, 755
boundaries, professional 142–143, 175
BPS *see* Brief Psychiatric Rating Scale
'brain fog' 159
Brief Psychiatric Rating Scale (BPS) 250, 387
bright light therapy 480
broker case management model 256
Brøset Violence Checklist (BVC) 264, 752
burden of caregiving 88
BVC *see* Brøset Violence Checklist

C

caffeine *411*, *417*
CAGE questionnaire *432*
cannabis (dagga) 383, 410, *411*, *417*, 440–441, *442–443*
Cape Support for Mental Health 396

carbamazepine 600
cardiovascular disease (CVD) 680, 681–682, 683, 685, 686, 688, 689–690
caregivers 86–93, 395–397, 483–487
case finding 72
case management 50, 255–259
catastrophising 292, 314–315, 329, 335
catatonia 385
CATIE study *see* Clinical Antipsychotic Trials of Intervention Effectiveness (CATIE) study
CBS *see* culture-bound syndromes
CBT *see* cognitive behavioural therapy
CC *see* community clinics
central nervous system stimulants 709
Centre for Epidemiological Studies Depression Scale (CES-D) 331, 332, 376–377
cerebrovascular disease 461
CES-D *see* Centre for Epidemiological Studies Depression Scale
CFI *see* cultural formulation interviews
chaining 525–526, 543
change talk 448
character ethics *see* virtue ethics
CHC *see* community health centres
Child Care Act 638
Childline 224, 656
children and adolescents 705–742
    abuse of 110, 638–656, *645*, *647*
    anxiety disorders 706, 716–719
    assessment of 724–736, *728–730*
    attention-deficit/hyperactivity disorder (ADHD) 706, 707–709, 713
    autism spectrum disorders 707
    behaviourally disturbed 737–739
    Children's Act 105, 111, 114, 125, 126, 134, 144
    Children's Amendment Act 110
    conduct disorder 707, 711–712
    consent to treatment 105
    disclosure of information 110, 650–651
    elimination disorders 712–716
    learning disorders 706
    major depressive disorder 719–722
    mental disorders in 706–724
    neglect 110, 639–640, 648
    oppositional defiant disorder 709–711
    post-traumatic stress disorder (PTSD) 723–724
    prevalence of mental disorders in 705–706
    rights of 144–145
    schizophrenia and 396–397
    services for 705–706, 739–740
    social disadvantage 739
    substance abuse 724
    suicide 721–722
    trauma and 614, 620, 638–656, *645*, *647*, 668–676
Children's Act 105, 111, 114, 125, 126, 134, 144
Children's Amendment Act 110
chlorpromazine 6, 402, *402*
Choice on Termination of Pregnancy Act 101, 105, 106–107
Choice on Termination of Pregnancy Amendment Act 633
cholesterol-lowering drugs 329
cholinesterase inhibitors 488
Christianity 130–131
Churchill, Winston 344
cigarette smoking *see* smoking
circumstantiality 394
CISM *see* critical incident stress management
clarifying 169
classification systems 176–177
clichés 230
Clinical Antipsychotic Trials of Intervention Effectiveness (CATIE) study 679, 683
clinical case management model 256
clinical mental health nursing formulations 206–207, *207*
clinical recovery 46
clock time 151
clonazepam *319*, *320*, 401, *412*
Clopixol 402, *403*
clozapine 354, 400, 402, *402*, 404
cluster A personality disorders 573–584, *575–576*, *581*
cluster B personality disorders 584–601, *585*, *590*, *594–598*

cluster C personality disorders 601–608, *602*, *604*, *606*
cocaine *413*, 440, 445, 446
codeine *412*, 447
codependence 414
cognitive behavioural perspective 289–292, *290*, *291*
cognitive behavioural therapy (CBT) 251, 307–311, *311*, 698, 718–719, 721
cognitive disorders *see* neurocognitive disorders
cognitive distortions, mood disorders 335–338
cognitive distraction techniques 307–309
cognitive impairment
    HIV/AIDS *694*, 699–700
    schizophrenia 386, 400
cohesion of groups 238
collaborative care 334–335
colonialism 17–18
Columbia Suicide Severity Rating Scale 362
communicable diseases *see* infectious diseases
communication
    anxiety disorders 301–303
    with children and adolescents 737
    culture and 150–151
    neurocognitive disorders (NCD) 474, *474*
    open 243
    skills 167–172, *168–169*
communities
    assertive community treatment (ACT) 256
    community clinics (CC) 65, *65–66*
    community health centres (CHC) 49, 65, *65–66*, 71
    district health system 63
    history of community services 9–10, *10*, 16–17
    Mental Health Care Act 113
    milieu therapy 244–245
    mood disorders 346, 369–370
    primary mental health care and 71–72
    primary prevention and 42, 215
    rehabilitation services in 49
    schizophrenia and 397–400, *398*
    trauma and 659–661
community clinics (CC) 65, *65–66*

community health centres (CHC) 49, 65, *65–66*, 71
comorbid medical conditions 678–692
    case studies 687–691
    definitions 678–679
    evidence-based practice 687–688
    medication compliance 688–691
    nursing interventions 686–691
    prevalence of 679–683
    screening 686–687
    substance-related disorders 418
    vulnerability factors 683–685
compassion 131, 631–633
'COMPETENCE' 157
complementary healing practices 8
complex post-traumatic stress disorder (PTSD) 622–623
comprehensive mental health care 37–60
    definition of 40–41
    disability-adjusted life year (DALY) 37–38
    epidemiology of mental illness 38–40, *38–39*
    global burden of disease (GBD) 37–38
    planning of programmes 50–57, *53–54*, *55*
    in primary health care (PHC) 68–69
    primary prevention (before illness) 40–43, *43–44*
    secondary prevention (during illness) 40–41, 44–46
    tertiary prevention (after illness) 40–41, 46–50, *47*, *48–49*
Concerta 709
conduct disorder 707, 711–712
confidentiality 134, 239, 360, 726
    see also disclosure of information
conflicting role of mental health nurses in forensic units 764–765
conflict resolution interviews 233–234
confrontation 169
    see also constructive confrontation interviews
congruence 166
consent to care and admission 104–107
conspicuous psychiatric morbidity (CPM) 44

constipation 714, 715
Constitution of South Africa 100, 138, 440
constructive confrontation interviews 233
consultation in multidisciplinary teams 72–73
consumers in mental health 80–99
    advocacy by 80–81, 95–96
    'carer' perspective 86–93
    definition of MHCUs 102
    family perspective 86–93
    involvement in policy, planning and evaluation 80–81, 96–97
    perceptions on recovery 84–86
    stigma 80, 81–84
    support groups 93–95
    types of MHCUs 114–121
contemporary issues in mental health nursing 14–18
contingency management 525
continuous traumatic stress 621–622
continuum of care model 256
contractual capacity 743
convulsions 434
coping 183, 225, 287, 486, *486*, 490–492, *491*, 494–495
corticosteroids 387
cortisol 329
counselling
    alcohol-related disorders 437–439
    crisis 222–226, *223–227*
    forensic mental health care users 761
    genetic 500
    group therapy 234–241, *235*, *241*, 761
    individual 229–234, *232*, 761
    medication 689–691
    for spouses 437–439
    trauma 623–627, 651–652
countertransference 561
CPM *see* conspicuous psychiatric morbidity
craving, definition of 414
crime 614, 744
criminal capacity *see* criminal responsibility/capacity
Criminal Law (Sexual Offences and Related Matters) Amendment Act 110

Criminal Procedure Act 101, 109, 119, 363, 744, 745, 748–749
criminal responsibility/capacity 746, *746*, 749–753, *751*
crises
    counselling 222–226, *223–227*
    definition of 222, 615
    intervention 221–229, *223–227*
    trauma vs 615
    types of 222–223, *223*
critical incident stress management (CISM) 221, 227–229
cultural diversity 149–161
    assessment and 24, 186
    cultural competence 153–155
    cultural formulation interviews (CFI) 186
    culture-bound syndromes (CBS) 158–159
    definitions 149–150
    diversity and 155–159
    ethics and 145
    Leininger Sunrise Model 156–157
    presentations of illness 158–159
    schizophrenia and 387
    Transcultural Assessment Model 150–153
    treatment and 159
    in workplace 157
cultural formulation interviews (CFI) 186
culture-bound syndromes (CBS) 158–159
curatorship 487
Cushing syndrome 387
custodial period 4, 6–7
CVD *see* cardiovascular disease
cycloserine *701*

D

dagga (cannabis) 383, 410, *411*, *417*, 440–441, 442–443
DALY *see* disability-adjusted life year
DASAIV *see* Dynamic Appraisal of Situational Aggression – inpatient version
debriefing 274, 627–630
    see also critical incident stress management
Declaration of Human Rights and Mental Health 143

decolonisation 17–18
de-escalation 264–266, *265*, 272, 762
defence mechanisms 558, *559–560*
degenerative disorders 387
dehydration 433–434
deinstitutionalisation 7, 9, 16, 25–26
deliberate self-harm, definition of 356
delirium
    causes of 459, *459*, *460*
    DSM-5 classification of 452, *461–462*
    major NCDs and 463, *463–464*
    nursing interventions 473, *473*
    prevalence of 453–454
    risk factors for 459, 467
    'sundown syndrome' 471
    urinary tract infection and 483
delirium tremens (DTs) 421, 433–434
delusional disorder 385, 418
delusions 90, 391–395, 416, 470, 787–788
dementia 452–453, *694*, 695, 699–700
democratisation of treatment process 242–243
denial 414, 585, 599
deontology 130
Department of Correctional Services 762
Department of Education 762
Department of Health 8, 9, 15, 61, 95, 100, 143, 272–273
Department of Labour 547–548, 549
dependent personality disorder 603–605, *604*
depersonalisation 619
depression
    in children and adolescents 706, 716–717
    comorbidity 681–682
    definitions 327
    depressive disorders 327–334
    diagnosis of 329–332, *331*
    HIV/AIDS and 693–698, *694*
    major depressive disorder (MDD) 283, 327, 469, *694*, 719–722
    neurocognitive disorders and 469–470, *470*
    nursing interventions 334–355, *341*, *342*, *344*, *349*
    tuberculosis and 695–698
derealisation 619

detoxification 426–427, 441, 446, 447, 448
developmental crises 223
Dexedrine *412*, 709
dhat 159
DHS *see* district health system
diabetes 350, 461, 679, 681, 683–685, 687–688
diagnoses, formulation of 207–208, *208*
Diagnostic and Statistical Manual of Mental Disorders (DSM-5) 185–186
    antisocial personality disorders 588
    anxiety disorders 293–301, *293*, 307
    avoidant personality disorder 601
    borderline personality disorder 598
    children and adolescents 706–710, 715, 717–719, 723
    cultural presentations of illness 158
    dependent personality disorder 603–604
    histrionic personality disorder 584
    intellectual disabilities 498–499, 502–503
    mood disorders 326, 367
    narcissistic personality disorder 593
    neurocognitive disorders (NCD) 452–453, 454, *459*, *461–463*, 470
    obsessive-compulsive personality disorder 605–606
    paranoid personality disorder 580
    personality disorders 557–558, *559–560*, 573–574, 579–580, 584, 588, 593, 598, 601, 603–606
    schizoid personality disorder 573–574
    schizophrenia *384–385*, 387
    schizotypal personality disorder 579–580
    substance-related disorders 411, 414, 415–416, 421
    trauma 617–621
diazepam *412*, 446, 447
dichotomous thinking 292
diet 323, 350, 434, 436
disability-adjusted life year (DALY) 37–38, 682
discernment 131
discharge of MHCUs 111, 248–249, 763–764
discipline 512–513
disclosure of information 110–111, 650–651
    see also confidentiality

discrimination 107
displacement 590, 606
distancing (defence mechanism) 574
distraction techniques 307–309
distributive justice 134–135
district health system (DHS) 61, 62–66, 65–66, 69, 71
diversity *see* cultural diversity
Dix, Dorothea Lynde 4
domestic violence 622, 633–637, 635–637, 705
Domestic Violence Act 633
'doors for intervention' 571–572, 571–572
dopamine 400
Down syndrome 500, 502
Down Syndrome South Africa (DSSA) 511, 550
drawings of children 736
dressing and undressing 542–543
driving capabilities 487
drug abuse *see* substance-related disorders
Drugs and Drug Trafficking Act 413
Drynamil 413
DSM-5 *see* Diagnostic and Statistical Manual of Mental Disorders
DSSA *see* Down Syndrome South Africa
DTs *see* delirium tremens
Dynamic Appraisal of Situational Aggression – inpatient version (DASAIV) 264
dyslipidaemia 679
dysphasia 471
dysthymia (persistent depressive disorder) 326, 327

E

EAPs *see* employee assistance programmes
early detection of intellectual disability 501
eating patterns *see* diet
ecocharts 210, 210
ECT *see* electroconvulsive therapy
education
    evaluation of 793–794
    for forensic mental health care users 762
    mental health education for public 49–50, 214–221, 793–794
    of persons with intellectual disabilities 502, 514–515
    psycho-education 49–50, 217–221
    on schizophrenia 396
    on substance-related disorders 423, 434–436, 435
    theatre programmes 217
    training in mental health nursing 12–14, 22, 62, 70–71, 706, 757, 766
Education for All Handicapped Children Act (USA) 502
efavirenz 329, 387, 695, 697, 699, 702
egoism 130
elderly, abuse of 467, 637–638
electroconvulsive therapy (ECT) 6, 108, 109, 140–141, 351–355
elimination disorders 712–716
emergency mental health care users 118
emotional abuse 639, 648
emotionality 585
emotionally disturbed children 737–739
empathy 166–167, 166
employee assistance programmes (EAPs) 439
employment *see* work-related activities
emtricitabine 702
enabling, definition of 414
encopresis 715–716
enuresis 713–714
environmental protectors 183
ephedrine 387, 413, 445
epilepsy 387, 489–495, 489, 491, 494
Epilepsy South Africa 495
EPS *see* extrapyramidal side effects
escape behaviour 551
Esidimeni tragedy *see* Life Esidimeni tragedy
ethambutol 701
ethical dilemmas 128–148
    committees 145–146
    culture sensitive care 145
    definitions 128–129
    neurocognitive disorders (NCD) 486–487
    principles 132–135
    review boards 145–146
    rights of patients 143–145

specific problems 139–143
structure of 135–138
theories 129–132
ethionomaide *702*
ethnicity 153
evaluation
    of group work 790–792
    of mental health education 793–794
    of programmes 56–57
    of services 96–97
Every Student Succeeds Act (USA) 502
evidence-based practice approach 35
exercise *see* physical activity
exploitation 107–109
external crises *see* situational crises
externalising of problems 29–30
extrapyramidal side effects (EPS) 400, 405–406

F
facilities for mental health care, types of 113
FAFOFS *see* Friends and Family of Schizophrenics
families
    assessment of 208–210, *209–211*
    case management models 256–257
    of children and adolescents 731–736, 738–739
    of children with intellectual disabilities 510–515
    counselling for spouses 437–439
    of forensic mental health care users 761, 762
    involvement of 244–245
    nurse–family relationship 175–176
    of persons with alcohol-related disorders 436–439
    of persons with anxiety disorders 317
    of persons with mood disorders 334–335
    of persons with neurocognitive disorders 483–487, *486*
    of persons with schizophrenia 395–398
    perspective of 86–93
    trauma in 656–658
fantasy *559*, 574, 643, 737
fear questionnaire 799–802

feeding skills 536–542, *537–540*
fidelity 135
fitness to stand trial 746–748, *746*, *747*
Fluanxol *402*, 601
fluorocarbons 442
fluoxetine 721
flupentixol *402*
fluphenazine 402, *402*
focusing
    as communication skill 170
    in group therapy 239
    on object 308
forensic mental health care users 743–769
    classification of 754–755
    conflicting role of nurses 764–765
    criminal responsibility/capacity 746, *746*, 749–753, *751*
    definitions 743–744, 765–766
    fitness to stand trial 746–748, *746*, *747*
    forensic nurses 765–766
    historical background 743–745, *746*
    legal provisions 746–753, *746*, *747*, *751*
    Mental Health Care Act 121–123
    nursing interventions 755–766
    observation units 755–757
    security units 757–764
    services provided for 753–754
forensic nurses, definition of 765–766
'Fragile X' 500
freedom 140
free time, utilisation of 399–400
Freud, Sigmund 6, 287
Friends and Family of Schizophrenics (FAFOFS) 396

G
games 546–547
gastrointestinal disorders 681, 685
gatekeeper approach 44, 215
GBD *see* global burden of disease
generalised anxiety disorder 298, *318*, 716, 718
genetic counselling 500
genograms for family assessment 208–209, *209*
gestures 151

global burden of disease (GBD) 37–38
greetings 150
Groote Schuur Hospital 13, 66
groups
    assessment of 208–211, *209–211*
    education of 215, 423
    evaluation of therapy 790–792
    forensic mental health care users 761
    intellectual disabilities 546
    mood disorders 346, 369–370
    neurocognitive disorders (NCD) 478, *479*
    personality disorders 577–578, 587–588, *597*, *598*, 603, 607
    schizophrenia 397–400
    support 93–95
    survivor 658
    therapy for 234–241, *235*, *241*
    trauma and 657–661
guilt 624–626, 658, 662

H

HAD *see* HIV-associated dementia
hallucinations 382, 385–386, 391–394, 416, 441, 470, 787
hallucinogens *411–412*, *417*, *444*, 446
haloperidol 401, 402, *402*
Halt Elder Abuse line (HEAL) 467
Hamilton Anxiety Rating Scale (HAM-A) 796–797
Hamilton Depression Rating Scale (HDRS) 331, 697
HAND *see* HIV-associated neurocognitive disorder
harmful use, definition of 414
hazardous use, definition of 414
HDRS *see* Hamilton Depression Rating Scale
head injuries 387
head of health establishment, definition of 103
HEAL *see* Halt Elder Abuse line
'healing environment' 247, *247–248*
health care system 61–79
    functions of mental health services 70, *70*
    human resources 70–71
    integration of mental health care into 61–62, 67–69
    legislation 61
    levels of structure and service 64–67, *65–66*
    multidisciplinary teams 72–76
    organisation of mental health services 62–64, *62*
    primary mental health care 71–72
    training 70–71
health establishment, definition of 102
Health Professions Act 100, 103
healthy lifestyle functioning 200–201, 389–390
heroin *412*, 440, 446–447
hero work with children 652
herpes simplex encephalitis 387
hidden psychiatric morbidity (HPM) 44–46
high-risk approach 42–43, 216
high-risk behaviours 390, 419, 684–685, 694, 695
Hippocrates 3
history of mental health nursing 3–21
    early period to Renaissance 3
    Reformation 4
    19th century 4, *5*
    20th and 21st century 5–6, 6–14, *10*
    contemporary issues 14–18
    establishment of psychiatric hospitals 5–6
histrionic personality disorder 584–588, *585*
HIV/AIDS 693–704
    HIV/TB co-infection and mental illness 693–695
    home visits 254
    intellectual disabilities and 500
    interrelationship between mental health disorders and 694, *694*
    neurocognitive disorders and 453, 460
    psychological conditions associated with 696–701
    psychotropic drug interactions with 701, *701–702*
    risk factors 694
    schizophrenia and 387
    serious mental disorders and 683, 684
HIV-associated dementia (HAD) 699–700

HIV-associated neurocognitive disorder (HAND) 699
holistic approach 180–182, 652–656
home visits 91, 113, 254–255, *254*
hospital discharge *see* discharge of MHCUs
hospitals *see* psychiatric hospitals
housing 50, 398–399, 549–550
HPM *see* hidden psychiatric morbidity
human immunodeficiency virus (HIV)/acquired immunodeficiency syndrome (AIDS) *see* HIV/AIDS
human resources 70–71
human rights *see* rights
Huntington's disease 387, 460
hyperlipidaemia 685, 690
hypertension 434, 453, 461, 679, 684–685
hyperthermia 434
hyperthyroidism 296, 387, 501
hypnotics *412*, *417*
hypoglycaemia 719
hypomanic episodes 367–368
hypothyroidism 329, 350, 387

I
ibuprofen 351, 447
ICD *see* International Classification of Diseases
ICNP *see* International Classification for Nursing Practice
idliso 158
imagery 310
'I-message' 167–168
imipramine 714
Immorality Act 11
implementation
    during crisis intervention 226
    of programmes 54–56, *55*
inactivity 91, 342–343, *342*
incoherence 394
indigenous knowledge 18, 150
inequality 11, 613–614
infectious diseases 500, 682–683
inhalants *412*, *417*, 442, *443–444*
innovations 85–86
Inpatient Evaluation Scale 773–781

inpatient model 256
insomnia 348–349, *349*, 433
    see also sleep-related problems
integrated drinking 422
Integrated National Disability Strategy 500
integration of mental health services 22–23, 67–69, 684, 686
integrity 132
intellectual disabilities 498–554
    adult persons with 547–550
    assessment of 505–510, *505–509*
    challenging behaviour 550–552
    development features of persons with *504*
    DSM-5 diagnostic criteria 498–499, 502–503
    ethical dilemmas 141–142
    institutional care 545–547
    Mental Health Care Act 102
    prevalence of 503
    prevention of 500–502
    rights of persons with 500
    self-care 524–544
    stimulation of development 515–524, *516–523*
    support for parents 510–515
    teaching of skills 524–544, *527*, *529–535*, *537–540*
    terminology 499
International Classification for Nursing Practice (ICNP) 176–177
International Classification of Diseases (ICD) 158, 185, 420
International Council of Nurses 9, 176
interpersonal relationships in mental health care 7, 25, 84, 166–172, *166*, *168–169*
interventions *see* nursing interventions
interviews
    with children 725–728, *728–730*
    conflict resolution interviews 233–234
    constructive confrontation interviews 233
    cultural formulation interviews (CFI) 186
    with families 731–736
    for mental health assessment 186–195, *188–195*

motivational interviews 251–252, 447–448
   with specific goals 233–234
intimate adult relationships 111
intoxication
   alcohol 421, 432–433
   substance 415, 416
involuntary mental health care users 116–118, 139–140
isolation, as defence mechanisms 559, 606
   see also seclusion
isoniazid 387, 701
isotretinoin (Accutane) 329

J
Japan 753
job skills see work-related activities
'judge' response in counselling 230
Jung, Karl 6
Jurgens vs the Attorney-General 750
justice 134–135, 138

K
Kant, Immanuel 130
Kernberg's model of narcissistic personality disorder 594–595, *595*, *596*, 597
ketamine *411*, 413
Khan vs the Commissioner of Mental Health 750
Kohut's model of narcissistic personality disorder 594–595, *594*, *595*, 597
koro 159
Kraepelin, Emil 6
kufungisisa 159

L
labelling 23, 29–30, 83–84
lamivudine (3TC) *702*
language usage 29–30, 474, *474*, 499
Largactil *402*
learning disorders 706
Legal Aid South Africa Act 111
legal structures in mental health care nursing 100–127
   Children's Act 105, 111, 114, 125, 126, 134, 144

forensic mental health care users 744–745, 746–753, *746*, *747*, *751*
   history of 10, 744–745
   Medicines and Related Substances Control Act 124
   Prevention of and Treatment for Substance Abuse Act 124–126
   see also Mental Health Care Act
Leininger Sunrise Model 156–157
Leponex *402*
Level 1 Cross Cutting Symptom Measure (1CCSM) 186
level 4 hospitals 66
levels in health care system 64–67, *65–66*
Life Esidimeni tragedy 16, 103, 137–138
life skills approach 43, 216–217, 762
life stories of mental health care users 184
light therapy 480
limit setting 259–260, 266, 369–370, 397, 600, 712, 738
Lipitor 329
listening 170
lithium 6, 600, 608
liver cirrhosis 434
loose associations 394
lorazepam 401, *412*
love, meaning of 131
lysergic acid diethylamide (LSD) *411*

M
magical thinking 395, 643, 651
major depressive disorder (MDD) 283, 327, 469, *694*, 719–722
   see also depression
major neurocognitive disorders
   carer liaison 484
   causes of *459*, 460–461
   delirium and 463, *463–464*
   DSM-5 classification of 452, *462–463*
   mild neurocognitive disorders and 464, 465–466
   nursing interventions 473–483
   prevalence of 453–454

risk factors for 467
social functioning problems 471
mandrax 439, 441–442, *443*
mania 698–699
manic episodes 366–367
MAOI *see* monoamine oxidase inhibitors
marijuana *see* cannabis
Marijuana Anonymous group 441
marital therapy 761
Marwick, Iris 8–9
maximum security facilities 123
MDD *see* major depressive disorder
mechanical restraint *see* restraint
medical aid schemes 83
medical practitioner, definition of 103
medication
    anxiety disorders 317–323, *318–321*, *322*
    assessment and 180–181
    attention-deficit/hyperactivity disorder (ADHD) 709
    comorbidity 685
    compliance 688–691
    ethical dilemmas 141, 144
    HIV/AIDS 701, *701–702*
    intellectual disabilities 551–552
    Mental Health Care Act 113
    mood disorders 329
    neurocognitive disorders (NCD) 467, 487, 488, *488–489*
    personality disorders 600–601, 607–608
    psychotropic 6–7, 64, 66–67, 487, 607–608, 683, 701, *701–702*
    schizophrenia 387, 400–406, *402–403*, *404*
    side effects of 400–406, *402–404*, *694*
    tuberculosis (TB) 701, *701–702*
Medicines and Related Substances Control Act 101, 124
Medicines and Related Substances Control Amendment Act 69
melatonin 348
memory 454, 461
MENDAMIND 459, *460*
meningitis 500
Menninger, Karl 244

'mental defect' vs 'mental illness' 745, *746*
Mental Disorder and Defective Persons Act 10
Mental Disorders Act 8
mental exercises 308
mental health, definition of 23–25
Mental Health Act 9–10, 101, 749–750
mental health assessment *see* assessment
Mental Health Care Act 101–123
    abuse 107–109
    definitions 101–103
    determinations of mental health status 109
    discharge reports 111
    disclosure of information 110–111
    duties relating to MHCUs 103–107
    ethical dilemmas 138, 139, 140, 143
    exploitation 107–109
    forensic mental health care users 748–750, 752, 753, 754, 756–758, 762, 765
    health care system and 61, 64
    history of 10, 15, 16, 25
    intellectual disabilities 499, 500
    intimate adult relationships 111
    mental health review boards 81, 103, 113–114
    personal property 112
    prisoners 121–123
    representation 111
    restraint 272, 273
    rights relating to MHCUs 103–107, 111, 112
    seclusion 272
    suicide 363
    types of facilities 113
    types of MHCUs 114–121
    unfair discrimination 107
mental health care nurses *see* nurses
mental health care nursing *see* nursing
mental health care practitioner, definition of 103
mental health care provider, definition of 103
mental health care users (MHCUs)
    definition of 102
    types of 114–121
    see also consumers in mental health
mental health review boards 81, 103, 113–114

mental health status, definition of 102
mental illness, definition of 102
'mental illness' vs 'mental defect' 745, *746*
'mental retardation', use of term 499
mescaline *412*
metabolic conditions 683
metabolic syndrome 400, 461, 683, 685
methadone *412*, 447, 448
methamphetamine 410, *413*, 440, 445–446
methaqualone *412*, 439, 441
methcathinone ('Cat') 410–411, *413*
methylphenidate *413*, 552
MHCUs *see* mental health care users
mild neurocognitive disorders
    carer liaison 484
    causes of *459*, 460–461
    depression and 469
    DSM-5 classification of 452
    major neurocognitive disorders and 464, 465–466
    nursing interventions 473–483
    prevalence of 453–454
    social functioning problems 471
milestone education 215, 423
milieu therapy 241–248, *245–248*
Mind that Found Itself, A 7
mini-mental state examination (MMSE) 466, 468–469, *468–469*
misuse, definition of 414
MMSE *see* mini-mental state examination
M'Naghten Rule 745
MOCA *see* Montreal Cognitive Assessment
Modecate 402, *402*
monoamine oxidase inhibitors (MAOI) 296
Montreal Cognitive Assessment (MOCA) 469
mood, definition of 185
mood disorders 326–381
    Beck's Suicide Intent Scale 378–380
    bipolar mood disorders 327–328, 366–371
    categories of 326–327
    Centre for Epidemiological Studies Depression Scale (CES-D) 376–377
    definitions 327
    depressive disorders 327–334
    diagnosis of 329–334, *331*, 367–368
    HIV/AIDS and 696–699
    nursing interventions 334–355, *341*, *342*, *344*, *349*, 368–371
    SAD PERSONS Scale (SPS) 362, 380–381
    screening tools 331–332, 376–381
    substance-related disorders and 418
    suicide 355–366, 378–381
    tuberculosis and 696–699
    WHO-five Well-being Index (WHO-5) 331, 332
mood stabilisers 552, 608
Moross, H 9
morphine *412*, 447
mortality rates 679
mothers of trauma victims 656
motivational interviews 251–252, 447–448
motor skills 526–536, *527*, *529–535*
Moya, Lily 81
multi-agency approach 752–753
multidisciplinary teams 72–76
multiple personality disorder 383
music therapy 480, 547

N

NAMI *see* National Alliance on Mental Illness
narcissistic personality disorder 593–597, *594–598*
narrative approach 28–30, 31, 344–346
National Alliance on Mental Illness (NAMI) 83, 93–94
National Council for Mental Health 8
National Development Plan 502
National Down Syndrome Society (NDSS) 502
National Health Act 61, 66, 100, 104, 138, 144
National Institute for Child Health and Human Development 498–499
National Mental Health Policy Framework and Strategic Plan 2013–2020
    advocacy by consumers and 95
    district health system and 63
    functions of mental health services 70
    history of 12
    primary health care and 15

psychotropic medication 66–67
stigmatisation 80, 83, 84
training and 14, 70–71
NCDLB *see* neurocognitive disorder with Lewy body disease
NDSS *see* National Down Syndrome Society
negative thoughts, questioning of 315–316
neglect 110, 639–640, 648
neurocognitive disorders (NCD) 452–497
    assessment 466–473, *468–469, 470*
    carer liaison 483–487
    causes of 459–461, *459, 460*
    clusters of 452, *452*
    differences between 463–464, *463–464, 465–466*
    DSM-5 diagnostic criteria 452–453, 454, *459, 461–463, 470*
    epilepsy 489–495, *489, 491, 494*
    family liaison 483–487, *486*
    with Lewy body disease (NCDLB) 461
    neurocognitive domains 454–455, *455, 456–458, 471*
    nursing interventions 473–483, *473–476, 478–479, 481–482, 489–495, 489, 491, 494*
    prevalence of 452–454
    social control 487–488, *488–489*
neurocognitive disorder with Lewy body disease (NCDLB) 461
neuroleptic malignant syndrome 406
neurosyphilis 387
nevirapine *702*
New Psychoactive Substances (NPS) 413
nicotine *413, 417*
    see also smoking
Nightingale, Florence 12
Nightingale pledge 134
nitrous oxide *412*
N-methyl-D-aspartate (NMDA) receptor antagonists 488
non-maleficence 133, 138
non-social behaviour 551
non-verbal communication 303, *474*
normalisation principle 545–546

normal post-traumatic stress response 616, *616*
normative behaviour 24
normative manipulation 422
norms of therapeutic groups 238–239
NPS *see* New Psychoactive Substances
nurses
    conflicting role of 764–765
    nurse–family relationship 175–176
    nurse–MHCU relationship 23, 26–35, *30, 32*, 165, 172–175, *173–174*, 263
    training for 12–14, 22, 62, 70–71, 706, 757, 766
nursing
    conceptual framework for 22–36, *26*
    definition of 25–26, *26*
    history of 7
    process of 176–177
Nursing Act 14, 69, 100
nursing interventions 214–279
    anger and aggression 260–274, *263, 265, 268–271*
    case management 255–259
    crisis intervention 221–229, *223–227*
    home visits 254–255, *254*
    hospital discharge planning 248–249
    individual counselling 229–234, *232*
    limit setting 259–260
    mental health education 214–221
    milieu therapy 241–248, *245–248*
    relapse prevention 249–253, *251*
    symptom management 249–253
    therapeutic groups 234–241, *235, 241*
nutrition *see* diet
nyaope *412*, 413

O

obesity 461, 681, 683
object constancy 589
observation of behaviour 306
observation units 755–757
obsessive-compulsive disorders 293, *293*, 298–301, *299–300, 320–321*
obsessive-compulsive personality disorder 605–607, *606*

obsessive type of violent offender 760
occupational activities *see* work-related activities
occupational therapy 738
ode-ori 159
olanzapine *319, 320, 402*, 551, 608
Older Persons Act 467
open communication 243
opioids *412*, 413, *417*, *445*, 446–447
oppositional defiant disorder 709–711
oral contraceptives 329
Orlando, Ida J 7
osteoporosis 685
outpatients 9–10, 16–17, 747–748
overgeneralisation 329, 335
over-sedation (snowing) 488
oxazepam *412*

P

painkillers *413*
pain sensitivity 684
panic disorders 283, 295–297, 316, *318–319*
paranoid personality disorder 580–584, *581*
paranoid type of violent offender 760
paraphrasing 170
parents
    of children with intellectual disabilities, support for 510–515
    mothers of trauma victims 656
parkinsonism-type syndrome 405
Parkinson's disease 387, 453, 460, 470
passive aggression *560*
pathic communication 174
patients *see* consumers in mental health
peer reviews 56
Peplau, Hildegard E 7, 214
persistent depressive disorder (dysthymia) 326, 327
personality changes (decline in social cognition) 454, 461, 472
personality disorders 555–609
    cluster A 573–584, *575–576, 581*
    cluster B 584–601, *585, 590, 594–598*
    cluster C 601–608, *602, 604, 606*
    common characteristics of 557

    DSM-5 diagnostic criteria 557–558, *559–560*
    forensic mental health care users 755, 764, 765
    reactions of mental health care professionals 560–561
    substance-related disorders and 418
    therapeutic principles 555–556
    transactional analysis model 561–572, *562–563, 565–569, 571–573, 595, 602, 604, 606*
    understanding persons with 555–561
personal property 112
personal protectors 183
personal recovery 46
personal space 151
pethidine *412*, 446–447
PHC *see* primary health care
phencyclidine (PCP) *411, 417, 459*
phobias 293–294
physical abuse 639, 648
physical activity 91, 342–343, *342*, 350, 480, 550
physical condition of mental health care users 199–200, *199*
physical restraint *see* restraint
Pinel, Philippe 4, 743–744
PL *see* provincial level
planning
    consumer involvement in 96–97
    during crisis intervention 226
    of programmes 50–57, *53–54, 55*
play 546–547
policies, consumer involvement in 96–97
polysubstance 411
positive psychology 350
post-traumatic stress disorder (PTSD) 222, *320*, 617–619, 620, 622–623, 696, 723–724
poverty 614, 739
powerlessness 642
'power of attorney' 486
pregnancy, termination of 105, 106–107
prejudicial responses 23
Premarin 329

prevention
- of alcohol-related disorders 421–425
- of child abuse 653–655
- of intellectual disabilities 500–502
- of mental ill health 25
- primary 40–43, *43–44*, 72, 215–217, 422–423, 500
- of relapse 249–253, *251*, 406–407
- secondary 40–41, 44–46, 217–221, 424–425, 501
- tertiary 40–41, 46–50, *47*, *48–49*, 217–221, 425, 501–502

Prevention of and Treatment for Substance Abuse Act 124–126, 363
primary health care (PHC) 14–16, 44–46, 49, 67–69, 71–72
primary prevention (before illness) 40–43, *43–44*, 72, 215–217, 422–423, 500
prisoners *see* forensic mental health care users
private health system 61
probing 170
problem-based programme planning 52–53
problem-solving techniques 397, 485
professional boundaries 142–143, 175
programme planning 50–57, *53–54*, *55*
Prohibition of Mixed Marriages Act 11
projection *559–560*, 581
projective identification *559*, 574, 581, 590, 594, 599
protective factors 32, 182, 183
provincial level (PL) 65–66, *66*
Prozac 721
psychiatric hospitals 4–6, *5–6*, 8–9, 113
'psychiatry', use of term 4
psychobiological vulnerability 31, *32*
psycho-education 49–50, 217–221
psycholegal, definition of 743
psychosis 698–699
psychosocial rehabilitation 16–17, 25–26, 48–50, *48–49*
psychosocial stress 31–32, *32*
psychotic disorders 385, 418
psychotropic medication 6–7, 64, 66–67, 487, 607–608, 683, 701, *701–702*

PTSD *see* post-traumatic stress disorder
pulmonary conditions 682
Pussin, Jean-Baptiste 4

Q

quality
- of care 8–9, 165
- of programmes 57

questioning, as communication skill 170–171
quetiapine *403*
quinolones *701*

R

race 153
racism 11–12
rape 614, 661–667, *665–666*
  see also sexual abuse
rating scales 362–363, 387–388, 796–802
rational planning 51
reality orientation (RO) 477–478, *478–479*
Reaven, G M 685
recovery
- -oriented rehabilitation paradigm 16–17
- perceptions on 84–86
- promotion of 25
- tertiary prevention 46–48, *47*

redecision therapy 569–572, *571*
re-experiencing 617
referral 73–74
reflection
- as communication skill 171–172, 447
- on experiences 32–35

reframing 308
refugees 153
refusal of treatment 91, 144
Regional Psychosocial Support Initiative (REPSSI) 652
regression 643
rehabilitation 16–17, 25–26, 48–50, *48–49*, 92–93, 102, 113
relapse prevention 249–253, *251*, 406–407
relational ethics 132
relaxation training 316–317
religion 88–89, 130–131, 346, 387

remotivation therapy 477–478, *479*
repetitive Transcranial Magnetic Stimulation (rTMS) 351
reports on discharge of MHCUs 111, 249
representation, right to 111
REPSSI *see* Regional Psychosocial Support Initiative
research ethics 145–146
resilience 222, 328
respiratory disease 681
restraint 108, 267–273, *268–271*, 487–488, 738
restrictive practices 266–273, *268–271*
review boards 145–146
rewards 482, *482*
rifampicin *701*
rights
    apartheid 11–12
    Constitution of South Africa 100
    Mental Health Care Act 103–107, 111, 112
    of MHCUs 103–107, 111, 112, 143–145
    of persons with intellectual disabilities 141–142, 500
    WHO *QualityRights tool kit* 245, *245–247*
risk–benefit medication counselling 689–691
risk factors for mental illness 41
Risperdal *403*
risperidone 354, 402, *403*
Ritalin 709
ritonavir *702*
RO *see* reality orientation
Robben Island 4
Roberts's model for crisis intervention 224
Rogers, Carl 166–167
'rolling with resistance' 448
'rootwork' 158
Royal College of Nursing 267
rTMS *see* repetitive Transcranial Magnetic Stimulation
rule-deontologists 130
rule-utilitarianism 129
Rumpff Commission of Inquiry into Criminal Responsibility of Mentally Disordered Persons and Related Matters 745
rural areas 16

S

SADAG *see* South African Depression and Anxiety Group
SAD PERSONS Scale (SPS) 362, 380–381
safety rituals 651
SAIL principle 401
SANC *see* South African Nursing Council
'sanctuaries', use of term 4
sangomas 158
SAPS *see* South African Police Service
SASH *see* South African Stress and Health
schizoaffective disorder 384
schizoid personality disorder 573–578, *575–576*
schizophrenia spectrum and psychotic disorders 382–409
    assessment of 386–388
    causes of 383
    definitions 382–383
    diagnosis of 384–386, *384*, 388, *388*
    medication management 400–406, *402–403*, *404*
    mortality rate in people with 679
    nursing interventions 389–407, *398*, *402–403*, *404*
    prevalence of 383
    prognosis of 383–384
    relapse prevention 250, 406–407
    stress–vulnerability framework *32*
Schizophrenics Anonymous 85–86
schizophreniform disorder 384
schizotypal personality disorder 579–580
schooling *see* education
Schultheiss, K 17
screening tools
    comorbidity 686–687
    intellectual disabilities 505–510, *505–509*
    mood disorders 331–332, 376–381
    neurocognitive disorders (NCD) 468–469, *468–469*
SDS *see* Self-rating Depression Scale
SE *see* supported employment
seclusion 108–109, 271–273
Seconal *412*

secondary prevention (during illness) 40–41, 44–46, 217–221, 424–425, 501
secondary traumatic stress disorder 631–633
security units 757–764
sedatives *412, 417*
selective abstraction 292, 329, 335
selective serotonin reuptake inhibitors (SSRI) *318–320*, 321, *322*, *694*, 697, 719
self-blame 624–626, 643, 651, 658, 662
self-care 395, 524–544, 551, 631–633
self-efficacy 41–42
self-esteem 41–42
self-harm 356, 550–552
self-monitoring 304–306, *305*, 309
Self-rating Depression Scale (SDS) 331
self-reporting questionnaire (SRQ) 45–46
sensory awareness 308
sensory stimulation 480, 516, *516–523*, 524
separation anxiety disorder 716–717
Serenace *402*
Seroquel XL *403*
service-based programme planning 53, *53–54*
service users, definition of 124–125
severe or profound intellectual disability, definition of 102
sexual abuse
    assessment 727
    in children 640–646, *645*, *647*, 649–656, *668–676*, 705, 723, 727
    developmental guidelines *668–676*
    forensic mental health care users 761
    physical symptoms of 649–650
    post-traumatic stress disorder (PTSD) 723
    preventative measures 653–656
    rape 614, 661–667, *665–666*
sexuality, children with intellectual disabilities 513–514
shared decision making 242–243
shared psychotic disorder 385
sheltered freedom 475
'Shin-Byung' 158
side effects of medication 400–406, *402–404*, *694*
situational crises 223, *223*

skills teaching 49, 50, 524–544, 762
sleep-related problems *203*, 348–349, *349*, 432, 433, 436, 471
smoking 681, 682, 685, 688
    see also nicotine
Snoezelen multisensory stimulation 524
snowing (over-sedation) 488
social anxiety disorder 295, *319*, 716, 718
social cognition, decline in (personality changes) 454, 461, 472
social determinants of health 39–40, 684, 739
social psychiatry 7
social skills 219–221, 551
social time 151
social withdrawal 338–340, *341*, 390–391
societal abuse 640
sociograms 210, *211*
sodium valproate 552, 608
South African Depression and Anxiety Group (SADAG) 93–94
South African Nursing Council (SANC) 13, 22, 68–69, 706, 765–766
South African Police Service (SAPS) 122–123, 655
South African Schools Act 142
South African Stress and Health (SASH) 11, 38
space perception 151
'spell', definition of 158
'split personality' vs schizophrenia 383
splitting *560*, 574, 581, 585, 590, 594, 599
spouses, counselling for 437–439
SPS *see* SAD PERSONS Scale
SRQ *see* self-reporting questionnaire
SSRI *see* selective serotonin reuptake inhibitors
standards of practice, for promotion of cultural competence 154–155
Stanford Panic Appraisal Inventory 797–798
state patients 119–121, 748–758, *751*, 762–765
stereotypes 23, 82, 139
sterilisation 107, 514
Sterilisation Act 101, 107
stigmatisation
    communication and 29
    definition of 23

833

ethical dilemmas 139
HIV/AIDS 693, *694*
of mental illness 80, 81–84
neurocognitive disorders (NCD) 453, 490
persons with intellectual disabilities 499
trauma 642
stimulants *412–413*, 552
stimulation of development, for children with intellectual disabilities 515–524, *516–523*
stimulus generalisation 292
Strattera 709
stress 89–90, 287–288
stress–vulnerability framework 30–32, *30, 32,* 182–184, 206–207, *207*
strokes 387, 460
substance-related disorders 410–450
 in adolescents 724
 amphetamines *412–413, 444,* 445, 446
 anabolic-androgenic steroids 413
 anxiety disorders and 323
 anxiolytics *412*, 417
 caffeine *411*, 417
 cannabis (dagga) 410, *411*, 417, 440–441, *442–443*
 cocaine *413*, 440, 445, 446
 commonly used substances 411–413, *411–413*
 comorbidity 411, 418, 685
 core concepts 414–417
 diagnostic criteria 411, 415–418, *417, 418*
 ethical dilemmas 141
 forensic mental health care users 755, 758
 hallucinogens *411–412, 417, 444,* 446
 history of 11
 HIV/AIDS and 693–694, 695, 700–701
 hypnotics *412, 417*
 inhalants *412, 417, 442, 443–444*
 mandrax 439, 441–442, *443*
 methamphetamine 410, *413*, 440, 445–446
 mood disorders and 330
 nicotine *413*, 417
 opioids *412, 417,* 445, 446–447
 painkillers 413
 phencyclidine *417*

 polysubstance 411
 prevalence of 410–411
 schizophrenia and 383, 385, 387
 sedatives *412*, 417
 stimulants *412–413*
 treatment 447–448
 tuberculosis and 700–701
 see also alcohol-related disorders
suicide
 in adolescents 721–722
 borderline personality disorder and 601
 definitions 356
 HIV/AIDS and 697
 mood disorders and 327–328, 355–366, 378–381
 nursing interventions 363–366
 prevention of 48, 357–359
 profiles 356–357
 risk assessment 360–363, 378–381
 schizophrenia and 388
 tuberculosis and 697
 warning signs 359–360
'sundown syndrome' 471
Sunshine Association 511
supported employment (SE) 50, 549–550
support groups 93–95
support systems 49, 225
survivor groups 658
survivor guilt 624–626
Sustainable Development Agenda 40
S vs Pretorius 747–748
symptom management 249–253
systemic lupus erythematosus 387

T
tangentiality 394
Tara Hospital 9, 12–13
tardive dyskinesia 405–406, 683
TB *see* tuberculosis
teams, multidisciplinary 72–76, 555–556
Technical Assistance Guidelines on the Employment of Persons with Disabilities 547–548
technology 8, 74–76, 85–86

telemental health 74–76
tenofivir *702*
teridazone *701*
termination of pregnancy 105, 106–107
tertiary prevention (after illness) 40–41, 46–50, *47*, *48–49*, 217–221, 425, 501–502
THC (9-delta-tetrahydrocannabinol) 440
theatre performances 217
thought disorders 394–395
thwasa 158
'tic' *see* methamphetamine
TIDE principle 401
'tik' *see* methamphetamine
time–event–symptom charts 204–205, *205*
time-out technique 397, 513
time perception 151
time-to-event charts 204, 304, 795
Tofranil 714
toilet training 543–544
tolerance, definition of 414
total population approach to education 215, 423
training in mental health nursing 12–14, 22, 62, 70–71, 706, 757, 766
transactional analysis model 561–572, *562–563*, *565–569*, *571–573*, *595*, *602*, *604*, *606*
Transcultural Assessment Model 150–153
trauma 613–677
    abuse of elderly 637–638
    anxiety disorders and 293, *293*
    children and 614, 620, 638–656, *645*, *647*, *668–676*
    complex post-traumatic stress disorder (PTSD) 622–623
    counselling 623–627
    debriefing 627–630
    definitions 614–615, *615*
    diagnosis of 617–623, *617–621*
    disclosure about abuse 650–651
    domestic violence 622, 633–637, *635*, *636*, *637*
    groups affected by 657–661
    impact of working with victims of 631–633, *631–633*
    normal response to 616–617, *616*
    nursing interventions 623–627, 651–661, 664–667, *665–666*
    rape 614, 661–667, *665–666*
    South African context 613–614
    types of 615
    see also abuse
traumagenic dynamics model 641–643
traumatised type of violent offender 760
treatment
    culture and 159
    refusal of 91
    rehabilitation vs *48–49*
tricyclic antidepressants 296
trigger symptoms 250–251
trustworthiness 131–132
truthfulness 133
tryptamines 413
tuberculosis (TB) 693–704
    HIV/TB co-infection and mental illness 693–695
    intellectual disabilities and 500
    psychological conditions associated with 696–701
    psychotropic drug interactions with 701, *701*–702
    risk factors 694
Tuke, William 4
type 2 diabetes 679, 681, 684, 685

U

Ubuntu 132, 151
ufunfunuana 158
UK *see* United Kingdom
umeqo 158
UN *see* United Nations
unconditional positive regard 167
unemployment 613–614
    see also work-related activities
unfair discrimination 107
UNFAS *see* University of Natal Functional Assessment Scale
United Kingdom (UK) 549, 750, 752–753
United Nations (UN) 40, 245
United States of America (USA) 217, 502, 753

University of Natal Functional Assessment Scale (UNFAS) 782-786
University of the Witwatersrand 12, 623
USA *see* United States of America
uthandazeli 158
utilitarianism 129-130

V

vagueness 394
validation therapy 477, 479
validity 184-185
Valium 329
VC *see* videoconferencing
venous thromboembolism 682
veracity 133
verbal communication 302
Verwoerd, H F, assassination of 745, 748
Vesperax *412*
vicarious traumatisation 631-633, *631-633*
videoconferencing (VC) 74-76
violence
    conduct disorder 712
    definition of 261
    domestic 622, 633-637, *635-637*, 705
    forensic mental health care users 752, 755, 757-762, 763
    managing violent behaviour 90-92
    paranoid personality disorder 583
    stereotypes 82
    trauma and 614
    see also aggression; anger
virtue ethics 131-132
visualisation techniques 308-309
Vitamin B12 deficiency 387
vocational rehabilitation *see* work-related activities
voluntary mental health care users 114, 124-125

W

Wachtel, Maximillian 757
wandering behaviour 480-481, *481*
Ware, Paul 562, 571-572
Washington State Early Learning and Development Guidelines 505, *505-509*
weight gain 683, 684, 685
Wellconal *412*, 446
Western Cape, prevalence of child mental disorders 38, *39*
WFMH *see* World Federation for Mental Health
WHO *see* World Health Organisation
witchcraft 89, 749
withdrawal
    alcohol 421, 433-434
    medications 321
    substance 415, 418
    see also social withdrawal
women, HIV infection among 695
work-related activities 50, 244, 346-347, 371, 399, 548-550, 762
World Federation for Mental Health (WFMH) 143
World Health Organisation (WHO)
    alcohol-related disorders 420, 422-423
    comorbidity 679-681, 683
    definition of mental health 24
    diagnostic system of 185
    Disability Assessment Schedule (WHODAS 2.0) 186
    -five Well-being Index (WHO-5) 331, 332
    on importance of mental health 40
    integration of mental health care 67-68
    intellectual disabilities 499
    Mental Health Action Plan (2013-2020) 328
    'mhGAP intervention guide' 186
    mood disorders 327-328
    primary health care (PHC) 14-15
    QualityRights tool kit 245, *245-247*

X

xenophobia 153, 613-614

Y

You Are Not Alone (YANA) 396

Z

zidovudine *702*
zuclopenthixol 401, 402, *403*
Zung's Self-rating Depression Scale (SDS) 331
Zyprexa 402

CPSIA information can be obtained
at www.ICGtesting.com
Printed in the USA
LVHW061905260222
712102LV00031B/479